# Spatially Fractionated, Microbeam and FLASH Radiation Therapy

A physics and multi-disciplinary approach

**Online at: https://doi.org/10.1088/978-0-7503-4046-5**

IPEM–IOP Series in Physics and Engineering in Medicine and Biology



### About the Series

The series in Physics and Engineering in Medicine and Biology will allow the Institute of Physics and Engineering in Medicine (IPEM) to enhance its mission to 'advance physics and engineering applied to medicine and biology for the public good'.

It is focused on key areas including, but not limited to:

- clinical engineering
- diagnostic radiology
- informatics and computing
- magnetic resonance imaging
- nuclear medicine
- physiological measurement
- radiation protection
- radiotherapy
- rehabilitation engineering
- ultrasound and non-ionising radiation.

A number of IPEM–IOP titles are being published as part of the EUTEMPE Network Series for Medical Physics Experts.

A full list of titles published in this series can be found here: https://iopscience.iop.org/bookListInfo/physics-engineering-medicine-biology-series.

www.ingramcontent.com/pod-product-compliance
Ingram Content Group UK Ltd.
Pitfield, Milton Keynes, MK11 3LW, UK
UKHW051041120926
8556IPUK00030B/696

9 780750 323505

# Spatially Fractionated, Microbeam and FLASH Radiation Therapy

A physics and multi-disciplinary approach

**Edited by**
**Hualin Zhang**
*Department of Radiation Oncology, Keck Medical School, University of Southern California, Los Angeles, CA, USA*

**Nina A Mayr**
*College of Human Medicine, Michigan State University, East Lansing, MI, USA*

**IOP** Publishing, Bristol, UK

ISBN 978-0-7503-4046-5 (ebook)
ISBN 978-0-7503-4044-1 (print)
ISBN 978-0-7503-4047-2 (myPrint)
ISBN 978-0-7503-4045-8 (mobi)

DOI 10.1088/978-0-7503-4046-5

Version: 20230601

IOP ebooks

British Library Cataloguing-in-Publication Data: A catalogue record for this book is available from the British Library.

Published by IOP Publishing, wholly owned by The Institute of Physics, London

IOP Publishing, No.2 The Distillery, Glassfields, Avon Street, Bristol, BS2 0GR, UK

US Office: IOP Publishing, Inc., 190 North Independence Mall West, Suite 601, Philadelphia, PA 19106, USA

*This book is dedicated to all those who have reached beyond the familiar to explore these new radiation therapy paradigms, to our patients who through their courage and their suffering help bring them into clinical reality, to our teachers for the knowledge and inspiration they give us, and to our students who will advance the field to the next level.*

*To my wife Yufen Wang, son Zhongqi 'Tom' Zhang for their support for my work on this book.*

# Contents

## Part II Physics of moderate dose rate SFRT

# Preface

**Hualin Zhang, Nina A Mayr and Mohammed Mohiuddin**

Spatially fractionated radiation therapy (SFRT), the concept of treating tumors by delivering a spatially modulated dose with highly non-uniform dose distributions, is an area of rapid development and high interest in radiation oncology, physics and tumor biology. Clinical experience in SFRT suggests high response and low toxicity in the treatment of challenging advanced and bulky tumors. Clinical outcome data are rapidly accumulating while SFRT technologies and techniques are continuously evolving. Initially limited to GRID therapy using block collimators, advanced and versatile multi-leaf collimators and volumetric modulated arc technologies have since broadened the capabilities and individualization of SFRT and expanded the clinical investigations of SFRT to various dosing regimens, multiple malignancies, tumor types and disease sites.

Meanwhile, the concepts of spatial fractionation are evolving and beginning to be applied to many different beam types. Microbeam radiation therapy that has recently emerged leverages rapid developments of synchrotron technologies, as does proton accelerator minibeam technology, and these technologies are expanding the SFRT platforms. In addition, FLASH therapy, a novel radiation therapy technique employing ultra-high dose rate, was recently used for the first time in human cancer treatment based on encouraging preclinical results.

However, the physics concept of SFRT, microbeam, minibeam and FLASH therapy, which are characterized by novel and unfamiliar heterogeneous and high-dose prescription parameters, is a profound departure from the current clinical concepts in radiation oncology. The understanding of SFRT physics in the context of treatment planning, delivery, clinical dose effects and biological underpinnings are critically important for this evolving field.

This textbook describes the physics of SFRT, microbeam, minibeam and FLASH therapy in the context of dose, dose effects, technology, clinical applications and biological concepts. While the book is primarily a physics text, SFRT cannot be comprehensively discussed without its interrelations to the clinical application and the underlying biology, which are intricately interconnected to the physical dose parameters. Therefore, the current status of heterogeneous-dose radiation is presented within a multi-disciplinary approach that is illustrated in figure 0.1.

The book reviews and discusses the current state-of-the-art understanding of SFRT physics principles, moderate dose rate GRID and Lattice SFRT techniques, and pertinent technologies applied in clinical patients. Standardization requirements and approaches for clinical application will be discussed. Novel concepts of the evolving minibeam, microbeam and ultra-high dose rate FLASH therapy modalities are explored. The biological basis and dose effect modeling as the ultimate essential link between physical parameters and clinical outcomes of tumor and normal tissue response are described.

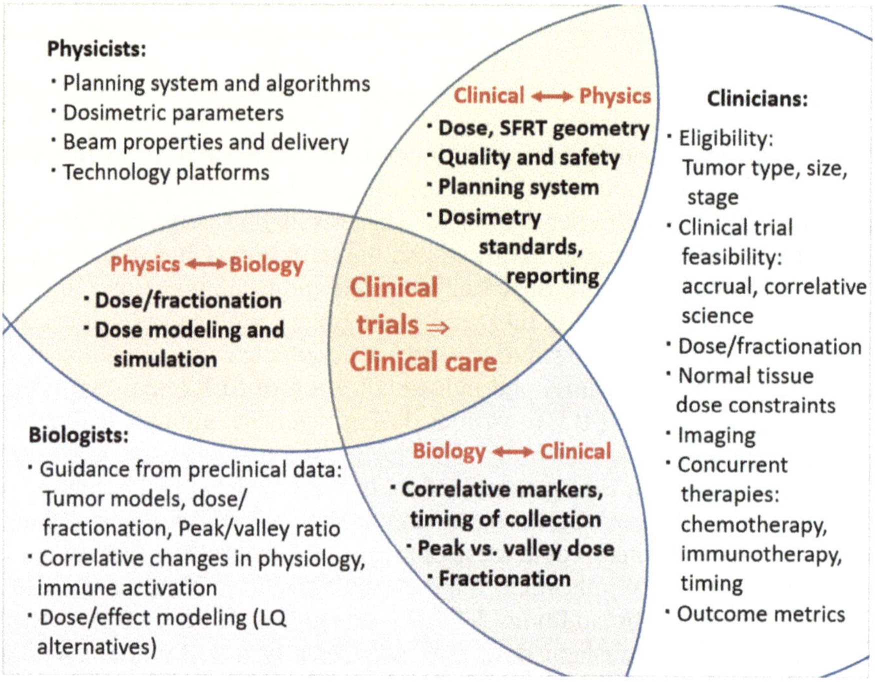


**Figure 0.1.** Examples for interdisciplinary conversation and collaboration in the emerging fields of heterogeneous dose irradiation.

The book contains three major parts:

Part I: **Biology and Clinical Use**

The underlying biology and clinical observations are closely linked to the physical properties of SFRT, and are reviewed in Part I. This section discusses *(1) the biological basis of SFRT, Microbeam and FLASH radiation, and (2) early and emerging clinical use with a critical appraisal of early outcome data.*

A comprehensive introduction and summary of physics/technical, clinical and biologic aspects of the various heterogeneous radiation modalities, GRID, Lattice, micro/minibeam and FLASH, are presented by Butterworth *et al* in chapter 1. In chapter 2, Johnsrud *et al* present a comprehensive overview and update on the biology of the heterogeneity dose domain from the bench to clinical translational aspects. In chapter 3, Marciscano *et al* focus on the immunologic effects of irradiation, provide an in-depth review of non-uniform dose induced immunomodulation, and explore clinical trial considerations and interpretation. Grilj and Vozenin critically appraise the technological basis, experimental data and emerging clinical investigations of FLASH therapy in chapter 4.

The clinical section focuses on the major SFRT modalities, GRID and Lattice therapy, that have entered the clinical domain. This discussion is held chronologically with a review of the early GRID experience at moderate dose rate in the palliative treatment of metastatic or recurrent disease and its more recent exploration into the definitive curative-intent treatment of bulky far-advanced tumors by Alexander *et al* in chapter 5. This is followed by Mohiuddin *et al* who provide a comprehensive review and update of the clinical GRID therapy experience in multiple primary disease entities in chapter 6. The clinical experience with Lattice therapy, a 3D form of SFRT that evolved from GRID therapy, is discussed by Amendola *et al* in chapter 7. Chow *et al* provide an overview of proton beam SFRT in chapter 8.

This comprehensive review of the relevant biological underpinnings and available clinical data provides an important and intricately intertwined framework and background for Parts II and III, that are dedicated to the physics of heterogeneous dose irradiation.

Part II: **Physics of Conventional-dose-rate SFRT**

The three subsections of Part II comprehensively review moderate dose rate SFRT with respect to *(1) methods, modalities and platforms, (2) dosimetric considerations and planning, and (3) Monte Carlo modeling of SFRT.*

Chapter 9 by H Zhang reviews the development of GRID based SFRT technologies, from the initial GRID block to current commercially available GRID collimators and MLC-based GRID technology and presents the dosimetric characteristics and planning strategies of the various platforms. The development of Lattice therapy, which uses advanced dose painting techniques and affords more individualized sparing of nearby normal structures, is summarized by Wu *et al*, along with the implementation steps and dosimetry and treatment planning guidelines for Lattice therapy in chapter 10.

Rotational arc SFRT, electron GRID and proton therapy offer additional modalities in the GRID radiation therapy domain that are in various stages of development. In chapter 11, X Zhang *et al* summarize key steps for the implementation and planning of rotational arc SFRT, including tomotherapy-based and volumetric modulated arc therapy based SFRT. While patient treatment has to date not been reported, electron GRID offers another type of SFRT, that may be advantageous for treating bulky shallow cancers. Several types of electron SFRT techniques are summarized by Monzen and Tamura in chapter 12. Concluding this part in chapter 13, Gao and Pankuch introduce proton beam SFRT techniques that have recently gained attention for their enhanced normal tissue sparing.

A profound understanding of dose response modeling of the putative biological effects of SFRT is fundamentally important for the clinical implementation of heterogeneity dose radiation approaches. In chapter 14, Bartzsch *et al* discuss the role of the linear quadratic model, equivalent uniform dose, and relative biological effectiveness to be able to account for and compare the biological effects of different types of beams and beam geometries used in SFRT. Further, for clinical implementation, comprehensive commissioning and quality assurance processes are paramount in SFRT. Grams and H Zhang provide an overview of GRID calibration, commissioning quality assurance for Lattice SFRT and suggested treatment workflows in chapter 15.

Practical aspects of SFRT dose prescription and a summary of current prescribing guidelines, which are important for the common understanding and communication among physicians and physicists, are presented in chapter 16 by Mayr *et al.*

The association of heterogeneity dose properties with treatment responses, a critically important area that has been explored experimentally and will require clinical translation along with potential concepts and challenges, is critically reviewed by Chang and Griffin in chapter 17. Monte Carlo simulation has and will continue to play a key role in developing, validating and expanding SFRT. Martínez-Rovira and Fernández-Varea introduce Monte Carlo techniques for photon SFRT simulations in chapter 18. Schneider *et al* discuss proton SFRT Monte Carlo simulations and provide unique insights into simulation techniques and practical approaches in chapter 19.

Part III: **Physics of microbeam, minbeam SFRT and ultra-high dose rate FLASH therapy**

This section focuses on the novel concepts and the potential and emerging applications of *microbeam, minibeam and FLASH therapy.*

Djonov *et al* provide a comprehensive assessment of the status of microbeam radiation, reviewing and discussing physics aspects, dose distribution properties, tumor and normal tissue effects, and potential underlying biologic mechanisms in chapter 20. Prezado gives a review of SFRT across the domains of photons through charged particle technologies and discusses the technological evolution of these domains from large synchrotrons to conventional compact systems in chapter 21.

The final two chapters are dedicated to ultra-high dose rate electron and photon FLASH radiation, the perhaps most profound departure from conventional radiation. Maxim *et al* review perspectives of ultra-high dose rate electron FLASH radiation therapy in chapter 22, which has entered human clinical trial efforts. Bouchet and Potez introduce SFRT and FLASH therapy using synchrotrons, discussed in conjunction with minibeam and microbeam radiation, provide a review of tissue response and biological considerations with synchrotron-based SFRT, and potential therapeutic application in chapter 23.

With such novel approaches at various stages of experimental and clinical progress, and many unanswered questions, each chapter includes a defined section on knowledge gaps that serves as a rigorous assessment of our current status of understanding and may provide potential direction for further investigative inquiry.

# Editor biographies

## Hualin Zhang

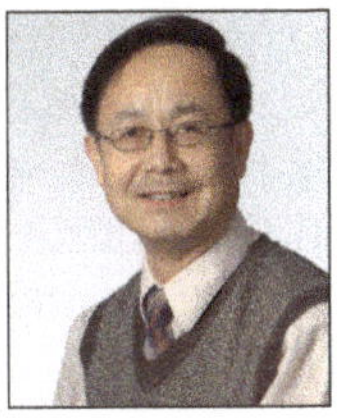

Hualin Zhang, PhD DABR, is an associate professor of the Department of Radiation Oncology at the University of Southern California. Prior to that he held the position of the chief physicist of brachytherapy in the Department of Radiation Oncology at Northwestern University Feinberg School of Medicine from 2013 to 2022. Previously, he was an assistant professor of the Department of Radiation Medicine at The Ohio State University after completing his medical physics residency from the Department of Radiation Medicine of University of Kentucky in 2005.

Dr Zhang's research interests are spatially fractionated (GRID) radiation therapy for bulky tumors, MRI image-guided low dose rate and high dose rate brachytherapy, intraoperative mesh brachytherapy, intraoperative balloon-based low energy x-ray source radiation therapy, and radiobiology modeling for all types of radiation therapy regimens. Dr Zhang has also done extensive research work on Monte Carlo simulation for external beam and brachytherapy dosimetry. Dr Zhang's early research interest was the physics of low energy ion–atom and ion–molecule collisions.

Dr Zhang's clinical focus is the implementation of advanced technologies, with emphasis on spatially fractionated radiation therapy for bulky tumors; MRI image-guided HDR and LDR brachytherapy, intraoperative radiation therapy (IORT), and stereotactic body radiation therapy (SBRT).

He has published over 50 scientific articles and given over 100 scientific presentations. He has served as an NIH reviewer on brachytherapy grants, the co-Chair of the American Association of Physicists in Medicine (AAPM) Intraoperative Mesh Brachytherapy Task Group (TG-222), member of AAPM Spatially Fractionated Radiation Therapy Working Group (SFRTWG), member of AAPM Brachytherapy Dosimetry Working Group (BDWG), member of the AAPM Brachytherapy Dosimetry Consensus Datasets Working Group (UN78), and member of AAPM Robotic Brachytherapy Working Group (RBWG). He currently serves as Chair of the Physics Working Group of the Radiosurgery Society GRID/Lattice, Microbeam and Flash Radiotherapy Working Groups.

Dr Zhang received the outstanding teacher award at Northwestern University Feinberg School of Medicine in 2018.

## Nina A Mayr

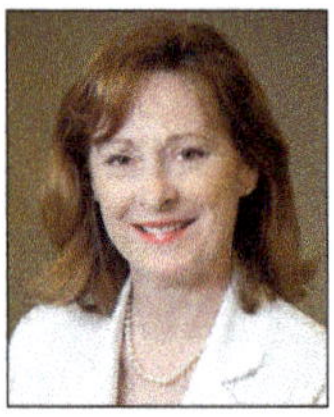

Dr Nina A Mayr, MD FAAAS FACR FASTRO FAAWR, is Professor and Senior Academic Advisor to the Executive Vice President for Health at Michigan State University. She previously served as endowed Professor of Radiation Oncology at the University of Washington School of Medicine, which she joined in 2013 after establishing the Department of Radiation Medicine at the Ohio State University and serving as its inaugural Chair. Prior to this position she was the Director of Radiation Oncology and Professor & Vice Chair of Radiological Sciences at the University of Oklahoma (OU), where she built OU's new radiation oncology facility.

Dr Mayr specializes in tumor imaging, women's cancers, neuro-radiation oncology, lung cancer, and advanced radiation therapy technologies, including stereotactic/ablative and spatially fractionated radiation therapy. For her research she has been awarded two NIH/NCI R01 grants for the study of functional/ molecular imaging as a predictor of cancer treatment outcome, and she has been co-investigator on numerous other awards. She has been focusing on image-guided treatment delivery and advanced technologies in radiation oncology, such as stereotactic radiotherapy and radiosurgery, leveraging advanced imaging for therapy planning, adaptive therapy and imaging-based response assessment.

She has published over 200 scientific articles, 13 book chapters, co-edited two books, and given over 200 scientific presentations and 134 invited lectures and presentations. She has served as NIH reviewer and in numerous capacities in professional societies in her field, including the Chair of the Funding and Advocacy Committee of the American Society for Radiation Oncology (ASTRO), Chair of International Education of ASTRO. She served as Chair of the Subcommittee for Radiation Oncology & Radiobiology of the Scientific Program Committee of the Radiological Society of North America (RSNA), Co-Director of the Instructional Education ('Refresher') Course Track in Radiation Oncology at RSNA, and as member of the Joint ASCO/SSO/ASTRO Expert Panel on Management of Hereditary Breast Cancer Guideline. She currently serves as member of the American College of Radiology (ACR) Human Resources Commission and the ACR Council of Affiliated Regional Radiation Oncology Societies (CARROS) Executive Committee, and as a Chair of the Clinical Working Group of the Radiosurgery Society GRID/Lattice, Microbeam and Flash Radiotherapy Working Groups.

Dr Mayr has been awarded the elected Fellowship by ASTRO in 2011 and has been an Elected Fellow of the American Association of the Advancement of Science (AAAS) since 2006 for her research in imaging and women's cancers. She received the Alice Ettinger Award of the American Association for Women Radiologists (AAWR) in 2013, the American Board of Radiology Lifetime Service Award in 2015, and the Fellow of AAWR in 2019 to recognize her contributions to Radiation Oncology education, mentorship and research, and was elected Fellow of the American College of Radiology in 2023.

# List of contributors

**Gregory S Alexander**
Department of Radiation Oncology, University of Maryland School of Medicine, Baltimore, MD, USA

**Beatriz E Amendola**
Innovative Cancer Institute, South Miami, FL, USA

**Marco A Amendola**
Innovative Cancer Institute, South Miami, FL, USA

**Stefan H Bartzsch**
School of Medicine, Klinikum rechts der Isar, Department of Radiation Oncology, Technical University of Munich, Munich, Germany
and
Institute for Radiation Medicine, Helmholtz Centre Munich, Munich, Germany

**Audrey Bouchet**
French Institute of Health and Medical Research

**Karl T Butterworth**
Patrick G Johnston Centre for Cancer Research, Queen's University Belfast, Northern Ireland

**Sha X Chang**
University of North Carolina, NC, USA

**Ronald Chow**
New York Proton Center, New York, NY, USA

**C Norman Coleman**
Radiation Research Program, Division of Cancer Treatment and Diagnosis, National Cancer Institute, NIH, Bethesda, MD, USA

**Ludovic De Marzi**
Institut Curie, Radiation Oncology Department, Proton Therapy Centre, PSL Research University, University Paris-Saclay, LITO, France

**Valentin Djonov**
University of Bern, Bern, Switzerland

**Cristian Fernández Palomo**
University of Bern, Bern, Switzerland

**José M Fernández-Varea**
Facultat de Física (FQA and ICC), Universitat de Barcelona, Barcelona, Catalonia, Spain

**Silvia C Formenti**
Department of Radiation Oncology, Weill Cornell Medical College, New York, NY, USA

and
Sandra and Edward Meyer Cancer Center, Weill Cornell Medical College, New York, NY, USA

**Mingcheng Gao**
Northwestern Medicine Proton Center, Warrenville, IL, USA

**Encouse B Golden**
Department of Radiation Oncology, Weill Cornell Medical College, New York, NY, USA

**Michael Grams**
Mayo Clinic, Rochester, MN, USA

**Robert J Griffin**
University of Arkansas for Medical Sciences, Little Rock, AR, USA

**Veljko Grilj**
Institute of Radiation Physics/Department of Radiology/CHUV, Lausanne University Hospital and University of Lausanne, Lausanne, Switzerland

**Georges F Hatoum**
JFK Comprehensive Cancer Institute, JFK Medical Center, Atlantis, FL, USA

**Samir V Jenkins**
University of Arkansas for Medical Sciences, Little Rock, AR, USA

**Andrew J Johnsrud**
Stanford University, Stanford CA, USA

**Minglei Kang**
New York Proton Center, New York, NY, USA

**Dan K Kunaprayoon**
Department of Radiation Oncology, University of Maryland School of Medicine, Baltimore, MD, USA

**Xiaobo Li**
Department of Radiation Oncology, Fujian Medical University Union Hospital, Fuzhou, China

**Charles L Limoli**
Department of Radiation Oncology, University of California, Irvine, CA, USA

**Simon S Lo**
Department of Radiation Oncology, University of Washington School of Medicine, Seattle, WA, USA

**Ariel E Marciscano**
Department of Radiation Oncology, Weill Cornell Medical College, New York, NY, USA

**Immaculada Martínez-Rovira**
Universitat Autònoma de Barcelona (UAB), Physics Department, Cerdanyola del Vallès, Barcelona, Catalonia, Spain

**Peter G Maxim**
University of California, Irvine, Orange, CA, USA

**Nina A Mayr**
College of Human Medicine, Michigan State University, East Lansing, MI, USA

**Juergen Meyer**
Department of Radiation Oncology, University of Washington School of Medicine, Seattle, WA, USA

**Majid Mohiuddin**
Northwestern Chicago Proton Center, Warrenville, IL, USA

**Mohammed Mohiuddin**
Radiation Oncology, Scottsdale, AZ, USA

**Hajime Monzen**
Department of Medical Physics, Graduate School of Medical Sciences, Kindai University, Osaka, Japan

**Eduardo G Moros**
Department of Radiation Oncology, Moffitt Cancer Center, Tampa, FL, USA

**Ramón Ortiz**
Institut Curie, University Paris-Saclay, CNRS UMR3347, Inserm U1021, Signalisation Radiobiologie et Cancer, France

**Mark Pankuch**
Northwestern Medicine Proton Center, Warrenville, IL, USA

**Paolo Pellicioli**
European Synchrotron Radiation Facility, Grenoble, France

**José Peñagarícano**
H. Lee Moffitt Cancer Center & Research Institute, Tampa, FL, USA

**Naipy C Perez**
Innovative Cancer Institute, South Miami, FL, USA

**Kristoffer Petersson**
University of Oxford, Oxford, UK

**Marine Potez**
Moffitt Cancer Center, Tampa, FL, USA

**Yolanda Prezado**
Institut Curie, University Paris-Saclay, CNRS UMR3347, Inserm U1021, Signalisation Radiobiologie et Cancer, France

**Kevin M Prise**
Patrick G Johnston Centre for Cancer Research, Queen's University Belfast, Northern Ireland

**William F Regine**
Department of Radiation Oncology, University of Maryland School of Medicine, Baltimore, MD, USA

**Tim Schneider**
Institut Curie, University Paris-Saclay, CNRS UMR3347, Inserm U1021, Signalisation Radiobiologie et Cancer, France

**Emil Schüler**
University of Texas MD Anderson Cancer Center, Houston, TX, USA

**Charles B Simone II**
New York Proton Center, New York, NY, USA

**James W Snider**
University of Alabama at Birmingham, Birmingham, AL, USA

**Robert D Stewart**
Department of Radiation Oncology, University of Washington School of Medicine, Seattle, WA, USA

**Mikoto Tamura**
Department of Medical Physics, Graduate School of Medical Sciences, Kindai University, Osaka, Japan

**Marie-Catherine Vozenin**
Department of Radiation Oncology/Department of Oncology/CHUV, Lausanne University Hospital and University of Lausanne, Lausanne, Switzerland

**James S Welsh**
Department of Radiation Oncology, Loyola University Stritch School of Medicine, Chicago, IL, USA
and
Radiation Oncology Service, Edward Hines Jr. VA Medical Center, Hines, IL, USA

**Xiaodong Wu**
Executive Medical Physics Associates, Miami, FL, USA
and
Innovative Cancer Institute, Miami, FL, USA
and
Department of Radiation Oncology, Fujian Medical University Union Hospital, Fuzhou, China
and
Department of R&D, Fudan University Shanghai Proton and Heavy Ion Center, Shanghai China

**Hualin Zhang**
Department of Radiation Oncology, Keck School of Medicine, University of Southern California, Los Angeles, CA, USA

**Benhua Xu**
Department of Radiation Oncology, College of Medical Technology and Engineering, Fujian Medical University, Fuzhou, China

**Xin Zhang**
Department of Radiation Oncology, Boston Medical Center, Boston University School of Medicine, Boston, MA, USA

# Introductory commentary

Spatially Fractionated Radiation Therapy (SFRT), FLASH, and Innovative Biologically Based New Radiation Therapy Technologies: Tribulations and Trials

**C Norman Coleman**[1, *]
[1]Radiation Research Program, Division of Cancer Treatment and Diagnosis, National Cancer Institute, NIH, Bethesda, MD, USA
*Disclaimer: this paper is the opinion of the author and does not represent the opinion or policy of the NCI, NIH, DHHS.

Conflicts: none

Acknowledgement: Alicia Livinski and Nina Mayr for editorial assistance and Drs Jeff Buchsbaum and Ceferino Obcemea for discussion of the physics and biology interface.

The occasion of this introductory commentary is the March 3, 2022, symposium 'Advancements in GRID/Lattice and FLASH Radiotherapy,' held in conjunction with the Radiosurgery Society's (RSS's) Annual Scientific Meeting in Carlsbad, CA [1]. For many participants, this was the first in-person workshop they had attended since the COVID-19 pandemic began. Face masks were sensibly worn indoors and hand shaking interspersed with elbow bumps as a greeting. This in-person meeting was dynamic and provided important opportunities for hallway and coffee break discussions between participants and colleagues. This 2022 symposium was an important update of the April 2018 workshop organized by the RSS and National Cancer Institute's Radiation Research Program (RRP), on 'Understanding High-Dose, Ultra-High Dose Rate and Spatially Fractionated Radiotherapy' at the NCI.

The invitation to prepare this commentary came from Drs Nina Mayr and Hualin Zhang who are the editors of this textbook *'Spatially Fractionated Microbeam and Flash Radiation Therapy: Physics and multidisciplinary approach'* which is a comprehensive appraisal of the states of these fields. This invitation was welcome, given my previous opinion regarding the need for caution before the clinical application of these therapies [2, 3]. My final question and admonition at that time (2018) for the SFRT field was whether a treatment prescription could be written for a GRID or Lattice treatment in one department (which would apply to microbeam treatments as well) that could readily be understood and duplicated at another. This is an essential question to address in order for a multicenter clinical trial to be able to apply the rigorous research methodology necessary to produce and collect credible results to address a null hypothesis of whether or not SFRT impacts treatment outcomes.

As a 'bottom line up-front,' the March 3, 2022 symposium demonstrated the important progress made by the RSS along with SFRT and FLASH researchers in better understanding the underlying biological and technological radiation dose delivery issues associated with the use of these therapies. Although Dr Nina Mayr was unable to attend, she was given well-deserved praise for her contributions in organizing this book together with Dr Hualin Zhang, and her efforts in developing a consensus on the components required for SFRT clinical trials [4]. The physics community has made important advances in defining criteria for prescriptions describing how to administer GRID and Lattice therapy to patients, which highlighted Dr Hualin Zhang's outstanding leadership efforts in this area, including the editorship of this book. Discussions with Dr Majid Mohiuddin on the proposed NRG Oncology sarcoma SFRT study that he led over the last few years demonstrated substantial efforts toward conducting a GRID randomized clinical trial. While many others are involved in these efforts to design and conduct rigorous clinical trials, these individuals are singled out for their leadership of the field.

The title of this commentary is a modification of the phrase 'trials and tribulations' defined in Merriam-Webster Online Dictionary as: 'trials and tribulations: difficult experiences, problems, etc' [5]. The altered sequence of tribulations and trials used here is a personal perspective on how one deals with treatments that are already in medical practice with varying results, but without a high level of evidence for their efficacy. Such is the case with GRID therapy and more recently with Lattice which have strong support for their use from practitioners based on their years of clinical experience. Their personal observations, enthusiasm, and experience have led to the RSS's interest in expanding the applications of SFRT. However, we do not have a high level of evidence of their efficacy; consequently, we have discussion, debate, and controversy within radiation oncology. Thus, we have *tribulations* (i.e. difficult experiences or problems) *before* the clinical *trials*. However, it is encouraging to see the efforts to provide standardization for GRID and Lattice treatments, and a consensus on the need to conduct clinical trials of these treatments.

At the US NCI, we support advances in radiation oncology [6] by strongly supporting the need to understand SFRT and FLASH and to carry out essential safety and efficacy trials before their widespread application to patients. Table I.1 is

**Table I.1.** NCI efforts stimulating interest in SFRT while working with the RSS.

1. Ahmed M M, Coleman C N, Mendonca M, *et al* 2018 Workshop report for cancer research: defining the shades of Gy: utilizing the biological consequences of radiotherapy in the development of new treatment approaches—meeting viewpoint [7].
2. Coleman C N and Ahmed M M 2019 Implementation of new biology-based radiation therapy technology: when is it ready so 'perfect makes practice?' [2].
3. Griffin R J, Ahmed M M, Amendola B, *et al* 2020 Understanding high-dose, ultra-high dose rate, and spatially fractionated radiation therapy [3].
4. Griffin R J, Limoli C L, Simone C B, 2nd 2020 Radiation research special issue: new beam delivery modalities are shaping the future of radiotherapy [8].
5. Demaria S, Guha C, Schoenfeld J, *et al* 2021 Radiation dose and fraction in immunotherapy: one-size regimen does not fit all settings, so how does one choose? [9].
6. Buchsbaum J C, Coleman C N, Espey M G, *et al* 2021 FLASH radiation therapy: new technology plus biology required. [10].

part of the symposium introduction by Drs Coleman and Mansoor Ahmed from NCI/RRP. It lists, in chronologic order, how the NCI and the RSS have worked together. The first paper by Ahmed, Coleman (equal first authors), *et al* [7] was a concept-changing paper from a 2017 NCI (not RSS) workshop 'Shades of Gy' which proposed that radiation therapy should define doses in biological as well as physical terms. Next, based on presentations on GRID therapy at that 2017 NCI workshop, the 2018 RSS workshop was held. The workshop commentary by Coleman and Ahmed [2] preceded the published workshop report due to the need for NCI to provide peer-reviewed information within a year of a workshop [3]. An extremely positive outcome of the 2018 RSS workshop was the effort made by the SFRT and FLASH communities to address the need for physical definitions of a treatment and biological mechanisms by which they work, as highlighted by Griffin *et al* [8] in the introduction to an outstanding issue of *Radiation Research Journal.* A few papers from that issue relating to clinical trials are included below, and overall, this *Radiation Research Journal* issue is an outstanding educational publication. The complexity of the dose effects of purposeful dose heterogeneity in SFRT is relevant to immunotherapy; thus, the paper by Demaria *et al* [9] was a spin-off relevant to the NCI–RSS efforts.

Again, I point out, as do some others, that the GRID radiotherapy of the early 20th century, which used grids to prevent normal tissue (skin) injury so that tumors could be treated at depth with kilovoltage radiation, was very different biologically than current SFRT, whose goal is to *purposely produce a heterogenous* dose at depth within a tumor using megavoltage radiation. The Buchsbaum *et al* [10] commentary from the NCI/RRP was in response to a now completed clinical trial 'Feasibility Study of FLASH Radiotherapy for the Treatment of Symptomatic Bone Metastases (FAST-01)' [11], which used FLASH with the three primary specified end points of work flow and treatment time, work flow and study treatment, and assessment of the toxicity of 8 Gy of FLASH for bone metastases. The secondary end points were the efficacy of pain control and analgesic use. However, one should interpret the efficacy and safety results cautiously at this dose, as discussed below.

An additional personal observation from the March 3, 2022 symposium is that *tribulations* remain, since there are as yet no prospective randomized efficacy trials. Notably, the work of the leaders and presenters of this symposium opens up the possibility of such studies [1]. The symposium participants showed substantial enthusiasm for the use of SFRT, as it is seemingly easier to write a prescription for GRID than for lattice. Wu *et al* [12] and Amendola *et al* [13] published a case series including the use of SFRT alone and SFRT followed by conventional external beam radiation. An 'encouraging result' was presented for a multi-institutional GRID trial for sarcomas [14]. Whether or not the available GRID devices provide the biological parameters attributed to SFRT as presented in the 2018 workshop, the spacing and configuration of the high and low dose 'peaks and valleys' appeared to be easier to replicate with GRID using standardized blocks, a few of which are available, than with Lattice. The ability to plan a Lattice treatment appears to be more complicated, but guidelines are available. The dose and fractionation appear to depend on clinicians' opinion and experience, which makes it more difficult to conduct clinical trials with Lattice. An assessment of the quality assurance used in the clinical application of these approaches remains to be reported and is a key missing piece of information. Efforts to develop standards are underway by the American Association of Physicists in Medicine (AAPM) through a committee [15] and the American College of Radiology's work on the Imaging and Radiation Oncology Core [16]. Hopefully, their work will be released soon and accepted and used by the community.

The enthusiasm for SFRT was obvious at the March 2022 symposium, and it may be that such enthusiasm, without a grounding in evidence, will make it difficult to conduct a randomized clinical trial. The following is my personal speculation and opinion (and does not in any way reflect the opinion or position of the NCI) that came from a discussion with Dr Majid Mohiuddin about how one might address an impasse over conducting the key randomized trials at the moment. Perhaps there may be biological, treatment timing/sequence, and clinical response end points that can be used if it is impossible at present to randomize a 'yes vs no' SFRT question—although it is likely that such a definitive trial will be necessary at some point. Certainly, the leaders in this field are currently wrestling with this issue (yes, a tribulation!). However, it must be remembered that *trials* test hypotheses and do not confirm or validate suppositions or preferences.

In addition, although there is much to be learned about the biology of SFRT, excellent presentations were given and very interesting potential biological end points were shared at the March 2022 symposium. Data were presented on the FAST-01 trial and progress on dosimetry made by Varian, including dose and dose-rate distributions with various types of beam, including protons. This is clearly an important essential effort in order to define the FLASH effect for clinical use. The incorporation of dose-rate distribution was very innovative in that the FLASH effect of proposed normal tissue sparing will be relevant in total dose ranges that are likely *to require* the FLASH effect to prevent injury. For this reason, the FAST-01 single dose of 8 Gy is a relatively safe dose, as single non-FLASH doses to peripheral bones greater than this are known to be effective with limited toxicity [10]. Thus, the use of FAST-01 for relevant safety signals is very limited in what can be concluded in terms of the demonstration of a FLASH effect in the clinic. Dr Charles Limoli presented information on the mechanisms of FLASH, showing that much is yet to be learned; however, there is clearly excellent research ongoing. He cautioned the audience that toxicity can occur based on specific tissues and doses with recent report from animal experiments [17]. In late 2021, an entire meeting (including virtual participants), 'FLASH Radiotherapy and Particle Therapy Conference,' was held to discuss FLASH [18]. The presentations available from this 2021 FLASH meeting were made available online and will likely appear in peer-reviewed publications in the not-too-distant future. I am grateful to Professor Marie-Catherine Vozenin for sharing her presentation with me, as it helped me prepare this piece.

In conclusion, the last few years have seen substantial efforts devoted to all aspects of SFRT and FLASH. These are very different therapies clinically and biologically, which was well recognized by the symposium attendees. They are potentially important contributions to the 'Shades of Gy' idea [7] of defining radiation doses in biological as well as physical terms. Therefore, keeping these new physical approaches together is useful, as it emphasizes the complexity of moving into the biological use of radiation when biological effects are required as the proposed benefit of novel radiation techniques. This requirement cannot be minimized; therefore, researchers and practitioners must carefully understand the *sine qua non* of the biological effects in order for the treatment to accomplish what is expected of it. There are many practitioners of GRID, as demonstrated by the symposium attendees. This is less the case for Lattice therapy, which is largely in the hands of expert practitioners. There is clearly intense interest in FLASH; progress in its biology and treatment application have made important strides. Yet, we remain in the *tribulations* stage of '*tribulations and trials.*'

I conclude here with praise for the extraordinary efforts of Dr Hualin Zhang in the creation of this textbook and for Dr Nina Mayr [4] in helping to lead and guide the field to be better positioned to conduct the necessary '*trials.*' This recognition was also echoed by many speakers at the March 3, 2022 symposium. The broad interest in moving these fields carefully forward led to an editorial published by Drs Coleman and Mayr based in part on this commentary to accelerate the exchange of information among academia, the NCI, and clinical practitioners [16]. The upcoming 2023 RSS symposium 'Advancements in GRID/Lattice and FLASH Radiotherapy' that will be held just before the publication of this book, is poised to take this discussion further and deeper into the multi-disciplinary 'cross-talk' across the intersections of biology, physics and clinical applications. Considering the complexity of these treatments, we may well go from '*tribulations to trials*' and when clinical data emerge that confound our expectations and biases [17] back to '*trials to tribulations.*' However, progress is made through well-designed and -conducted clinical studies and all with the goal of providing the best patient-centered cancer care.

## References and further reading


[1] *Advancements in GRID, LATTICE and FLASH Radiotherapy Symp., 2022 Radiosurgery Society® Scientific Meeting (March 4–6, 2022, Carlsbad, CA)*

[2] Coleman C N and Ahmed M M 2019 Implementation of new biology-based radiation therapy technology: when is it ready so 'perfect makes practice?' *Int. J. Radiat. Oncol. Biol. Phys.* **105** 934–7

[3] Griffin R J, Ahmed M M and Amendola B *et al* 2020 Understanding high-dose, ultra-high dose rate, and spatially fractionated radiation therapy *Int. J. Radiat. Oncol. Biol. Phys.* **107** 766–78

[4] Mayr N A, Snider J W and Regine W F *et al* 2022 An international consensus on the design of prospective clinical–translational trials in spatially fractionated radiation therapy *Adv. Radiat. Oncol.* **7** 100866

[5] Merriam-Webster.com Dictionary. 'Trials and Tribulations' (accessed 15 March 2022) https://merriam-webster.com/dictionary/trials%20and%20tribulations

[6] Coleman C N, Buchsbaum J C and Prasanna P G S *et al* 2021 Moving forward in the next decade: radiation oncology sciences for patient-centered cancer care *JNCI Cancer Spectr.* **5** pkab046

[7] Ahmed M M, Coleman C N and Mendonca M *et al* 2018 Workshop report for cancer research: defining the shades of Gy: utilizing the biological consequences of radiotherapy in the development of new treatment approaches—meeting viewpoint *Cancer Res.* **78** 2166–70

[8] Griffin R J, Limoli C L and Simone C B 2nd 2020 Radiation research special issue: new beam delivery modalities are shaping the future of radiotherapy *Radiat. Res.* **194** 567–70

[9] Demaria S, Guha C and Schoenfeld J *et al* 2021 Radiation dose and fraction in immunotherapy: one-size regimen does not fit all settings, so how does one choose? *J. Immunother. Cancer* **9** e002038

[10] Buchsbaum J C, Coleman C N and Espey M G *et al* 2021 FLASH radiation therapy: new technology plus biology required *Int. J. Radiat. Oncol. Biol. Phys.* **110** 1248–9

[11] Feasibility Study of FLASH Radiotherapy for the Treatment of Symptomatic Bone Metastases (FAST-01): NCT04592887. 2021; https://clinicaltrials.gov/ct2/show/NCT04592887 (accessed 14 March 2022)

[12] Wu X, Perez N C and Zheng Y *et al* 2020 The technical and clinical implementation of LATTICE radiation therapy (LRT) *Radiat. Res.* **194** 737–46

[13] Amendola B E, Perez N C, Mayr N A, Wu X and Amendola M 2020 Spatially fractionated radiation therapy using lattice radiation in far-advanced bulky cervical cancer: a clinical and molecular imaging and outcome study *Radiat. Res.* **194** 724–36

[14] Snider J W, Molitoris J and Shyu S *et al* 2020 Spatially fractionated radiotherapy (GRID) prior to standard neoadjuvant conventionally fractionated radiotherapy for bulky, high-risk soft tissue and osteosarcomas: feasibility, safety, and promising pathologic response rates *Radiat. Res.* **194** 707–14

[15] American Association of Physicists in Medicine. AAPM Committee: Task Group No. 359 – FLASH (ultra-high dose rate) radiation dosimetry (TG359). https://aapm.org/org/structure/default.asp?committee_code=TG359 (accessed 15 March 2022)

[16] American College of Radiology. Imaging and Radiation Oncology Core. https://irocqa.org/ (accessed 15 March 2022)

[17] Rohrer Bley C *et al* 2022 Dose and volume limiting late toxicity of FLASH radiotherapy in cats with squamous cell carcinoma of the nasal planum and in mini-pigs *Clin. Cancer Res.* **28** 3814–23

[18] *Flash Radiotherapy and Particle Therapy Conf.*, December 1–3, 2021. 2021; https://2021.frpt-conference.org/ (accessed 15 March 2022)

[19] Coleman C N and Mayr N 2022 Tribulations and Trials: The Implementation of Biologically Dependent Radiation Therapy Technologies *Int. J. Radiat. Oncol. Biol. Phys.* **113** 701–4

[20] National Cancer Institute, National Institutes of Health. Radiation Research Program. https://rrp.cancer.gov/default.htm (accessed 15 March 2022)

# Part I

## Biology and clinical use

# Chapter 1

## Introduction to the principles of spatially fractionated radiotherapy

**Karl T Butterworth, Yolanda Prezado and Kevin M Prise**

For several decades, it has been recognized that spatially fractionated radiation fields can be used to improve the therapeutic index of radiotherapy (RT) by reducing normal tissue toxicity. The concept of spatially fractionated radiotherapy (SFRT) was first demonstrated in the clinic using macroscale GRID therapy and has since led to the development of several related spatial fractionation techniques. The dose administered by SFRT can be modulated at several scales; on the micron scale, this has led to the development of microbeam radiotherapy (MRT), and on the millimeter scale it has led to the development of minibeam radiotherapy (MBRT). These approaches have also progressed to three-dimensional irradiation, which allows for the delivery of high dose vertices inside bulky tumors, known as lattice radiotherapy (LRT). Despite increasing evidence from preclinical and clinical studies supporting the role of SFRT, significant challenges remain in optimizing the use of these techniques (including their technical delivery) and the lack of a mechanistic understanding of the responses of tumors and normal tissues.

In this chapter, we provide a brief historical perspective on the development of SFRT and define different forms of SFRT based on their beam properties and dose delivery characteristics. We examine the current preclinical and clinical evidence bases supporting the use of these techniques and discuss the current knowledge gaps that may limit their successful translation to the clinic.

### 1.1 Introduction

RT remains the most effective non-surgical cancer treatment modality that is delivered with curative intent in more than 40% of all cancer cases [1]. RT is most frequently delivered as high energy x-ray photons but can also be delivered as particles in the form of electrons or charged particles including protons. The biological effects of radiation exposure result from the direct or indirect ionization

doi:10.1088/978-0-7503-4046-5ch1

of target molecules, predominantly DNA, in the nucleus of cells. The central clinical concept of RT is to deliver a total tolerable dose that maximizes the difference between the competing tumor control probability (TCP) and the normal tissue complication probability (NTCP), defined as the therapeutic index. Advances in imaging, RT treatment planning, and conformal delivery techniques have significantly improved the therapeutic index of RT, yet the most significant contribution has been the use of fractionated RT, in which the total dose is delivered as a series of smaller doses over the treatment time according to a particular regimen. Conventionally, fractionated RT has been delivered using daily fractions of 2 Gy to allow sufficient time between fractions for normal tissue recovery.

Our current understanding of RT response is predicated on the principle of achieving uniform dose distributions in tumor target volumes. However, evidence from the last century has shown that nonuniform dose distributions achieved by alternating high- and low-dose regions can allow for the delivery of higher integral doses that exceed the tolerance of normal tissues. These approaches are collectively known as SFRT and were originally developed in the early 1900s as a strategy to reduce skin injury during low-energy x-ray exposures by placing an attenuating grid directly onto the patient's skin [2]. This approach directly reduced the exposed volume of skin directly under the grid, resulting in reduced toxicity. Since then, the field of SFRT has continued to evolve through the development of several different techniques that have been explored across different beam geometries ranging from micrometer- to centimeter-scale beams and using two-dimensional or three-dimensional beam patterns. Evidence from both clinical and preclinical studies has clearly demonstrated that dividing the target volume into discrete subvolumes can limit normal tissue damage whilst obtaining levels of tumor control similar to those obtained using broad field exposures. However, the complex interplay between dose distributions and time factors in SFRT remains to be fully understood. Despite evidence supporting the involvement of multiple radiobiological mechanisms in SFRT, the relative contributions of these processes in different SFRT techniques await full definition.

In this introductory chapter, we provide a brief historical perspective on the development and general principles of SFRT. We consider the radiation exposure parameters of conventional RT techniques and compare these characteristics with different types of SFRT currently under investigation. Finally, we highlight the current gaps in knowledge and identify future research opportunities in the field of SFRT.

## 1.2 The historical development of spatially fractionated radiotherapy techniques

The spatial modulation of x-ray fields was first demonstrated over a century ago by Alban Köhler (1874–1947), a pioneering German radiologist who developed GRID RT [2]. Kohler's early GRID approaches involved placing 1 mm square iron wires woven into a 3.0–3.5 mm GRID onto the surface of the skin to deliver around ten times the total dose usually delivered by conventional uniform fields. In contrast to conventional RT, this approach allows high doses to be delivered to tumor subvolumes whilst avoiding the skin toxicities that were usually manifested when delivering large, uniform fields across the entire tumor volume during the orthovoltage era.

The establishment of megavoltage sources in the 1950s limited the development of GRID due to improvements in dose distributions and skin sparing. Major advances in imaging and conformal delivery techniques limited the development of GRID but also offered new opportunities for its delivery at megavoltage energies. In 1990, Mohiuddin and colleagues adapted the principles of GRID therapy to megavoltage photon beams to treat patients with large or recurrent tumors after tolerance doses had been delivered [3]. A 50:50 (open to closed area) GRID was delivered using a custom hexaboard array composed of lucite plates. A dose of 1000–1500 cGy was delivered to the open areas of the GRID using a single 6 MV photon field. Of the 22 patients recruited to the study, eighteen patients had no acute side effects, three patients had minimal effects and only two patients treated for massive liver disease showed any significant nausea or vomiting. None of the patients developed any long-term complications. Since then, GRID has been applied to treat patients with large or recurrent tumors; it has demonstrated encouraging clinical outcomes in both palliative and curative settings and has been recently reviewed by Yan *et al* [4].

GRID therapy is most commonly delivered using physical GRID blocks placed in front of the x-ray head to form alternating high- and low-dose regions. However, these may not be available and can be challenging for routine use. GRID may also be delivered using multileaf collimators (MLCs) or helical tomotherapy systems [5, 6]. These approaches are often more widely available and also offer improved dosimetry due to reduced lateral scattering of the radiation fields. Despite these advances, two-dimensional GRID remains challenging, as normal tissues are still exposed to high radiation doses and the highest doses are delivered to superficial tissues outside of the target volume.

The limitations of two-dimensional GRID can be overcome by delivering SFRT in three dimensions. This approach is termed LRT and uses three-dimensional beam geometries to generate localized high-dose spheres within the target volumes whilst minimizing doses in the peripheral regions. This approach was first conceptualized by Wu *et al* who demonstrated the feasibility of a 3D peak-to-valley dose falloff from 100% to 20%–30% with a greater ability to place dose peaks within the radiation target volume and to deliver minimal doses to the surrounding normal tissues using non-coplanar focused beams and MLC-based or aperture-modulated arc approaches [7]. LRT has translated to the clinic, and several studies demonstrating safety and efficacy in lung and cervical cancers and recurrent gynecologic cancers have been reported by Amendola and colleagues [8–11].

Both GRID and LRT achieve nonuniform dose distributions on the mm–cm scale and have used dose rates of typically 2 Gy $min^{-1}$. In addition, SFRT techniques have been developed using different beam sizes and dose rates. MRT was proposed in 1992 by Slatkin and colleagues [12] and refers to the use of parallel microbeams approximately 25–50 μm wide separated by center-to-center (ctc) distances of 200–400 μm. MRT requires the delivery of very high doses which must be delivered at very high dose rates within a very narrow time window to prevent blurring of the minibeam (MB) tracks due to organ motion, so that the irradiation of an entire organ can be performed in a fraction of a second [13]. Despite decades of preclinical research demonstrating the reduced probabilities of normal tissue complications in different models and tissues, MRT has yet to translate to the clinic due to the requirements for high doses, high-dose-rate synchrotron-generated x-rays, accurate patient positioning, and treatment planning uncertainties. MRT is also limited by the use of x-rays, which still deposit a considerable dose behind the tumor target.

To overcome these limitations whilst still providing a very high therapeutic index, Dilmanian and colleagues proposed the use of minibeam radiotherapy (MBRT) and demonstrated the tissue-sparing advantage of MBRT in the rat brain following exposure to 0.68 mm beams spaced 4 mm on-center at an in-beam depth dose of 400 Gy [14]. MBRT can use higher x-ray energies, offering better sparing of the skin and superficial tissues while maintaining a distinct peak-and-valley pattern [15]. These advantages make MBRT more accessible for widespread implementation using conventional, widespread, and less expensive x-ray equipment compared to MRT, yet MBRT has also not progressed to clinical trials.

The increased establishment of proton therapy in the clinic has led to the development of SFRT using protons. The feasibility of GRID using protons was first demonstrated in a treatment planning study for two patients with abdominal cancer [16]. The first clinical use of pencil beam scanning (PBS) GRID was reported by Gao and colleagues who showed that the treatment was well tolerated and caused no significant skin toxicity in two sarcoma patients [17]. More recently, Mohiuddin and colleagues reported the clinical outcomes of ten patients treated with a single-proton GRID field who were unsuitable for photon GRID due to adjacent critical organs [18].

The use of proton minibeam radiotherapy (pMBRT) was first explored by Prezado and Fois who used simulations to demonstrate that equivalent or higher peak–valley dose ratios (PVDRs) could be achieved using 105 MeV and 1 GeV protons than those obtained using a GammaKnife beam [19]. In contrast to x-ray MBRT, in which multiple interlacing fields are required to achieve target dose homogenization, pMBRT enables the simultaneous achievements of homogenous tumor dose coverage and highly modulated spatial dose distributions in normal tissues [20, 21]. The first implementation of pMBRT was achieved at the Proton Therapy Centre at the Institute Curie in Paris. A schematic representation of the major landmarks in the development of SFRT is shown in figure 1.1.

## 1.3 Current definitions of spatially fractionated radiotherapy

By definition, SFRT divides treatment volumes into fractional subvolumes of high and low doses that alternate between the subvolumes. Whilst no formal definitions have been proposed for the different SFRT modalities, SFRT techniques can be subdivided into main four delivery types based on beam characteristics: GRID, LRT, MBRT, and MRT. A summary of the main beam characteristics of the

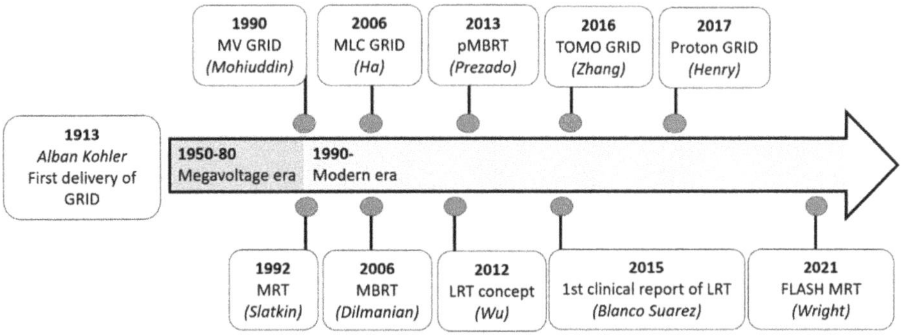


**Figure 1.1.** A time line showing the major landmark developments in SFRT. MRT: microbeam radiotherapy; MBRT: minibeam radiotherapy; pMBRT: proton minibeam radiotherapy; LRT: lattice radiotherapy; TOMO GRID: tomotherapy GRID; FLASH MRT: ultrahigh-dose-rate microbeam radiotherapy.

different forms of SFRT is presented in table 1.1. A schematic representation of the lateral dose profiles for different SFRT techniques is shown in figure 1.2.

The most obvious difference between the four types of SFRT is the irradiation geometry used, which includes the scale and beamlet width. Beamlet widths typically range from 1–2 cm in GRID and LRT to 0.3–1.0 mm in MBRT and micron-sized beams in MRT. The level of spatial modulation also differs: the PVDRs range from two to five in GRID to higher than 50 in MRT. The main characteristics of these different forms of SFRT are summarized in table 1.1 [23]. Both GRID and LRT have been translated to the clinic, whilst MBRT and MRT have not yet been evaluated in clinical trials. Whilst all four types have been mainly explored using x-rays thus far, the delivery of SFRT using charged particles continues to develop and is discussed in chapter 21.

### 1.3.1 GRID radiotherapy

GRID is the oldest form of SFRT that has been used in the clinic. It is typically delivered using beamlets of 1–2 cm with peak doses of <15 Gy. GRID is delivered at conventional dose rates of 2 Gy $min^{-1}$ and can be delivered using GRID blocks, MLCs, helical tomotherapy systems, or flattening filter-free (FFF) accelerators [24]. Compared to conventional GRID approaches, FFF accelerators allow the use of thinner beams in the range of 3 $mm^2$. The prescription doses in GRID are commonly peak doses of between 10 and 20 Gy, usually in one but sometimes up to three fractions, and are usually delivered preceding conventional RT.

The most common indications that have been treated with GRID include mainly palliative treatments of head and neck cancers, soft-tissue sarcomas, and other bulky tumors. In the palliative setting, GRID has shown response rates of over 70% (pain reduction and mass effect) in patients with bulky tumors [25, 26]. Mohuiddin and colleagues [27] reported promising improvements in local control and limb salvage in patients with locally advanced high-grade extremity soft-tissue sarcoma. Penagaricano *et al* [28] also reported an overall control rate of 79%

**Table 1.1.** Summary of the main beam characteristics for different spatially fractionated radiotherapy (SFRT) techniques.

| SFRT Technique | Radiation sources | Beamlet widths | Typical peak dose | Level of spatial modulation (Peak valley dose ratio) | Dose/fraction (Gy) | Dose rates | Intended use |
|---|---|---|---|---|---|---|---|
| GRID | x-rays (MV), gamma rays, protons | 1–2 cm | 10–15 | Low (2–5) | 15–20 | 1–6 Gy $min^{-1}$ | Mainly palliative |
| Lattice | x-rays, protons | 1–2 cm | 10–15 | Low (2–5) | 15–20 | 2 Gy $min^{-1}$ | Mainly Palliative |
| Minibeam | x-rays (MV), protons | 0.3–1 mm | 50–100 | Medium (10–20) | 15–20 | 2 Gy $min^{-1}$ | Preclinical (potentially radical treatments) |
| Preclinical | Microbeam (potentially radical treatments) | x-rays | 50–100 μm | 300–600 | High (> 50) | 50–1000 | 50–1000 Gy $sec^{-1}$ |

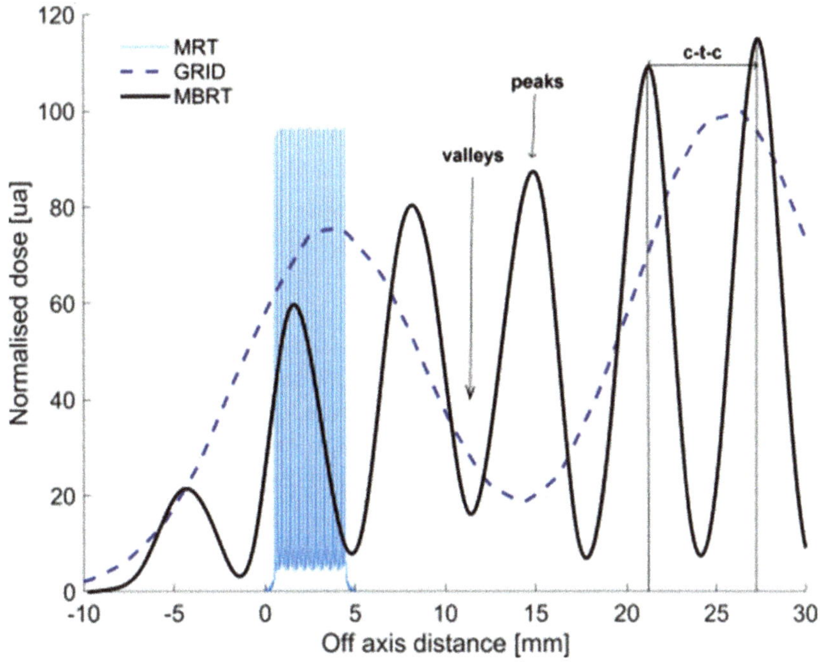


**Figure 1.2.** A schematic illustration of the lateral dose profiles for spatially fractionated radiotherapy techniques. MRT: microbeam radiotherapy; MBRT: minibeam radiotherapy; ctc: center-to-center distance. Reprinted from [22], Copyright (2019), with permission from Elsevier.

(11 of 14 patients) for the GRID gross tumor volume in patients with bulky (⩾6 cm) tumors from locally advanced squamous cell carcinoma of the head and neck.

Despite the high therapeutic index observed in difficult-to-treat cases, these studies did not include a control arm and treated heterogeneous patient groups. However, the most critical point in these studies is the dose prescription point, which was usually placed at the surface or the depth of the maximum dose deposition in the peak region. Consequently, the same GRID geometry and prescription may result in very different doses both to the target and organs at risk, depending on the patient-specific anatomical context. An extensive review of clinical GRID studies has been recently been reported [29], and GRID therapy is discussed in more detail in chapters 5 and 6.

GRID therapy has been commonly performed with photon beams; however, the use of other particles such as protons, carbon ions, and electrons has also been proposed. Proton GRID therapy uses beamlets of around 1 cm in diameter and is currently limited to palliative treatments in bulky tumors. The use of protons results in a more uniform dose within the tumor (lower PVDR) and helps in the sparing of normal tissues located beyond the tumor. Early clinical results from ten patients with large and bulky tumors refractory to prior treatments reported tumor regression/local control improvement rates of 80%, and only 50% of patients showed acute grade one or grade two toxicities [18]. As a result of the tolerance of normal tissues to proton GRID, it may enable the treatment of patients unsuitable for conventional RT or photon GRID. A more detailed evaluation of SFRT using protons and other heavy ions is presented in chapter 21.

### 1.3.2 Lattice radiotherapy

LRT is a novel form of SFRT that builds on conventional two-dimensional GRID to deliver high doses of radiation to small vertices distributed within the central areas of the gross tumor volume (GTV) whilst minimizing the dose administered to the peripheral areas adjacent to normal tissues [7, 8].

LRT has been used in the clinic to treat indications including cervical squamous cell carcinoma, ovarian cancer, and non-small cell lung cancer [8–10]. These approaches have typically used macroscale beam geometries to deliver a single fraction in which the lattice vertices received high doses of up to 18 Gy delivered using 6 MeV photons. LRT is further discussed in chapters 7 and 10.

### 1.3.3 Minibeam radiotherapy

MBRT involves the delivery of planar minibeams typically ranging from 0.3 to 1 mm with ctc distances of a few millimeters. Beams of these sizes are less affected by dose smearing due to cardio-synchronous pulsations, thereby lowering the requirements for the high dose rates associated with MRT. Despite the larger beam sizes, many experiments have found that MBRT can still lead to substantial increases in the doses tolerated by normal tissue as compared to standard uniform irradiation [14, 30–32]. Preclinical studies have demonstrated significant increases in normal tissue tolerance in the rat brain to single-fraction peak doses of >100 Gy following exposure to 600–700 μm wide beams [32, 33]. MBRT has also been shown to deliver equivalent levels of tumor control to those delivered by broad beam sources in rat models of glioma [33, 34].

Whilst MBRT has yet to be translated to humans, it has been trialed in veterinary radiation oncology. Kundapour [35] reported a Phase III study of *de novo* brain tumors in pet dogs. Dogs were randomized to standard stereotactic RT (9 Gy × 3 fractions) or single-fraction MBRT with synchrotron-generated 6 MV 1 mm beams (a mean dose of 26 Gy). All of the dogs showed almost complete response on follow-up by magnetic resonance imaging (MRI) at the time of the report. Four out of seven dogs showed a complete pathological response and one dog was still on follow-up at the time of reporting. Fewer long-term toxicities were observed in MBRT-treated dogs compared to those treated using standard RT.

The high therapeutic index of MBRT can be further enhanced by exploiting the superior relative biological effectiveness and dose distributions of charged particles. The use of charged particles opens new possibilities for the generation of magnetically focused and scanned minibeams. pMBRT is the most explored experimental form of SFRT based on charged particles. This idea has recently been conceptualized using a minibeam nozzle with a clinical proton linear accelerator to achieve beams of 0.6–0.9 mm full width at half maximum [36].

In contrast to MBRT delivered using x-rays, in which multiple interlacing fields are required to achieve target dose homogenization, pMBRT simultaneously offers homogenous tumor dose coverage and highly modulated spatial dose distributions in normal tissues [20]. A series of radiobiological studies has already shown that pMBRT offers a very high therapeutic ratio for radioresistant tumors such as high-grade gliomas together with a significant reduction in normal tissue damage (skin and brain) compared to standard proton therapy, while offering equivalent or superior tumor control [20, 37–40]. These data expand the evidence base for the use of pMBRT and support its future translation to Phase I clinical trials. Finally, the use of heavier particles such as neon ions is being reconsidered in the context of MBRT, and light ions such as helium ions have been explored as a potential alternative to protons. Further details are discussed in chapter 21.

### 1.3.4 Microbeam radiotherapy

MRT was first defined in 1992 by Slatkin and colleagues [12] to refer to the use of parallel 50–150 keV micron-sized x-ray beams for potential therapeutic use, specifically in the treatment of pediatric brain tumors. This concept was developed from earlier approaches introduced by Curtis using deuteron beams that were restricted into 25 mm circular or rectangular incident beams [41]. In contrast to macroscopic beam exposures, much higher doses were required to produce tissue necrosis in the mouse brain with these deuteron beams.

The development of MRT approaches has been driven by this observation of reduced normal tissue toxicity. A key factor in the use of MRT is the ability to deliver very high doses (up to 1000 Gy) at high dose rates (300–600 Gy $s^{-1}$). Therefore, these approaches have been limited to using the large synchrotron facilities available at the European Synchrotron Facility (ESRF) and the Brookhaven National Laboratory (BNL). These microbeams are defined by key physical parameters including the peak dose of each microbeam (50–1000 Gy), the width of each beam (typically 25–100 μm), and the peak-to-peak spacing (i.e. the interbeam spacing, typically 50–200 μm). Extensive preclinical work has validated the approach for extensive sparing of normal tissue damage, not only in the brain [42] but also in the lungs [43], skin [44], and vasculature [45]. Under these conditions, significant cell killing is observed in tumor cells, leading to a significant increase in the therapeutic ratio. Although studies were initially undertaken with unidirectional beams, today's studies involve bidirectional beams, or in the most advanced studies, multiple beam arrays directed at the target. To date, no clinical trials of MRT have been undertaken.

### 1.3.5 Implications of dose rate

With the exception of MRT, most forms of SFRT involve beam delivery at conventional dose rates of 2–6 Gy $min^{-1}$. MRT typically involves the delivery of high dose rates (50–1000 Gy $s^{-1}$) and in most cases high peak dose exposures (100–1000 Gy). In conventional RT, a wide range of dose rates have been explored, ranging from 0.1 Gy $h^{-1}$ to several Gy $min^{-1}$. In this range, the fraction of cells killed by a given dose decreases with decreasing dose rate, which is principally due to the repair of sublethal damage [46]. However, this paradigm is being challenged by new data at higher dose rates (typically >40 Gy $s^{-1}$) showing remarkable protection of normal tissues via the FLASH effect [47–49]. While previous studies in the 1970s and 1980s suggested that increased dose rates may potentially have protective effects in normal tissues [47], it is only recently that these effects have been better defined and are beginning to translate to the clinic [50].

The potential interplay between dose rate effects and spatial fractionation remains to be understood. However, given the observations of the dose-sparing effects in MRT, it is plausible that the underlying mechanisms responsible for the responses to MRT and FLASH exposures may be related. To date, only one study has evaluated the impact of spatially fractionated MRT at ultrahigh dose rates. A recent study by Wright *et al* demonstrated the tissue-sparing efficacy of FLASH MRT with 50 μm beams at an average dose rate of 1.4 $\times 10^4$ Gy $s^{-1}$. The study showed that FLASH MRT provided an order of magnitude reduction in pulmonary fibrosis in male Fischer-344 rats 12 months after irradiation [51]. Whilst this study did not include a direct comparison between FLASH MRT or conventional FLASH and low-dose-rate broad field exposures, it raises intriguing hypotheses concerning the interplay between dose rate and dose distribution and the potential to optimize these parameters for some indications.

## 1.4 Knowledge gaps and future perspectives

The successful translation and implementation of SFRT techniques to the clinic is limited due to due to a lack of specialist centers with the required technologies and physics expertise to deliver high-quality SFRT and a lack of understanding of the biological mechanisms that mediate response. Also, it is not clear for which tumor sites SFRT techniques are likely to deliver the largest improvement in therapeutic ratio. The majority of preclinical studies of MRT and MBRT have been performed using glioma models, yet other sites may be equally suited to these techniques. It is not clear how SFRT can be exploited in a precision medicine context, i.e. one based on tumor and normal tissue biomarkers. This question is equally applicable across all RT modalities, but is an important consideration as we move towards realizing this treatment paradigm in radiation oncology.

From a technological perspective, the use of MRT with sufficiently low beam divergence currently relies on large infrastructure synchrotron sources that are not optimized for patient treatments. There is continued interest in the development of alternative beam sources for SFRT including, for example, modular multilevel converters (MMCs) from high-voltage direct-current transmission technologies for line-focused x-ray tubes [52]. In addition, an improved understanding and consensus are needed to define the optimum treatment parameters for different SFRT techniques, including dose prescriptions and constraints, fractionation schedules, and perhaps also for dose rates.

From a biological perspective, an improved understanding of the mechanisms underpinning response in preclinical SFRT can provide important information to inform the design of clinical trials. The steep dose gradients associated with SFRT generally suggest significantly greater than expected out-of-field effects and unexpected increases in survival infield. These data indicate that the observed dose–response relationships for high modulated fields cannot be predicted from uniform exposures based on the standard radiobiological DNA damage and repair model. On a basic level, this concept has been explored extensively in a series of *in vitro* studies and modeling studies [53, 54]. Additional biological mechanisms including radiation-induced bystander responses, microvascular effects, and immune modulation play a role in mediating responses to SFRT and may potentially increase tumor cell death or reduce normal tissue damage. To date, the relative contributions and interrelationship of these mechanisms in response to different SFRT modalities have remained unclear. The biological basis of SFRT has been reviewed extensively [11, 29, 55, 56] and is discussed in detail in chapter 2.

An area that has yet to be extensively explored is how best to optimize the combination of SFRT with other systemic therapies. Classically, RT has been combined with cytotoxic chemotherapy, yet there is clear potential to combine RT with molecularly targeted agents. As only relatively small tumor volumes receive high doses in SFRT, curative treatments may require the use of other systemic therapies. SFRT may also play a key role in the metastatic disease setting if abscopal effects play a role. Given the well-established effects of RT on the immune system, a case study recently reported the combined use of LRT and immune checkpoint blockade using anti-PD1 immunotherapy in a non-small cell lung cancer (NSCLC) patient with multiple metastases [57]. The patient showed a 77.84% regression in metastatic mass one month after the treatment with a complete local response five months after the treatment; no treatment-related side effects were observed during follow-up. These data support the further investigation and exploration of SFRT combined with immune checkpoint blockade.

## 1.5 Summary

SFRT challenges the conventional RT paradigm by aiming to deliver a highly heterogeneous dose to the tumor target volume and normal tissues using subvolumes of high and low doses. The unique spatial dose patterns associated with SFRT can be achieved using several different approaches and have unique features that protect normal tissues at high dose exposures while achieving equivalent levels of tumor control. Both GRID and LRT have translated to the clinic; however, further studies are needed to better define the most effective beam characteristics for these treatments and potential biological opportunities for treatment optimization.

## References

[1] Ringborg U, Bergqvist D, Brorsson B, Cavallin-Ståhl E, Ceberg J and Einhorn N *et al* 2003 The Swedish Council on Technology Assessment in Health Care (SBU) systematic overview of radiotherapy for cancer including a prospective survey of radiotherapy practice in Sweden 2001—summary and conclusions *Acta Oncol.* **42** 357–65

[2] Laissue J A, Blattmann H and Slatkin D N 2012 Alban Köhler (1874–1947): inventor of grid therapy *Z. Med. Phys.* **22** 90–9

[3] Mohiuddin M and L CD W T G L K 1990 Palliative treatment of advanced cancer using multiple nonconfluent pencil beam radiation. A pilot study *Cancer* **1** 114–8

[4] Yan W, Khan M K, Wu X, Simone C B, Fan J and Gressen E *et al* 2020 Spatially fractionated radiation therapy: history, present and the future *Clin. Transl. Radiat. Oncol.* **20** 30–8

[5] Ha J K, Zhang G, Naqvi S A, Regine W F and Yu C X 2006 Feasibility of delivering grid therapy using a multileaf collimator *Med. Phys.* **33** 76–82

[6] Zhang X, Penagaricano J, Yan Y, Liang X, Morrill S and Griffin R J *et al* 2016 Spatially fractionated radiotherapy (GRID) using helical tomotherapy *J. Appl. Clin. Med. Phys.* **17** 396–407

[7] Wu X, Ahmed M M, Wright J, Gupta S and Pollack A 2012 On modern technical approaches of three-dimensional high-dose lattice radiotherapy (LRT) *Cureus* **2** e9

[8] Amendola B E, Perez N C, Wu X, Amendola M A and Qureshi I Z 2019 Safety and efficacy of lattice radiotherapy in voluminous non-small cell lung cancer *Cureus* **11** e4263

[9] Blanco Suarez J M, Amendola B E, Perez N, Amendola M and Wu X 2015 The use of lattice radiation therapy (LRT) in the treatment of bulky tumors: a case report of a large metastatic mixed mullerian ovarian tumor *Cureus* **7** e389

[10] Amendola B E, Perez N C, Wu X, Blanco Suarez J M, Lu J J and Amendola M 2018 Improved outcome of treating locally advanced lung cancer with the use of Lattice Radiotherapy (LRT): a case report *Clin. Transl. Radiat. Oncol.* **9** 68–71

[11] Griffin R J, Ahmed M M, Amendola B, Belyakov O, Bentzen S M and Butterworth K T *et al* 2020 Understanding high-dose, ultra-high dose rate, and spatially fractionated radiation therapy *Int. J. Radiat. Oncol. Biol. Phys.* **107** 766–78

[12] Slatkin D N, Spanne P, Dilmanian F A and Sandbora M 1992 Microbeam radiation therapy *Med. Phys.* **19** 1395–400

[13] Grotzer M A, Schültke E, Bräuer-Krisch E and Laissue J A 2015 Microbeam radiation therapy: clinical perspectives *Phys. Medica* **31** 564–7

[14] Dilmanian F A, Zhong Z, Bacarian T, Benveniste H, Romanelli P and Wang R *et al* 2006 Interlaced x-ray microplanar beams: a radiosurgery *Proc. Natl Acad. Sci. USA* **103** 9709–14

[15] Prezado Y, Thengumpallil S, Renier M and Bravin A 2009 X-ray energy optimization in minibeam radiation therapy *Med. Phys.* **36** 4897–902

[16] Henry T, Ureba A, Valdman A and Siegbahn A 2017 Proton grid therapy: a proof-of-concept study *Technol. Cancer Res. Treat.* **16** 749–57

[17] Gao M, Mohiuddin M M, Hartsell W F and Pankuch M 2018 Spatially fractionated (GRID) radiation therapy using proton pencil beam scanning (PBS): feasibility study and clinical implementation *Med. Phys.* **45** 1645–53

[18] Mohiuddin M, Lynch C, Gao M and Hartsell W 2020 Early clinical results of proton spatially fractionated GRID radiation therapy (SFGRT) *Br. J. Radiol.* **93** 20190572

[19] Prezado Y and Fois G R 2013 Proton-minibeam radiation therapy: a proof of concept *Med. Phys.* **40** 031712

[20] Zlobinskaya O, Girst S, Greubel C, Hable V, Siebenwirth C and Walsh D W M *et al* 2013 Reduced side effects by proton microchannel radiotherapy: study in a human skin model *Radiat. Environ. Biophys.* **52** 123–33

[21] Gil S, Prezado Y and Sabés M 2014 Double-strand breaks on F98 glioma rat cells induced by minibeam and broad-beam synchrotron radiation therapy *Clin. Transl. Oncol.* **16** 696–701
[22] De Marzi L, Nauraye C, Lansonneur P, Pouzoulet F, Patriarca A and Schneider T *et al* 2019 Spatial fractionation of the dose in proton therapy: proton minibeam radiation therapy *Cancer Radiother.* **23** 677–81
[23] Prezado Yolanda 2022 Divide and conquer: spatially fractionated radiation therapy *Expert Rev. Mol. Med.* **24** E3
[24] Martínez-Rovira I, Puxeu-Vaqué J and Prezado Y 2017 Dose evaluation of grid therapy using a 6 MV flattening filter-free (FFF) photon beam: a Monte Carlo study *Med. Phys.* **44** 5378–83
[25] Mohiuddin M, Fujita M, Regine W F, Megooni A S, Ibbott G S and Ahmed M M 1999 High-dose spatially-fractionated radiation (GRID): a new paradigm in the management of advanced cancers *Int. J. Radiat. Oncol. Biol. Phys.* **45** 721–7
[26] Neuner G, Mohiuddin M M, Vander Walde N, Goloubeva O, Ha J and Yu C X *et al* 2012 High-dose spatially fractionated GRID radiation therapy (SFGRT): a comparison of treatment outcomes with cerrobend vs. MLC SFGRT *Int. J. Radiat. Oncol. Biol. Phys.* **82** 1642–9
[27] Mohiuddin M, Memon M, Nobah A, Elsebaie M, Suhaibani A L and Pant R A *et al* 2014 Locally advanced high-grade extremity soft tissue sarcoma: response with novel approach to neoadjuvant chemoradiation using induction spatially fractionated GRID radiotherapy (SFGRT) *J. Clin. Oncol.* **32** 10575
[28] Peñagarícano J A, Moros E G, Ratanatharathorn V, Yan Y and Corry P 2010 Evaluation of spatially fractionated radiotherapy (GRID) and definitive chemoradiotherapy with curative intent for locally advanced squamous cell carcinoma of the head and neck: initial response rates and toxicity *Int. J. Radiat. Oncol. Biol. Phys.* **76** 1369–75
[29] Billena C and Khan A J 2019 A current review of spatial fractionation: back to the future? *Int. J. Radiat. Oncol. Biol. Phys.* **104** 177–87
[30] Prezado Y, Dos Santos M, Gonzalez W, Jouvion G, Guardiola C and Heinrich S *et al* 2017 Transfer of Minibeam Radiation Therapy into a cost-effective equipment for radiobiological studies: a proof of concept *Sci. Rep.* **7** 17295
[31] Deman P, Vautrin M, Stupar V, Barbier E L, Elleaume H and Esteve F *et al* 2011 Monochromatic minibeam radiotherapy: theoretical and experimental dosimetry for preclinical treatment plans *Phys. Med. Biol.* **56** 4465–80
[32] Prezado Y, Deman P, Varlet P, Jouvion G, Gil S and Le Clec' H C *et al* 2015 Tolerance to dose escalation in minibeam radiation therapy applied to normal rat brain: long-term clinical, radiological and histopathological analysis *Radiat. Res.* **184** 314–21
[33] Deman P, Vautrin M, Edouard M, Stupar V, Bobyk L and Farion R *et al* 2012 Monochromatic minibeams radiotherapy: from healthy tissue-sparing effect studies toward first experimental glioma bearing rats therapy *Int. J. Radiat. Oncol. Biol. Phys.* **82** E693–E700
[34] Prezado Y, Sarun S, Gil S, Deman P, Bouchet A and Le Duc G 2012 Increase of lifespan for glioma-bearing rats by using minibeam radiation therapy *J. Synchrotron Radiat.* **19** 60–5
[35] V K 2019 New kid on the block-mini beam radiation treatment – final report of a randomized phase III study of treating canine denovo brain tumors *Int. J. Radiat. Oncol. Biol. Phys.* **105** 683–4

[36] Schneider T, Patriarca A, Degiovanni A, Gallas M and Prezado Y 2021 Conceptual design of a novel nozzle combined with a clinical proton linac for magnetically focussed minibeams *Cancers (Basel)* **13** 1–15
[37] Lamirault C, Brisebard E, Patriarca A, Juchaux M, Crepin D and Labiod D *et al* 2020 Spatially modulated proton minibeams results in the same increase of lifespan as a uniform target dose coverage in F98-glioma-bearing rats *Radiat. Res.* **194** 715–23
[38] Prezado Y, Jouvion G, Guardiola C, Gonzalez W, Juchaux M and Bergs J *et al* 2019 Tumor control in RG2 glioma-bearing rats: a comparison between proton minibeam therapy and standard proton therapy *Int. J. Radiat. Oncol. Biol. Phys.* **104** 266–71
[39] Prezado Y, Jouvion G, Hardy D, Patriarca A, Nauraye C and Bergs J *et al* 2017 Proton minibeam radiation therapy spares normal rat brain: long-term clinical, radiological and histopathological analysis *Sci. Rep.* **7** 1–7
[40] Girst S, Greubel C, Reindl J, Siebenwirth C, Zlobinskaya O and Walsh D W M *et al* 2016 Proton minibeam radiation therapy reduces side effects in an *in vivo* mouse ear model *Int. J. Radiat. Oncol. Biol. Phys.* **95** 234–41
[41] Curtis H J 1967 The use of a deuteron microbeam for simulating the biological effects of heavy cosmic-ray particles *Radiat. Res. Suppl* **7** 250–7
[42] Laissue J A *et al* 2001 Weanling piglet cerebellum: a surrogate for tolerance to MRT (microbeam radiation therapy) in pediatric neuro-oncology *Penetrating Radiation Systems and Applications III International Symposium on Optical Science and Technology Proc. SPIE* 4508 (Bellingham, WA: SPIE) 65–73
[43] Schültke E, Bayat S, Bartzsch S, Bräuer-Krisch E, Djonov V and Fiedler S *et al* 2021 A Mouse model for microbeam radiation therapy of the lung *Int. J. Radiat. Oncol. Biol. Phys.* **110** 521–5
[44] Crosbie J C, Anderson R L, Rothkamm K, Restall C M, Cann L and Ruwanpura S *et al* 2010 Tumor cell response to synchrotron microbeam radiation therapy differs markedly from cells in normal tissues *Int. J. Radiat. Oncol. Biol. Phys.* **77** 886–94
[45] Van Der Sanden B, Bräuer-Krisch E, Siegbahn E A, Ricard C, Vial J C and Laissue J 2010 Tolerance of arteries to microplanar X-ray beams *Int. J. Radiat. Oncol. Biol. Phys.* **77** 1545–52
[46] Hall E J and Brenner D J 1991 The dose-rate effect revisited: radiobiological considerations of importance in radiotherapy *Int. J. Radiat. Oncol. Biol. Phys.* **21** 1403–14
[47] Vozenin M C, Hendry J H and Limoli C L 2019 Biological benefits of ultra-high dose rate FLASH radiotherapy: sleeping beauty awoken *Clin. Oncol.* **31** 407–15
[48] Favaudon V, Caplier L, Monceau V, Pouzoulet F, Sayarath M and Fouillade C *et al* 2014 Ultrahigh dose-rate FLASH irradiation increases the differential response between normal and tumor tissue in mice **6** 1–10
[49] Friedl A A, Prise K M, Butterworth K T, Montay-Gruel P and Favaudon V 2021 Radiobiology of the FLASH effect *Med. Phys.* **49** 1993–2013
[50] Bourhis J, Sozzi W J, Jorge P G, Gaide O, Bailat C and Duclos F *et al* 2019 Treatment of a first patient with FLASH-radiotherapy *Radiother. Oncol.* **139** 18–22
[51] Wright M D, Romanelli P and Bravin A *et al* 2021 Non-conventional ultra-high dose rate (FLASH) microbeam radiotherapy provides superior normal tissue sparing in rat lung compared to non-conventional ultra-high dose rate (FLASH) radiotherapy *Cureus* **13** e19317

[52] Winter J, Galek M, Matejcek C, Wilkens J J, Aulenbacher K and Combs S E *et al* 2020 Clinical microbeam radiation therapy with a compact source: specifications of the line-focus X-ray tube *Phys. Imaging Radiat. Oncol.* **14** 74–81

[53] Butterworth K T, Ghita M, McMahon S J, McGarry C K, Griffin R J and Hounsell A R *et al* 2017 Modelling responses to spatially fractionated radiation fields using preclinical image-guided radiotherapy *Br. J. Radiol.* **90** 20160485

[54] Butterworth K T, Trainor C, O'Sullivan J M, Hounsell A R and Prise K M 2011 Out-of-field cell survival following exposure to intensity-modulated radiation fields *Int. J. Radiat. Oncol.* **79** 1516–22

[55] Asur R, Butterworth K T, Penagaricano J A, Prise K M and Griffin R J 2013 High dose bystander effects in spatially fractionated radiation therapy *Cancer Lett.* **356** 52–7

[56] Fukunaga H, Butterworth K T, McMahon S J and Prise K M 2021 A brief overview of the preclinical and clinical radiobiology of microbeam radiotherapy *Clin. Oncol.* **33** 705–12

[57] Jiang L, Li X, Zhang J, Li W, Dong F and Chen C *et al* 2021 Combined high-dose LATTICE radiation therapy and immune checkpoint blockade for advanced bulky tumors: the concept and a case report *Front. Oncol.* **10** 1–8

# Chapter 2

## General principles of SFRT biology

**Andrew J Johnsrud, Samir V Jenkins and Robert J Griffin**

While the radiobiologic effects leading to tumor responses after spatially fractionated radiotherapy (SFRT) are incompletely understood, accumulating evidence supports the involvement of local bystander and abscopal effects, vascular damage and angiogenic responses, and radiation-induced immune modulation as important events that occur after nonuniform dose exposures. These are likely generated and maintained by complex interactions between the interspersed areas of unequal heterogeneous dose distribution and highly dependent on peak (high dose) to valley (low dose) dose ratios. The biologic mechanisms are not mutually exclusive, and their relative impact may vary between different SFRT techniques. Similarly, the coordination of these unique properties may lead to tremendous antitumor responses beyond those attributable to traditional radiobiologic properties and may also promote early abscopal phenomena outside of the radiation field. The latter are likely immune mediated, as supported by multiple studies describing increased cytokine production that results in broad systemic effects. While the exact mechanisms of antitumor immune effects remain unknown, they likely originate from initial changes to the local immune microenvironment after SFRT that may derive from heterogeneous sparing of vascular integrity and lymphocyte viability due to unequal dose distribution inside the radiation field. Unique alterations in vascular architecture and enhanced reoxygenation of the tumor may further contribute to tumor control following SFRT. Here, we review emerging concepts from the nascent field of SFRT, with an emphasis on preclinical studies that highlight biologic principles and their translational potential.

### 2.1 Introduction

In this chapter, we review the general principles of SFRT biology with an emphasis on accumulating evidence supporting multifactorial non-target (bystander) effects, microvascular alterations, and radiation-induced immune modulation as important

doi:10.1088/978-0-7503-4046-5ch2

sequelae of SFRT. Importantly, these mechanisms are not mutually exclusive of one another, and their relative impact may vary among different techniques (GRID/LRT, FLASH, MRT). Advanced or bulky tumors for which these methods have historically been applied may also be radio- and chemotherapy-resistant due to poor blood flow, hypoxia, or low pH in the tumor, features which may influence the degree to which these biologic responses occur. Ultimately, the continued exploration of how these and other distinct biologic processes during SFRT can synergize with one another and in combination with novel immunotherapy schemes holds promise for translation into significant clinical benefits.

### 2.1.1 Defining the biologic characteristics of spatially fractionated radiotherapy

By definition, SFRT divides treatment volumes into interspersed areas of inhomogeneous dose distribution, whereas more traditional external beam radiation methods deliver whole-tumor exposures. Historically, this was developed using grid pattern or multileaf collimators with the goal of achieving better tumor control with reduced normal tissue toxicity after high doses of radiation. Today, emerging methods of SFRT use increasingly sophisticated, highly conformal techniques which have been established at various stages of development. These include GRID, FLASH, lattice radiation therapy (LRT), microbeam radiation therapy (MRT) and minibeam radiation therapy (MBRT) (figure 2.1). The more novel SFRT techniques (i.e. MRT, FLASH) share common spatial distribution characteristics but are distinct in that they occur on the scale of micron- and centimeter-wide beam parameters and at remarkably different dose rates.

The notion that SFRT might generate unique biological effects was established after early reports demonstrating successful palliation of otherwise intractable, deep-seated tumors with minimal toxicity despite relatively high dose levels [1–4] (further reviewed in chapter 5), followed by mechanistic studies implicating the reoxygenation and modulation of growth factor or systemic cytokine production as important features of SFRT. While the specific radiobiologic effects leading to tumor responses after SFRT remain incompletely understood, the molecular underpinnings are likely driven by modulation of the spatial dose distribution, which leads to dramatic peak–valley differences inside the radiation field. Importantly, optimal peak–valley gradients and their defining downstream biologic events are incompletely understood. Likewise, the way in which such gradient definitions correspond to newer, variable beam parameters is an area of active investigation. As our insight into these processes broadens, it will be important to refine our model of the clinical responses that occur after SFRT. In this chapter, we review the basic concepts of SFRT and their defining biologic characteristics as they are currently understood.

## 2.2 Mechanisms of response to SFRT—current concepts

### 2.2.1 The bystander response

*2.2.1.1 Historical view of the bystander effect*

The distinction of DNA as the solitary target of radiation has been challenged by mounting examples demonstrating radiobiologic effects in cells not directly exposed

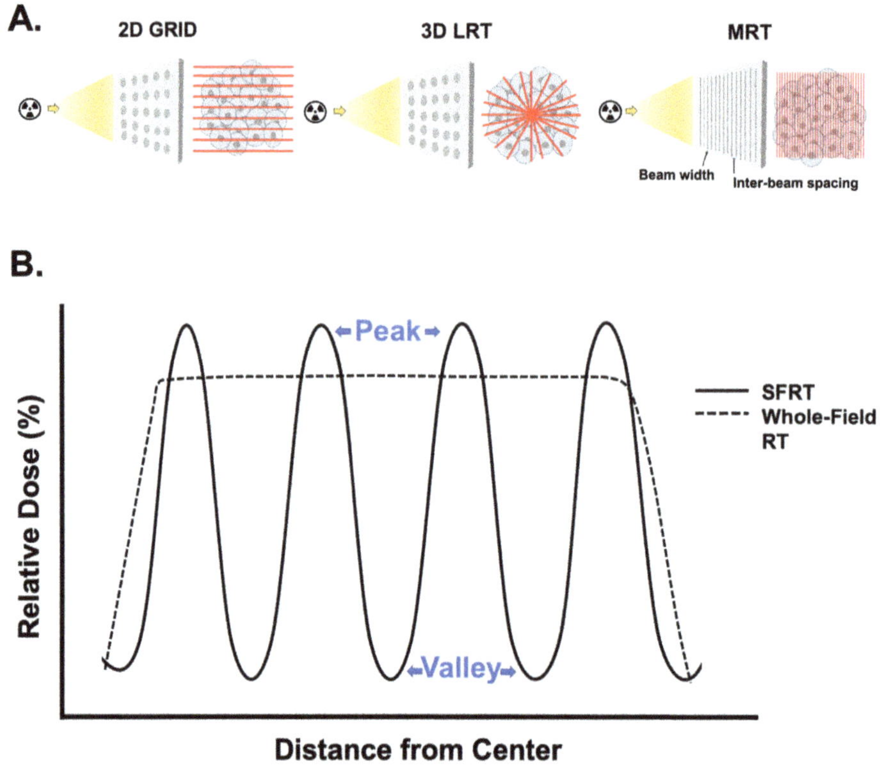


**Figure 2.1.** A schematic representation of the different SFRT delivery methods. (A) Representative configurations of spatial fractionation including a variable two-dimensional GRID design which can be obtained using a cerrobend block or multileaf collimator. A three-dimensional dose distribution can be achieved using a LATTICE simulation approach. Microbeam radiation utilizes interspersed microscale radiation beams which generate distinct biologic effects based on the dose rate, the width of the microbeam, and the spacing between beams. (B) Each method shares basic characteristics involving unequal dose distribution and steep dose gradients, whereas traditional external beam radiation methods deliver whole-tumor exposures with more homogeneous distributions. *Abbreviations*: SFRT, spatially fractionated radiotherapy; LRT, lattice radiation therapy; MRT, microbeam radiotherapy.

to the radiation field, which are broadly defined as radiation-induced bystander effects (RIBEs). These were first identified in 1992 by Nagasawa and Little who observed an increased frequency of sister chromatid exchange occurring in the nuclei of many cells not actually traversed by α particles [5]. In addition, the observation that soluble factors obtained from serum in irradiated patients can confer transferable clastogenic (chromosome breaking) activity also provided early *in vivo* evidence of potential RIBEs [6, 7]. The mechanisms responsible for RIBEs are incompletely understood, but appear to be mediated through secretion of soluble mediators, signaling by cell–cell contact via gap junctions, and/or through inflammatory cell networks. These signals may include ions such as calcium, reactive oxygen or nitrogen species, cytokine or chemokine mediators, and most recently, exosomes, which are nanoscale vesicles that may be packaged with various cargoes including protein mediators, miRNA, or other metabolites [8–10].

RIBEs may be further classified as 'abscopal effects' occurring outside the radiation field (i.e. distant sites of disease) and 'cohort effects,' defined as interactions between irradiated cells within a field of nonuniform dose distribution. According to convention, RIBEs may contribute to radiation-induced toxicity in skin and other regional organs at risk. A variety of other adverse effects have been described, including but not limited to impaired wound healing [11], cognitive impairment [12], and impaired hematopoietic reconstitution after hematopoietic cell transplantation (HCT), which are all directly attributable to bystander effects [13]. Conversely, as the complexities of bystander responses are increasingly recognized, it appears that RIBEs may modulate responses to radiation in more favorable ways which can increase the therapeutic window and minimize toxicity.

In general, local bystander signaling leads to damaging effects in bystander cell(s) through reduction in clonogenic survival, genomic instability, increased cell stress signaling, or apoptosis [14]. However, it is clear that RIBEs vary substantially depending on the dose, source ($\alpha$, $\beta$, $\gamma$, protons, etc.), radiation delivery method, and the biologic characteristics of both the irradiated and non-irradiated cell types involved. It is also critical to note that increased survival may occur in non-irradiated cells [15, 16], which remains poorly characterized but could have important consequences, particularly in the peritumoral immune microenvironment (PIM). It is likely that in some instances, reciprocal or bidirectional dialog from bystander to irradiated cells may modulate responses to radiation, which requires further study but could be viewed as a rescue effect, mitigating damage in directly irradiated cells [17, 18]. Finally, host immune responses are increasingly recognized as a critical component of RIBEs, which may rely on macrophage-generated bystander signaling, enhanced T-cell trafficking, or other heretofore unknown elements that regulate the complex interplay between inflammation, signaling mediators, apoptosis, necrosis, and immunogenic cell death within the tumor microenvironment [8]. The use of advanced sequencing techniques and the application of *in vivo* models allowing the study of dynamic microenvironmental changes will be crucial to make continued progress in understanding the radiobiology of RIBEs. To date, the immunologic interplay with conventionally described bystander effects is largely agreed upon as a source for systemic immune activation and a critical component of abscopal responses, making this a crucial area of study in modern radioimmunotherapy regimens.

#### *2.2.1.2 Distinction of bystander effects after SFRT*

While traditional RIBEs occur in non-irradiated cells, SFRT represents a unique circumstance in which bystander areas may be exposed, albeit to dramatically lower doses (valley dose regions) with variable peak-to-valley dose ratios, depending on the technique and delivery methods used. Due to complex interactions between interspersed areas of unequal dose distribution, high-dose RIBEs in SFRT appear to

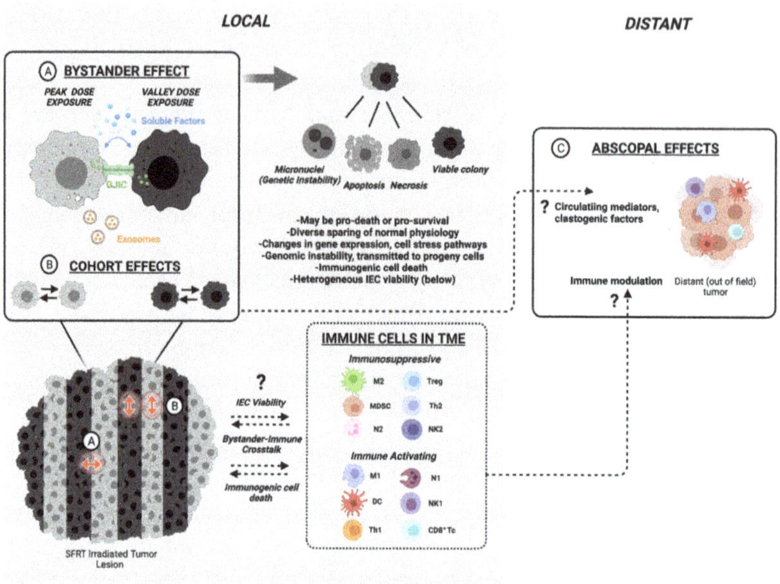


**Figure 2.2.** The current model of local and distant non-targeted effects in spatially fractionated radiotherapy. Non-targeted effects can be classified into three categories, defined by the relationship between peak- and valley-exposed cells and their proximity to the radiation field. Bystander effects (A) occur at the primary tumor, generated by steep dose gradients in areas of peak and valley dose exposure. These are mediated through soluble factors, gap junction intercellular communication, or inflammatory networks within the microenvironment. Cohort effects (B) may occur between cells in areas of similar exposure within a field of heterogeneous dose distribution. Bystander and cohort effects may be bidirectional and can lead to pro-death or pro-survival outcomes. The impact of local non-targeted effects in relation to the peritumoral immune microenvironment remains unknown and may influence the radiobiological response to SFRT. Distant abscopal effects (C) occur outside of the radiation field, mediated by systemic changes which may include circulating clastogenic factors and the promotion of tumor-specific immune responses. Figure created with BioRender.com. *Abbreviations*: SFRT, spatially fractionated radiotherapy; GJIC, gap junction intercellular communication; IEC, immune effector cell; Tc, T-cell; M2, M2 polarized macrophage; Treg, T-regulatory cell; Th2, type 2 helper T-cell; NK2, natural killer type 2 cell; N2, N2 polarized neutrophil; MDSC, myeloid derived suppressor cell; M1, M1 polarized macrophage; N1, N1 polarized neutrophil; DC, dendritic cell; NK1, natural killer type 1 cell; Th1, type 1 helper T-cell.

be distinct from more conventional delivery methods and are likely mediated by molecular changes in bystander cells in valley regions, cytotoxic effects, and/or local immune modulation (figure 2.2). Perhaps most indicative of this has been the consistent demonstration of differential bystander cell survival after heterogenous dose distribution compared to uniform exposures, which cannot be accounted for by scattered dose effects alone [19–22]. Others have likewise demonstrated decreased out-of-field cell survival using various techniques with different proportions of tumor shielding [19, 20, 23–25] and have made similar observations across a variety of cell types (fibroblasts, human breast, prostate, and glioma cell lines) with 50% shielding of radiation fields [26]. In a pivotal study using murine mammary carcinoma (SCK) and head and neck sarcoma (SCCVII) cells treated with GRID therapy, *in vitro* analysis demonstrated increased bystander killing in cells adjacent to irradiated areas when exposed to a medium obtained from cells exposed to 10 Gy. Here, bystander cells showed increased expression of DNA damage response genes as well as antioxidant, heat shock, and chaperone genes following the exposure of adjacent cells to GRID, highlighting their nature as a possible cell-stress-related phenomenon [27]. In contrast, others have shown that p53-related genes exhibit minimal activation in bystander cells, while the genes involved in the NFkB pathway were equally activated in bystander and directly irradiated cells [28, 29], suggesting that the true nature of gene expression alterations following SFRT remains to be fully elucidated.

While it has been demonstrated that RIBEs may occur after SFRT without direct physical contact, it does appear they are dramatically enhanced by gap junction intercellular communication (GJIC) [22, 23, 30]. It has also been indicated that bystander responses after GRID therapy might be more pronounced in radioresistant cell lines [22, 23], a finding that may explain the observed efficacy of SFRT in bulky or treatment-resistant tumors. Of note, it has also been demonstrated in preclinical and clinical models that the targeted irradiation of hypoxic, radioresistant tumor segments with ablative doses (SBRT-PATHY; SBRT-based partial tumor irradiation of hypoxic segment) may be more adept at generating bystander effects with immunogenic potential [31, 32]. While comparable similar findings have not been directly observed for other methods, SFRT has been consistently shown to generate abscopal effects across various experimental models and hence may be well suited to generate clinically relevant abscopal phenomena owing to unique bystander effects attributable to complex spatial and temporal dose distributions. Ultimately, bystander responses following SFRT likely depend not only on steep dose gradients but also oxygen tension, beam energy, and temporal dose distribution. Further investigations are therefore needed before their full translational potential will be reached [33]. By the same token, while experimental approaches such as media transfer and cell co-culture have provided clear evidence of RIBEs, they may not accurately represent the tumor microenvironment or *in vivo* radiation exposures as encountered clinically.

### 2.2.2 Microvascular alterations

#### *2.2.2.1 Traditional concepts of vascular normalization*

Vascular normalization may occur after conventional radiation, which contributes greatly to the control of tumor growth or evolution and may also improve responses to concurrent systemic therapies [34]. While the changes in microvascular networks may be secondary to tumor shrinkage, it has been theorized that endothelial cell apoptosis serves as an independent mechanism which ultimately determines radiation sensitivity [35] (figure 2.3). This may explain observations that adequate tumor control can be achieved with radiation doses that would not otherwise be mathematically predicted to do so and is also indirectly supported by multiple examples of synergy resulting from the combination of angiogenesis inhibitors and radiotherapy [36].

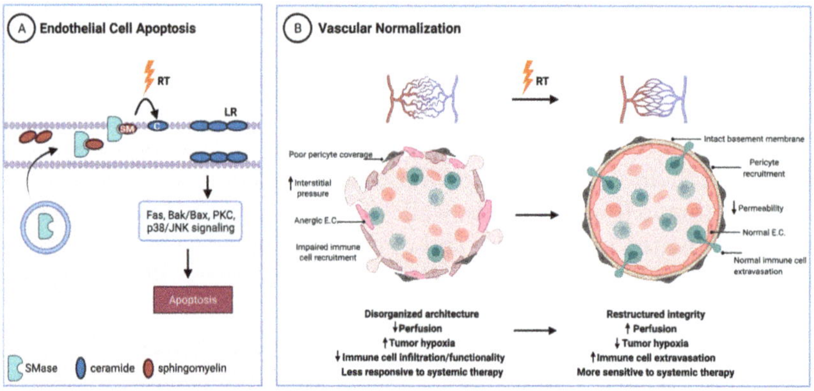


**Figure 2.3.** Microvascular alterations in response to radiotherapy. Endothelial cell apoptosis (A) may be an independent mechanism in the biologic response to radiotherapy, which is followed by the normalization of tumor vasculature (B). This involves the restoration of tumor vascular networks, increased endovascular integrity, increased oxygen tension, and improvement in the response to systemic therapies. Sphingomyelinase activity and ceramide levels may represent useful biomarkers for effective tumor responses to radiotherapy. Figure created with BioRender.com. *Abbreviations*: SMase, sphingomyelinase; SM, sphingomyelin; C, ceramide; LR, lipid raft; EC, endothelial cell.

### *2.2.2.2 The vascular response to spatial fractionation*

Multiple studies utilizing various SFRT methods have demonstrated vascular perturbations, damage, and inflammation [36–39]. Ceramide generated by activated sphingomyelinase in the plasma membrane appears to sensitize endothelial cells to radiation-induced apoptosis and provides an important marker for microvascular responses to radiation [40]. Interestingly, it has been shown in patients receiving GRID therapy that an increase in sphingomyelinase activity and ceramide levels correlated with objective responses, which was not observed in non-responders, lending support to the notion that endothelial cell apoptosis may be a critical component in the biologic response to SFRT [41]. Subsequent changes in the microvascular network likely distinguish responses to SFRT from whole-beam exposures, and there are, perhaps counterintuitively, indications that angiogenesis or vasculogenesis may even be potentiated when the tumor is partially spared. Ultimately, the dynamics of tumor microvascular networks are acknowledged to be increasingly complex, often making it difficult to discern the exact consequences of vascular normalization on the tumor microenvironment. This suggests that temporal and spatial monitoring of vascular function will be critical in defining the response to SFRT and maximizing its subsequent therapeutic opportunities—particularly with the combined use of chemotherapy, nanoparticles, or immune therapy, which require vascular access in conjunction with radiotherapy.

### *2.2.2.3 Dynamic angio-disruptive effects observed after microbeam radiotherapy*

Microbeam radiotherapy (MRT) is increasingly recognized as a novel angio-disruptive treatment strategy, which relies on the inherent resistance of normal, mature vessels which specifically limits vascular disruption to the more immature tumor vasculature. This permits higher dose delivery while minimizing normal tissue toxicity, which has been particularly effective in brain tumor models. However, it is clear that the angio-disruptive effects of MRT do not depend on dose alone, as beam width and spatial distribution have been identified as crucial factors impacting growth delay. Specifically, a narrow beam appears to be more effective than a wide beam [42]. In a landmark study, Griffin *et al* compared the effects of MRT on vascular normalization using multiple treatment parameters, and demonstrated that the lowest peak dose (75 Gy) combined with widest beam spacing (2000 μm center-to-center (c-t-c)) resulted in inferior tumor responses, while the highest peak dose (150 Gy) combined with the closest spacing (200 μm c-t-c) resulted in optimal tumor control [36]. The observation that the beam width and spatial distribution of dose exposures are crucial in order to optimize vascular effects and subsequent tumor responses should be emphasized in future studies. However, it remains unclear precisely how these interactions are coordinated. While unopposed interbeam tumor growth (i.e. between beams) or diminished surface areas for beneficial bystander effects may be responsible, future efforts should also investigate changes to stromal cells and immune populations in the microenvironment as well as unique ways in which normal versus tumor cells might react to ultrahigh dose rates.

In contrast to vascular normalization, other experimental models have demonstrated the growth or potentiation of tumor vasculature after MRT, which have important implications for the current modeling of SFRT biology and its clinical applications. Conceptually, this phenomenon may be compared in part to wound healing processes, in which angiogenic responses are expected to occur after periods of vascular stress. Using a single (non-parallel) beam, Fontanella *et al* identified unique patterns of vascular remodeling and pronounced angiogenic effects after MRT within non-irradiated regions along the radiation path, associated with increases in circumferential hypoxia-inducible factor (HIF-1) expression [39]. It is postulated that in this scenario, HIF-1-related genes may promote angiogenesis and/or vasculogenesis as a protective response after MRT. It has also been shown that a transient 'vascular permeability window' may be induced within the immediate 4 h after high-dose MRT, represented morphologically by partially fragmented endothelial walls [43]. This suggests MRT or possibly other SFRT methods may provide a novel avenue for improved delivery and accumulation of therapeutic agents (e.g. chemotherapy, antibodies, or nanoparticles) within tumors. Though speculative, they may also provide an opportunity for regional or circulating immune cells to modulate antitumor immune responses. Leukocyte recruitment into the tumoral space has indeed been demonstrated after MRT [44–46], and it will be important for future studies of SFRT to account for the interplay between local vascular and immune responses. More broadly, these early studies suggest that the radiation treatment scheme may have more significant effects on microvessel stability and the subsequent biological consequences than previously thought.

### 2.2.3 Immunomodulation

*2.2.3.1 Overview of radioimmunological interactions*

While radiotherapy has historically been intended primarily for local disease control, emerging evidence suggests it may have both immune suppressive and immune stimulatory effects, including the capacity to elicit systemic, tumor-specific responses [47–49]. The mechanisms responsible for these effects are multifactorial and incompletely understood. At cytotoxic doses, radiation may behave as an *in situ* vaccination by causing immunogenic tumor cell death and the release of neo-antigens, which are subsequently presented to T-cells by antigen-presenting cells (APCs), generating an adaptive immune response. Indirectly, radiation may also modify the tumor microenvironment by promoting vascular permeability, endothelial cell adhesion molecule expression (i.e. VCAM-1, ICAM-1), and chemokine or cytokine production, all of which enhance leukocyte trafficking and infiltration into tumors. The loss of MHC-I expression, a common immune-evasive mechanism utilized by tumors, may also be overcome at even lower doses of radiation which upregulate MHC-I receptors on tumor cells and re-establish active host immunity by disinhibiting endogenous antigen exposure. Radiotherapy may also promote apoptosis through increased surface expression of cell death receptors, including Fas/Fas ligand pathway receptors and tumor necrosis factor-related apoptosis-inducing ligand (TRAIL) signaling pathways. Based on a growing appreciation for the interactions between radiobiology and immunology, it is generally agreed that historically rare observations of out-of-field (abscopal) responses in the clinic are likely driven by immunostimulatory radiation mechanisms [50, 51]. Importantly, most tumors have acquired one or more mechanisms of immune tolerance prior to being diagnosed, making radiotherapy an attractive way to re-establish effective local and/or distant anti-tumoral immune responses. By the same token, this makes radiotherapy an enticing partner in combination with currently approved immune therapies including immune checkpoint inhibitors, monoclonal antibodies, bispecific T-cell engagers, and cellular therapy (chimeric antigen receptor T-cell therapy (CAR T) and allogeneic HCT) [52, 53].

*2.2.3.2 Proposed immunogenic effects of SFRT*

In view of these novel radioimmunological interactions, it is of immense interest that unique immunologic sequelae appear to occur following SFRT, which are likely paramount to the dramatic tumor responses that have been observed (as suggested by the clinical experience reviewed in chapters 4–7). While whole-tumor exposures are hypothesized to trigger abscopal effects by causing extensive vascular damage and inflammation, SFRT may allow a more intact physiological response due to the heterogeneous distribution of peak dose exposures interspersed with areas of valley dose exposures, which may contain more viable vascular networks or immune populations.

As details of the radiation-induced immune response emerge, it has become clear that local, immunogenic effects are critical for the induction of systemic antitumor effects, including abscopal immune responses. These require forms of immunogenic cell death (ICD) which generate danger signals including damage-associated molecular patterns (DAMPs) such as calreticulin (CRT), adenosine triphosphate (ATP), and high-mobility group box 1 (HMGB1), which promote the infiltration of monocytic cells and their maturation into antigen-presenting cells (APCs). Among these, fragmented DNA (particularly double-strand DNA breaks) appear to be crucial in facilitating immune responses after radiotherapy by activating the cytosolic cyclic GMP–AMP synthase/stimulator of interferon genes (cGAS/STING) pathway, ultimately leading to the amplification of type I interferons which are essential for the development of effective downstream cellular immunity. It should be emphasized that this cytosolic DNA sensing pathway is highly modulated by the DNAase three prime repair exonuclease 1 (TREX1), which is upregulated after higher dose exposures (generally between 12 and 18 Gy) and appears to dictate whether stimulation of these pathways will ultimately occur [54, 55]. It follows that the heterogenous dose distribution achieved with SFRT would have distinct, dramatic effects on downstream immune pathways due to spatial variations in the regulation of interferon-stimulatory dsDNA sensing pathways, which are distributed throughout the tumor in a manner that is unachievable after high-dose open-field exposures. Importantly, spatial distribution of the dose has also been demonstrated to cause a variety of sparing effects in the peritumoral microenvironment (PIM), which are likely required to facilitate such responses and would differ substantially from the more uniform whole-tumor exposures which are known to cause radiation-induced lymphopenia or at times even global immune suppression [56–58].

Multiple preclinical studies have indeed demonstrated robust bystander killing in valley regions following the use of various SFRT methods along with control of both local and distant (non-irradiated) tumors in comparison to open-field radiation [27, 32, 59–65]. Others have demonstrated that the abscopal responses observed after SFRT appear to be associated with systemic inflammatory cytokine production and immune activation [60, 66]. When compared with whole-tumor irradiation, LRT with varying tumor volume exposures has been shown to induce robust IFN$\gamma$ and IL-2 production as well as T-cell infiltration into both irradiated and non-irradiated tumors [64]. Markovsky *et al* similarly demonstrated both local and distant control using partial tumor irradiation, showing that tumors with 50% field exposure achieved the same treatment effect as whole-tumor exposures, which was associated with increased T-cell infiltration and was abrogated in athymic mice or by the use of anti-CD8 or anti-intercellular adhesion molecule (ICAM) antibodies [65]. The authors of this study also demonstrated an effective immunologic memory response when reimplanted breast cancer cells failed to produce tumors. Using FTY720, a compound that inhibits the egress of T-cells from lymph nodes and depletes circulating lymphocytes, they also provided evidence which suggested that the likely origin of infiltrating $CD8^+$ T-cells was from the tumor periphery, irradiated portion, or both, as opposed to regional nodes or the systemic circulation [65]. This has important ramifications for the understanding of radiation-induced immunogenicity, as it suggests that a primary barrier exists within the local T-cell compartment, perhaps instigated by tumor-induced T-cell exhaustion or poor effector function via mechanisms such as PD-L1 expression rather than barriers to leukocyte recruitment and infiltration. This is further supported by multiple preclinical studies showing synergistic immune responses when SFRT is combined with immune checkpoint inhibitors [60, 67–69] and may also imply that the radiosensitivity or viability of within-field immune populations may be a crucial factor, which would certainly distinguish SFRT from conventional delivery methods. Emerging clinical data also suggests that using partially irradiated tumor volumes directly targeted to hypoxic segments (SBRT-PATHY) can be immunogenic, which is attributed to the observation in preclinical models that hypoxic tumor cells are more likely to generate non-targeted or bystander effects compared to normoxic cells and may also promote more functional immune activation through preservative or favorable effects within the PIM [31, 32, 70].

In summary, it has been demonstrated in both preclinical and clinical settings that effective immune responses may be augmented after SFRT. Ultimately, better elucidation of the determinants of the radiosensitivity of intratumoral lymphocytes, their susceptibility to bystander effects, and interactions with the tumor microenvironment (TME) after immunogenic cell death is expected to precede monumental gains in our understanding of how different SFRT methods can evoke a protective immune response. Likewise, it may also guide dosing strategies and the development of rational combinatorial approaches using modern immune therapy regimens.

### 2.2.4 Knowledge gaps and future perspectives

Despite our growing understanding of the underlying principles of SFRT, many questions remain, particularly regarding its biologic mechanisms. As summarized in figure 2.4, RIBEs, microvascular alterations, and immune modulation all appear to contribute to the promising clinical results observed. Precisely how these variable responses occur conjointly with one another and the scenarios in which they occur independently remain undefined.

#### *2.2.4.1 What are the key components orchestrating favorable or immunogenic bystander responses after SFRT?*

While *in vitro* studies have identified important concepts, including the elucidation of key bystander responses, *in vivo* studies, which more accurately account for the environmental variables necessary to understand the full impact of spatial fractionation, are lacking. When possible, *in vitro* investigations should utilize 3D tumor models, which can better emulate the tumor microenvironment and may also contain endogenous immune cells. In these studies, the molecular mechanisms responsible for response should be reported, and the relevant immune repertoires should be identified using cytometry or advanced sequencing techniques. Furthermore, currently established SFRT parameters are generally designed and modeled for experiments in the laboratory that may fail to implicate and quantify the multifactorial radiobiologic response mechanisms that seem to occur. Therefore, emphasis should be given to unifying patterns used in preclinical studies with those

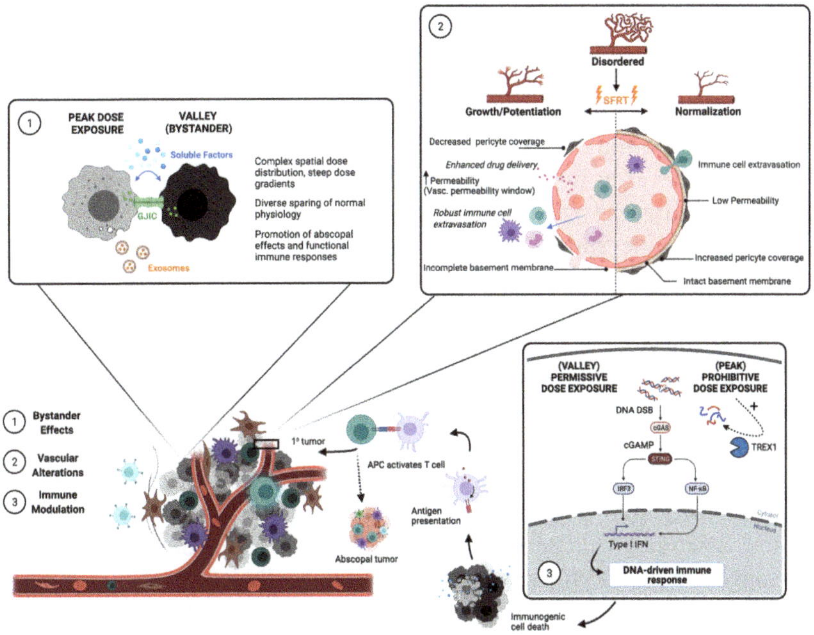


**Figure 2.4.** A summary of the proposed biologic response mechanisms in SFRT. (1) Bystander effects maintained by complex interactions between the interspersed areas of unequal dose distribution are highly dependent on peak (high dose) to valley (low dose) dose ratios. These may lead to spatiotemporally diverse sparing of normal physiological processes and promote the development of distant antitumor responses. (2) Vascular alterations include vascular normalization or potentiation, which leads to tumor shrinkage. Such alterations may exhibit spatiotemporal variation within tumor vascular networks, depending on the dose rate and spatial distribution. In the immediate postradiotherapy period, a 'vascular permeability window' may exist which has the potential to improve the delivery of adjunctive therapies such as chemotherapy or immune therapy. (3) Immunostimulatory effects originate from changes to the local (irradiated tumor) microenvironment after SFRT, defined by heterogeneous dose distribution with unique bystander effects and modulation of vascular integrity. The activity of cytosolic DNA sensing pathways regulates type I interferon production and may vary according to steep dose gradients; when promoted, it may lead to immunogenic cell death with subsequent adaptive immune responses. Figure created with BioRender.com. *Abbreviations*: SFRT, spatially fractionated radiotherapy; GJIC, gap junction intercellular communication; APC, antigen-presenting cell; DSB, double-strand break; cGAS, cytosolic cyclic GMP–AMP synthase; cGAMP, cyclic guanosine monophosphate–adenosine monophosphate; STING, stimulator of interferon genes; TREX1, three prime repair exonuclease 1; IRF3, interferon regulatory factor-3; NF-κB, nuclear factor kappa-light-chain-enhancer of activated B cells; IFN, interferon.

which are commonly used in clinical practice. The precise way in which peritumoral immune cells, including lymphocyte subsets and antigen-presenting cells, are impacted by exposure to nonuniform dose distributions may be crucial to defining the immunologic sequelae of bystander responses attributable to SFRT. Studies focusing on intercellular communication between neighboring cells in the exposed and unexposed areas (cohort effects) might also provide valuable information about the bystander response involved, which should include an analysis of tissue-specific effects and their dependency on functional or viable host immune populations.

#### *2.2.4.2 What physical parameters are needed to elicit the desired biological responses to SFRT?*

In all future studies, it is imperative that the physical definitions of treatment techniques, including the size/volume of peak and valley dose exposures are included, in the hope that this will identify the key physical elements distinguishing bystander responses after nonuniform dose distributions are administered. This will also better delineate the true dose gradients needed to generate beneficial host responses and provide standardization for emerging biologic endpoints in study protocols.

As novel SFRT methods are emerging (i.e. MRT, FLASH), the importance of defining the optimal dose rates and beam parameters needed to elicit beneficial responses should be emphasized. Regarding FLASH, current evidence suggests that higher dose-rate thresholds are required. While most clinical conventional radiotherapy doses (which are commonly combined with GRID and lattice SFRT) are fractionated, the majority of studies using FLASH have utilized a stand-alone large single-fraction scheme. Therefore, demonstrating responses to FLASH using fractionated schedules will be important for future translational studies. While it has been suggested that a physicochemical effect (the depletion of oxygen at FLASH dose rates) occurs, the modulation of immunologic responses between tumor and normal tissues has also been described, which could be due to either the downstream consequences of FLASH or independent response mechanisms.

#### *2.2.4.3 What biologic principles are needed for the successful translation of SFRT to the clinic?*

To date, a limited number of clinical trials have been developed to investigate SFRT. Retrospective analyzes are also lacking; these could provide guiding principles for clinical trial development. These should include an analysis of specific physical dosimetric properties, such as peak and valley dose exposures, dose gradients, and volumetric measurements of tumor exposures. They might also include the identification of tumor types that may be more amenable to SFRT as well as the potential impact of different concurrent therapies on patient outcomes. Specifically, different classes of chemotherapy are commonly used alongside radiation and may promote immune suppression, stimulation, or lymphodepletion before or after SFRT delivery, which would be relevant for future clinical trial design.

As more in-human studies are developed, a consensus will be needed on the types of biomarker to be studied and their timing in relation to radiation delivery. Prospective studies should include correlatives which may be instrumental in defining key features of the response to SFRT, particularly those of immunologic nature. This may include broad cytokine profiling, both systemic and within irradiated and non-irradiated tumors when possible. Detailed analyses of lymphocyte repertoires as well as clinical T-cell, B-cell, and natural killer cell subsets will help us to understand global immune changes in the host. They may also help to identify patients who are likely to respond or not respond. Considering that immune responses can vary among different target tissues, including the vasculature, the timing and distribution of SFRT may have a critical impact on its immunogenic potential, and these parameters should be clearly defined.

## 2.3 Summary

Due to complex interactions between interspersed areas of unequal heterogeneous dose distribution, SFRT has been shown to be effective in bulky and advanced tumors and may provide adequate local control as well as a unique nidus for the generation of distant tumor responses outside the radiation field. As summarized here, the radiobiologic consequences of inhomogeneous dose distribution include unique bystander effects, changes to microvascular networks, and novel ways to stimulate local and systemic immune responses. It is unlikely that these observed mechanisms are mutually exclusive, and their relative contributions may vary with different dose-delivery schemes. At present, the optimal peak–valley dose ratios, beam energies, and temporal dose variations best suited to promote these effects also remain incompletely understood. Moreover, it is expected that oxygen tension within the tumoral space also has implications in determining radiosensitivity and therapeutic responses after SFRT. Considering the current key findings in this nascent field, optimism exists that future studies will further delineate the biologic sequelae of spatial fractionation and lead to dramatic improvements in novel radioimmunotherapy treatment regimens.

## References


[1] Laissue J A, Blattmann H and Slatkin D N 2012 [Alban Köhler (1874–1947): inventor of grid therapy] *Z. Med. Phys.* **22** 90–9

[2] Marks H 1952 Clinical experience with irradiation through a grid *Radiology* **58** 338–42

[3] Mohiuddin M, Curtis D L, Grizos W T and Komarnicky L 1990 Palliative treatment of advanced cancer using multiple nonconfluent pencil beam radiation. A pilot study *Cancer* **66** 114–8

[4] Shirato H, Gupta N K, Jordan T J and Hendry J H 1990 Lack of late skin necrosis in man after high-dose irradiation using small field sizes: experiences of grid therapy *Br. J. Radiol.* **63** 871–4

[5] Nagasawa H and Little J B 1992 Induction of sister chromatid exchanges by extremely low doses of alpha-particles *Cancer Res.* **52** 6394–6 https://aacrjournals.org/cancerres/article/52/22/6394/498591/Induction-of-Sister-Chromatid-Exchanges-by

[6] Emerit I 1994 Reactive oxygen species, chromosome mutation, and cancer: possible role of clastogenic factors in carcinogenesis *Free Radic. Biol. Med.* **16** 99–109

[7] Lindholm C, Acheva A and Salomaa S 2010 Clastogenic plasma factors: a short overview *Radiat. Environ. Biophys.* **49** 133–8

[8] Daguenet E, Louati S, Wozny A S, Vial N, Gras M and Guy J B *et al* 2020 Radiation-induced bystander and abscopal effects: important lessons from preclinical models *Br. J. Cancer* **123** 339–48

[9] Du Y, Du S, Liu L, Gan F, Jiang X and Wangrao K *et al* 2020 Radiation-induced bystander effect can be transmitted through exosomes using mirnas as effector molecules *Radiat. Res.* **194** 89–100

[10] Elbakrawy E, Kaur Bains S, Bright S, Al-Abedi R, Mayah A and Goodwin E *et al* 2020 Radiation-induced senescence bystander effect: the role of exosomes *Biology (Basel)* **9** 191
[11] Suzuki K and Yamashita S 2014 Radiation-induced bystander response: mechanism and clinical implications *Adv. Wound Care (New Rochelle)* **3** 16–24
[12] Yang X, Ma L, Ye Z, Shi W, Zhang L and Wang J *et al* 2021 Radiation-induced bystander effects may contribute to radiation-induced cognitive impairment *Int. J. Radiat. Biol.* **97** 329–40
[13] Hu L, Yin X, Zhang Y, Pang A, Xie X and Yang S *et al* 2021 Radiation-induced bystander effects impair transplanted human hematopoietic stem cells via oxidative DNA damage *Blood* **137** 3339–50
[14] Rzeszowska-Wolny J, Przybyszewski W M and Widel M 2009 Ionizing radiation-induced bystander effects, potential targets for modulation of radiotherapy *Eur. J. Pharmacol.* **625** 156–64
[15] Goldberg Z and Lehnert B E 2002 Radiation-induced effects in unirradiated cells: a review and implications in cancer *Int. J. Oncol.* **21** 337–49
[16] Mackonis E C, Suchowerska N, Zhang M, Ebert M, McKenzie D R and Jackson M 2007 Cellular response to modulated radiation fields *Phys. Med. Biol.* **52** 5469–82
[17] Chen S, Zhao Y, Han W, Chiu S K, Zhu L and Wu L *et al* 2011 Rescue effects in radiobiology: unirradiated bystander cells assist irradiated cells through intercellular signal feedback *Mutat. Res* **706** 59–64
[18] Widel M, Przybyszewski W M, Cieslar-Pobuda A, Saenko Y V and Rzeszowska-Wolny J 2012 Bystander normal human fibroblasts reduce damage response in radiation targeted cancer cells through intercellular ROS level modulation *Mutat. Res* **731** 117–24
[19] Suchowerska N, Ebert M A, Zhang M and Jackson M 2005 In vitro response of tumour cells to non-uniform irradiation *Phys. Med. Biol.* **50** 3041–51
[20] Konopacka M and Rzeszowska-Wolny J 2006 The bystander effect-induced formation of micronucleated cells is inhibited by antioxidants, but the parallel induction of apoptosis and loss of viability are not affected *Mutat. Res* **593** 32–8
[21] Alexandre J, Hu Y, Lu W, Pelicano H and Huang P 2007 Novel action of paclitaxel against cancer cells: bystander effect mediated by reactive oxygen species *Cancer Res.* **67** 3512–7
[22] Pakniyat F, Nedaie H A, Mozdarani H, Mahmoudzadeh A, Salimi M and Griffin R J *et al* 2020 Enhanced response of radioresistant carcinoma cell line to heterogeneous dose distribution of grid; the role of high-dose bystander effect *Int. J. Radiat. Biol.* **96** 1585–96
[23] Butterworth K T, McGarry C K, Trainor C, O'Sullivan J M, Hounsell A R and Prise K M 2011 Out-of-field cell survival following exposure to intensity-modulated radiation fields *Int. J. Radiat. Oncol. Biol. Phys.* **79** 1516–22
[24] Trainor C, Butterworth K T, McGarry C K, McMahon S J, O'Sullivan J M and Hounsell A R *et al* 2012 DNA damage responses following exposure to modulated radiation fields *PLoS One* **7** e43326
[25] Butterworth K T, McGarry C K, Trainor C, McMahon S J, O'Sullivan J M and Schettino G *et al* 2012 Dose, dose-rate and field size effects on cell survival following exposure to non-uniform radiation fields *Phys. Med. Biol.* **57** 3197–206
[26] Trainor C, Butterworth K T, McGarry C K, Liberante F, O'Sullivan J M and Hounsell A R *et al* 2012 Cell survival responses after exposure to modulated radiation fields *Radiat. Res.* **177** 44–51

[27] Asur R S, Sharma S, Chang C W, Penagaricano J, Kommuru I M and Moros E G *et al* 2012 Spatially fractionated radiation induces cytotoxicity and changes in gene expression in bystander and radiation adjacent murine carcinoma cells *Radiat. Res.* **177** 751–65

[28] Ghandhi S A, Ming L, Ivanov V N, Hei T K and Amundson S A 2010 Regulation of early signaling and gene expression in the alpha-particle and bystander response of IMR-90 human fibroblasts *BMC Med. Genom.* **3** 31

[29] Ghandhi S A, Yaghoubian B and Amundson S A 2008 Global gene expression analyses of bystander and alpha particle irradiated normal human lung fibroblasts: synchronous and differential responses *BMC Med. Genom.* **1** 63

[30] Autsavapromporn N, Suzuki M, Funayama T, Usami N, Plante I and Yokota Y *et al* 2013 Gap junction communication and the propagation of bystander effects induced by microbeam irradiation in human fibroblast cultures: the impact of radiation quality *Radiat. Res.* **180** 367–75

[31] Tubin S, Ahmed M M and Gupta S 2018 Radiation and hypoxia-induced non-targeted effects in normoxic and hypoxic conditions in human lung cancer cells *Int. J. Radiat. Biol.* **94** 199–211

[32] Tubin S, Popper H H and Brcic L 2019 Novel stereotactic body radiation therapy (SBRT)-based partial tumor irradiation targeting hypoxic segment of bulky tumors (SBRT-PATHY): improvement of the radiotherapy outcome by exploiting the bystander and abscopal effects *Radiat. Oncol.* **14** 21

[33] Asur R, Butterworth K T, Penagaricano J A, Prise K M and Griffin R J 2015 High dose bystander effects in spatially fractionated radiation therapy *Cancer Lett.* **356** 52–7

[34] Magnussen A L and Mills I G 2021 Vascular normalisation as the stepping stone into tumour microenvironment transformation *Br. J. Cancer* **125** 324–36

[35] Garcia-Barros M, Paris F, Cordon-Cardo C, Lyden D, Rafii S and Haimovitz-Friedman A *et al* 2003 Tumor response to radiotherapy regulated by endothelial cell apoptosis *Science* **300** 1155–9

[36] Griffin R J, Koonce N A, Dings R P, Siegel E, Moros E G and Bräuer-Krisch E *et al* 2012 Microbeam radiation therapy alters vascular architecture and tumor oxygenation and is enhanced by a galectin-1 targeted anti-angiogenic peptide *Radiat. Res.* **177** 804–12

[37] Serduc R, Christen T, Laissue J, Farion R, Bouchet A and Sanden B *et al* 2008 Brain tumor vessel response to synchrotron microbeam radiation therapy: a short-term *in vivo* study *Phys. Med. Biol.* **53** 3609–22

[38] Serduc R, van de Looij Y, Francony G, Verdonck O, van der Sanden B and Laissue J *et al* 2008 Characterization and quantification of cerebral edema induced by synchrotron x-ray microbeam radiation therapy *Phys. Med. Biol.* **53** 1153–66

[39] Fontanella A N, Boss M K, Hadsell M, Zhang J, Schroeder T and Berman K G *et al* 2015 Effects of high-dose microbeam irradiation on tumor microvascular function and angiogenesis *Radiat. Res.* **183** 147–58

[40] Kolesnick R and Fuks Z 2003 Radiation and ceramide-induced apoptosis *Oncogene* **22** 5897–906

[41] Sathishkumar S, Boyanovsky B, Karakashian A A, Rozenova K, Giltiay N V and Kudrimoti M *et al* 2005 Elevated sphingomyelinase activity and ceramide concentration in serum of patients undergoing high dose spatially fractionated radiation treatment: implications for endothelial apoptosis *Cancer Biol. Ther.* **4** 979–86

[42] Uyama A, Kondoh T, Nariyama N, Umetani K, Fukumoto M and Shinohara K *et al* 2011 A narrow microbeam is more effective for tumor growth suppression than a wide microbeam: an *in vivo* study using implanted human glioma cells *J. Synchrotron Radiat.* **18** 671–8

[43] Sabatasso S, Fernandez-Palomo C, Hlushchuk R, Fazzari J, Tschanz S and Pellicioli P *et al* 2021 Transient and efficient vascular permeability window for adjuvant drug delivery triggered by microbeam radiation *Cancers (Basel)* **13** 2103

[44] Bouchet A, Lemasson B, Le Duc G, Maisin C, Bräuer-Krisch E and Siegbahn E A *et al* 2010 Preferential effect of synchrotron microbeam radiation therapy on intracerebral 9L gliosarcoma vascular networks *Int. J. Radiat. Oncol. Biol. Phys.* **78** 1503–12

[45] Serduc R, Bräuer-Krisch E, Siegbahn E A, Bouchet A, Pouyatos B and Carron R *et al* 2010 High-precision radiosurgical dose delivery by interlaced microbeam arrays of high-flux low-energy synchrotron X-rays *PLoS One* **5** e9028

[46] Brönnimann D, Bouchet A, Schneider C, Potez M, Serduc R and Bräuer-Krisch E *et al* 2016 Synchrotron microbeam irradiation induces neutrophil infiltration, thrombocyte attachment and selective vascular damage *in vivo Sci. Rep.* **6** 33601

[47] Gandhi S J, Minn A J, Vonderheide R H, Wherry E J, Hahn S M and Maity A 2015 Awakening the immune system with radiation: optimal dose and fractionation *Cancer Lett.* **368** 185–90

[48] Ludgate C M 2012 Optimizing cancer treatments to induce an acute immune response: radiation abscopal effects, PAMPs, and DAMPs *Clin. Cancer Res.* **18** 4522–5

[49] Merrick A, Errington F, Milward K, O'Donnell D, Harrington K and Bateman A *et al* 2005 Immunosuppressive effects of radiation on human dendritic cells: reduced IL-12 production on activation and impairment of naive T-cell priming *Br. J. Cancer* **92** 1450–8

[50] Demaria S, Ng B, Devitt M L, Babb J S, Kawashima N and Liebes L *et al* 2004 Ionizing radiation inhibition of distant untreated tumors (abscopal effect) is immune mediated *Int. J. Radiat. Oncol. Biol. Phys.* **58** 862–70

[51] Yilmaz M T, Elmali A and Yazici G 2019 Abscopal effect, from myth to reality: from radiation oncologists' perspective *Cureus* **11** e3860

[52] Hauth F, Ho A Y, Ferrone S and Duda D G 2021 Radiotherapy to enhance chimeric antigen receptor T-cell therapeutic efficacy in solid tumors: a narrative review *JAMA Oncol.* **7** 1051–9

[53] Jagodinsky J C, Harari P M and Morris Z S 2020 The promise of combining radiation therapy with immunotherapy *Int. J. Radiat. Oncol. Biol. Phys.* **108** 6–16

[54] Vanpouille-Box C, Alard A, Aryankalayil M J, Sarfraz Y, Diamond J M and Schneider R J *et al* 2017 DNA exonuclease Trex1 regulates radiotherapy-induced tumour immunogenicity *Nat. Commun.* **8** 15618

[55] Vanpouille-Box C, Formenti S C and Demaria S 2017 TREX1 dictates the immune fate of irradiated cancer cells *Oncoimmunology* **6** e1339857

[56] Wild A T, Ye X, Ellsworth S G, Smith J A, Narang A K and Garg T *et al* 2015 The association between chemoradiation-related lymphopenia and clinical outcomes in patients with locally advanced pancreatic adenocarcinoma *Am. J. Clin. Oncol.* **38** 259–65

[57] Venkatesulu B P, Mallick S, Lin S H and Krishnan S 2018 A systematic review of the influence of radiation-induced lymphopenia on survival outcomes in solid tumors *Crit. Rev. Oncol. Hematol* **123** 42–51

[58] Sun G Y, Wang S L, Song Y W, Jin J, Wang W H and Liu Y P *et al* 2020 Radiation-induced lymphopenia predicts poorer prognosis in patients with breast cancer: a post hoc analysis of a randomized controlled trial of postmastectomy hypofractionated radiation therapy *Int. J. Radiat. Oncol. Biol. Phys.* **108** 277–85

[59] Matthew E P, Mohammed M S, Seema G, Marianna Z-S, Munira K, Mohammed M and Mansoor M A 2007 Potential utilization of bystander / abscopal-mediated signal transduction events in the treatment of solid tumors *Curr. Signal Transduct. Ther.* **2** 129–43 https://benthamscience.com/article/23184

[60] Johnsrud A J, Jenkins S V, Jamshidi-Parsian A, Quick C M, Galhardo E P and Dings R P M *et al* 2020 Evidence for early stage anti-tumor immunity elicited by spatially fractionated radiotherapy–immunotherapy combinations *Radiat. Res.* **194** 688–97

[61] Prasanna A, Ahmed M M, Mohiuddin M and Coleman C N 2014 Exploiting sensitization windows of opportunity in hyper and hypo-fractionated radiation therapy *J. Thorac. Dis* **6** 287–302

[62] Wattenberg M M, Fahim A, Ahmed M M and Hodge J W 2014 Unlocking the combination: potentiation of radiation-induced antitumor responses with immunotherapy *Radiat. Res.* **182** 126–38

[63] Billena C and Khan A J 2019 A current review of spatial fractionation: back to the future? *Int. J. Radiat. Oncol. Biol. Phys.* **104** 177–87

[64] Kanagavelu S, Gupta S, Wu X, Philip S, Wattenberg M M and Hodge J W *et al* 2014 In vivo effects of lattice radiation therapy on local and distant lung cancer: potential role of immunomodulation *Radiat. Res.* **182** 149–62

[65] Markovsky E, Budhu S, Samstein R M, Li H, Russell J and Zhang Z *et al* 2019 An antitumor immune response is evoked by partial-volume single-dose radiation in 2 murine models *Int. J. Radiat. Oncol. Biol. Phys.* **103** 697–708

[66] Sathishkumar S, Dey S, Meigooni A S, Regine W F, Kudrimoti M S and Ahmed M M *et al* 2002 The impact of TNF-alpha induction on therapeutic efficacy following high dose spatially fractionated (GRID) radiation *Technol. Cancer Res. Treat.* **1** 141–7

[67] Jiang L, Li X, Zhang J, Li W, Dong F and Chen C *et al* 2020 Combined high-dose LATTICE radiation therapy and immune checkpoint blockade for advanced bulky tumors: the concept and a case report *Front. Oncol.* **10** 548132

[68] Buchwald Z S, Wynne J, Nasti T H, Zhu S, Mourad W F and Yan W *et al* 2018 Radiation, immune checkpoint blockade and the abscopal effect: a critical review on timing, dose and fractionation *Front. Oncol.* **8** 612

[69] Chandra R A, Wilhite T J, Balboni T A, Alexander B M, Spektor A and Ott P A *et al* 2015 A systematic evaluation of abscopal responses following radiotherapy in patients with metastatic melanoma treated with ipilimumab *Oncoimmunology* **4** e1046028

[70] Tubin S, Gupta S, Grusch M, Popper H H, Brcic L and Ashdown M L *et al* 2020 Shifting the immune-suppressive to predominant immune-stimulatory radiation effects by SBRT-PArtial Tumor Irradiation Targeting HYpoxic Segment (SBRT-PATHY) *Cancers (Basel)* **13** 50

# Chapter 3

# The immunologic effects of nonuniform dose irradiation

**Ariel E Marciscano, Encouse B Golden and Silvia C Formenti**

The immunologic effects of nonuniform dose irradiation are largely uncharacterized in both preclinical models and in humans. The immunologic consequences of ionizing radiation can be broadly conceptualized as immunogenic, immunosuppressive/tolerogenic, or immune-depleting. In addition to the distinct immunologic consequences of ionizing radiation, the irradiated volume and irradiated anatomic/biologic compartment are also likely to modify radiation response. Nonuniform dose irradiation has the potential to expand the therapeutic window by enhancing local responses and/or reducing normal tissue toxicity; this advantage may be explained, at least in part, by immune-based mechanisms. Herein, we provide an overview of the current understanding of the radiation-induced mechanisms of immunomodulation and describe how different ionizing radiation dose distributions, dose qualities, and delivery techniques may alter radiobiology through immunological mechanisms. We discuss preclinical and clinical studies supporting the notion that nonuniform dose irradiation yields distinct immunomodulatory effects relative to conventional radiotherapy approaches. We explore future considerations for clinical trial design with a specific emphasis on implications for radiation–immunotherapy combinations and translational immune-based readouts that will help to refine our current understanding of the way in which the manipulation of ionizing radiation doses, quality, and distribution/delivery can be leveraged for clinical benefit.

## 3.1 Introduction/overview

Over the last two decades, there has been substantial interest in understanding the immunologic response to ionizing radiation. A growing body of preclinical data and clinical studies suggest that ionizing radiation can yield potent immunomodulatory

doi:10.1088/978-0-7503-4046-5ch3  

effects that are context dependent and may vary with changes in radiobiological and physical parameters. This has led to the notion that the immune response to ionizing radiation may be harnessed to enhance irradiated tumor control, promote antitumor immunity, and ultimately improve clinical outcomes. Therefore, understanding and optimizing the delivery of ionizing radiation to potentiate immunogenicity as well as limit deleterious effects has become a subject of intense investigation, particularly given the emergence of immunotherapy and of various radiotherapy–immunotherapy combinations in the clinic [1, 2].

To date, most efforts to exploit the immunostimulatory effects of ionizing radiation have focused on purported differences in immunobiology between distinct radiation dose-fractionation schedules (i.e. 'immunogenic' hypo-fractionated regimens), while others have focused on technological advances that facilitate highly conformal radiation dose delivery that permits dose escalation and normal tissue sparing (i.e. image-guided radiation therapy and stereotactic body radiation therapy) [3, 4]. Preclinical work has now provided mechanistic insight into the way in which ionizing radiation governs immunogenicity, and efforts have more recently shifted towards testing and validation in human studies [5]. It has become clear that alterations in both radiation dose and targeting yield different immunologic effects—these areas of investigation have opened novel research questions pertaining to how nonuniform dose distributions of ionizing radiation may differentially impact the host immune response and consequently tumor and disease control.

It is plausible that the promising clinical outcomes thus far observed with spatially fractionated radiation therapy (SFRT), further described in chapters 5–8, are, in part, a consequence of radiation-induced immune modulation. Nonuniform dose distributions may be particularly immunogenic and favorably tilt the balance toward immune-mediated tumor control. Herein, we review our current understanding of the relevant immunologic and radiobiologic mechanisms and explore how these principles might be relevant to SFRT and other evolving approaches such as FLASH radiotherapy. We further speculate on how different radiation dose spatial distributions, qualities, and delivery techniques might elicit distinct biological consequences that can be exploited therapeutically [6].

## 3.2 The mechanisms of radiation-induced immunomodulation

Ionizing radiation provokes a complex molecular and cellular response in target tissues that has consequent local, bystander, and potentially distant effects [7, 8]. It has long been recognized that ionizing radiation induces DNA damage, primarily via lethal double-stranded DNA (dsDNA) breaks, which results in tumor cell death [9]. The more recent recognition that the biophysical damage induced by ionizing radiation can directly trigger an inflammatory tumor-specific immune response is a critical step in our understanding of radiation-induced immunomodulation [10]. Therefore, a direct link between radiation-induced DNA damage and radiation-induced immunomodulation provides a foundation to understand how different permutations of ionizing radiation dose, quality, fractionation, and distribution might yield different immunological consequences [11, 12]. More broadly, effective antitumor immunity is dependent on the ability to recognize and present antigens in the context of proper activation signals (adjuvant) which facilitate the downstream priming and amplification of tumor-specific immune responses. Ionizing radiation has been shown to induce antigenicity and alter adjuvanticity through distinct effects on both the innate and adaptive arms of the host immune response. It has been postulated that ionizing radiation can potentially convert an irradiated tumor into an immunogenic hub that functions as an *in situ* vaccine through various coordinated actions, including the exposure of tumor-associated antigens, the induction of immunogenic cell death (ICD), and the cross-priming of antigen-specific T-cells [13, 14]. In addition, ionizing radiation can remodel the tumor microenvironment via the local production of chemokines and/or cytokines and alter tumor-associated stroma, lymphatic and endothelial cells to influence the recruitment, trafficking, and access of immune cells into irradiated tissues [15, 16].

### 3.2.1 DNA damage and innate immune sensing

Ionizing radiation has been shown to drive a type I interferon (IFN) response and an IFN-stimulated gene (ISG) program which closely resembles the antiviral immune response of the host. Accordingly, radiation has been described as enacting a form of 'viral mimicry' which activates innate and adaptive immune [17]. Plausible mechanisms for radiation-induced innate immune sensing via DNA damage have recently been described (see figure 3.1). Genotoxic stress incited by ionizing radiation results in the production of dsDNA breaks that leak through the ruptured nuclear envelope and/or mitochondrial outer membrane [10, 18]. The accumulation of dsDNA (and other nucleic acid species) within the cytosol is a robust inflammatory stimulus and is interpreted as foreign or as a 'danger' signal. The presence of foreign nucleic acid species in the cytosol elicits a conserved molecular response similar to that observed when viral RNA or DNA are detected within a host cell. Thus, radiation-induced cytosolic nuclei acids and micronuclei are considered to be damage-associated molecular patterns (DAMPs) that are sensed by pattern recognition receptors (PRRs) and trigger a signaling cascade that mounts a prototypical antiviral-like IFN-driven innate immune response [10]. The cyclic GMP–AMP synthase/stimulator of IFN genes (cGAS–STING) axis is a well-characterized cytosolic dsDNA sensing pathway and has been shown to be activated by ionizing radiation. Further, preclinical studies have demonstrated that radiation-driven antitumor immunity is dependent on the cGAS–STING axis [4, 19], while other studies have also implicated additional nucleic acid sensing PRR pathways that are activated in response to ionizing radiation [20]. Interestingly, TREX1, a DNA exonuclease which degrades cytoplasmic dsDNA, has been shown to be induced in response to radiotherapy [4, 5]. Thus, TREX1 may antagonize the activation of innate immune sensing pathways by clearing radiation-induced DNA damage byproducts and may ultimately impact radiation response. Preclinical work has described a radiation-dose-dependent induction of TREX1 in which high dose-per-fraction regimens robustly induce TREX1, while lower dose-per-fraction

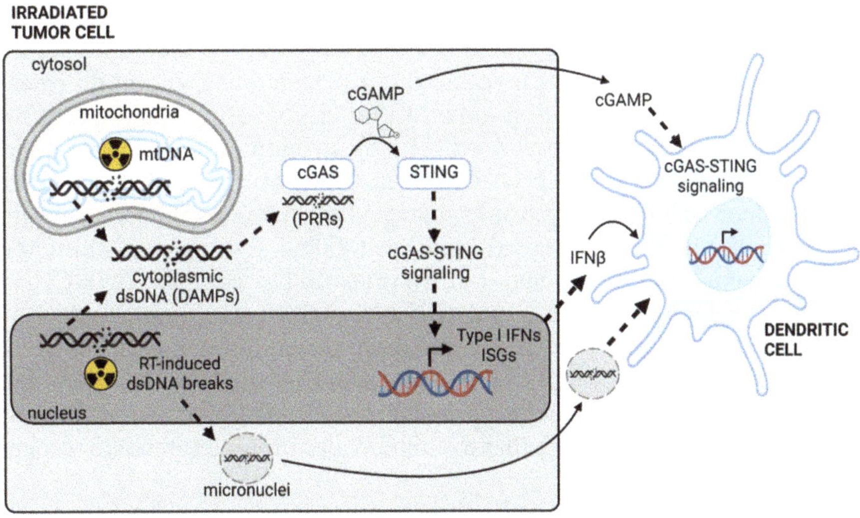


**Figure 3.1.** Radiation-induced DNA damage is inflammatory. Radiation therapy (RT) induces double-stranded DNA (dsDNA) breaks and micronuclei which leak from nuclear DNA or mitochondrial DNA (mtDNA) compartments. Cytoplasmic localization of dsDNA is inflammatory and functions as damage-associated molecular patterns (DAMPs) which bind to pattern recognition receptors (PRRs). cGAS is an innate immune sensor and PRR for dsDNA that binds dsDNA, triggering the production of cGAMP and the subsequent activation of cGAS–STING signaling. cGAS–STING signaling results in the expression of Type I IFN production and IFN-stimulated genes (ISGs). Dendritic cells also engulf dsDNA, bind secreted IFN-beta (IFNβ), and take up extracellular cGAMP which can trigger cGAS–STING pathway activation and IFN signaling, ultimately resulting in dendritic cell activation, antigen uptake, and the cross-priming of T-cells.

hypo-fractionated regimens (approximately up to 8–12 Gy per fraction) circumvent TREX1 induction and therefore may be relatively more immunogenic [4]. These findings require validation in clinical studies, but support the critical concept that the modulation of physical radiation dose parameters can have profound immunological consequences.

### 3.2.2 Immunogenic modulation and adaptive immunity

Beyond innate immune activation, ionizing radiation modulates antitumor immunity through additional mechanisms. Ionizing radiation has been shown to induce ICD and trigger hallmark molecular events associated with ICD, including the translocation of calreticulin, extracellular release of HMGB1, and ATP release [21]. These molecular hallmarks as well as cytoplasmic nucleic acids (see section 3.2.1) function as DAMPs or adjuvants that recruit and activate dendritic cells and other antigen-presenting cells (APCs). In the context of appropriate stimuli, 'licensed' dendritic cells (and other APCs) engulf and process antigens for presentation to naïve T-cells that possess antigen specificity. The cross-presentation of antigens by activated and mature dendritic cells is a critical step that links the innate and adaptive arms of the antitumor immune response and facilitates the generation of antigen-specific effector T-cells [3, 22].

Ionizing radiation promotes the release of tumor-associated neoantigens and the exposure of neoepitopes, thus augmenting antigenicity [23, 24]. Indeed, radiation has been demonstrated to enhance the intracellular peptide pool, and more recently a novel mechanism for the radiation-induced transcriptional upregulation of immunogenic neoantigens has been described [25, 26]. In addition to ICD, the notion of immunogenic modulation has been described, whereby the surviving fraction of irradiated tumor cells is modified in a manner that enhances immune recognition and susceptibility to T-cell-mediated tumor cell killing. Examples of immunogenic modulation include increased major histocompatibility complex (MHC) class I expression via STING-dependent and IFN-independent mechanisms which facilitate antigen presentation as well as increased expression of immune checkpoint and co-stimulatory molecules [27–29]. In addition, ionizing radiation has been demonstrated to upregulate retinoic acid early inducible-1 (RAE-1) expression, a ligand for the NKG2D receptor, suggesting that irradiation also promotes immune recognition by natural killer cells [30].

Upon antigen capture and activation, mature dendritic cells migrate to the tumor-associated draining lymph nodes (TdLNs). Dendritic cells are trafficked via chemotactic gradients within the lymphatic endothelium to the TdLNs, where they interact and prime naïve antigen-specific T-cells. In particular, it has been shown that IFN-β (which is induced by ionizing radiation and ligates the IFN-α/β receptor, IFNAR) is critical for licensing BATF3-dependent conventional type I dendritic cells—a subset that has superior capacity for the cross-priming of T-cells relative to other APCs (see figure 3.1) [2]. Cross-presentation of exogenous tumor-associated antigen via the MHC class I is critically important for radiation-driven immunity, as this facilitates the direct priming and activation of CD8+ T-cells [22]. These activated T-cells undergo clonal expansion and are subsequently trafficked into the peripheral circulation and the tumor microenvironment in order to carry out tumoricidal effector functions. This spatiotemporal separation of antigen uptake and T-cell cross-priming carries significant implications for locoregional therapies such as radiotherapy. Irradiation of the tumor microenvironment incites a robust inflammatory milieu in which various chemokines and cytokines attract and potentiate immune cell infiltration and function, respectively. Chemotactic gradients dictate immune cell trafficking; thus, ionizing radiation can help to guide and instruct effector T-cells and other immune subsets towards sites of inflammation that harbor malignant cells. Further, irradiation of the TdLN, a critical site of immunological synapse and generation of the adaptive tumor-specific immune responses, has been shown to hamper tumor control through immune-based mechanisms [31, 32].

As such, the establishment of nonuniform ionizing radiation dose gradients and the application of SFRT in tumors relative to adjacent tissues might be leveraged to potentiate antitumor immunity via an intentional induction of chemotactic gradients across tumoral tissues and/or by minimizing the irradiation of anatomic compartments that harbor reservoirs of immune cells or sites of immunological crosstalk (see section 3.3.4) [33]. For example, in the setting of partial volume irradiation, it is plausible that steep chemokine gradients and remodeled tumor stroma and vasculature provoke robust immune infiltration that underlies tumor control, particularly in the nonirradiated or adjacent segments that receive lower doses of radiation. This may require a recalibration of the conventional dogma of a linear relationship between radiation dose and tumor control. Harnessing immune-based mechanisms to augment tumor control may be necessary to achieve optimal outcomes—particularly in bulky tumors or in scenarios in which it is infeasible to administer definitive doses to the entire tumor volume.

### 3.2.3 Local and systemic radiation responses

Achieving irradiated tumor control (i.e. local control) is often a primary goal of radiation therapy and is also dependent on host immunity [34]. However, the notion that focal radiotherapy can induce systemic antitumor immunity responses that contribute to distant disease control in nonirradiated lesions remains intriguing. This is increasingly relevant with expanding indications for radiotherapy in the metastatic setting and increasing options for life-prolonging systemic therapies, in which the intent of local therapies may shift from short-term palliation towards more durable disease control. Preclinical models have provided substantial evidence that radiation can induce abscopal responses in nonirradiated lesions, particularly when combined with immune-modulating agents [35]. However, translating these findings to human disease remains elusive with generally underwhelming findings in trials rigorously evaluating the ability of radiotherapy–immunotherapy combinations to enhance the overall response rate relative to immunotherapy alone [36, 37]. Alternatively, the importance of local control and irradiated tumor control is emerging as an investigational predictive marker of survival outcomes; several recent clinical studies have demonstrated impressive pathological responses when combining radiotherapy with immunotherapy [5, 38, 39]. Nevertheless, a uniform approach with radiotherapy–immunotherapy combinations cannot be adopted, since different histologies, disease stages, and clinical settings have shown divergent results. While the addition of immunotherapy following chemoradiation-based primary therapy has transformed the standard of care in inoperable locally advanced lung cancers [40], it has failed to improve outcomes in locally advanced head and neck cancers, albeit tested in a different sequence [41]. There is increasing appreciation that radiation-specific parameters including target volumes (i.e. elective nodal irradiation) and relative sequencing with systemic immune-modulators can dramatically impact outcomes [42]. Biomarkers and correlative analyses from clinical studies and human tissues have started to identify potential biomarkers of radiation-associated local and systemic responses, including increased serum IFN-β levels in systemic responders [25], upregulated IFN-ɣ-associated gene expression signatures in irradiated lesions that positively correlate with treatment response in nonirradiated tumors [43], *TREX1* expression inversely correlated with irradiated tumor controls, and *DNASE1* expression positively correlated with irradiated tumor control [5].

The majority of preclinical and clinical studies that have evaluated local and systemic radiation-induced immune responses have largely explored ionizing radiation in the context of conventional field design and dose-fractionation schemes, often in combination with established concurrent chemotherapy regimens. Nevertheless, the preclinical data and translational data provide insight into radiation factors that may dictate outcomes and thus may be modifiable with SFRT and other evolving radiation techniques [2].

## 3.3 The immunologic effects of ionizing radiation

Understanding the duality of radiation-induced immunomodulation whereby ionizing radiation can simultaneously promote potent immune suppression and activation is critical to optimizing outcomes. The critical steps necessary to induce and sustain radiation-mediated antitumor immunity have been described (see sections 3.2.1 and 3.2.2). Ionizing radiation also carries several deleterious effects ranging from the induction and activation of immunosuppressive cytokines and immunometabolites which can directly and indirectly limit immune cell function to direct damage to immune cells or tissues critical for the generation of immune responses [44].

### 3.3.1 The immunogenic effects of ionizing radiation

As discussed, ionizing radiation impacts both the innate and adaptive aspects of antitumor immunity. In alignment with preclinical studies, peripheral blood analyses have fairly consistently demonstrated the capacity for ionizing radiation to modulate the T-cell repertoire and expand tumor-specific T-cell clones in patients responding to radiotherapy–immunotherapy combinations [25, 45, 46]. Among responders, baseline or dynamic on-treatment enrichment of effector T-cells (or natural killer cells) as well as the reversal of an 'exhausted' phenotype have been associated with favorable outcomes [47–50]. Taken together, these findings suggest that T-cell responses are critical mediators of radiation-induced immunogenicity. Nevertheless, given the capacity for ionizing radiation to activate innate immune sensing pathways, preclinical studies have suggested that poorly immunogenic tumors that are devoid of dendritic cells might be sensitized to immune-based approaches by applying radiotherapy as a focal adjuvant [51, 52]. This alludes to the concept that in the proper context, ionizing radiation may help to convert immunologically 'cold' tumors into immune-infiltrated 'hot' or 'inflamed' tumors [53].

### 3.3.2 The immunosuppressive and tolerogenic effects of ionizing radiation

Central to our understanding of immunity is the concept of homeostasis, whereby the host counteracts and suppresses excessive inflammation after 'foreign' antigen and danger signals are cleared to limit immune-mediated damage to normal tissues and suppress autoimmune disease. These coordinated actions taken to suppress or tolerize immune responses are often hijacked in the context of cancer, in which tumor cells evade immune recognition or inhibit antitumor immune responses.

In addition, the injury and inflammatory remodeling induced by radiotherapy upregulates suppressive and homeostatic cytokines and metabolites (TGF-beta, IL-10, IDO, adenosine), recruits suppressive immune populations (myeloid-derived suppressor cells, regulatory T-cells) into the tumor microenvironment, and/or polarizes/skews resident populations towards a suppressive phenotype or functional state (tolerogenic dendritic cells, M2-like tumor-associated macrophages) [11, 20, 31, 54–60]. These immunosuppressive or tolerogenic activities induced by radiation therapy can directly or indirectly block dendritic cell activation/maturation and T-cell priming or effector functions, thus restraining innate immune activation and the potentiation of antigen-specific antitumor responses.

### 3.3.3 The immune-depleting effects of ionizing radiation

Immune cells are generally considered to be radiosensitive. This property of ionizing radiation has been exploited clinically in the use of total body irradiation as a myeloablative conditioning regimen for stem cell transplantation. Notably, a range of radiosensitivity likely exists across immune cell types; naïve circulating T-cells are particularly sensitize to low doses of ionizing radiation, whereas tissue-resident memory T-cells appear to be relatively more radioresistant [61]. It is known that low absolute lymphocyte count (ALC) at baseline is a poor prognostic factor for cancer outcomes, and similar findings apply for associated metrics such as the neutrophil-to-lymphocyte (NLR) ratio [62]. The development of severe radiation-induced lymphopenia (RIL) and/or treatment-related lymphopenia has also consistently been shown to carry a significant adverse prognostic impact on overall survival across multiple solid tumors [63, 64]. Interestingly, preclinical work has suggested that the immune-depleting effects of ionizing radiation extend beyond the direct targets of irradiation, as circulating irradiated cells migrate to the bone marrow and, in addition to RIL, appear to potentiate immune suppression by suppressing hematopoiesis in nonirradiated bone marrow [65]. Other researchers have suggested that the absence of a homeostatic IL-7 response to RIL may drive poor outcomes [66–68]. Post-hoc analyses of three prospective clinical trials exploring radiation–immunotherapy combinations have corroborated that abscopal response rates were substantially higher among patients with high post-radiotherapy ALCs and that higher than median ALCs were associated with superior overall survival [69].

### 3.3.4 The irradiation of anatomic/biologic compartments on radiation response

Because radiation-induced lymphopenia and immunosuppression contribute to poor oncological outcomes, it has been suggested that the ionizing radiation dose administered to biologic/anatomic compartments important to immune function should be minimized. The concept of the immune system as an organ at risk (OAR) is a novel approach to optimizing the delivery of ionizing radiation to enhance immunogenicity and mitigate deleterious effects [70]. Accordingly, researchers see potential in SFRT and other emerging approaches for the delivery of ionizing radiation that effectively spare immune OARs. The circulating blood volume which

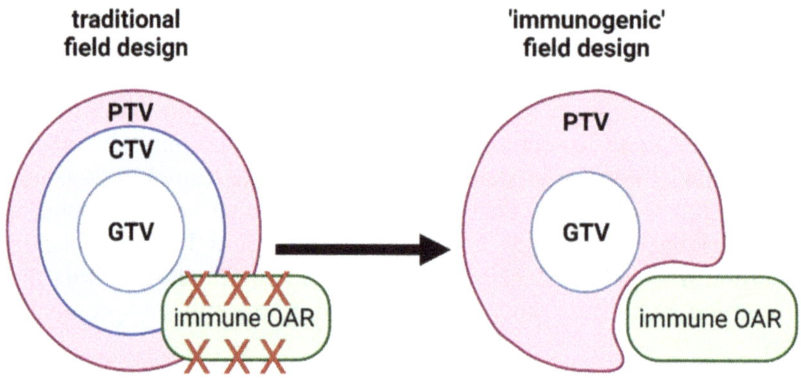


**Figure 3.2.** Target volume considerations for optimizing the immunogenicity of ionizing radiation. Radiotherapy can promote immunogenic or immunosuppressive effects, depending on the context. Traditional fields (left) generally do not consider the sparing of certain organs and tissues that are important reservoirs of immune cell populations (i.e. the spleen, bone marrow, or circulating blood pool) or important sites for immune function (i.e. tumor-draining lymph nodes) and thus may lead to radiation-induced tolerance or immune depletion (i.e. radiation-induced lymphopenia). Immunogenic field design (right) may account for the sparing of immune organs at risk (OARs) to potentiate immunogenic effects and mitigate the deleterious effects of ionizing radiation.

harbors peripheral blood mononuclear cells (PBMCs) is relatively radiosensitive; thus, even low-dose exposure to large proportions of the blood volume can yield substantial RIL and immune-depleting effects. Various physical, temporal, and radiobiological parameters modulate the exposure of circulating PBMCs to radiation, and various models have been developed to estimate the radiation doses administered to various components of the host immune system [71, 72]. In addition to PBMCs, other important hematopoietic tissues (i.e. bone marrow) and lymphoid organs, including the TdLNs and spleen, are critical for initiating or sustaining host immunity. Radiation-induced damage or exposure to these immune OARs may deplete, suppress, or tolerize immune cells. Irradiation of the TdLN has been shown to abrogate adaptive immune response in preclinical models; given recent negative studies combining immunotherapy with chemoradiation to treat head and neck cancer, it has been speculated that the use of elective nodal irradiation may have contributed to suboptimal antitumor immunity [31, 41]. Incidental bone marrow (i.e. in the pelvis or vertebral body) or splenic irradiation, for which the radiation dose is often not constrained, has also been implicated as a potential predictor of RIL and associated poor outcomes [73]. The development of radiation target volumes that specifically account for and spare 'immune OARs' may be necessary to fully harness radiation-induced immunogenicity (see figure 3.2). It has been demonstrated that reducing the volume of the irradiated field as well as hypofractionation result in significantly less exposure to circulating immune populations and lymphoid organs, resulting in reduced RIL [74]. Stereotactic body radiation therapy (SBRT) in pancreatic cancer as well as early-stage lung cancers has been demonstrated to result in superior lymphocyte sparing relative to conventionally fractionated regimens [75, 76]. Treatment volume reduction, such as the omission of contralateral neck elective nodal irradiation, has also been shown to have a favorable impact on immune parameters [77, 78].

## 3.4 Understanding the potential immunologic consequences of nonuniform dose irradiation

Fraction size and target volume modulation are proof of the concept that altering irradiation parameters has immunological consequences. Recent preclinical and clinical data evaluating nonuniform dose irradiation techniques and other emerging ionizing radiation delivery methods, including ultrahigh-dose-rate FLASH radiotherapy, warrant more investigation to define their immunomodulatory effects and potential synergy with immunotherapy.

### 3.4.1 The integration of nonuniform irradiation and immunomodulation

Partial volume irradiation is often utilized by necessity for bulky tumors in order to limit the damage to adjacent normal tissues. Nevertheless, response rates and irradiated tumor control appear favorable, suggesting that both cytotoxic and immunological mechanisms are at play. Preclinical studies of hemi-tumor irradiation suggest that partial volume irradiation activates intratumoral T-cells and upregulates adhesion molecules that facilitate immune infiltration into the non-irradiated portion of the tumor; similar tumor control is observed for partial and complete tumor irradiation [79]. Similarly, a phase I study of multi-site SBRT followed by pembrolizumab only permitted SBRT prescribed to a maximum volume of 65 mL, and a proportion of tumors received only partial volume irradiation. A comparison of one-year treated metastasis control showed there was no significant difference between partially versus completely irradiated tumors. These findings should be considered in the context that partially irradiated tumors were by definition larger, yet achieved similar irradiated tumor control [5]. Preclinical studies of lattice radiation therapy in an abscopal model also corroborated these findings. Kanagavelu *et al* tested a range of partial volume treatments (20% as one or two lattice vertices and one 50% lattice vertex) as well as complete tumor irradiation, noting similar irradiated tumor control across groups (favoring complete and 20% in two vertices) [80]. However, response in 'distant' abscopal nonirradiated tumors was most pronounced among partially irradiated tumors, which was mechanistically linked to robust IFN-γ expression and T-cell infiltration [80]. Collectively, these data suggest that nonuniform dose irradiation in both mice and humans (specifically as partial volume or lattice irradiation) appears immunomodulatory and may augment both local and systemic immune responses to high-dose radiation. A more biologically guided approach to nonuniform dose irradiation that targets hypoxic segments of tumors has yielded impressive clinical results, resulting in a bulky tumor control rate of 95% [81, 82]. The rationale for this SBRT-based partial tumor irradiation targeting hypoxic segments (SBRT-PATHY) is that targeting the hypoxic segments with high-dose ionizing radiation circumvents the lymphopenia associated with total tumor volume irradiation and spares the peritumoral immune microenvironment, thereby exploiting radiation-induced immunogenic shifts in both local and distant sites [83]. While this requires more rigorous validation through prospective, randomized clinical testing, it alludes to the potential to develop a more immunologically centered approach to target volume design and treatment delivery as we continue to improve our understanding of the mechanistic basis for immunomodulation induced by nonuniform dose irradiation. Akin to the use of spatially modulated intratumoral dose gradients with SFRT, other investigators are exploring the combination of high-dose ionizing radiation with non-ablative low-dose radiation at additional metastatic sites. This concept was developed based on unplanned clinical findings that non-targeted lesions that received 'incidental' low-dose radiation had significantly improved response rates compared to the response rates of non-targeted lesions that received no low-dose radiation [84, 85]. Formalizing this concept, preclinical work has suggested that the low-dose radiation remodels the immunosuppressive stroma, permitting immunogenic repolarization and enhanced infiltration of these irradiated sites and thus leading to improved systemic disease control [86]. The results of a phase II trial combining high-dose and non-ablative low-dose radiotherapy in immunotherapy refractory patients reported a four-month disease control rate of 42% and an objective response rate of 19%—notably, there was an improved lesion-specific response rate in patients who received both high- and low-dose radiotherapy as compared with those receiving high-dose radiotherapy alone [87].

There is a distinct rationale for immunomodulatory combinations involving FLASH radiotherapy (which is reviewed in more detail in chapters 4 and 8), given the hypothesis that ultrahigh-dose-rate radiotherapy preferentially spares the normal tissue compartment while preserving tumoricidal effects. While the biological mechanisms involved are yet to be fully worked out, this rationale can be extended to the concept of immune OARs. It is plausible that traditionally radiosensitive immune cells may have different sensitivities to ultrahigh-dose-rate ionizing radiation—therefore, FLASH may be relatively less immunosuppressive or less tolerogenic compared with more conventional approaches. Further, if validated, rather than anatomically sculpting the dose away from immune OARs, this approach might allow the simultaneous targeting of subclinical disease in lymphoid organs while preserving immune function. Thus, the unique biology of FLASH radiotherapy might be exploited to promote the immunogenic effects of ionizing radiation. To this end, in an advanced ovarian cancer preclinical model, the combination of abdominopelvic FLASH radiotherapy combined with anti-PD-1 immunotherapy demonstrated encouraging safety and tumor control; intriguingly, it was also associated with adaptive T-cell infiltration and a reduction in suppressive regulatory T-cells [88].

## 3.5 Knowledge gaps and future perspectives

Our understanding of immunomodulation in the context of nonuniform dose irradiation remains in its infancy. Critical areas for the field to focus on are: (1) the development of improved and robust preclinical irradiation platforms that reliably model the radiation dosimetry and dose distribution of SFRT (or the ultrahigh dose rate of FLASH radiotherapy); (2) the design of clinical studies that robustly and prospectively test these techniques using embedded blood-based, imaging-based, and tissue-based (when feasible) correlatives; (3) the preclinical modeling of combination treatments with SFRT or other modalities with immunomodulators that have potentially synergistic/complementary mechanisms of action. Leveraging the successes, learning from the tribulations, and rationally applying the knowledge gained from the last decades of preclinical and clinical research in radiation-induced immunity will help to accelerate progress in this space. It is clear that ionizing radiation is a highly efficacious therapy with a complex underlying immunobiology that can be modulated based on radiation-specific parameters.

## 3.6 Conclusions

Radiation-induced immunomodulation is highly context dependent and yields both immunostimulatory and immunosuppressive effects. Nonuniform dose irradiation appears to have unique immunologic effects relating to cytokine induction, immune cell trafficking, adaptive immunity, and remodeling of the local (irradiated) and distant tumor microenvironment. Additional preclinical and clinical work is needed to better understand these mechanisms and how they can be exploited to promote antitumor immunity.

## References

[1] Demaria S, Golden E B and Formenti S C 2015 Role of local radiation therapy in cancer immunotherapy *JAMA Oncol* **1** 1325–32

[2] Vanpouille-Box C, Formenti S C and Demaria S 2018 Toward precision radiotherapy for use with immune checkpoint blockers *Clin. Cancer Res.* **24** 259–65

[3] Marciscano A E *et al* 2021 Immunomodulatory effects of stereotactic body radiation therapy: preclinical insights and clinical opportunities *Int. J. Radiat. Oncol. Biol. Phys.* **110** 35–52

[4] Vanpouille-Box C *et al* 2017 DNA exonuclease Trex1 regulates radiotherapy-induced tumour immunogenicity *Nat. Commun.* **8** 15618

[5] Luke J J *et al* 2020 Improved survival associated with local tumor response following multisite radiotherapy and pembrolizumab: secondary analysis of a phase I trial *Clin. Cancer Res.* **26** 6437–44

[6] Petroni G *et al* 2021 Radiotherapy as a tool to elicit clinically actionable signalling pathways in cancer *Nat. Rev. Clin. Oncol.* **19** 114–31

[7] Hall E 2019 *Radiobiology for the Radiologist* 8th edn (Philadelphia, PA: Wolters Kluwer)

[8] Becker D and Sevilla M D 1993 The chemical consequences of radiation damage to DNA *Adv. Radiat. Biol.* **17** 121–80

[9] Hutchinson F 1961 Molecular basis for action of ionizing radiations *Science* **134** 533–8

[10] Harding S M *et al* 2017 Mitotic progression following DNA damage enables pattern recognition within micronuclei *Nature* **548** 466–70

[11] McLaughlin M *et al* 2020 Inflammatory microenvironment remodelling by tumour cells after radiotherapy *Nat. Rev. Cancer* **20** 203–17

[12] Wilkins A C *et al* 2019 The immunological consequences of radiation-induced DNA damage *J. Pathol.* **247** 606–14
[13] Golden E B, Marciscano A E and Formenti S C 2020 Radiation therapy and the *in situ* vaccination approach *Int. J. Radiat. Oncol. Biol. Phys.* **108** 891–98
[14] Formenti S C and Demaria S 2012 Radiation therapy to convert the tumor into an *in situ* vaccine *Int. J. Radiat. Oncol. Biol. Phys.* **84** 879–80
[15] Weichselbaum R R *et al* 2017 Radiotherapy and immunotherapy: a beneficial liaison? *Nat. Rev. Clin. Oncol.* **14** 365–79
[16] Matsumura S *et al* 2008 Radiation-induced CXCL16 release by breast cancer cells attracts effector T cells *J. Immunol.* **181** 3099–107
[17] McGee H M *et al* 2021 Parallels between the antiviral state and the irradiated state *J. Natl. Cancer Inst.* **113** 969–79
[18] Yamazaki T *et al* 2020 Mitochondrial DNA drives abscopal responses to radiation that are inhibited by autophagy *Nat. Immunol.* **21** 1160–71
[19] Deng L *et al* 2014 STING-dependent cytosolic DNA sensing promotes radiation-induced type I interferon-dependent antitumor immunity in immunogenic tumors *Immunity* **41** 843–52
[20] Widau R C *et al* 2014 RIG-I-like receptor LGP2 protects tumor cells from ionizing radiation *Proc. Natl. Acad. Sci. USA* **111** E484–91
[21] Golden E B *et al* 2014 Radiation fosters dose-dependent and chemotherapy-induced immunogenic cell death *Oncoimmunology* **3** e28518
[22] Sharabi A B *et al* 2015 Stereotactic radiation therapy augments antigen-specific PD-1-mediated antitumor immune responses via cross-presentation of tumor antigen. *Cancer Immunol. Res.* **3** 345–55
[23] Sharabi A B *et al* 2015 Stereotactic radiation therapy combined with immunotherapy: augmenting the role of radiation in local and systemic treatment *Oncology (Williston Park)* **29** 331–40
[24] Lhuillier C *et al* 2019 Radiation therapy and anti-tumor immunity: exposing immunogenic mutations to the immune system *Genome Med.* **11** 40
[25] Formenti S C *et al* 2018 Radiotherapy induces responses of lung cancer to CTLA-4 blockade *Nat. Med.* **24** 1845–51
[26] Reits E A *et al* 2006 Radiation modulates the peptide repertoire, enhances MHC class I expression, and induces successful antitumor immunotherapy *J. ExMed.* **203** 1259–71
[27] Gameiro S R *et al* 2014 Radiation-induced immunogenic modulation of tumor enhances antigen processing and calreticulin exposure, resulting in enhanced T-cell killing *Oncotarget* **5** 403–16
[28] Wattenberg M M *et al* 2014 Unlocking the combination: potentiation of radiation-induced antitumor responses with immunotherapy *Radiat. Res.* **182** 126–38
[29] Zebertavage L K *et al* 2020 Transcriptional upregulation of NLRC5 by radiation Drives STING- and interferon-independent MHC-I expression on cancer cells and T cell cytotoxicity *Sci. Rep.* **10** 7376
[30] Ruocco M G *et al* 2012 Suppressing T cell motility induced by anti-CTLA-4 monotherapy improves antitumor effects. *J. Clin. Invest.* **122** 3718–30
[31] Marciscano A E *et al* 2018 Elective nodal irradiation attenuates the combinatorial efficacy of stereotactic radiation therapy and immunotherapy *Clin. Cancer Res.* **24** 5058–71

[32] Buchwald Z S *et al* 2020 Tumor-draining lymph node is important for a robust abscopal effect stimulated by radiotherapy *J. Immunother. Cancer* **8** e000867 Corrected in http://dx.doi.org/10.1136/jitc-2020-000867corr1

[33] Griffin R J *et al* 2020 Understanding high-dose, ultra-high dose rate, and spatially fractionated radiation therapy *Int. J. Radiat. Oncol. Biol. Phys.* **107** 766–78

[34] Stone H B, Peters L J and Milas L 1979 Effect of host immune capability on radiocurability and subsequent transplantability of a murine fibrosarcoma *J. Natl. Cancer Inst.* **63** 1229–35

[35] Park S S *et al* 2015 PD-1 restrains radiotherapy-induced abscopal effect. *Cancer Immunol. Res.* **3** 610–9

[36] Schoenfeld J D *et al* 2022 Durvalumab plus tremelimumab alone or in combination with low-dose or hypofractionated radiotherapy in metastatic non-small-cell lung cancer refractory to previous PD(L)-1 therapy: an open-label, multicentre, randomised, phase 2 trial *Lancet Oncol.* **23** 279–91

[37] McBride S *et al* 2021 Randomized phase II trial of nivolumab with stereotactic body radiotherapy versus nivolumab alone in metastatic head and neck squamous cell carcinoma *J. Clin. Oncol.* **39** 30–7

[38] Altorki N K *et al* 2021 Neoadjuvant durvalumab with or without stereotactic body radiotherapy in patients with early-stage non-small-cell lung cancer: a single-centre, randomised phase 2 trial. *Lancet Oncol.* **22** 824–35

[39] Leidner R *et al* 2021 Neoadjuvant immunoradiotherapy results in high rate of complete pathological response and clinical to pathological downstaging in locally advanced head and neck squamous cell carcinoma *J. Immunother. Cancer* **9** e002485

[40] Antonia S J *et al* 2017 Durvalumab after chemoradiotherapy in stage III non-small-cell lung cancer *N. Engl. J. Med.* **377** 1919–29

[41] Lee N Y *et al* 2021 Avelumab plus standard-of-care chemoradiotherapy versus chemoradiotherapy alone in patients with locally advanced squamous cell carcinoma of the head and neck: a randomised, double-blind, placebo-controlled, multicentre, phase 3 trial. *Lancet Oncol.* **22** 450–62

[42] Wei J *et al* 2021 Sequence of αPD-1 relative to local tumor irradiation determines the induction of abscopal antitumor immune responses. *Sci. Immunol.* **6** eabg0117

[43] Luke J J *et al* 2018 Safety and clinical activity of pembrolizumab and multisite stereotactic body radiotherapy in patients with advanced solid tumors *J. Clin. Oncol.* **36** 1611–18

[44] Wennerberg E *et al* 2017 Barriers to radiation-induced *in situ* tumor vaccination *Front. Immunol.* **8** 229

[45] Twyman-Saint Victor C *et al* 2015 Radiation and dual checkpoint blockade activate non-redundant immune mechanisms in cancer *Nature* **520** 373–7

[46] Dovedi S J *et al* 2017 Fractionated radiation therapy stimulates antitumor immunity mediated by both resident and infiltrating polyclonal T-cell populations when combined with PD-1 blockade. *Clin. Cancer Res.* **23** 5514–26

[47] McGee H M *et al* 2018 Stereotactic ablative radiation therapy induces systemic differences in peripheral blood immunophenotype dependent on irradiated site *Int. J. Radiat. Oncol. Biol. Phys.* **101** 1259–70

[48] Hammerich L *et al* 2019 Systemic clinical tumor regressions and potentiation of PD1 blockade with *in situ* vaccination *Nat. Med.* **25** 814–24

[49] Seung S K *et al* 2012 Phase 1 study of stereotactic body radiotherapy and interleukin-2—tumor and immunological responses. *Sci. Transl. Med.* **4** 137ra74

[50] Yu J *et al* 2021 Liver metastasis restrains immunotherapy efficacy via macrophage-mediated T cell elimination. *Nat. Med.* **27** 152–64

[51] Hegde S *et al* 2020 Dendritic cell paucity leads to dysfunctional immune surveillance in pancreatic cancer *Cancer Cell* **37** 289–307.e9

[52] Blair T C *et al* 2020 Dendritic cell maturation defines immunological responsiveness of tumors to radiation therapy *J. Immunol.* **204** 3416–24

[53] Theelen W *et al* 2021 Pembrolizumab with or without radiotherapy for metastatic non-small-cell lung cancer: a pooled analysis of two randomised trials *Lancet Respir. Med.* **9** 467–75

[54] Akkari L *et al* 2020 Dynamic changes in glioma macrophage populations after radiotherapy reveal CSF-1R inhibition as a strategy to overcome resistance. *Sci. Transl. Med.* **12** eaaw7843

[55] Hardee M E *et al* 2012 Resistance of glioblastoma-initiating cells to radiation mediated by the tumor microenvironment can be abolished by inhibiting transforming growth factor-β *Cancer Res.* **72** 4119–29

[56] Monjazeb A M *et al* 2016 Blocking indolamine-2,3-dioxygenase rebound immune suppression boosts antitumor effects of radio-immunotherapy in murine models and spontaneous canine malignancies. *Clin. Cancer Res.* **22** 4328–40

[57] Wennerberg E *et al* 2020 CD73 blockade promotes dendritic cell infiltration of irradiated tumors and tumor rejection *Cancer Immunol. Res.* **8** 465–78

[58] Xu J *et al* 2013 CSF1R signaling blockade stanches tumor-infiltrating myeloid cells and improves the efficacy of radiotherapy in prostate cancer *Cancer Res.* **73** 2782–94

[59] Muroyama Y *et al* 2017 Stereotactic radiotherapy increases functionally suppressive regulatory t cells in the tumor microenvironment *Cancer Immunol. Res.* **5** 992–1004

[60] Liang H *et al* 2017 Host STING-dependent MDSC mobilization drives extrinsic radiation resistance *Nat. Commun.* **8** 1736

[61] Arina A *et al* 2019 Tumor-reprogrammed resident T cells resist radiation to control tumors *Nat. Commun.* **10** 3959

[62] Thor M *et al* 2022 Pre-treatment immune status predicts disease control in NSCLCs treated with chemoradiation and durvalumab *Radiother. Oncol.* **167** 158–64

[63] Jing W *et al* 2021 Prognosis of severe lymphopenia after postoperative radiotherapy in non-small cell lung cancer: results of a long-term follow up study *Clin. Transl. Radiat. Oncol.* **28** 54–61

[64] Damen P J J *et al* 2021 The influence of severe radiation-induced lymphopenia on overall survival in solid tumors: a systematic review and meta-analysis *Int. J. Radiat. Oncol. Biol. Phys.* **111** 936–48

[65] Kapoor V *et al* 2020 Radiation induces iatrogenic immunosuppression by indirectly affecting hematopoiesis in bone marrow *Oncotarget* **11** 1681–90

[66] Byun H K *et al* 2021 Effect of interleukin-7 on radiation-induced lymphopenia and its antitumor effects in a mouse model. *Int. J. Radiat. Oncol. Biol. Phys.* **109** 1559–69

[67] Piotrowski A F *et al* 2018 Systemic depletion of lymphocytes following focal radiation to the brain in a murine model *Oncoimmunology* **7** e1445951

[68] Ellsworth S *et al* 2014 Sustained CD4(+) T cell-driven lymphopenia without a compensatory IL-7/IL-15 response among high-grade glioma patients treated with radiation and temozolomide. *Oncoimmunology* **3** e27357

[69] Chen D *et al* 2020 Absolute lymphocyte count predicts abscopal responses and outcomes in patients receiving combined immunotherapy and radiation therapy: analysis of 3 phase 1/2 trials. *Int. J. Radiat. Oncol. Biol. Phys.* **108** 196–203
[70] Jin J Y *et al* 2020 A framework for modeling radiation induced lymphopenia in radiotherapy *Radiother. Oncol.* **144** 105–13
[71] Ladbury C J *et al* 2019 Impact of radiation dose to the host immune system on tumor control and survival for stage iii non-small cell lung cancer treated with definitive radiation therapy *Int. J. Radiat. Oncol. Biol. Phys.* **105** 346–55
[72] Jin J Y *et al* 2021 Higher radiation dose to the immune cells correlates with worse tumor control and overall survival in patients with stage III NSCLC: a secondary analysis of RTOG0617 *Cancers (Basel)* **13** 6193
[73] Chadha A S *et al* 2017 Does unintentional splenic radiation predict outcomes after pancreatic cancer radiation therapy? *Int. J. Radiat. Oncol. Biol. Phys.* **97** 323–32
[74] Ellsworth S G 2018 Field size effects on the risk and severity of treatment-induced lymphopenia in patients undergoing radiation therapy for solid tumors *Adv. Radiat. Oncol.* **3** 512–19
[75] McLaughlin M F *et al* 2020 Stereotactic body radiation therapy mitigates radiation induced lymphopenia in early stage non-small cell lung cancer *PLoS One* **15** e0241505
[76] Wild A T *et al* 2016 Lymphocyte-sparing effect of stereotactic body radiation therapy in patients with unresectable pancreatic cancer *Int. J. Radiat. Oncol. Biol. Phys.* **94** 571–9
[77] Rudra S *et al* 2018 Effect of radiation treatment volume reduction on lymphopenia in patients receiving chemoradiotherapy for glioblastoma *Int. J. Radiat. Oncol. Biol. Phys.* **101** 217–25
[78] Lin A J *et al* 2018 Post-operative radiation effects on lymphopenia, neutrophil to lymphocyte ratio, and clinical outcomes in palatine tonsil cancers *Oral Oncol.* **86** 1–7
[79] Markovsky E *et al* 2019 An antitumor immune response is evoked by partial-volume single-dose radiation in 2 murine models *Int. J. Radiat. Oncol. Biol. Phys.* **103** 697–708
[80] Kanagavelu S *et al* 2014 In vivo effects of lattice radiation therapy on local and distant lung cancer: potential role of immunomodulation *Radiat. Res.* **182** 149–62
[81] Tubin S *et al* 2020 Shifting the immune-suppressive to predominant immune-stimulatory radiation effects by SBRT-PArtial Tumor Irradiation Targeting HYpoxic Segment (SBRT-PATHY) *Cancers (Basel)* **13** 50
[82] Tubin S, Popper H H and Brcic L 2019 Novel stereotactic body radiation therapy (SBRT)-based partial tumor irradiation targeting hypoxic segment of bulky tumors (SBRT-PATHY): improvement of the radiotherapy outcome by exploiting the bystander and abscopal effects *Radiat. Oncol.* **14** 21
[83] Tubin S *et al* 2019 Mono-institutional phase 2 study of innovative Stereotactic Body RadioTherapy targeting PArtial Tumor HYpoxic (SBRT-PATHY) clonogenic cells in unresectable bulky non-small cell lung cancer: profound non-targeted effects by sparing peri-tumoral immune microenvironment *Radiat. Oncol.* **14** 212
[84] Welsh J W *et al* 2019 Phase II trial of ipilimumab with stereotactic radiation therapy for metastatic disease: outcomes, toxicities, and low-dose radiation-related abscopal responses *Cancer Immunol. Res.* **7** 1903–9
[85] Menon H *et al* 2019 Influence of low-dose radiation on abscopal responses in patients receiving high-dose radiation and immunotherapy *J. Immunother. Cancer* **7** 237

[86] Barsoumian H B *et al* 2020 Low-dose radiation treatment enhances systemic antitumor immune responses by overcoming the inhibitory stroma *J. Immunother. Cancer* **8** e000537

[87] Patel R R *et al* 2021 High-dose irradiation in combination with non-ablative low-dose radiation to treat metastatic disease after progression on immunotherapy: results of a phase II trial *Radiother. Oncol.* **162** 60–7

[88] Eggold J T *et al* 2022 Abdominopelvic FLASH irradiation improves PD-1 immune checkpoint inhibition in preclinical models of ovarian cancer *Mol. Cancer. Ther.* **21** 371–81

# Chapter 4

# The biology of FLASH—a critical appraisal for clinical translation

**Veljko Grilj and Marie-Catherine Vozenin**

The field of radiation oncology is engaged in a continuous effort to improve the difference between the responses to radiation of tumors and healthy tissues. In this context, the development of novel radiotherapy (RT) approach named FLASH-RT might soon dramatically change the standard practice in RT and positively affect patients' quality of life in the short and long terms. FLASH-RT utilizes high-intensity radiation beams to reduce the delivery time of a treatment dose to less than a few hundred milliseconds, which results in remarkable healthy tissue sparing but retains tumor killing in comparison with conventional RT at isodose. The so-called FLASH effect has been confirmed using electron, photon, and proton beams in various tissues (the lung, brain, gut, and skin) and animal models (mice, pigs, cats, and zebrafish), leading to the initiation of clinical trials in domestic animals and human patients. However, the research was conducted with preclinical beams and small radiation fields (<3 cm diameter) and was mainly delivered in the form of a single dose. The widespread clinical transfer of FLASH-RT in this form is not feasible. Today, the technology of FLASH irradiators still does not meet the clinical requirements to treat relevant target volumes and has not been proven to offer acceptable treatment quality. In addition, it is unclear whether the validated FLASH parameters used in preclinical settings are readily translatable into clinical situations.

## 4.1 Introduction

RT remains a powerful tool in the fight against cancer, as more than half of all cancer patients are treated using RT at some point in the management of their disease [1]. When administered with curative intent, RT remains (along with surgery) a successful and cost-effective form of cancer treatment [2]. Over the last few decades, technological and biological advances have transformed RT into a

doi:10.1088/978-0-7503-4046-5ch4  

precise and personalized treatment; nevertheless, the treatment of radio-resistant tumors is still restricted by normal tissue complications, the occurrence of unintended side effects, and the frequent development of metastases that ultimately kill patients. Therefore, enhancing the differential effect of RT by selective tumor radio sensitization to avoid the development of metastases and enhance normal tissue protection remains the overarching goal for radiobiologists/oncologists. In this context, our team conceptualized and implemented FLASH-RT, an irradiation modality with extreme temporal properties.

## 4.2 FLASH-RT

FLASH-RT presents a paradigm-shifting approach in radiation oncology that relies on the use of high-intensity beams that can shorten the treatment time to a fraction of a second (typically less than 100 ms) as opposed to the minutes required by conventional (CONV) RT protocols [3–8]. Such rapid irradiations can elicit the FLASH effect, which is characterized by its capability to control tumors without normal tissue complications. FLASH-RT is now recognized as one of the most promising ways to resolve issues related to the protection of normal tissues, as its ubiquitous nature has been confirmed in numerous preclinical studies involving various animals and organs/tissues [9, 10]. With a dose modifying factor (DMF) ranging between 10% [11] and 50% [12] depending upon the model used, the organ targeted, the type of beam, and the dose used, the therapeutic index achieved by FLASH-RT far exceeds that of any known radio-mitigating agent. FLASH-RT has primarily been investigated with pulsed electron beams [12–14]. Later studies were successful at reproducing the FLASH effect with protons accelerated by medical cyclotron machines at dose rates surpassing several tens of Gy $s^{-1}$ [15, 16]. Moreover, initial experiments using synchrotron light sources yielded similar results in terms of reduced normal tissue toxicity following high-intensity x-ray irradiation [17]. Electron and x-ray FLASH technologies are reviewed in more detail in chapters 22 and 23. Today, it seems that once the temporal requirements are met, all types of radiation commonly used to treat oncology patients are suitable for FLASH-RT.

Interestingly, normal tissue preservation with high-dose-rate electron irradiation was first described in the seventies [18–20]. The potential for clinical application was not pursued because of the (wrong) assumption that tumors would be protected as well. It took more than three decades before the first *in vivo* evidence of the isoefficiency of FLASH and conventional beams in killing tumors emerged [12]. This finding marked the beginning of the FLASH-RT era.

Finally, the extremely short treatment time of FLASH-RT has the added benefit of eliminating problems related to organ or tumor motion, provided that the targeting is accurate. This is not trivial, since significant efforts have been made to resolve the organ motion problem during RT; for example, in the case of proton therapy, motion mitigation strategies are needed during pencil beam scanning delivery in order to alleviate motion-induced dose disruption [21, 22]. As such, the capability to eliminate the concerns caused by motion alone would already constitute a sufficient rationale to pursue the clinical translation of FLASH-RT.

### 4.2.1 The FLASH effect

The most appealing benefit of FLASH-RT results from the FLASH effect, which spares normal tissues while preserving tumor kill [9, 10]. As an example, well-documented tissue hallmarks of the FLASH effect in a glioblastoma-bearing mouse brain are displayed in figure 4.1. Today, the exploration of the mechanistic basis for normal tissue protection by FLASH-RT is an ongoing collective effort. While significant work remains to be done, some important biological concepts have recently emerged, such as reductions in DNA damage [23], apoptosis [12, 24], vascular damage [25], and fibrotic and inflammatory molecules [12, 24, 26, 27]. At the radiochemical level, one popular hypothesis involves the transient local oxygen depletion induced by the fast oxygen consumption by irradiation at high dose rates [28, 29], an idea that was already suggested 40 years ago [18, 20]. Nevertheless, it was challenged by recent publications showing that oxygen depletion is marginal at the doses known to trigger the FLASH effect *in vivo* and that very high doses (>80 Gy) would be required to induce oxygen depletion corresponding to only 2% of atmospheric pressure [30, 31]. Although these recent measurements refute the local depletion hypothesis, the contributions of oxygen, reactive oxygen species (ROS), and redox metabolism to the FLASH effect are still worth investigating. Oxygen supplementation reverses normal tissue sparing, while ROS production and/or mutual radical interactions seem to be altered after the exposure of pure water to FLASH-RT [27].

Apart from normal tissue sparing, no data has been generated showing that FLASH protects tumors from the sterilizing effects of radiation. Results derived

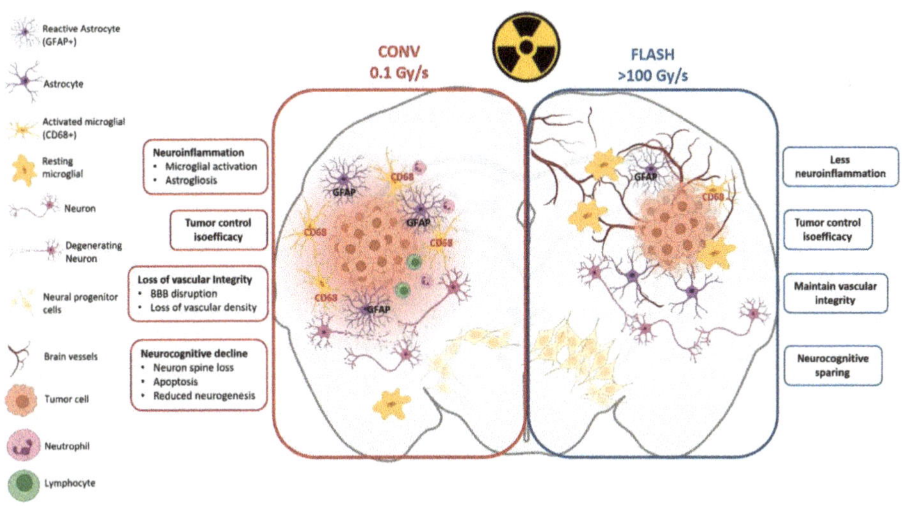


**Figure 4.1.** Hallmarks of the FLASH effect in the normal mouse brain and glioblastom multiforme (GBM) tumor. Whole-brain irradiation with a CONV beam results in the early loss of vascular integrity, followed by chronic neuroinflammation, finally leading to the loss of neurons and decreased neurogenesis. FLASH-RT does not trigger these pathogenic processes and therefore protects the brain from the cognitive disorders caused by CONV RT. Both radiation modalities are equally effective in killing of the GBM tumor cells [9] (2021), reprinted by permission of the publisher (Taylor & Francis Ltd, https://www.tandfonline.com).

from single-dose studies provide convincing evidence that in various xenografts (breast, prostate, lung, GBM) [12], orthotopic tumor (lung, GBM) models [32, 33], as well as in genetically engineered mouse models, FLASH-RT is isoefficient at delaying tumor growth compared to CONV irradiation. As fractionated RT regimens are the standard of care for the treatment of solid tumors, it was important to evaluate whether dose fractionation would alter the FLASH effect reported after single doses. To address this directly, the neuroprotective effects and antitumor efficacy of several hypofractionated regimens were investigated simultaneously. Fractionation schedules ranging from 4×3.5 Gy to 2×7 Gy and 3 ×10 Gy were found to be indistinguishable in terms of overall survival and tumor growth delay when FLASH-RT was compared to CONV irradiation at isodose [32]. Importantly, hypofractionated (>7 Gy) and single-fraction (10 Gy) FLASH regimens were still found to protect normal tissues. However, to date, no experiments have been performed to investigate the benefit of FLASH-RT using conventional fractionation (2 Gy fractions). These long-term tumor control studies will be necessary to promote the clinical implementation of FLASH-RT.

## 4.3 The physical characteristics of FLASH beams

Today, multidisciplinary teams are collaborating to explore and understand the physicochemical and biological bases of the FLASH effect. In addition, the development of a suitable technology to generate radiation beams with sufficient intensity is urgently needed. In this context, the terminology 'FLASH beam' has been a frequent overstatement for radiation beams capable of exceeding an average dose rate ($DR_{av}$) of 40 Gy $s^{-1}$ without any prior validation of the biological effect [24]. Although the temporal beam characteristics indisputably play a key role in FLASH-RT, this overly simplistic practice raises some concerns for a few reasons:

(1) It implies that $DR_{av}$ is the only critical beam parameter that determines the tissue response to FLASH-RT.
(2) It assumes a universal $DR_{av}$ threshold, regardless of any other circumstances.

The characterization of FLASH beams is actually much more complex. The $DR_{av}$ values that lead to observations of the FLASH effect are not fully delimited, since some publications have shown negative results with similar $DR_{av}$ values [34–36]. The situation is complicated further by the case of pulsed beams whose temporal structure cannot be defined solely by the $DR_{av}$, but requires the specification of parameters such as the dose per pulse ($D_p$), the pulse width ($w$), and the pulse repetition frequency (*PRF*). Other factors, such as the type of radiation beam, the size of the irradiated target, the organ/tissue exposed, and the total dose administered might all affect the optimal beam parameters for eliciting the FLASH effect. Finally, possible differences in individual sensitivity to FLASH-RT might exist at both the normal tissue and tumor levels, as recently suggested by Chabi *et al* [37].

Despite of a growing number of reports confirming the occurrence of the FLASH effect in various biological models, systematic investigations of the beam parameters required to elicit the effect have been barely performed. So far, a single dose-rate escalation study has been reported for the use of a FLASH-validated irradiator [13]. Thus, the precise FLASH beam requirements remain unknown, meaning that any beam intended for FLASH-RT should first undergo a rigorous *in vivo* validation that includes both healthy tissue and tumor responses. However, some general characteristics of FLASH beams can be deduced from the literature.

### 4.3.1 FLASH beams in preclinical studies

Preclinical research on FLASH-RT has predominantly been conducted using two types of radiation beam: (1) electron beams produced by experimental prototype or modified clinical linacs at energies of 4–20 MeV and (2) proton beams accelerated by cyclotrons to energies of 230–250 MeV. In both cases, the unique nature of the FLASH mode follows from extremely fast delivery of the dose. This is commonly expressed by $DR_{av}$ values surpassing tens of Gy $s^{-1}$, in contrast to clinical RT treatments which are rarely administered at rates of more than a few Gy $min^{-1}$. However, the inherent temporal structures of the two types of beam are substantially different, as reviewed below. Additionally, one publication reported the sparing part of the FLASH effect after high-dose-rate x-ray irradiation [17], but did not look at the tumor response. Other chapters of this book review synchrotron light sources, whose limited availabilities and expensive beam times prevent their more extensive use for FLASH-RT. A suitable source of FLASH x-ray beams is currently missing, while the new generation of brighter linacs is still under development.

Electron linac beams consist of 1–4 μs pulses separated by tens or hundreds of milliseconds (figure 4.1). In the CONV mode, they operate by delivering a large number of pulses, each carrying a small portion of the total dose ($D_p \leqslant 0.01$ Gy). The transition to the FLASH mode is made by increasing $D_p$ by at least two orders of magnitude, which drastically reduces the number of pulses required for an equivalent total dose and shortens the irradiation time. Other parameters such as $w$ and $PRF$ are sometimes scaled up as well. The $DR_{av}$ of such beams is strongly dependent on the underlying pulse structure, and the various parameters cannot be analyzed independently when considering the critical FLASH beam properties. The authors of the abovementioned dose-escalation study, Montay-Gruel *et al*, looked at the sparing of memory in mice as a function of the $DR_{av}$ of a pulsed electron beam produced by the eRT6/Oriatron linac [13]. $PRF$ and $w$ were fixed at 100 Hz and 1.8 μs, respectively, so that the value of $DR_{av}$ was raised by a gradual increase in $D_p$. The number of pulses was adjusted accordingly to deliver a dose of 10 Gy in all cases. The study reported that the threshold conditions required to evoke the FLASH effect in the mouse brain were a $DR_{av}$ of between 20–60 Gy $s^{-1}$ paired with a $D_p$ of 0.2–0.6 Gy. The magnitude of the effect varied abruptly from full memory sparing at $DR_{av}/D_p$ values larger than 100 Gy $s^{-1}$ and 1 Gy, respectively, to complete loss of sparing below a $DR_{av}$ of 20 Gy $s^{-1}$ and a $D_p$ of 0.2 Gy. Because both $DR_{av}$ and $D_p$ were altered together, it was impossible to separately evaluate their individual contributions to the observed biological outcomes. Interestingly, the

$DR_{av}$ and $D_p$ thresholds set by this work are still applicable, even if the data generated by other electron machines are taken into account. Figure 4.2 depicts all reported cases of reduced normal tissue injury with both FLASH-validated and non-validated electron beams in a parameter space spanned by $DR_{av}$ and $D_p$. Conditions under which the toxicity was equal to the CONV level are shown as well. In only one case were the protective effects of a pulsed electron beam observed with a $DR_{av}$ value of less than 100 Gy $s^{-1}$ and a $D_p$ of less than 1 Gy [20]. We recently reproduced a similar dose-rate escalation study of zebrafish (ZF) embryos using the exact same parameters and a fixed total dose of 10 Gy [9]. The embryos were irradiated at 4 h post-fertilization and the outcome was evaluated using the fish body length at five days post-irradiation. The development of the fish notably followed the same dependency on beam parameters as that observed in data from the mouse brain, showing remarkable consistency. The results of dose escalation on the mouse brain and zebrafish embryos are shown in figure 4.3. Therefore, despite major differences between the biological models (i.e. late responding organs vs acute responding systems), the following combination of parameters was found to reproducibly trigger normal tissue sparing: a *PRF* of 100 Hz, a *w* of 1.8 µs, a $DR_{av}$ of 100 Gy $s^{-1}$, a $D_p$ of 1 Gy $s^{-1}$ and a dose of 10 Gy .

Further studies are ongoing to investigate the respective relevance of, and interrelation between, these physics parameters. We should also keep in mind that correlation is not causality. However, we have already identified that the dose is the most critical parameter. In the same two models (the mouse brain and the zebrafish embryo), increasing the dose by 40% (up to 14 Gy) while keeping the other parameters the same abrogated the protective effects of FLASH irradiation. However, the fact that a dose of 10 Gy was used in both models does not imply that a dose of 10 Gy is mandatory to trigger the FLASH effect. Rather, the total dose of 10 Gy is dictated by the specific organ or system itself (i.e. the level of radiation-induced normal tissue complication measurable in the CONV regime). In the mouse brain, a whole brain irradiation (WBI) at 10 Gy is needed to obtain

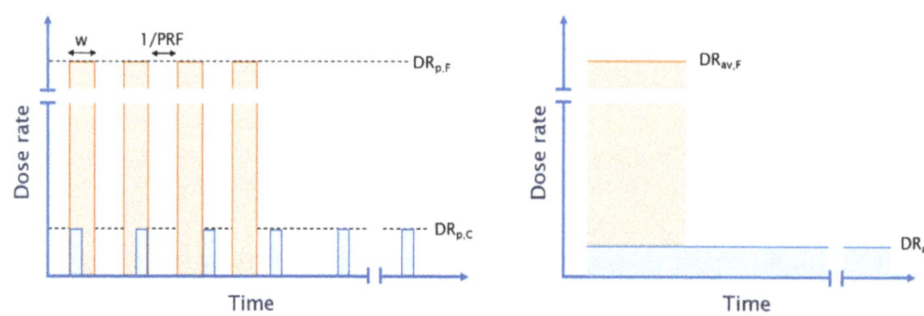


**Figure 4.2.** The temporal structures of pulsed (left) and continuous (right) FLASH (orange) and CONV (blue) beams. Here, *w* stands for the duration of the pulse (typically 1–4 µs); *PRF* stands for the number of pulses per unit time (typically 10–250); $DR_{p,F}$ and $DR_{p,C}$ stand for the doses carried in a single pulse of the FLASH and CONV beams, respectively; $DR_{av,F}$, and $D_{av,C}$ stand for the average dose rates of continuous FLASH and CONV beams, respectively.

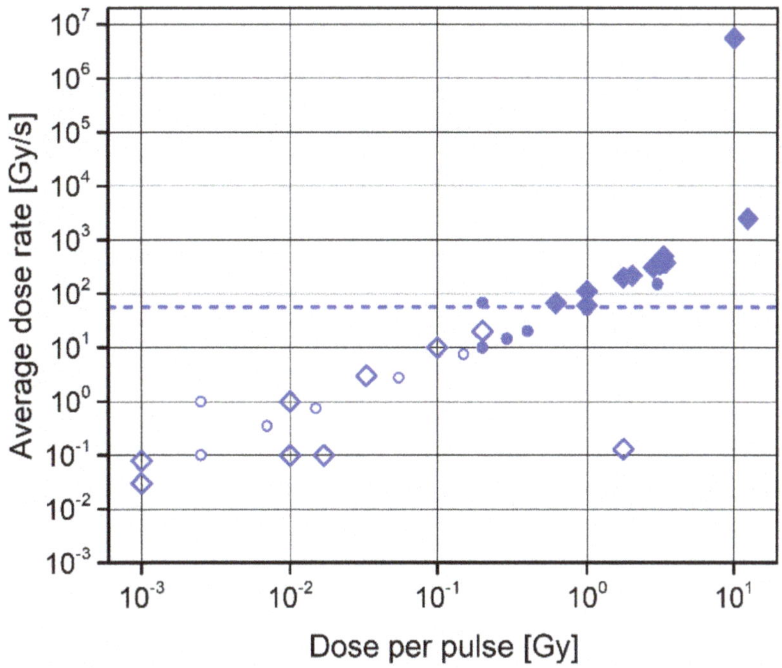


**Figure 4.3.** Combinations of $D_p$ and $D_{av}$ from different electron irradiators leading to normal tissue sparing (filled symbols) or no sparing (empty symbols) in regard to CONV radiation. Diamonds represent data generated by FLASH-validated irradiators, while circles represent data from electron irradiators that have not been validated for the full FLASH effect (normal tissues and tumors) [ref]. The intermittent line indicates the lowest reported $DR_{av}$ value that produces the FLASH effect with proton beams [38] John Wiley & Sons. © 2022 The Authors. Medical Physics published by Wiley Periodicals LLC on behalf of American Association of Physicists in Medicine.

cognitive decrements two months post-RT. In ZF (irradiated at 4 h post-fertilization), a dose of 10 Gy is needed to induce a measurable 30% decrease in fish length.

In contrast, cyclotron-generated proton beams are considered to deliver the dose continuously over time (down to the level of ns bunches generated at the RF frequency of the cyclotron). The FLASH mode is obtained by ramping up the beam current extracted from the accelerator, which effectively elevates $DR_{av}$. In the absence of a pulsed beam structure, $DR_{av}$ remains the main beam parameter determining the temporal characteristics of continuous proton beams. Unfortunately, no systematic dose-rate escalation study has been performed to date using protons. Diffenderfer *et al* observed the FLASH effect in the gut using a double scattered proton beam at 78 Gy $s^{-1}$ [15]. The same group later demonstrated the feasibility of FLASH-RT inside the spread-out Bragg peak (SOBP) region at a $DR_{av}$ of slightly more than 100 Gy $s^{-1}$ [39]. Finally, the FLASH effect was reproduced by Cunningham *et al* using a pencil beam scanning (PBS) technique at $DR_{av}$ values of 57 and 115 Gy $s^{-1}$ [16]. However, those numbers should be treated with some caution. The time for which each small part of the target volume is exposed to the beam produced by PBS is drastically shorter than the total irradiation time. This means that the actual dose rates in the target were higher than the reported overall averages. Furthermore, PBS creates an inhomogeneous dose-rate distribution over the irradiated volume as a consequence of the overlap between neighboring irradiation spots. Several attempts have been made to establish a novel FLASH-relevant metric with which to evaluate the dose-rate distributions created by PBS treatment plans without reaching a final consensus [40, 41].

Despite many positive results to date, it is important to note that some studies have reported the absence of the FLASH effect using synchrotron photon [34], proton [36], and electron [35] beams. Although performed at high $DR_{av}$, these studies might have been conducted outside the necessary beam parameters required to observe a robust FLASH effect. Together with the general complexity of defining the FLASH beam requirements, this demonstrates the necessity to carefully document and control experimental conditions (both physical and biological parameters) to enable reproducible and comparable experimental results. These will be the conditions that ultimately promote the safe and reliable transfer of FLASH-RT into the clinic.

## 4.4 The technological level of existing FLASH systems

The production of FLASH beams creates significant technical hurdles for medical accelerators initially designed to deliver more than two orders of magnitude lower beam intensities. Usually, the characteristics of such machines can be adjusted to meet the needs of preclinical FLASH studies, but they fall short for more demanding clinical requirements. The realization of FLASH radiation fields larger than several squared centimeters has proven to be particularly challenging. In addition, the existing electron FLASH devices suffer from limited beam energies, making them suitable only for superficial and intraoperative treatments.

### 4.4.1 The feasibility of performing FLASH-RT using electron linacs

Experimental electron linacs have been the true 'workhorses' of preclinical FLASH research. Prototype machines such as the Kinetron [42] and the Oriatron eRT6 [43] were specifically manufactured to generate high-intensity pulsed electron beams, whose temporal characteristics can easily reach $DR_{av}$ values of several hundreds of Gy $s^{-1}$ and $D_p$ values of more than 1 Gy. In turn, these machines have been extensively used as FLASH-RT sources in research studies and remain the most productive FLASH irradiators to date. Moreover, the quick adjustment and high variability of all beam-defining parameters makes them ideal tools with which to study the rather complex relationship between the FLASH effect and the pulsed beam structure.

As opposed to experimental devices, clinical linac systems are not intended to generate ultrafast irradiations, but still can achieve the FLASH conditions after certain modifications [44, 45]. They are primarily used to generate photon beams by stopping the electrons in the photon conversion target located inside the linac head; they also use beam shaping and monitoring equipment. Standard photon treatment plans are delivered at rates of a few Gy $min^{-1}$. Even in the flattening filter-free (FFF) configuration, the $DR_{av}$ can barely exceed 40 Gy $min^{-1}$. The situation can be

**Table 4.1.** Typical FLASH beam parameters used by electron linacs validated for the FLASH effect.

| | Kinetron | Oriatron eRT6 | Modified Clinac 21EX |
|---|---|---|---|
| Manufacturer | CGRMeV | PMB Alcen | Varian |
| Energy (MeV) | 4.5 | 4.9 | 16 |
| Pulse width (μs) | 1 | 1.8 | 5 |
| Pulse repetition frequency (Hz) | 150 | 100 | 108 |
| Dose per pulse (Gy) | 1 | 1–10 | 2 |
| Dose rate in pulse (Gy $s^{-1}$) | 1E6 | 5.6E5–5.6E6 | 4E5 |
| Average dose rate (Gy $s^{-1}$) | 60 | >100 | >180 |
| 90% Beam radius (cm) | NA | 3–9 | ~4 |

improved by roughly an order of magnitude by switching to the electron mode and avoiding the substantial beam losses caused by photon conversion. Finally, by tuning the linac control parameters and positioning the target inside or in close proximity to the linac head, it is possible to achieve beam characteristics similar to those of FLASH-validated experimental irradiators. In fact, one of the modified clinical linacs, the Varian Clinac 21EX from Stanford University, passed the *in vivo* biological FLASH validation, becoming the third electron irradiator ever (after the Kinetron and the Oriatron eRT6) to reproduce the FLASH effect [46]. A comparison of the FLASH beam parameters of all three FLASH-validated electron linacs is given in table 4.1.

A common feature of all electron linacs is proportionality between the radiation field size and the source-to-surface distance (SSD). On the other hand, due to the power limitations of RF-generating technology, large $D_\mathrm{p}$ and $DR_\mathrm{av}$ values require the target to be positioned in close proximity to the linac, i.e. at small SSDs. Therefore, the size is often traded off to obtain the required temporal beam characteristics. Another limitation of FLASH systems based on electron linacs is the low penetration of their beams in tissue. Electrons with energies of 4–20 MeV stop within the first few centimeters of tissue, making them unsuitable to reach deep-seated tumors. However, they can be still applied in intraoperative RT (IORT) settings. This opportunity was immediately recognized by the manufacturers of dedicated IORT machines. The two companies involved in IORT, IntraOp and Sordina IORT Technologies, produced special versions of their systems [47, 48]. Apart from the conventional mode, these devices have been engineered to operate in an ultrahigh-dose-rate (UHDR) mode that closely resembles the characteristics of the Oriatron eRT6 FLASH beam. The UHDR versions of these devices have successfully been commissioned, although the *in vivo* FLASH validation has not been reported yet.

### 4.4.2 The feasibility of FLASH-RT with medical proton accelerators

The three sources of energetic proton beams used by modern proton therapy centers are isochronous cyclotrons, synchrocyclotrons, and synchrotrons. Even though all of these fall into the category of circular accelerators, their working principles are quite different, which affects the temporal properties of the generated beams. The isochronous cyclotron is the most abundant of the three types of machine and the only one so far that has been confirmed to reproduce the FLASH effect. The first cyclotron-based FLASH experiments were performed with a unidirectional passively scattered proton beam using the entrance portion of the proton depth dose profile [15]. This arrangement leads to increased $DR_{av}$ by saving the time lost in energy modulation and beam scanning in standard proton RT. However, it can only be applied in the preclinical setting because of the potentially unacceptable degradation of the dose conformity as well as the restricted FLASH beam size (<10 $cm^2$). The team from the Cincinnati Children's Hospital Medical Center subsequently proved that isochronous cyclotrons are capable of supplying enough beam current to keep the $DR_{av}$ above 100 Gy $s^{-1}$ even in the case of PBS dose delivery [16]. It should be kept in mind, nevertheless, that the size of the scanned area in this research study was only 2.5 cm × 2.3 cm and required 30 individual spots. Clinical targets would necessitate coverage of an area more than an order of magnitude larger, which would prolong the irradiation time and drag down the $DR_{av}$ to less than 10 Gy $s^{-1}$. It follows that as in the case of passive scattering, PBS delivery of cyclotron-generated proton beams is well suited for experimental FLASH studies on small animal models, but falls short of the clinical requirements for larger volumes.

The applicability of synchrocyclotrons and synchrotrons as FLASH-RT sources has been discussed on several occasions. Based on purely theoretical considerations, Farr *et al* [38] and Jolly *et al* [49] concluded that given small technical adjustments, the two types of accelerator should be able to deliver FLASH-RT, at least to small target volumes of several $cm^3$. However, both reports assumed a $DR_{av}$ value of 40 Gy $s^{-1}$ over the fraction dose of 2 Gy as the specification of a FLASH beam. In fact, it is still not clear whether there is a dose threshold for the production of the FLASH effect. If such a threshold exists, then the relevance of 2 Gy fractions in producing the FLASH effect urgently needs to be investigated. A higher fraction dose would proportionally affect the presented considerations, which might have underestimated the required number of protons. In addition, synchrocyclotrons generate proton pulses of a few μs at repetition rates of around 1 kHz. As with pulsed electron beams, the FLASH beam characteristics in this case are likely to include not only $DR_{av}$ but also an inter-dependent combination of several other parameters such as $D_p$, $w$, and $PRF$.

## 4.5 The clinical implementation of FLASH-RT

In the last seven years, over 230 peer-reviewed scientific publications (based upon a simple PubMed search) have addressed various aspects of FLASH-RT. The reported DMF along with the ubiquitous nature of the FLASH effect strongly support the rationale to implement FLASH-RT in the clinic. In fact, the field is already moving in that direction, and several clinical trials in domestic animals and humans are currently in progress worldwide. However, the existing body of research was almost exclusively conducted on small targets (rodents) and in simple geometries using radiation beams that do not meet the high quality standards desired in the clinical setting (figure 4.4).

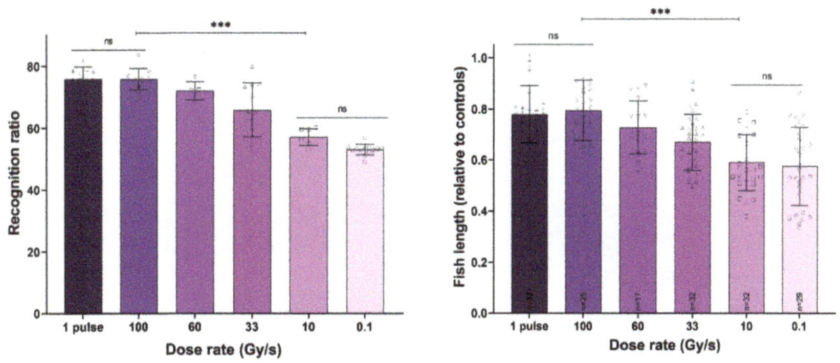


**Figure 4.4.** Dose-rate dependency of the recognition ratio (RR) obtained by novel object recognition (NOR) tests that were used to evaluate the memory in mice after 10 Gy whole-brain irradiation [13] (left). Dose-rate dependency of the length of zebrafish on day five after irradiation with a 10 Gy dose [9] (right). The length is normalized to the value of the sham irradiated controls. Both the RR score and the fish length exhibit the same dependency on dose rate, with a Pearson's correlation coefficient of 0.99 between the two datasets.

### 4.5.1 Ongoing clinical trials

Clinical trials using electron and proton FLASH beams in domestic animals are ongoing [4, 50, 51], and the first late toxicity issues are now being discovered and reported [52] while tumor response post-FLASH-RT in one of the cats treated within the phase I clinical trial at the Centre Hospitalier Universitaire Vaudois (CHUV) [14] was good and is shown in figure 4.5. The first feasibility study in a human patient with superficial cutaneous lymphoma was performed in 2019 at CHUV using an intermediate-energy electron beam produced by an eRT6/Oriatron machine [53]. In 2021, the same institution started the Impulse Trial, a phase I dose-escalation study of high-dose-rate radiotherapy with electrons in patients with skin metastases from melanoma using the Mobetron device.

In 2019, encouraged by the ability of the existing proton accelerators to deliver FLASH-RT, Varian launched the FlashForward consortium with twenty participating institutions (nearly half from the US and others from all over the world) to establish preclinical study designs, develop technical solutions, and share research protocols that will advance the translation of proton FLASH-RT into clinics. This global effort led to the first-ever clinical trial of proton FLASH-RT, started by one of the consortium members, the Cincinnati Children's Hospital. The pilot phase I study (FAST-01 trial, NCT04592887), which aimed to evaluate the feasibility and safety of proton FLASH treatment in patients with painful bone metastases of the extremities is now completed; more clinical trials are expected to be launched by this team in the near future.

### 4.5.2 What still needs to be resolved?

In order to secure the clinical transfer of FLASH-RT, the quality of preclinical FLASH beams has to be substantially improved. In particular, the following solely technological issues should be addressed:

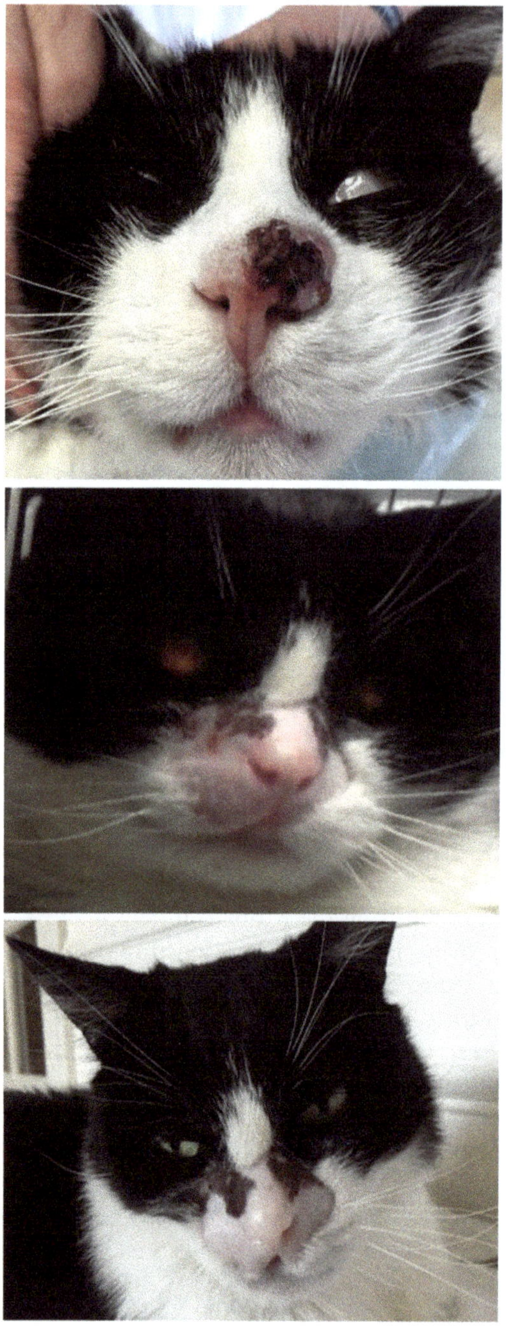

**Figure 4.5.** Tumor response on a cat patient treated with a single FLASH dose of 27 Gy (with a radiation field size of 25×34 mm$^2$). Top—before irradiation, middle—seven months post-FLASH-RT, bottom—14 months post-FLASH-RT. The cat participated in the phase I dose-escalation trial of FLASH-RT conducted at CHUV using an eRT6/Oriatron machine. Adapted from [14] with permission from the American Association for Cancer Research.

1. What are the critical FLASH beam requirements/parameters required to obtain the FLASH effect in human patients?

   More work is required to define the precise temporal beam structure needed to elicit the FLASH effect in various organs and volumes. It is noteworthy that investigating the dependency of the FLASH effect on beam parameters is time-consuming and requires a large number of animals (mice). In addition, such systematic studies are not easily approved by ethical committees in Western countries. On the other hand, the clinical transfer of FLASH-RT is currently based upon the assumption that the beam requirements applicable in small-volume murine studies will be directly transferable to humans. Apart from all biological differences, the administration of FLASH-RT in the clinic will require drastically larger radiation fields. Our data obtained using mini-pigs reveals that increasing the volume is not without consequences. In our previously published paper [14], we showed that irradiating a 2.6 cm diameter spot with a single dose of 31 Gy FLASH (10 pulses of 3.1 Gy, 1.8 μs, 100 Hz) induced no acute nor long-term damage (>3 y follow up) to the skin, whereas 31 Gy delivered at the conventional dose rate resulted in the development of a severe fibronecrosis nine months post-irradiation [14]. However, increasing the field to $8 \times 8$ cm$^2$ and performing FLASH irradiation at 31 Gy resulted in the development of telangiectasia four months post-RT in the center of the field, followed by ulceration of the epidermis and skin necrosis over the entire field of irradiation at six months post-RT. This large lesion was essentially superficial and spontaneously resolutive. It resulted in a stable fibrotic scar after 12 months (figure 4.6). We want to emphasize here that in order to irradiate an 8×8 cm$^2$ field with a flat FLASH beam, $D_p$ had to be halved and the dose of 31 Gy was delivered in 20 pulses of 1.55 Gy (1.8 μs, 100 Hz). Notably, the irradiation duration was doubled compared to that used for the field 2.6 cm in diameter (190 ms vs 90 ms). Therefore, it is possible that the beam parameters were outside the range for the optimal FLASH effect, even though a smaller $D_p$ of 1 Gy has been proven to give full FLASH protection to the memory in mice [13]. This suggests that the magnitude of the FLASH effect may be reduced by large irradiation fields or that large fields impose more restrictive FLASH beam requirements in order to maintain the tissue protection observed with smaller fields. In any case, the results obtained call for caution when applying FLASH-RT over large volumes.
2. How should FLASH-RT be delivered to larger volumes?

   Both types of preclinical FLASH irradiator, i.e. electron and proton irradiators, suffer from small radiation fields which make them unsuitable for the treatment of larger, clinically relevant volumes. A logical step to enlarge the area irradiated by proton beams is to implement PBS, which necessarily leads to prolonged irradiation times compared to the double-scattering configuration. The first results indicated that PBS is compatible with the FLASH effect if the total irradiation time is kept well under a second [16].

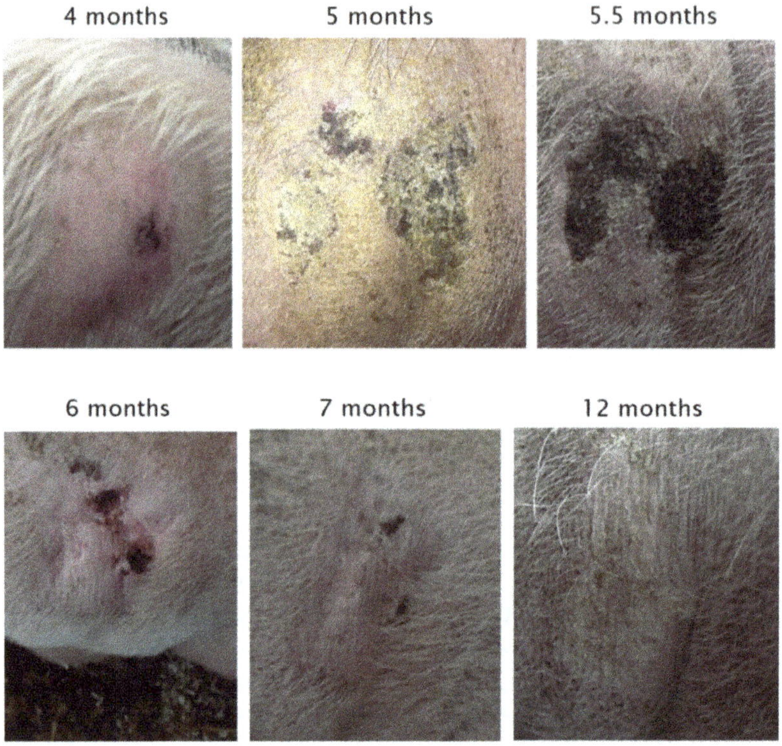


**Figure 4.6.** Evolution of a mini-pig's skin over time after large-field ($8 \times 8$ cm$^2$) FLASH irradiation at 31 Gy (20 pulses, $D_p = 1.55$ Gy, PRF = 100 Hz, $w = 1.8$ μs).

However, the number of 4 mm spots used was only 30, covering an area of less than 6 cm$^2$. Maintaining the irradiation time at the same level would be much more demanding if PBS FLASH were to be applied to targets requiring several hundreds of pencil beam spots, as is typically the case in the clinic. It remains thus unclear whether PBS is indeed a feasible delivery method for clinical proton FLASH-RT.

In addition to the radiation field size issues shared with protons, existing electron FLASH beams are limited by their shallow penetration in tissue, which makes them only suitable for the treatment of superficial lesions or intraoperative exposures. This limitation might be soon overcome by advances in high-gradient linac and laser wakefield acceleration, which have brought the idea of a compact very-high-energy electron (VHEE; > 50 MeV) machine for tumor treatment closer to realization than ever before [54]. In comparison with intermediate-energy electrons (4–20 MeV), VHEE beams provide superior depth dose profiles and deeper ranges in tissue, and are sufficient to reach targets located more than 20 cm below the surface (figure 4.7). Another advantage of VHEE is its small lateral penumbra, which is essential for conformal dose delivery. The lateral penumbras of VHEE beams that have energies above 100 MeV are comparable to, or even

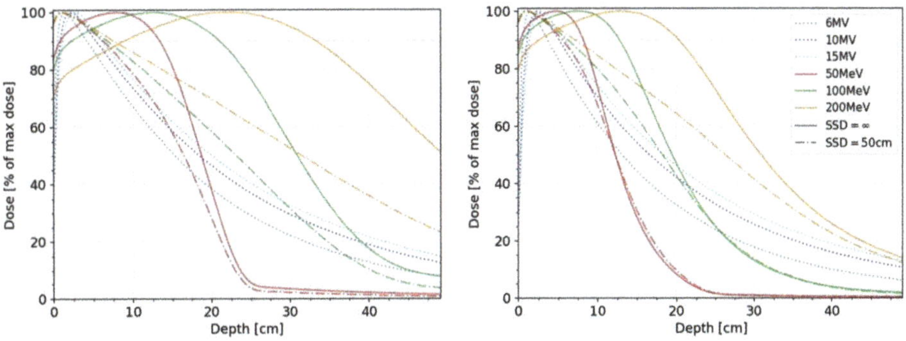


**Figure 4.7.** Comparison of the percentage depth dose (PDD) profiles of VHEE and MV photon beams for field sizes of 10 × 10 $cm^2$ (left) and 3 × 3 $cm^2$ (right). VHEE profiles are shown for energies of 50 MeV, 100 MeV, and 200 MeV with the assumption of parallel (SSD = ∞, solid lines) or divergent beams (SSD = 50 cm, dash–dotted lines). MV photon beams are shown with dotted lines [55] John Wiley & Sons. © 2021 American Association of Physicists in Medicine.

better (at smaller depths) than those of megavoltage (MV) photon beams applied in the clinic [55]. Nevertheless, VHEE technology is still developing and the capability of VHEE beams to operate at dose rates compatible with the FLASH effect needs to be further investigated [54].

3. How to monitor the doses produced by FLASH beams in real time.

   The standard practice for online dose monitoring in the clinic relies on the use of transmission ionization chambers (TICs). When exposed to pulsed (electron) FLASH beams, TICs experience significant charge recombination [56, 57] and require the introduction of saturation correction factors that greatly surpass those recommended by the IAEA International Code of Practice for the Dosimetry of External Electron Beams (IAEA TRS-398 [58]). While the lack of an appropriate dose-monitoring device presents a severe problem for the clinical implementation of FLASH-RT using electrons (and photons in the future), continuous proton FLASH beams do not experience the same problems, and the use of standard TICs remains valid in this case [15, 59]. Nevertheless, several groups are working on the optimization of TICs to overcome the saturation issues. At the same time, the application of unconventional monitoring devices, such as AC current transformers (ACCT) [60], has already been proposed; if proven beneficial, this might potentially result in the replacement or supplementation of traditional TICs.
4. How can conformity be achieved using FLASH-RT?

FLASH-RT reduces normal tissue injury and allows for dose escalation to the tumor. Still, the effect of 10%–50% reported in preclinical studies might fall short of securing an overall advantage of FLASH-RT over the standard-of-care RT if the former were to suffer from severely degraded dose conformity. In order to translate the benefits of the FLASH effect to the clinic, the treatment plans for FLASH-RT have to be of comparable quality to the CONV plans. This is very difficult to achieve with the single static field configuration used in the preclinical FLASH research. However, due to the very short irradiation time, there is no possibility to change the direction of the FLASH beam by the rotation of either the gantry or the patient. One possible solution is to use multiple beams positioned at different angles around the patient, firing either simultaneously or sequentially. An advanced concept for multidirectional FLASH beam delivery was recently proposed by the Pluridirectional High-energy Agile Scanning Electron Radiotherapy (PHASER) project [61]. Based on an array of 16 stationary linacs aligned in a conical geometry around the patient together with full-ring CT imaging, PHASER is supposed to provide near-instantaneous delivery of highly conformal image-guided radiotherapy without requiring gantry rotation. The project is still in an early developmental phase and is building a fully integrated single beamline as a stepping stone toward the full sixteen-beamline version. However, the compatibility of this or any other type of multibeam setup with the FLASH effect is yet to be investigated.

## 4.6 Conclusion

We are currently standing at a crossroads in the development of FLASH-RT. The differential FLASH response between normal tissue and tumors creates a unique opportunity for the field of radiation oncology to enhance tumor control in a safe and more efficacious manner. While precise FLASH beam requirements are still unknown, any beam intended for the clinical use of FLASH-RT should first undergo *in vivo* validation that includes both healthy tissue and tumor responses. In addition, technological rigor should be applied in terms of physical parameters, the stability and robustness of the beam, dose monitoring, and dose conformity. We have at our disposal a methodology that could significantly change oncology practice at a reasonable cost, and care should be taken to preserve this opportunity for the benefit of all cancer patients. The feasibility of using standard fractionation for FLASH-RT remains to be investigated, but it should not be overlooked that as the RT practice moves toward hypofractionated regimens to treat a variety of tumor types, the capability to escalate doses using FLASH-RT facilitates these approaches and minimizes the number of patient visits, ultimately reducing the cost of healthcare.

## References


[1] Rosenblatt E, Izewska J and anacak Y *et al* 2013 Radiotherapy capacity in European countries: an analysis of the Directory of Radiotherapy Centres (DIRAC) database *Lancet Oncol.* **14** e79–e86

[2] Lievens Y, Dunscombe P and Defourny N *et al* 2015 HERO (Health Economics in Radiation Oncology): a pan-European project on radiotherapy resources and needs *Clin. Oncol. (R. Coll. Radiol.)* **27** 115–24

[3] Lin B, Gao F and Yang Y *et al* 2021 FLASH radiotherapy: history and future *Front. Oncol.* **11** 644400

[4] Hughes J R and Parsons J L 2020 FLASH radiotherapy: current knowledge and future insights using proton-beam therapy *Int. J. Mol. Sci.* **21** 6492

[5] de Kruijff R M 2020 FLASH radiotherapy: ultra-high dose rates to spare healthy tissue *Int. J. Radiat. Biol.* **96** 419–23
[6] Marcu L G, Bezak E, Peukert D D and Wilson P 2021 Translational research in FLASH radiotherapy-from radiobiological mechanisms to *in vivo* results *Biomedicines* **9** 181
[7] Wilson J D, Hammond E M, Higgins G S and Petersson K 2020 Ultra-high dose rate (FLASH) radiotherapy: silver bullet or fool's gold *Front. Oncol.* **9** 1563
[8] Vozenin M C, Hendry J H and Limoli C L 2019 Biological benefits of ultra-high dose rate FLASH radiotherapy: sleeping beauty awoken *Clin. Oncol. (R Coll. Radiol.)* **31** 407–15
[9] Kacem H, Almeida A, Cherbuin N and Vozenin M C 2021 Understanding the FLASH effect to unravel the potential of ultra-high dose rate irradiation *Int. J. Radiat. Biol.* **98** 506–16
[10] Friedl A A, Prise K M, Butterworth K T, Montay-Gruel P and Favaudon V 2021 Radiobiology of the FLASH effect *Med. Phys.* **49** 1993–2013
[11] Ruan J L, Lee C and Wouters S *et al* 2021 Irradiation at ultra-high (FLASH) dose rates reduces acute normal tissue toxicity in the mouse gastrointestinal system *Int. J. Radiat. Oncol. Biol. Phys.* **111** 1250–61
[12] Favaudon V, Caplier L and Monceau V *et al* 2014 Ultrahigh dose-rate FLASH irradiation increases the differential response between normal and tumor tissue in mice *Sci. Transl. Med.* **6** 245ra93–245ra93 Corrected in https://doi.org/10.1126/scitranslmed.aba4525
[13] Montay-Gruel P, Petersson K and Jaccard M *et al* 2017 Irradiation in a flash: unique sparing of memory in mice after whole brain irradiation with dose rates above 100Gy/s *Radiother. Oncol.* **124** 365–9
[14] Vozenin M C, De Fornel P and Petersson K *et al* 2019 The advantage of FLASH radiotherapy confirmed in mini-pig and cat-cancer patients *Clin. Cancer Res.* **25** 35–42
[15] Diffenderfer E S, Verginadis I I and Kim M M *et al* 2020 Design, implementation, and *in vivo* validation of a novel proton FLASH radiation therapy system *Int. J. Radiat. Oncol. Biol. Phys.* **106** 440–8
[16] Cunningham S, McCauley S and Vairamani K *et al* 2021 FLASH proton pencil beam scanning irradiation minimizes radiation-induced leg contracture and skin toxicity in mice *Cancers (Basel)* **13** 1012
[17] Montay-Gruel P, Bouchet A and Jaccard M *et al* 2018 X-rays can trigger the FLASH effect: ultra-high dose-rate synchrotron light source prevents normal brain injury after whole brain irradiation in mice *Radiother. Oncol.* **129** 582–8
[18] Hornsey S and Bewley D K 1971 Hypoxia in mouse intestine induced by electron irradiation at high dose-rates *Int. J. Radiat. Biol. Relat. Stud. Phys. Chem. Med.* **19** 479–83
[19] Field S B and Bewley D K 1974 Effects of dose-rate on the radiation response of rat skin *Int. J. Radiat. Biol. Relat. Stud. Phys. Chem. Med.* **26** 259–67
[20] Hendry J H, Moore J V, Hodgson B W and Keene J P 1982 The constant low oxygen concentration in all the target cells for mouse tail radionecrosis *Radiat. Res.* **92** 172–81
[21] Gut P, Krieger M and Lomax T *et al* 2021 Combining rescanning and gating for a time-efficient treatment of mobile tumors using pencil beam scanning proton therapy *Radiother. Oncol.* **160** 82–9
[22] Krieger M, Giger A and Jud C *et al* 2021 Liver-ultrasound-guided lung tumour tracking for scanned proton therapy: a feasibility study *Phys. Med. Biol.* **66** 035011
[23] Fouillade C, Curras-Alonso S and Giuranno L *et al* 2020 FLASH irradiation spares lung progenitor cells and limits the incidence of radio-induced senescence *Clin. Cancer Res.* **26** 1497–506

[24] Simmons D A, Lartey F M and Schüler E *et al* 2019 Reduced cognitive deficits after FLASH irradiation of whole mouse brain are associated with less hippocampal dendritic spine loss and neuroinflammation *Radiother. Oncol.* **139** 4–10
[25] Allen B D, Acharya M M and Montay-Gruel P *et al* 2020 Maintenance of tight junction integrity in the absence of vascular dilation in the brain of mice exposed to ultra-high-dose-rate FLASH irradiation *Radiat. Res.* **194** 625–35
[26] Buonanno M, Grilj V and Brenner D J 2019 Biological effects in normal cells exposed to FLASH dose rate protons *Radiother. Oncol.* **139** 51–5
[27] Montay-Gruel P, Acharya M M and Petersson K *et al* 2019 Long-term neurocognitive benefits of FLASH radiotherapy driven by reduced reactive oxygen species *Proc. Natl Acad. Sci. USA* **116** 10943–51
[28] Pratx G and Kapp D S 2019 A computational model of radiolytic oxygen depletion during FLASH irradiation and its effect on the oxygen enhancement ratio *Phys. Med. Biol.* **64** 185005
[29] Petersson K, Adrian G, Butterworth K and McMahon S J 2020 A quantitative analysis of the role of oxygen tension in FLASH radiation therapy *Int. J. Radiat. Oncol. Biol. Phys.* **107** 539–47
[30] Cao X, Zhang R and Esipova T V *et al* 2021 Quantification of oxygen depletion during FLASH irradiation in vitro and *in vivo Int. J. Radiat. Oncol. Biol. Phys.* **111** 240–8
[31] Jansen J, Knoll J and Beyreuther E *et al* 2021 Does FLASH deplete oxygen? Experimental evaluation for photons, protons, and carbon ions *Med. Phys.* **48** 3982–90
[32] Montay-Gruel P, Acharya M and Jorge P G *et al* 2021 Hypofractionated FLASH-RT as an effective treatment against glioblastoma that reduces neurocognitive side effects in mice *Clin. Cancer Res.* **27** 775–84
[33] Bourhis J, Montay-Gruel P and Gonçalves Jorge P *et al* 2019 Clinical translation of FLASH radiotherapy: why and how *Radiother. Oncol.* **139** 11–7
[34] Smyth L M L, Donoghue J F and Ventura J A *et al* 2018 Comparative toxicity of synchrotron and conventional radiation therapy based on total and partial body irradiation in a murine model *Sci. Rep.* **8** 12044
[35] Venkatesulu B P, Sharma A and Pollard-Larkin J M *et al* 2019 Ultra high dose rate (35 Gy/sec) radiation does not spare the normal tissue in cardiac and splenic models of lymphopenia and gastrointestinal syndrome *Sci. Rep.* **9** 17180
[36] Beyreuther E, Brand M and Hans S *et al* 2019 Feasibility of proton FLASH effect tested by zebrafish embryo irradiation *Radiother. Oncol.* **139** 46–50
[37] Chabi S, To T H V and Leavitt R *et al* 2021 Ultra-high-dose-rate FLASH and conventional-dose-rate irradiation differentially affect human acute lymphoblastic leukemia and normal hematopoiesis *Int. J. Radiat. Oncol. Biol. Phys.* **109** 819–29
[38] Farr J, Grilj V and Malka V *et al* 2022 Ultra-high dose rate radiation production and delivery systems intended for FLASH *Med. Phys.* **49** 4875–911
[39] Kim M M, Verginadis I I and Goia D *et al* 2021 Comparison of FLASH proton entrance and the spread-out bragg peak dose regions in the sparing of mouse intestinal crypts and in a pancreatic tumor model *Cancers (Basel)* **13** 4244
[40] van de Water S, Safai S and Schippers J M *et al* 2019 Towards FLASH proton therapy: the impact of treatment planning and machine characteristics on achievable dose rates *Acta Oncol.* **58** 1463–9

[41] van Marlen P, Dahele M and Folkerts M *et al* 2020 Bringing FLASH to the clinic: treatment planning considerations for ultrahigh dose-rate proton beams *Int. J. Radiat. Oncol. Biol. Phys.* **106** 621–9
[42] Lansonneur P, Favaudon V and Heinrich S *et al* 2019 Simulation and experimental validation of a prototype electron beam linear accelerator for preclinical studies *Phys. Med.* **60** 50–7
[43] Jaccard M, Durán M T and Petersson K *et al* 2018 High dose-per-pulse electron beam dosimetry: commissioning of the Oriatron eRT6 prototype linear accelerator for preclinical use *Med. Phys.* **45** 863–74
[44] Schüler E, Trovati S and King G *et al* 2017 Experimental platform for ultra-high dose rate FLASH irradiation of small animals using a clinical linear accelerator *Int. J. Radiat. Oncol. Biol. Phys.* **97** 195–203
[45] Lempart M, Blad B and Adrian G *et al* 2019 Modifying a clinical linear accelerator for delivery of ultra-high dose rate irradiation *Radiother. Oncol.* **139** 40–5
[46] Levy K, Natarajan S and Wang J *et al* 2020 Abdominal FLASH irradiation reduces radiation-induced gastrointestinal toxicity for the treatment of ovarian cancer in mice *Sci. Rep.* **10** 21600
[47] Moeckli R, Gonçalves Jorge P and Grilj V *et al* 2021 Commissioning of an ultra-high dose rate pulsed electron beam medical LINAC for FLASH RT preclinical animal experiments and future clinical human protocols *Med. Phys.* **48** 3134–42
[48] Felici G, Barca P and Barone S *et al* 2020 Transforming an IORT linac into a FLASH research machine: procedure and dosimetric characterization *Front. Phys.* **8** 374
[49] Jolly S, Owen H, Schippers M and Welsch C 2020 Technical challenges for FLASH proton therapy *Phys. Med.* **78** 71–82
[50] Konradsson E, Arendt M L and Bastholm Jensen K *et al* 2021 Establishment and initial experience of clinical FLASH radiotherapy in canine cancer patients *Front. Oncol.* **11** 658004
[51] Velalopoulou A, Karagounis I V and Cramer G M *et al* 2021 FLASH proton radiotherapy spares normal epithelial and mesenchymal tissues while preserving sarcoma response *Cancer Res.* **81** 4808–21
[52] Rohrer Bley C, Wolf F, Gonçalves Jorge P, Grilj V, Petridis I, Petit B, Böhlen T T, Moeckli R, Limoli C, Bourhis J, Meier V and Vozenin M-C 2022 Dose- and volume-limiting late toxicity of FLASH radiotherapy in cats with squamous cell carcinoma of the nasal planum and in mini pigs *Clin. Cancer Res.* **28** 3814–23
[53] Bourhis J, Sozzi W J and Jorge P G *et al* 2019 Treatment of a first patient with FLASH-radiotherapy *Radiother. Oncol.* **139** 18–22
[54] Ronga M G, Cavallone M and Patriarca A *et al* 2021 Back to the future: very high-energy electrons (VHEEs) and their potential application in radiation therapy *Cancers (Basel)* **13** 4942
[55] Böhlen T T, Germond J F and Traneus E *et al* 2021 Characteristics of very high-energy electron beams for the irradiation of deep-seated targets *Med. Phys.* **48** 3958–67
[56] Petersson K, Jaccard M and Germond J F *et al* 2017 High dose-per-pulse electron beam dosimetry—a model to correct for the ion recombination in the advanced Markus ionization chamber *Med. Phys.* **44** 1157–67
[57] McManus M, Romano F and Lee N D *et al* 2020 The challenge of ionisation chamber dosimetry in ultra-short pulsed high dose-rate very high energy electron beams *Sci. Rep.* **10** 9089

[58] IAEA 2000 *Absorbed Dose Determination in External Beam Radiotherapy* 398 1–229 https://www.iaea.org/publications/5954/absorbed-dose-determination-in-external-beam-radiotherapy

[59] Patriarca A, Fouillade C and Auger M *et al* 2018 Experimental set-up for FLASH proton irradiation of small animals using a clinical system *Int. J. Radiat. Oncol. Biol. Phys.* **102** 619–26

[60] Oesterle R, Gonçalves Jorge P and Grilj V *et al* 2021 Implementation and validation of a beam-current transformer on a medical pulsed electron beam LINAC for FLASH-RT beam monitoring *J. Appl. Clin. Med. Phys.* **22** 165–71

[61] Maxim P G, Tantawi S G and Loo B W Jr 2019 PHASER: a platform for clinical translation of FLASH cancer radiotherapy *Radiother. Oncol.* **139** 28–33

# Chapter 5

# SFRT experience in multi-disease studies of voluminous and metastatic tumors

**Gregory S Alexander, Dan K Kunaprayoon and William F Regine**

Spatially fractionated radiotherapy (SFRT) with GRID therapy is a technique that utilizes high-dose radiation distributed in a planned heterogeneous grid-like pattern to deliver alternating areas of high doses and low doses of radiation within a target. GRID therapy has a long history of use as a modality predating the megavoltage era and has been associated with a rapid and dramatic response, resulting in a reduction in tumor size while sparing normal tissues. Substantial clinical experience with GRID radiotherapy has been reported for the palliative treatment of bulky tumors in incurable patients, and this experience has gradually expanded into the treatment of bulky, advanced but non-metastatic, potentially curable head and neck cancers, sarcomas, and other malignancies. The delivery and understanding of GRID radiotherapy continues to evolve alongside concurrent technological advances in radiation therapy delivery. Improvements in other therapies including chemotherapy, immunotherapy, and surgery as well as an understanding of the mechanisms underlying the biology of these tumors have ignited a resurgence in spatially fractionated GRID radiotherapy. This chapter explores the clinical rationale for GRID therapy and summarizes the published clinical experience in the palliation of patients with bulky disease as well as in definitive settings for large soft-tissue sarcomas or locally advanced head and neck cancers.

## 5.1 Introduction

Megavoltage GRID radiotherapy has been delivered with both palliative and curative intent. Initial clinical reports demonstrated its feasibility and safety for patients who were already heavily pretreated with conventional radiotherapy and multiple other treatment modalities in cases of refractory disease. This experience was largely accumulated in the palliative setting with mixed tumor types, histologies, and disease sites [1–4]. After the initial observations of unexpectedly high response

doi:10.1088/978-0-7503-4046-5ch5

rates with low rates of toxicity, this foundational experience has more recently also been applied to patients with bulky poor-prognosis *primary* tumors that are non-metastatic and therefore potentially curable. The expansion of GRID therapy into the domain of advanced primary tumors has included head and neck cancer and sarcoma in particular, though the use of SFRT continues to expand into other tumor sites. The treatment of both large metastases and bulky, locally advanced primary tumors stands to benefit from the collective experience that has been generated by the early palliative GRID therapy studies.

Improvements in systemic therapy and advanced surgical techniques have greatly extended survival in patients with historically poor prognoses, which can alter the optimal radiotherapy approach. With improved survival, the need for effective palliation becomes more critical. The treatment of refractory, progressive, and symptomatic tumor growth in patients with otherwise responding or controlled disease continues to be frequently hampered by the dose limits of prior radiation and/or patients' inability to tolerate further systemic therapy. The GRID therapy summarized in this chapter provides the historical context and encouraging clinical experiences for SFRT in both palliative and definitive settings.

## 5.2 Palliative treatment with GRID radiotherapy

While radiotherapy is often used definitively to treat patients with curative intent, palliative treatment is one of the most common indications for radiation. Metastatic or recurrent cancer can cause pain, bleeding, malodor, hemoptysis, dyspnea, dysphagia, edema, bronchial or intestinal obstruction, or other symptoms that may be related to the tumor's mass effect. These symptoms may pose extraordinary challenges for clinicians trying to manage them and they may also greatly diminish the patient's quality of life.

Historically, delivering tumoricidal doses to tumors without unacceptable normal tissue damage was technologically challenging due to the limitations of low-energy, poorly penetrating orthovoltage beams; this led to the rise of SFRT techniques over 100 years ago. The recognition that small areas of normal tissues could tolerate high doses of radiotherapy spawned the development of the first GRID device to overcome this challenge [5]. GRID therapy could deliver high tumoricidal doses with orthovoltage radiotherapy to achieve rapid palliation while maintaining a much improved toxicity profile. This initial SFRT approach was largely abandoned following the rise of cobalt units in the 1950s and subsequent megavoltage technology, whose beam properties allowed for better skin and normal sparing and thereby enabled tolerable dose escalation; however, despite vast improvements in the delivery of radiation therapy, delivering an effective dose of radiotherapy to large, bulky, and recurrent tumors without violating accepted radiation tolerances remains challenging.

As a result of the longer survival achieved through advancements in surgical techniques and systemic therapies, the modern high-energy linac era has faced a renewed and at times more complex challenge of reducing normal tissue dose, particularly in advanced, radioresistant, refractory, and recurrent tumors that occur in patient populations that are now experiencing improved survival due to improvements in systemic therapy.

These renewed challenges fueled the technical development of megavoltage GRID therapy (as described in more detail in chapter 9) in the 1980s, which used similar principles to those that allowed SFRT to provide more successful treatment delivery 100 years earlier. The first clinical application of GRID therapy was in the palliation of patients with refractory large-volume tumors, and the fundamental principles learned from this experience remain highly relevant for SFRT's subsequent expansion into the treatment of advanced primary tumors along with its technological advances.

The first megavoltage GRID device was developed by designing a Cerrobend block that contained 0.8 mm wide holes arranged in a lattice pattern and following the beam divergence; this was fitted into the alloy tray of a linear accelerator (as described in more detail in chapter 9). This GRID configuration resulted in a field that was 50% open and 50% blocked. The initial clinical experience with the megavoltage GRID was obtained with patients who had undergone extensive pretreatment (six of whom had already received external beam radiotherapy doses in excess of 50 Gy). Mohuiddin *et al* [1] reported this pilot study of 22 patients with mixed histology who underwent palliative GRID therapy at Thomas Jefferson University at a dose of 10–15 Gy in a single fraction. The results were impressive—20 of 22 patients (91%) achieved successful palliation despite the large volumes of their tumors, whose sizes ranged from 6 cm to 25 cm. Based on a follow-up time of 1–18 months, acute toxicities were limited to nausea and diarrhea in two patients treated for liver disease and skin erythema which was transient and self-resolved. Only one late toxicity occurred in a patient who developed a small bowel obstruction requiring surgery for lysis of adhesions. This toxicity occurred in the setting of cumulative radiotherapy doses in excess of 70 Gy. The major studies of GRID radiation therapy for palliative treatment are summarized in table 5.1.

Based on this encouraging experience, Mohiuddin *et al* published a report of an independent cohort of 61 patients with 72 tumor sites treated in the early 1990s at the University of Kentucky [4]. Patients were treated with GRID therapy at a dose of 10–25 Gy (median: 15 Gy) in one fraction administered to primarily large, soft-tissue masses. The disease primary sites included gastrointestinal tumors (30%), sarcomas (20%), gynecological tumors (15%), genitourinary tumors (15%), melanomas (8%), and head and neck tumors (5%). Of all tumors, 64% were located in the abdomen or pelvis, and 24% had received prior radiation (at doses of 12.6–79 Gy). Follow-up ranged between two and 28 months. The symptomatic response rates were high (91%) and toxicity was minimal, validating the initial results of the Thomas Jefferson University pilot study.

A third cohort of 71 patients treated by the same group from 1995 to 1998 [2] further validated the prior results. In this series, 87 sites of bulky tumors measuring >8 cm were treated with the same Cerrobend-based GRID technique. GRID doses ranged from 10 to 20 Gy (median: 15 Gy) in one fraction, and two thirds of patients also received conventional external beam radiation therapy (cERT). Symptomatic responses were again impressive and without appreciable increases in toxicity.

**Table 5.1.** Clinical reports of patients' palliative treatment with GRID therapy.

| Authors | Patient numbers | Follow-up, median (range) (mo.) | GRID dose | Partial response | Complete response rate | Overall response rate | Significant complications |
|---|---|---|---|---|---|---|---|
| Mohiuddin *et al* [1] | 22 | 1–18 | 10–15 Gy | 12/22 (54%) | 23% (5/22) | 91% (20/22) | One small bowel obstruction requiring surgical intervention |
| Mohiuddin *et al* [4] | 61 (72 sites)* | 1–18 | 10–20 Gy | 64% (41/64) | 27% (17/64) | 91% (58/64) | No grade 2 or greater acute morbidity |
| Mohiuddin *et al* [2]** | 71 patients (87 sites)** | 7 (3–42) | 10–20 Gy | 58.5% (pain) | 20% (pain) | 78% (pain) | No grade 3 or higher late toxicities |
| Neuner *et al* [3]** | 79** | 2 (0–51.6) | 10–20 Gy (median 15 Gy) | 47.5% (pain) | 27.5% (pain) | 75% (pain) | Eight cases of acute grade 3–4 dermatitis; one acute grade 3–4 fatigue; Three late cases of grade 3–4 dermatitis |
| Kudrimoti *et al* [6]† | 19 | n/r | 12–20 Gy | 9/19 (47%)$ | 36% (7/19)¥ | 80% (local control rate); >50% reduction in pain (assessment within 48 h of treatment) | No late grade 3–4 toxicities |

*Notes*: CR = complete response; n/r = not reported; PR = partial response.
* 64 of which were evaluable.
** Included patients treated with curative intent; also included conventional external beam radiation therapy (cERT). †Abstract only.
$ PR and local control.
¥ CR and local control.

The patient cohort had a variety of symptoms. For pain, the response rate was 78%, and almost 20% achieved complete remission of pain. Improvement of bleeding occurred in all patients, 50% of whom had complete resolution. Similarly, for those treated for dyspnea, 40% had complete resolution. No grade 3 late toxicities were observed in this cohort, despite high cumulative doses. These results suggest that combining SFRT with conventionally fractionated radiotherapy in patients with bulky tumors is feasible and effective in a patient cohort for whom standard external beam radiotherapy would likely have suboptimal results.

This study also set the pace for an expansion of SFRT from the palliative domain to the definitive treatment of bulky advanced primary tumors. Among the cohort, eight patients with locally advanced non-metastatic tumors in the head and neck region were treated *definitively* with GRID, followed by cERT with doses ranging from 50 to 70 Gy. All patients responded to the radiation treatment; five of them (62.5%) achieved a clinical complete response. Radiation therapy was followed by surgical resection in four of the eight patients, all of whom had a pathologic complete response (pCR). One acute grade 3 mucositis (without significant late effect) was observed, and one grade 5 complication (carotid blowout after rapid tumor lysis). These results suggested that GRID could be used in the definitive setting, particularly for head and neck cancers.

While these results are impressive, they were obtained using a physical Cerrobend GRID which has to be manually loaded into the machine, and many departments do not have access to this technology. GRID can also be delivered by multileaf collimator (MLC), which can improve convenience and access. Neuner *et al* [3] reported their comparative experience with both Cerrobend and MLC-based SFRT approaches at the University of Maryland. Between 2003 and late 2005, 39 patients were treated with a GRID dose of 10–20 Gy (median 15 Gy) in one fraction, using a Cerrobend GRID block; the institution then transitioned to an MLC-based GRID delivery system which was used to treat 40 patients between late 2005 and 2008. The GRID fraction was followed by a cERT dose in the range of >35–40 Gy in 80% of patients.

This cohort included both patients receiving palliative-intent treatment for symptomatic relief and those receiving curative-intent treatment (23%). The subset of 18 definitively treated patients largely consisted of patients with advanced bulky head and neck and lung cancers, for whom a GRID dose of 15 Gy was followed after a one- or two-day break by cERT at definitive doses (for example, 70.2 Gy for head and neck cancer) and definitive chemotherapy as indicated.

For those receiving SFRT for palliation, the response rates were again favorable. There were no statistically significant differences in pain response, with 75% pain response among patients treated with the Cerrobend block, and 74% in those treated with an MLC-based technique. Response outcomes were similar for mass effects (67% and 73%, respectively), and variable for bleeding (50% and 80%, respectively).

In addition to establishing the efficacy of an MLC-based GRID technique, Neuner *et al*'s study is important because it is one of the largest clinical reports of GRID radiotherapy. Toxicities were acceptable for the entire cohort, as the vast majority of patients experienced only grade 1–2 toxicities, although there were three patients who developed late grade 3 skin toxicities. All of these patients had initial skin involvement of their tumor and were treated to high doses of external beam radiotherapy following their GRID treatment. While they had favorable clinical responses, they also had persistent skin ulceration, suggesting a need for caution in dosimetric planning with respect to minimizing skin toxicity in SFRT.

*Summary.* Over the course of these four studies, which spanned three institutions, important dose response relationships were established and the approach to the combination of SFRT with cERT and the management of the normal tissue dose were refined. While the patient cohorts were heterogeneous, these studies established SFRT with GRID therapy as a modality that can rapidly palliate symptoms with minimal toxicity in challenging and refractory tumors for patients with short expected survival times. This strategy can expeditiously provide at least short-term symptomatic relief while minimizing the number of fractions and thereby reducing the economic burden and the time spent in therapy and transportation for a patient population with short survival times. In those with longer expected survival times, SFRT combined with cERT can lead to durable symptom control and objective tumor responses.

These studies demonstrate a gradual expansion of SFRT beyond the palliative domain towards an exploration of definitive treatment by generating early experience in patients with voluminous advanced primary tumors that are potentially curable. This paved the way for more detailed study of SFRT in specific disease sites using a curative approach that included GRID therapy and subsequent forms of SFRT.

Reports in other more disease-specific palliative GRID therapy studies have also shown promising results. Kudrimoti *et al* [6] reported a small experience of 19 patients with 20 recurrent bulky >8 cm melanomas measured after prior failed chemo- or immunotherapy. Patients were treated with GRID radiotherapy, and ten patients also received cERT to doses in excess of 40 Gy. Ten of the 19 patients experienced rapid relief, reporting a subjective reduction in pain within 48 h of receiving GRID therapy. Ten patients survived for more than a year, and six patients had survived for two years at the time of the study's last follow-up. There were no reports of unacceptable or unanticipated toxicity, and no grade 3 or 4 long-term toxicities were seen. In addition to this series, there are dramatic case reports in the literature demonstrating clinical responses beyond what would be expected with standard fractionated radiotherapy [6].

While it may be difficult to conduct randomized trials in this patient population, given the poor prognosis of most patients with bulky metastatic disease, growing clinical experience suggests that large randomized trials are needed to rigorously study SFRT in larger comparative cohorts.

## 5.3 Transition to the definitive treatment of primary tumors

The favorable responses to GRID therapy in palliation have spawned an extension and exploration of SFRT beyond the palliative domain into the treatment of advanced but non-metastatic primary tumors. These tumors currently present a continuous and significant challenge in terms of local control and metastatic failure. The next two sections of this chapter provide examples that illustrate this transition and the outcomes obtained using GRID therapy in definitive treatment regimens. A comprehensive and detailed review of GRID therapy for the definitive treatment of the non-metastatic tumors studied to date is provided in chapter 6.

### 5.3.1 Head and neck cancer

Palliative GRID therapy series have long included selected patients with very advanced primary tumors [3], and the experience derived from these SFRT series on local control and toxicity outcomes has informed the transition from the palliative to the definitive domain. Advanced head and neck cancer is such an example and has been among the first primary tumor types to be treated with SFRT.

Despite the recent trend toward dose de-escalation with the rise of human papillomavirus (HPV)-associated oropharyngeal cancer and its higher cure rates, patients with large and bulky tumors of the head and neck still present a difficult challenge regardless of HPV status. Many studies have demonstrated that increasing size and bulk are associated with inferior outcomes in head and neck cancer [7–9]. In one single-institution retrospective cohort, tumor volume was the best predictor of overall survival and progression-free survival, even when compared to T and N staging. For primary tumor volumes measuring >35 cc, progression-free survival at five years was 33% versus 61% for lower-volume tumors [7]. Given the historically worse outcomes for those with bulky disease, treatment intensification with SFRT is an attractive option, although published clinical experience is still limited.

A number of small case series have reported outcomes for patients who were treated with GRID radiotherapy for cancers of the head and neck (table 5.2) with promising results compared to those achieved via historic controls. While these series all appear favorable when compared to historic results, prospective randomized clinical trials are needed to validate and quantify the benefits of SFRT. Figure 5.1 illustrates a GRID treatment plan for bulky lymph node involvement in head and neck cancer.

Huhn *et al* [10] reported their experience with the first such series (table 5.2). They applied GRID in 27 cases of non-metastatic stage IV head and neck primaries in which GRID (prescribed at $D_{max}$ and off-cord) was directed to bulky lymph node disease. The combination of conventional full-dose external radiation with GRID—as distinct from the more variable palliative approach—is a hallmark of SFRT in the treatment of potentially curative patients. This was illustrated in Huhn *et al*'s series. Following GRID therapy, patients were treated with cERT via a variety of schemes (most with conventional fractionation, six with hyperfractionation and one with accelerated hyperfractionation/concomitant boost), and seven received concurrent chemotherapy. The GRID dose was 15 Gy in one fraction, except for one patient who received 20 Gy.

This early series was remarkable, as it explored both definitive and preoperative combined GRID and cERT regimens. Half of the cohort (13 patients) had a planned neck dissection following completion of cERT. Impressively, the pCR was 85%,

**Table 5.2.** Clinical reports of squamous cell carcinoma (SCC) of the head and neck treated with GRID therapy.

| Authors | Number of patients | Follow-up, median (range) (mo.) | GRID dose | GRID target | Control rate | Significant complications |
|---|---|---|---|---|---|---|
| Huhn *et al* [10] | 27 | 10 (3–44) | 15 Gy* | LN | 93% | Acute grade 2–3 skin toxicity, ten cases of late grade 2 soft-tissue and muscle fibrosis, three cases of poor post-operative wound healing, four cases of fibrosis that limited neck movement |
| Penagaricano *et al* [11] | 14 | 19.5 (2–38) | 20 Gy | P (6), LN (8) | 79% | Eleven acute grade 2–3 skin reactions, 13 acute grade 2–3 mucosal reactions, four late cases of grade 2–3 skin fibrosis; **one grade 5 carotid blowout** |
| Edwards *et al* [12]† | 53 | mean 34 (1–239) | 15 Gy | P or LN | 81% | Two late toxicities requiring feeding tubes |
| Choi *et al* [13] | 21 (9 definitive) | Definitive: 7 (4–16) Palliative: 2 (0.5–9) | 15–20 Gy | n/r | Definitive: CR 4.4%(4/9) Palliative:response 54%(6/11) | Five grade 3 or 4 skin toxicities, no grade 3 or higher mucous membrane toxicity, late toxicities not reported |

*Notes*: LN = lymph node; P = primary; n/r = not reported. †Abstract only.
*One patient treated to 20 Gy.

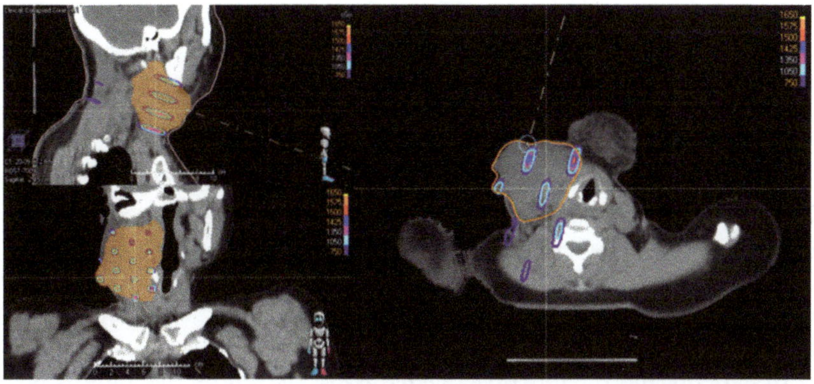

**Figure 5.1.** GRID treatment plan for a patient with bulky right-side cervical adenopathy from head and neck cancer. Dosimetry is shown for a GRID therapy plan in a 58 year old male with massive right neck lymph node involvement from oral cavity squamous cell carcinoma. The GRID prescription dose is 15 Gy in one fraction. The heterogeneity dose pattern is distributed regularly within the tumor's gross tumor volume (GTV) (orange color wash) and along the beam path, which excludes the spinal cord and the aerodigestive tract. Steep dose gradients can be seen between the prescription dose (red isodose line), the dose gradient (dark blue through aqua isodose lines) and the low-dose remainder of the GTV.

much higher than the reported historical pCR rates of approximately 40% [14]. Of note, however, significant wound healing complications were reported in three cases. The other half (14 patients) had definitive cERT following the GRID fraction. Results were also impressive: neck control was achieved in 93% of patients and the disease-specific survival was 50%, which compare favorably to historic controls. Acute and late toxicities were limited to grade 2–3 for patients undergoing radiotherapy alone. For patients undergoing surgery, there was no acute grade 5 toxicity nor late grade 4–5 toxicity.

These results were confirmed by Penagaricano *et al* [11] who reported 14 head and neck cancer patients with bulky neck nodes or bulky (⩾6 cm) primaries. In an overall more intensified regimen, a higher GRID dose of 20 Gy in one fraction was directed at bulky neck nodes or the bulky primary, followed by intensity-modulated radiation therapy (IMRT) with curative intent. Concurrent chemotherapy was given; and this was also the only study that administered concurrent chemotherapy on the same day as the GRID fraction. Penagaricano *et al*'s [11] study marks a transition in the definition of gross tumor volume (GTV) for SFRT. The GTV was defined as the gross nodal or primary tumor mass without any CTV expansion. Further, Penagaricano *et al*'s study expanded GRID therapy to include the primary tumor. In their cohort of 14 patients, six received GRID at their primary disease site, whereas in Huhn *et al*'s initial experience, GRID therapy was limited to nodal involvement. Ten of Penagaricano *et al*'s patients went on to receive a planned neck dissection. The impressive 80% (8/10) pCR rate mirrored and confirmed Huhn *et al*'s earlier results. Of note, there was one grade 5 toxicity from carotid blowout [11].

Choi *et al* [13] published another small, single-institution series of 21 patients, nine of whom had definitive treatment with curative intent. GRID therapy (most commonly 15 Gy in one fraction) was combined with definitive IMRT. For the nine patients with definitive treatment, the complete clinical response was 44%, accompanied by acceptable rates of toxicity. The follow-up time, however, was very suboptimal, as the median follow-up was only seven months in surviving patients, which limited the interpretation of the findings.

Edwards *et al* [12] reported their GRID experience in abstract form. Patients with stage T4 or N3 non-metastatic head and neck cancer with a large primary tumor or lymph node measuring >6 cm received GRID therapy in a single fraction of 15 Gy followed by definitive cERT. The three-year local regional failure rate was 19%, and the five-year overall survival rate was 23%, with only 9% developing distant metastases. While these results must be interpreted with caution given the small number of patients and the retrospective nature of the study, the authors postulated that the lower-than-expected rate of distant metastases could be related to a GRID abscopal effect on micrometastases [6].

Despite the fact that the dose administered by spatially fractionated radiotherapy is inhomogeneous, tumor regression is generally uniform after GRID. Several studies have demonstrated the ability of spatially fractionated radiotherapy to induce systemic effects such as increased levels of tumor necrosis factor alpha as well as decreased levels of TGF beta 1 [15]. Determination of whether or not these changes can result in improved oncologic outcomes would require prospective evaluation in a randomized clinical trial.

As the clinical benefit of spatially fractionated radiotherapy has yet to be demonstrated in randomized trials, and while dosimetry and planning standards and optimal dosing and delivery of SFRT are still evolving, careful GRID therapy planning and close monitoring during radiotherapy are important to avoid excess toxicity in a definitively treated population with potential long-term survival.

### *5.3.2 Sarcoma*

Sarcomas represent another major disease entity in the transition from palliative to definitive GRID therapy. Sarcomas comprise a rare and highly diverse group of tumors arising from cells of mesenchymal origin with a myriad of molecular and histological subtypes [16].

Despite the improvement in limb preservation [17] achieved through the use of preoperative radiation therapy, bulky (>8 cm) sarcomas continue to pose a major challenge for both local control and survival. In such cases, pCR rates, a major predictor of overall survival based on RTOG 0630 and RTOG 9514 [18], are suboptimal and survival is poor [19]. As sarcomas are a relatively rare disease site, trial accrual is difficult; thus, some have suggested utilizing the pCR rate as a surrogate for patient outcomes [18].

In addition, sarcoma is considered to be a relatively radioresistant tumor for which both local control and distant metastases present common challenges. Therefore, GRID radiotherapy is considered a promising modality to augment existing treatment paradigms.

The initial work in sarcoma (published largely in abstract form) applied both radiation alone and preoperative radiation with concurrent chemotherapy in patients with voluminous bulky soft-tissue sarcomas (table 5.3) [20, 21]. An example of a GRID treatment plan in an extremity sarcoma is shown in figure 5.2. The initial series documented by Mohiuddin *et al* [20] included 33 patients with recurrent and/or unresectable soft-tissue sarcomas (44 lesions) treated with GRID doses of 12–20 Gy. These were prescribed at $D_{\max}$, and the majority were combined with cERT. The response rate was high (76%), and the results demonstrated that cERT was needed after GRID therapy to improve response. The toxicity was acceptable. Mohiuddin *et al*'s subsequent study of 14 patients combined GRID therapy of 18 Gy in one fraction followed by 50 Gy cERT with concurrent ifosfamide in a preoperative regimen. Among the 14 patients, 13 underwent successful limb salvage surgery. Twelve of the 13 had negative margins, and 78% had >80% tumor necrosis, which are both of paramount prognostic importance in sarcoma. In addition to the high response rates frequently observed in these small case series, dramatic tumor regression with GRID therapy has been demonstrated in a case report [22], which is further illustrated in figure 5.3.

In both series, the preoperative approach of GRID therapy combined with the standard dose of preoperative cERT was introduced for another definitively treated tumor, and an initial understanding of the effect of this regimen on the important prognostic parameters of tumor necrosis and margin status in sarcoma was gained.

These early results in sarcoma were recently confirmed independently. In 2020 Snider *et al* [23] published a retrospective analysis of 26 patients with bulky (>8 cm) sarcomas, largely soft-tissue sarcomas with a variety of histologies, but also including four osteosarcomas and one chondrosarcoma (table 5.3). A GRID dose of 15 Gy in one fraction was followed by 45–50.4 Gy in cERT prior to surgery. With a pCR threshold of 80%, they demonstrated an impressive 35.3% pCR rate, despite the unusually high median tumor size of 14.2 cm. Despite a major wound healing complication rate of 34.6%, or nine out of 26 patients (defined per the NCIC definition as needing secondary operations for wound treatment, hospital readmission for wound care, invasive procedures for wound care, prolonged dressing changes, repeat surgery, or prolonged care for a skin graft), the complication rate was similar to that of the original NCIC sarcoma trial [24], which included patients who had substantially lower tumor sizes (<10 cm in two thirds of the patients).

In aggregate, the preceding studies have evaluated SFRT in both the definitive and preoperative settings in two curatively treated tumor types. As in the studies of head and neck cancer, the studies of sarcoma further suggest that SFRT-based dose escalation can improve the necrosis rate (when compared to historic controls), the important predictor of survival in sarcomas, and can result in high resectability with negative margins. Larger prospective clinical trials are required to verify these findings and elucidate their relevance to longer-term clinical endpoints, including local control and overall survival.

## 5.4 Knowledge gaps and future perspectives

An increased understanding of the biological mechanisms underlying GRID radiation therapy has fueled continued interest in this modality. GRID radiation therapy has been shown *in vitro* and *in vivo* to be associated with the bystander

**Table 5.3.** Clinical reports of sarcoma treated with GRID therapy.

| Authors | Patient population | Follow-up (mo.) | Size | GRID dose | pCR rate* | Control rate | Significant toxicities |
|---|---|---|---|---|---|---|---|
| Mohiuddin *et al* [20]† | 33 recurrent/ unresectable disease (44 sites) | n/r Survival: median 9 (range: 2–44) | Median 13 cm (6–32 cm) | 15 Gy median (range: 10–20 Gy) | n/r | Response rate 76% | Two grade 3 skin reactions |
| Mohuiddin *et al* [21]† | 14 neoadjuvant radiotherapy | Median 14 (range: 3–43) | Median 11.5 cm (8–26 cm) | 18 Gy** | 84.6% | Local control 100% | One grade 3 skin reaction; two patients had delayed wound healing; one patient underwent an amputation of the foot mid treatment |
| Snider *et al* [23] | 26 neoadjuvant radiotherapy | Median 25 (range n/r) | Median 14.2 cm (range: 8.8–40 cm) | 15 Gy | 35.3% | Local control 84.6% | 34.6% major wound healing complications |

*Notes*: n/r = not reported; pCR = pathologic complete response rate.
† Abstract only.
* Defined as >80% necrosis.
** Concurrent ifosfamide and mesna during standard external beam fractionated radiotherapy.

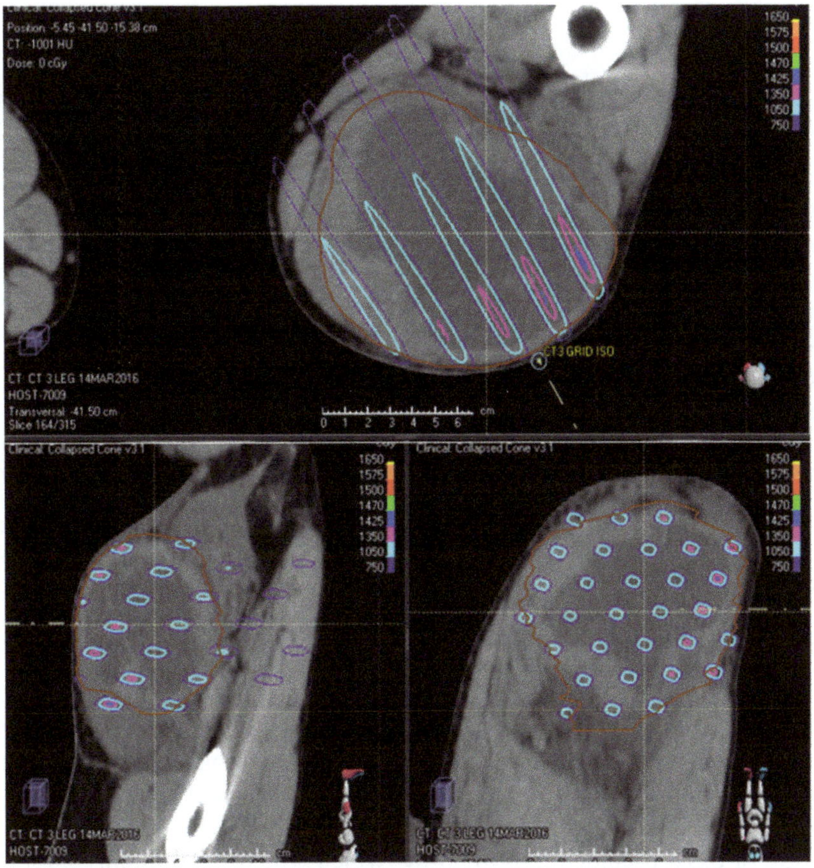


**Figure 5.2.** GRID treatment plan for a bulky lower extremity sarcoma. Dosimetry of GRID therapy in a large bulky soft-tissue high-grade pleomorphic sarcoma of the thigh is shown in a 51-year-old male. Simulation CT shows the bulky centrally necrotic tumor mass. The GRID prescription dose is 15 Gy in one fraction. The heterogeneous dose pattern is shown within the GTV (brown contour). The beam path traverses muscle but excludes bone.

effect, vascular damage, and the abscopal effect, as laid out in more detail in chapters 2 and 3. Cumulatively, these associations support an effect for GRID radiotherapy greater than the expected response under the conventional model of radiotherapy. In particular, the interplay between GRID radiotherapy and the immune system provides an opportunity to combine the modalities of SFRT and immunotherapy. This combination using checkpoint inhibitors against PD1 and CTLA-4 has been postulated and studied in mouse models and has shown evidence of an abscopal immune response, suggesting a role for GRID radiotherapy in instigating immune responses outside the irradiated target [25]. Clinically, the first case report suggested that SFRT combined with anti-PD1 immunotherapy can elicit complete local regression without side effects in a patient with non-small cell lung cancer with multiple metastases [26].

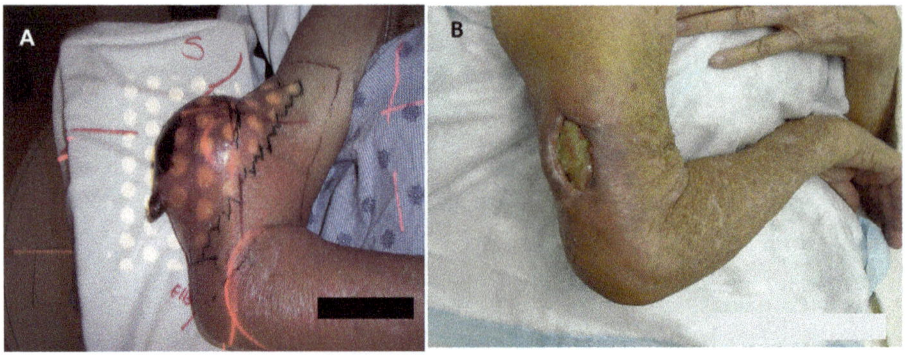


**Figure 5.3.** Clinical response of an upper extremity sarcoma before and after GRID therapy. This case illustrates high response to GRID therapy in a bulky extremity sarcoma with high-grade spindle cell histology in an 82-year-old female reported by Kaiser *et al* [22]. The tumor progressed rapidly with fast growth during conventionally fractionated radiation therapy (cERT) and developed finger-like tumor projections breaking through the skin (at a cERT dose of 10 Gy in five fractions). (A) The massive tumor is seen distorting the right upper extremity prior to GRID therapy. (B) Six weeks after a GRID dose of 18 Gy in one fraction, followed by additional 11 fractions of cERT (total cERT dose: 32 Gy in 16 fractions), drastic volume reduction is seen with only a tissue defect remaining. The patient underwent resection. Pathology showed a 99% necrosis rate. She experienced no wound complications [22] (2012) (Copyright © 2012, Springer-Verlag). With permission of Springer.

GRID radiotherapy intentionally prescribes heterogeneous doses of radiotherapy based on a preset pattern, but bulky tumors are also heterogeneously oxygenated as a result of irregular growth, irregular blood supply, and local demand for nutrients. Hypoxic areas within tumors are more radioresistant. This notion leads to the suggestion of oxygen-guided radiotherapy, which would differentially target radiation toward the hypoxic areas [27]. This concept coincides with GRID radiotherapy in that this need not take place in a preset fashion, but would instead be adapted to areas of hypoxia. As in the case of GRID radiotherapy, this would offer the ability to escalate treatment with high doses of radiotherapy heterogeneously distributed to areas of hypoxia to enhance hypoxic tumor cell kill while avoiding normal tissue complications, ultimately increasing the therapeutic ratio.

Moreover, it is unknown to what degree the oxygenation profiles of tumors change with radiotherapy and how this might be used as an advantage to overcome radioresistant hypoxic cells. Advanced imaging may provide an insight in this regard. Magnetic resonance (MR) sequences can serve as surrogates for oxygenation, including dynamic contrast-enhanced sequences that can identify areas of tumor with inadequate blood flow and perfusion, which have been shown to correlate with experimental hypoxia [28]. Diffusion-weighted imaging which utilizes water movement depends on the density of tumor cells; areas of lower cell density may be due to relative hypoxia. Blood oxygen-level-dependent (BOLD) MRI and tissue oxygen-level-dependent (TOLD) MRI also correlate with tumor pO2. Other methods are also being developed to map oxygenation, including electron paramagnetic resonance, which is being studied in pre-clinical models, and positron emission tomography (PET)-based hypoxia tracers such as 18F-fluoromisonidazole, 18F-flortanidazole, and 18F-fluoroazomycin arabinoside. Such an approach is currently being tested for image-guided dose escalation in hypoxic head and neck cancer (DAHANCA 33, NCT02976051) [29].

Much work remains to be done to guide the optimal use of GRID radiotherapy and other SFRT modalities. The standardization of treatment planning parameters, including the prescription dose, beam energy, beam angle, peak-to-valley ratio, peak-to-peak distance, aperture size, GRID pattern, treatment time, collimation method, dose heterogeneity properties, and other dosimetric parameters can help facilitate data sharing between institutions and clinical trial development. Equally important is standardization of the measurement of clinical outcomes, including acute and late toxicities. This can be especially challenging given the variety of differing clinical scenarios and goals of SFRT in individual disease entities. As an intermediate step, data collected prospectively under an international registry can form the basis for the development of randomized controlled trials that may help elucidate unanswered clinical questions. A registry approach would also address the still uncommon clinical use and sparse published SFRT experience that provide a relatively low level of evidence.

While there is a strong biologic rationale and intriguing first reports, spatially fractionated radiotherapy is not widely utilized. The safety profile appears to be well established based on retrospective reports, but this is a relatively low level of evidence that has limitations. If improved meaningful clinical outcomes are not demonstrated prospectively, then critics of SFRT may argue that the addition of GRID to cERT merely increases the doses administered to normal tissues and overall toxicity risk without a meaningful clinical benefit at the patient level, particularly for patients who are being treated definitively. To address this criticism and increase the utilization of SFRT, well-designed prospective trials are desperately needed.

In terms of clinical trial strategy, in the case of bulky soft-tissue sarcomas, a prospective trial using a surrogate endpoint such as the pCR rate may be more feasible than a randomized trial. For bulky head and neck cancers, improvement in local control or freedom from salvage neck dissection, compared to historic controls, may serve as a good surrogate outcome. For large, bulky tumors needing palliation, determination of an appropriate endpoint is more challenging, given the inherently subjective nature of the outcomes, but the early GRID studies provide valuable guidance. In addition, the selection of experimental arms poses a challenge, as one could compare cERT to GRID or cERT with and without GRID. The selection of an appropriate cERT fractionation scheme would also present a challenge.

In conclusion, the available clinical reports show the development of GRID-based SFRT from a palliative modality toward the treatment of advanced primary tumors along with advancements in technical capability and dosimetric planning. The better-than-expected results reported for patients with large tumor volumes provide the rationale and demonstrate the need for well-designed prospective clinical trials.

## References


[1] Mohiuddin M, Curtis D L, Grizos W T and Komarnicky L 1990 Palliative treatment of advanced cancer using multiple nonconfluent pencil beam radiation. A pilot study *Cancer* **66** 114–8

[2] Mohiuddin M, Fujita M, Regine W F, Megooni A S, Ibbott G S and Ahmed M M 1999 High-dose spatially-fractionated radiation (GRID): a new paradigm in the management of advanced cancers *Int. J. Radiat. Oncol. Biol. Phys.* **45** 721–7

[3] Neuner G, Mohiuddin M M, Walde N V, Goloubeva O, Ha J and Yu C X *et al* 2012 High-dose spatially fractionated GRID radiation therapy (SFGRT): a comparison of treatment outcomes with cerrobend vs. MLC SFGRT *Int. J. Radiat. Oncol. Biol. Phys.* **82** 1642–9

[4] Mohiuddin M, Stevens J H, Reiff J E, Huq M S and Suntharalingam N 1996 Spatially fractionated (GRID) radiation for palliative treatment of advanced cancer *Radiat. Oncol. Invest.* **4** 41–7

[5] Köhler A 1909 Zur Röntgentiefentherapie mit Massendosen *Münchener Medizinische Wochenschrift* **56** 2314–6

[6] Kudrimoti M, Regine W F, Huhn J L, Meigooni A S, Ahmed M and Mohiuddin M 2002 Spatially fractionated radiation therapy (SFR) in the palliation of large bulky (>8 cm) melanomas *Int. J. Radiat. Oncol. Biol. Phys.* **54** 342–3

[7] Strongin A, Yovino S, Taylor R, Wolf J, Cullen K and Zimrin A *et al* 2012 Primary tumor volume is an important predictor of clinical outcomes among patients with locally advanced squamous cell cancer of the head and neck treated with definitive chemoradiotherapy *Int. J. Radiat. Oncol. Biol. Phys.* **82** 1823–30

[8] Johnson C R, Thames H D, Huang D T and Schmidt-Ullrich R K 1995 The tumor volume and clonogen number relationship: tumor control predictions based upon tumor volume estimates derived from computed tomography *Int. J. Radiat. Oncol. Biol. Phys.* **33** 281–7

[9] Dubben H H, Thames H D and Beck-Bornholdt H P 1998 Tumor volume: a basic and specific response predictor in radiotherapy *Radiother. Oncol.* **47** 167–74

[10] Huhn J L, Regine W F, Valentino J P, Meigooni A S, Kudrimoti M and Mohiuddin M 2006 Spatially fractionated GRID radiation treatment of advanced neck disease associated with head and neck cancer *Technol. Cancer Res. Treat.* **5** 607–12

[11] Peñagarícano J A, Moros E G, Ratanatharathorn V, Yan Y and Corry P 2010 Evaluation of spatially fractionated radiotherapy (GRID) and definitive chemoradiotherapy with curative intent for locally advanced squamous cell carcinoma of the head and neck: initial response rates and toxicity *Int. J. Radiat. Oncol. Biol. Phys.* **76** 1369–75

[12] Edwards J M, Shah P H, Huhn J L, Clair W S, Regine W F and Mohiuddin M *et al* 2015 Definitive GRID and fractionated radiation in bulky head and neck cancer associated with low rates of distant metastasis. *Int. J. Radiat. Oncol. Biol. Phys.* **93** E334

[13] Choi J I, Daniels J, Cohen D, Li Y, Ha C S and Eng T Y 2019 Clinical outcomes of spatially fractionated grid radiotherapy in the treatment of bulky tumors of the head and neck *Cureus* **11** e4637

[14] Adelstein D J, Lavertu P, Saxton J P, Secic M, Wood B G and Wanamaker J R *et al* 2000 Mature results of a phase III randomized trial comparing concurrent chemoradiotherapy with radiation therapy alone in patients with stage III and IV squamous cell carcinoma of the head and neck *Cancer* **88** 876–83

[15] Sathishkumar S, Dey S, Meigooni A S, Regine W F, Kudrimoti M S and Ahmed M M *et al* 2002 The impact of TNF-alpha induction on therapeutic efficacy following high dose spatially fractionated (GRID) radiation *Technol. Cancer Res. Treat.* **1** 141–7

[16] Schaefer I-M, Cote G M and Hornick J L 2018 Contemporary sarcoma diagnosis, genetics, and genomics *J. Clin. Oncol.* **36** 101–10
[17] Rosenberg S A, Tepper J, Glatstein E, Costa J, Baker A and Brennan M *et al* 1982 The treatment of soft-tissue sarcomas of the extremities: prospective randomized evaluations of (1) limb-sparing surgery plus radiation therapy compared with amputation and (2) the role of adjuvant chemotherapy *Ann. Surg.* **196** 305–15
[18] Wang D, Harris J, Kraybill W G, Eisenberg B L, Kirsch D G and Kane J M *et al* 2017 Pathologic complete response and survival outcomes in patients with localized soft tissue sarcoma treated with neoadjuvant chemoradiotherapy or radiotherapy: long-term update of NRG Oncology RTOG 9514 and 0630 *J. Clin. Oncol.* **35** 11012
[19] Kepka L, DeLaney T F, Suit H D and Goldberg S I 2005 Results of radiation therapy for unresected soft-tissue sarcomas *Int. J. Radiat. Oncol. Biol. Phys.* **63** 852–9
[20] Mohiuddin M, Miller T, Ronjon P and Malik U 2009 Spatially fractionated grid radiation (SFGRT): a novel approach in the management of recurrent and unresectable soft tissue sarcoma. *Int. J. Radiat. Oncol. Biol. Phys.* **75** S526
[21] Mohiuddin M, Memon M, Nobah A, Elsebaie M, Suhaibani A L and Pant A R *et al* 2014 Locally advanced high-grade extremity soft tissue sarcoma: response with novel approach to neoadjuvant chemoradiation using induction spatially fractionated GRID radiotherapy (SFGRT) *J. Clin. Oncol* **32** 10575
[22] Kaiser A, Mohiuddin M M and Jackson G L 2013 Dramatic response from neoadjuvant, spatially fractionated GRID radiotherapy (SFGRT) for large, high-grade extremity sarcoma *J. Radiat. Oncol.* **2** 103–6
[23] Snider J W, Molitoris J, Shyu S, Diwanji T, Rice S and Kowalski E *et al* 2020 Spatially fractionated radiotherapy (GRID) prior to standard neoadjuvant conventionally fractionated radiotherapy for bulky, high-risk soft tissue and osteosarcomas: feasibility, safety, and promising pathologic response rates *Radiat. Res.* **194** 707–14
[24] O'Sullivan B, Davis A M, Turcotte R, Bell R, Catton C and Chabot P *et al* 2002 Preoperative versus postoperative radiotherapy in soft-tissue sarcoma of the limbs: a randomised trial *Lancet* **359** 2235–41
[25] Johnsrud A J, Jenkins S V, Jamshidi-Parsian A, Quick C M, Galhardo E P and Dings R P M *et al* 2020 Evidence for early stage anti-tumor immunity elicited by spatially fractionated radiotherapy-immunotherapy combinations *Radiat. Res.* **194** 688–97
[26] Jiang L, Li X, Zhang J, Li W, Dong F and Chen C *et al* 2021 Combined high-dose LATTICE radiation therapy and immune checkpoint blockade for advanced bulky tumors: the concept and a case report *Front. Oncol* **10** 548132
[27] Ferini G, Valenti V, Tripoli A, Illari S I, Molino L and Parisi S *et al* 2021 Lattice or oxygen-guided radiotherapy: what if they converge? Possible future directions in the era of immunotherapy *Cancers (Basel)* **13** 3290
[28] Ellingsen C, Egeland T A M, Gulliksrud K, Gaustad J-V, Mathiesen B and Rofstad E K 2009 Assessment of hypoxia in human cervical carcinoma xenografts by dynamic contrast-enhanced magnetic resonance imaging *Int. J. Radiat. Oncol. Biol. Phys.* **73** 838–45
[29] DAHANCA 33: image guided dose-escalated radiotherapy to patients with hypoxic HNSCC https://clinicaltrials.gov/ct2/show/NCT02976051

# Chapter 6

# GRID spatially fractionated radiation therapy: definitive radiation therapy in bulky primary tumors

**Majid Mohiuddin, James W Snider and José Peñagarícano**

GRID spatially fractionated radiation therapy (SFRT) has been used in definitive settings for a variety of tumors, including melanomas and also head and neck, lung, breast, and cervical cancers. The greatest experience has been gained in the treatment of head and neck cancer, for which multiple academic centers have independently verified and reported the clinical efficacy of GRID. Neoadjuvant GRID enhances the response rate in T4/N2/N3 type tumors that would otherwise be refractory. As experience and technology have advanced, it has become possible to easily incorporate GRID into the current treatment paradigm without foregoing the prevailing standard of care.

## 6.1 Introduction/overview

Spatially fractionated GRID radiation therapy was initially reintroduced in the modern era for the treatment of palliative cases involving very large and bulky tumors that were expected to have poor responses to conventional radiation therapy [1, 2].

### 6.1.1 Early experience in palliation at Thomas Jefferson University Hospital

The initial experience at Thomas Jefferson University Hospital described by Mohiuddin *et al* showed very favorable symptomatic response rates—in excess of 90%—to even a single dose of GRID, while toxicity was unexpectedly low [3]. These initial results were independently validated in subsequent larger case series at the University of Kentucky [4, 5]. These established the early dose–response relationship for the GRID dose and the need to add conventional external beam radiation (cERT) to achieve more durable consolidation of the palliative response, while

doi:10.1088/978-0-7503-4046-5ch6

expanding the response outcome measures from symptomatic responses to objective tumor regression. The palliative application of GRID therapy is reviewed in detail in chapter 5.

### 6.1.2 Early University of Kentucky experience: early transition to definitive therapy

Building on the experience gained at the Thomas Jefferson University Hospital, Mohiuddin *et al* at the University of Kentucky noted in two subsequent cohorts of 61 and 71 patients that a GRID dose of ⩾15 Gy provided better response and, if followed by ⩾40 Gy of cERT, led to more durable control of the local tumor with minimal toxicity [4, 5]. The lack of acute side effects beyond those that would be expected from a conventional radiation treatment regimen soon led to the concept that GRID therapy could be used not just in palliative settings but also with curative intent in patients in definitive settings to treat advanced, bulky, but non-metastatic primary tumors. It was theorized that GRID could represent a safer form of dose escalation as well as a different radiobiological strategy with which to attack these bulkier, more radioresistant tumors.

Within the second series of 71 patients, eight patients (11%) were treated definitively with GRID therapy to the head and neck region, and four of these treatments were followed by surgical resection. The external beam radiation dose ranged from 50–70 Gy. All eight patients responded to the radiation treatment, and five of them achieved a clinical complete response (62.5%). No moderate to severe late toxicities were seen. The pathological complete response (pCR) rate was 50% (corresponding to the four out of eight patients who underwent resection). This early result suggested that GRID could be used in definitive and preoperative settings, particularly for head and neck cancers.

### 6.1.3 University of Maryland

Subsequent work included palliative cohorts that increasingly contained definitively treated patients, while reporting refinements in GRID technology and technique. Neuner *et al* shared the University of Maryland experience gained from 79 patients, comparing Cerrobend block GRID with the more recently developed multileaf collimator (MLC)-based GRID technique [6]. The various GRID techniques are further described in chapter 9. Of Neuner *et al*'s patients, 18 (23%) were treated with definitive curative intent, and overall 80% of all patients received additional cERT, suggesting a more aggressive treatment intent. Four of the 18 were treated neoadjuvantly prior to surgical intervention. However, the impact on survival for these 'curative' patients was not assessed due to the heterogeneity of their presentations. Interestingly, the majority of body sites treated were the head and neck (37%) and the thorax (26%). The most common primaries were lung (23%) and head and neck (18%) cancers. No differences in outcome were seen between treatment with the newly developed MLC-based GRID technique and the Cerrobend block technique.

### 6.1.4 University of Kentucky

Kudrimoti *et al* summarized the very large University of Kentucky experience in 2001 [7]. Three hundred and seven patients were treated at 357 body sites with a median GRID dose of 15 Gy (10–20 Gy) using Cerrobend GRID. All types of tumor and disease site were treated, including sites in the abdomen/pelvis (39%), head and neck (24%), thorax (18%), and extremities (19%). Ninety-five patients received GRID alone, while 262 received GRID in combination with cERT. Of these latter patients, 76 patients were treated as part of a definitive treatment course that combined high-dose cERT (dose range: 50–70 Gy) with surgery. The authors noted that the response rate for GRID alone was 73%, the response rate for GRID plus cERT was 82%, and the response rate for GRID combined with cERT at a dose of ⩾50 Gy was 95%. This experience further refined the dose–response relationship for cERT, first reported in Mohiuddin *et al*'s palliative series, toward higher cERT doses and has guided the cERT dose schedules that are used today [4, 5]. Of the patients in the group with the >50 Gy cERT dose, 38% were complete responders and 58% were partial responders. Almost one third of the patients ($n$=99) were alive at one year and 18 patients were alive at five years. No late grade 3 toxicities of the subcutaneous or mucosal areas or the skin were noted in any patient.

In regards to histology, a relatively higher complete response rate was observed in patients with soft-tissue sarcomas (20%) and melanomas (35%) as compared to those with squamous cell carcinomas (20%) and adenocarcinomas (15%), ($p$=0.003). This was surprising, considering that sarcoma and melanoma have historically been considered to be more radioresistant tumors. This supported the hypothesis that GRID treatment holds particular promise for the treatment of large radioresistant primary tumors that do not have good existing conventional treatments.

In the literature published to date, the most commonly described tumors for which GRID has been used in definitive (non-palliative) settings with intent to cure have been primary bulky sarcomas, bulky melanomas, and locally advanced head and neck cancers. As sarcoma was addressed in chapter 5, we focus here on melanoma and head and neck cancer; we also provide an overview of GRID experience gained with other tumors and disease sites, such as lung, breast, and cervical cancers.

## 6.2 Melanoma

### 6.2.1 The advantage of hypofractionation for adjuvant melanoma

Melanomas are traditionally considered to be radioresistant or radio-insensitive tumors, as *in vitro* studies suggest that they have a large capacity for the repair of sublethal damage. To overcome this radiobiology, external beam treatments would require higher total doses and higher doses per fraction than those typically utilized. However, larger doses per fraction introduce the risk of potentially increasing short- and long-term side effects.

Several hypofractionated dose regimens have informed the dosing strategies used for GRID therapy in melanoma. In cases of melanoma, a common radiation schedule proposed by the MD Anderson Cancer Center is 6 Gy per fraction for five fractions of *en face* electrons prescribed at $D_{max}$ to the head and neck region above the clavicle [8]. The patients in this published study were all treated electively and adjuvantly after wide local excision with or without limited or full neck dissection because they had a predicted local–regional failure rate of 50% with surgery alone. With the addition of hypofractionation, the five-year local–regional control rate was 88%. Patients with more than three involved nodes had a lower survival rate. In order to minimize some of the potential acute and long-term side effects, the 6 Gy per fraction regimen was only delivered twice weekly.

Another study at MD Anderson using the same dose of 30 Gy at 6 Gy per fraction looked at adjuvant radiation for axillary metastasis originating from malignant melanoma. All patients underwent axillary dissection and postoperative radiation treatment. If microscopic residual disease was present, a single boost of 4–6 Gy was also given to a reduced field. Based on risk factors such as lymph nodes $\geqslant$3 cm in size and $\geqslant$4 positive lymph nodes, these patients had a 30%–50% predicted risk of subsequent axillary recurrence. The actuarial axillary control rate at five years was 87%. On univariate analysis, the probability of axillary control was inferior when the axillary disease measured $\geqslant$6 cm in size, 72% vs 93% ($p$=0.02). This size threshold was the factor most closely associated with subsequent axillary failure. Ballo *et al* did suggest that improvements were needed for tumors with bulky nodal masses greater than 6 cm in size and that mild to moderate arm edema was common but manageable [9].

These two classic MD Anderson studies suggest that hypofractionation can overcome the high local–regional recurrence of melanoma in the subclinical disease setting of residual microscopic disease after a tumor has already been surgically debulked. For larger tumor sizes or more extensive lymph node involvement, the chance of local control or cure is much decreased. To apply these principles to situations involving bulky melanomas, particularly in the case of large or conglomerated matted lymph nodes for which surgical resection is not an option, moderately hypofractionated regimens in the range of 6 Gy in five fractions are insufficient for dose escalation. Higher dose hypofractionation, such as a treatment of 15 Gy in one fraction, may be needed to overcome the tumor resistance and tumor bulk.

### 6.2.2 Modeling hypofractionated GRID for primary melanoma

Zhang *et al* investigated the impact of single-fraction dose size in SFRT with GRID therapy for melanoma using mathematical modeling [10]. Their aim was to determine whether there was a therapeutic advantage at different dose levels for the cell killing of interspersed cancer cells for melanomas of varying sizes located at different depths and within various types of normal tissue. The Monte Carlo technique was used to calculate the 3D dose distribution administered by a 6 MV beam passing through a GRID collimator. Linear–quadratic (LQ) and modified linear–quadratic (MLQ) models were used separately to evaluate the therapeutic ratio (TR) of a series of single fractions of 1, 2, 3, 5, 7.5, 10, 15, 20, and 30 Gy per fraction. The therapeutic advantage of the GRID therapy was evaluated at these different dose levels for the treatment of melanomas of varying spherical sizes from 2 cm to 10 cm at depths from the surface to 3 cm deep. The 10 cm tumor was actually ellipsoid, being 6 cm along the beam path and 10 cm perpendicular to it. The alpha/beta ($\alpha/\beta$) ratios of nine different melanoma cell lines were varied from 1.15 to 8.68 to model different levels of acute or late response, and three types of normal tissue, all with $\alpha/\beta$ ratios of 3.1 but SF2 values of 0.3, 0.5, and 0.7, were interspersed with the melanoma tumors as part of the model. Surviving fractions of <0.3 at 2 Gy (SF2) were considered radiosensitive and those >0.7 were considered radioresistant. The equivalent uniform dose (EUD) was calculated for open fields so that GRID therapy could be compared to open-field therapy based on the same tumor cell killing ability or EUD.

The results suggested that acutely responding melanoma cells ($\alpha/\beta > 6$) that are surrounded by radiosensitive normal tissues (SF2 of 0.3 or 0.5) are more suitable for GRID therapy and have a higher TR. Melanomas for which $\alpha/\beta < 6$ or any tumor cells that are located in radioresistant normal tissue (SF >0.7) would not benefit from the highly nonuniform GRID field compared to open-field therapy. In order to take advantage of the therapeutic ratio of GRID, the clinician therefore needs to consider the radiobiology of both the tumor and the normal tissues that the tumor inhabits. The GRID field effectively increases the normal cell survival ratio (needed for recovery), while maintaining the same cancer cell killing rate at the same equivalent uniform dose (EUD) as that of an open field. In effect, GRID therapy is clinically advantageous since it delivers a large dose to a significant portion of the tumor volume and selectively kills melanoma cells (if they are acutely responding cells).

The results also indicated that GRID therapy does not provide any additional therapeutic advantage and sparing of interspersed normal tissue cells compared to open-field therapy if the GRID dose is <15 Gy. The radiation response is enhanced at the threshold dose of approximately 15 Gy and reaches a TR as high as 1.3 at 30 Gy, at which extensive tumor cell killing is achieved by high-dose zones with concomitant sparing of interspersed normal cells in relatively low-dose zones. In addition, a 20 Gy GRID nominal dose has the same EUD as a 4.1 Gy open field, which is insufficient to fully control tumor growth. Zhang *et al*'s study therefore confirms the requirement for subsequent cERT with open fields to provide tumor control in melanoma and supports a GRID dose in the range of 15–20 Gy for melanoma. Their model is consistent with the clinical data.

### 6.2.3 Melanoma experience gained at the University of Kentucky

Kudrimoti *et al* reported on 19 patients with advanced bulky melanoma (defined as greater than 8 cm in size) [11]. Five of these patients had progressed on vaccine therapy and 16 had failed chemotherapy. Twenty sites were treated, most commonly the chest wall/axilla (45%) or the groin/lower extremity (35%), but one patient was treated at the head/neck (5%) and another at the abdomen/pelvis (5%). A single dose at a median value of 15 Gy (12–20 Gy) was prescribed at $D_{max}$ using 6–20 MV photons; this was delivered via the classic Cerrobend GRID with a 50:50 open-to-closed ratio (further described in chapter 9) with a single field. Five of these patients received GRID only due to the prior use of radiation, while ten patients received GRID followed by ⩾40 Gy cERT.

The palliation of pain and mass effect was experienced within 48 h of the GRID therapy in over half of the patients. While the intent was palliative, the response rate for some patients was much better than expected. The overall response rate in terms of local control was 80% (16/20), among which seven patients achieved a complete response and nine a partial response. Three had no response and one was non-evaluable. Of the ten patients who received more than 40 Gy of cERT after GRID, five out of ten (50%) had a complete response versus two out of ten (20%) in the group that received less than 40 Gy; three out of ten (30%) had a partial response versus six out of ten (60%). This finding further confirms the need for cERT that was seen in the early palliative GRID studies [3–5] (chapter 5) and Zhang *et al*'s [10] modeling study described above. Of the 19 patients, 15 have died; six were alive at two years, and four were alive beyond two years.

### 6.2.4 Immunological indications of GRID in melanoma

Current treatments for advanced melanoma attempt to enhance the patient's own immune response to invasive cancer cells. Considerable progress has been made (compared to earlier cytokines such as interleukin-2 regimens) in novel immune checkpoint inhibitors in the form of specific human monoclonal antibodies. These newer drugs, such as ipilimumab, nivolumab, and pembrolizumab, target and inhibit proteins on T cells such as CTLA-4 or PD-1. By removing a suppressive checkpoint on the immune response, the immune response against cancer cells is enhanced. These drugs have offered increased progression-free survival as compared to chemotherapy.

Beyond the dose fractionation advantage as proposed by Zhang *et al* [10] above, GRID therapy may also function as an immunological primer by causing tumor lysis. The fragmented tumor cells can then be processed as radiation-specific antigens by the immune system, creating an *in situ* vaccine that can now potentiate the immune response against the tumor [12, 13]. The high dose may also release cytokines that upregulate cell-mediated immunity, such as T cell migration. Thus, GRID may recruit and enhance the body's innate immune response.

Mohiuddin *et al* published a case report of a 53-year-old male with a right axillary melanoma which had become refractory to immunotherapy after four cycles of ipilimumab, two cycles of interleukin-2 (IL-2), and five cycles of pembrolizumab [14]. The tumor had progressed on treatment when he presented with an 18 × 15 × 8 cm large painful left posterior neck mass. He was treated with 20 Gy using parallel opposed GRID through a brass block. He also received 50 Gy in 25 fractions of cERT with concurrent pembrolizumab. The neck mass had resolved by 75% at two months and then completely resolved at five months without any substantial side effects. The neck remained clear of any disease for one year of follow-up. Figure 6.1 shows the dosimetry and the treatment response.

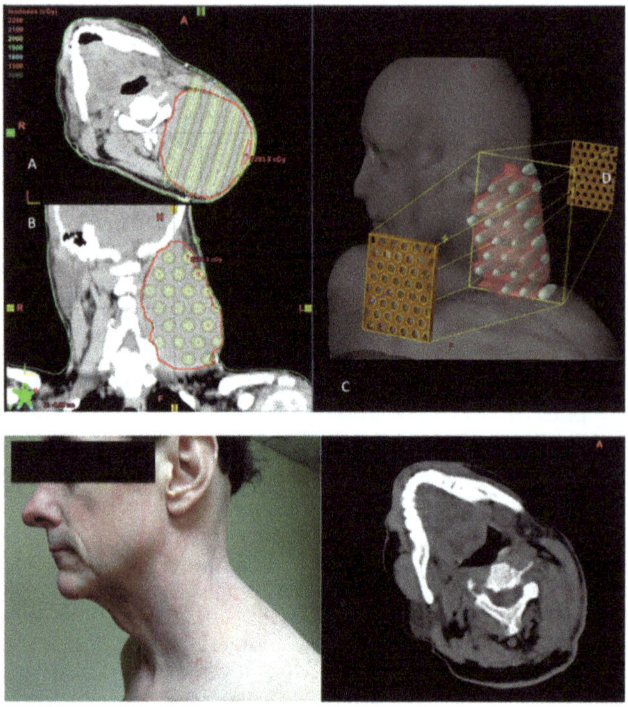


**Figure 6.1.** Images of a patient before treatment (above left) with a parallel opposed GRID planning dose (upper right) and after treatment (below). Reprinted from [14] with permission of Cureus.

Most interestingly, the patient was then able to continue on pembrolizumab for another 18 cycles with efficacy. He had previously been refractory to the drug and was now susceptible again. If the tumor-specific immune response is strong enough, it can also enable systemic regression in areas outside the local radiation field; this is known as the abscopal effect [15], which is further described in chapters 2 and 3. At the urging of medical oncology, Mohiuddin has routinely used GRID in the clinic as a single priming dose prior to the initiation of immunologic drugs in order to potentiate the immune response to systemic therapy delivered with curative intent (unpublished data).

## 6.3 Experience with bulky primary head and neck cancers

### 6.3.1 Introduction

Local control and survival of bulky and locally advanced head and neck cancers continues to be challenging in definitive settings. Alternate fractionation schemes have been utilized, such as hyperfractionation and delayed concomitant boost. Chemotherapy is also standardly added to radiation treatment.

Radiation therapy alone using conventional fractionation provides local–regional control at a rate of 30%–50%. RTOG 90-03 was a very large randomized trial that investigated altered fractionation, namely hyperfractionation or accelerated fractionation with a boost. The two-year locoregional control was reported to be 54% in patients who received the altered fractionation [16]. Most of these patients are now treated with chemotherapy and radiation treatment in a standardized fractionation as per RTOG 91-11, which had a local control rate of 78% [17].

N3 disease treated using conventional radiation results in a pCR rate of 30%–60%. As the nodal disease becomes larger in size, the chance of achieving a pCR decreases steeply. Achieving a pCR is very important, as the locoregional control in those who achieve pCR can be as high as 90%–100%, compared to the range of about 25%–65% in those who do not. The addition of chemotherapy to radiation treatment can increase the pCR rate to as much as 75%, but this causes additional toxicity [18]. With larger necrotic lymph nodes and tumors that outstrip their vascular supply, the delivery of chemotherapy to the tumor is non-optimal, and the clinical response rate falls to 40%. Even salvage surgical debulking may not be a viable option in bulky N3 disease due to morbidity. These tumors often present with frank ulceration, carotid or jugular vessel invasion, or taut, compromised skin that heals poorly. The tumor bed may result in a defect that is too large for flap reconstruction. T4 primaries often locally invade the bone, including the mandible and skull base.

GRID therapy offers promise for the definitive treatment of these bulky advanced head and neck cancers and can easily be incorporated into the current treatment paradigm without foregoing the current standard of care. In addition, head and neck cancers have a relatively higher response rate to GRID (23% complete response, 60% partial response) compared to the responses of other tumors [5].

### 6.3.2 Early University of Kentucky experience

As previously described in sections 6.1.3, eight patients in a palliative series were treated with definitive intent using GRID treatments of 10 Gy (one patient), 15 Gy (six patients), and 18 Gy (one patient) for primary head and neck cancer from 1995 to 1998. These patients then received a median dose of 60 Gy of cERT (46.4–64 Gy). The primary tumor sites included the tonsils (two patients), the skin (two patients), Merkel cells, the parotid gland, the gingiva, and an unknown site. The neck was targeted 75% of the time, and the skull or face was targeted in the other instances. Two patients who had a clinical complete response and two partial responders were not surgically evaluated. Interestingly, one patient with a clinical partial response had a leiomyosarcoma of the parotid and was found to have had a complete pathological response on surgical resection of the neck.

### 6.3.3 University of Kentucky

The University of Kentucky published its head and neck cancer experience gained from 27 patients with bulky N2–N3 disease treated between 1995 and 2002 [19]. This was the first study to investigate the impact of GRID in a definitive treatment setting for head and neck cancer as a separate cohort. None of the patients were metastatic. All patients had N2–N3 disease at a size ⩾6 cm; the median nodal size was 7 cm. All patients received the GRID treatment as a single dose of ⩾15 Gy. The patients were divided into two groups, taking the approach that bulky-tumor patients with N2 disease were treated definitively with radiation alone and those with N3 disease were also given planned combined surgery. Group 1 consisted of 14 patients who received the GRID treatment followed by cERT at a median dose of 69 Gy (range 54–79 Gy). Group 2 consisted of 13 patients who received GRID treatment followed by a median dose of 59 Gy (range 54–72 Gy) followed by planned neck dissection four to six weeks later.

GRID therapy was delivered through a Cerrobend block with holes that projected to a 1 cm diameter at the isocenter; the center-to-center spacing between the holes was 1.8 cm. GRID technologies and configurations are described in more detail in chapter 9. The dose was prescribed at a depth of approximately 1.5 cm, which approximates the $D_{max}$ for 6 MV beams; 100% of the total dose was prescribed for the open areas (peak dose) and the closed area (valley) dose was 15%–40%. The GRID treatment was delivered to encompass the nodal mass only, and the spinal cord and mandible were excluded. It did not treat the primary tumor. Twenty-six of 27 patients received 15 Gy and only one patient received 20 Gy.

All patients received cERT using the standard three-field head and neck technique. Importantly, the cERT dose was not reduced from the common definitive dose regimens used for head and neck cancer, despite the GRID dose contribution. For the 3D conformal cERT in the era prior to the implementation of intensity-modulated radiation therapy (IMRT), $\geqslant$6 MV photons were generally delivered to the upper neck mass via parallel opposed photon portals and a single anterior yoke portal. The spinal cord was limited to a maximum of 45 Gy, after which electron fields were used to supplement the posterior cervical nodes, or used as a boost if the tumor/nodal area overlaid the spinal cord. Out of 27 patients, 20 (74%) were treated with once-a-day fractionation, six with hyperfractionation, and one with an accelerated concomitant boost. Seven patients received concurrent chemotherapy with the cERT.

Twenty-three patients were male and four were female. Their median age was 65 years (range 44–85). All patients except for one had squamous cell carcinoma. The head and neck subsites included: 14 at the oropharynx, five at the oral cavity, one nasopharynx, one hypopharynx, and five unknown primary sites. One patient had both hypopharynx and oral cavity treatment synchronously.

The patients in group 1 (14 patients with radiation, no surgery) had a median tumor size of 7 cm (range 6–10 cm). Eight of the 14 patients were treated definitively at a full median dose of 70 Gy. Of the other six for whom full doses were intended, four received a lesser dose (median: 59 Gy, range: 54–60 Gy) because of the progression of systemic disease, loss to follow-up, progression at the primary site accompanied by death (one), and treatment refusal (one). Twelve of the 14 received a full dose to the primary at least.

The overall neck control was 93% (13/14). Seven patients died of systemic disease, only one of whom had regional failure. The patient that had a regional failure did so outside the GRID field and also had a new primary ten months post-therapy. Four died of unrelated disease. Two continued to have no evidence of disease at 39 and 44 months post-therapy. One patient was lost to follow-up. Disease-specific survival was 50%, with a local–regional control rate of 86% at a median follow-up time of ten months (3–44 months).

The patients in group 2 (13 patients, radiation and neck dissection) had a median tumor diameter of 8 cm (range 6–13 cm). These patients received a median dose of 59.4 Gy (range 54–72 Gy) to the involved neck followed by a planned neck dissection. Twelve of the 13 received a full dose to the primary tumor. One patient received less because the primary was also resected at the time of neck dissection. The patients receiving surgery had a younger median age of 55 years as compared to the other group, whose median age was 70 years.

The pCR rate was 85% (11/13). The N3 neck control rate was 92% (12/13). Among all 13 patients, 62% (8/13) had no evidence of disease, and all of these had achieved a pCR. Two did not have local–regional recurrence, but eventually died of distant metastatic disease. Three died of intercurrent medical disease with one local failure at the primary, not the nodal region.

The overall survival, disease-specific survival, and local–regional control were 62% (8/13), 85%, and 92%, respectively at a median follow-up of 38 months (range: 5–116 months).

The side effects reported for group 1 (radiation, no surgery) were mostly grade 2–3 acute skin reactions without any grade 4 toxicities. The long-term side effects in this group were mostly grade 2 soft-tissue muscle fibroses that restricted full neck mobility. In group 2 (radiation and neck dissection), one third (4/12) of patients had some fibrotic soft-tissue changes. Acute surgical toxicities were limited to three patients with postoperative wound healing requiring debridement of flap necrosis, flap closure due to wound breakdown, and delayed wound healing which was managed without surgical intervention as an outpatient.

The lack of major long-term wound healing complications after GRID and full-dose preoperative cERT supports the feasibility of this regimen and suggests that surgical techniques and standard definitive radiation do not need to be modified.

In the study by Huhn *et al*, GRID radiation treatment followed by cERT without chemotherapy resulted in an 88% local–regional control rate [19]. These favorable pathologic CR outcomes of the preoperative subgroup, the local control results in the subgroup without surgery, and in the overall cohort suggest that GRID therapy combined with full-dose cERT results in higher-than-expected tumor response and control in patients with bulky advanced head and neck cancer.

### 6.3.4 University of Kentucky updated experience

A report of an updated series of 53 patients was published by the University of Kentucky in 2015 [20]. Patients with non-metastatic squamous cell carcinoma of the head and neck region with large primary tumors (T4) or lymph nodes greater than 6 cm (N3) were treated with curative intent between 1991 and 2014. The primary tumor sites were the oropharynx (49%), the oral cavity (34%), the sinonasal area (11%), and the larynx (6%). Patients with N3 nodes most commonly had tumors of the oropharynx (81%), followed by the larynx (66%), the oral cavity (50%), and then sinonasal (32%) sites. The median maximal tumor diameter was 8 cm. All patients were treated with 15 Gy of GRID therapy followed by a median cERT dose of 60 Gy (48–79.2 Gy). The local–regional control, including the areas outside the GRID treatment volume, was 81% at three years. The distant metastasis rate was only 9% (five patients) at three years. Only two patients (4%) became feeding tube dependent, representing grade 3+ long-term toxicity. The overall survival rate was 23% at five years. In addition to its excellent local control, an intriguing finding of this study was the much lower distant metastasis rate compared to that obtained via historical controls, despite the advanced bulky head and neck tumors of T4 or N3 disease. The expected distant metastasis rate for radiation alone in this population is 20%–30% [16]. Even with the use of induction chemotherapy, such as cisplatin–5-fluoruracil (PF) or TPF (the addition of paclitaxel to PF), the distant metastasis rate is 10%–13% [21]. The unexpectedly low metastasis rate achieved using GRID and cERT suggests that GRID therapy may induce an abscopal effect (beyond local control) on micrometastasis without compromising primary treatment [15]. If this finding is confirmed by future studies, the toxicities caused by currently used induction chemotherapies which do not have a clear overall survival (OS) or progression-free survival (PFS) benefit [21, 22] or concurrent therapies might be avoided in the future. This is clinically significant because in head and neck cancer patients, induction chemotherapy often introduces significant hematological toxicity and the inability to complete the concurrent chemoradiation regimen in up to one third of patients.

### 6.3.5 University of Arkansas experience

Peñagarícano *et al* reported 14 patients with bulky (⩾6 cm) locally advanced squamous cell carcinomas of the head and neck region in 2010 [23]. These patients were treated at the University of Arkansas and participated in the first study to administer GRID therapy followed by definitive chemotherapy and IMRT. All patients underwent CT planning and were treated with a single field using MLC-based GRID at 20 Gy in one fraction using 6 MV photons. The GRID treatment was provided on the first day, followed by concomitant chemotherapy and cERT on the subsequent treatment day. Simultaneous integrated boost IMRT (SIB-IMRT) was utilized for the cERT course. The GRID field was always directed away from critical structures such as the spinal cord or brainstem. The MLC GRID pattern used at the University of Arkansas had holes 1 cm in diameter with a 1 cm center-to-center spacing at 100 cm from the photon source. This created a valley-to-peak ratio of 22%–29% for a 10 × 10 cm field at 1.5 cm, a ratio of 27%–32% at 5 cm, or a ratio of 29%–38% at a distance of 10 cm. The GRID field was prescribed at $D_{\text{max}}$ or 1.5 cm for 6 MV for the first 12 patients, but then shifted to $D_{\text{max}}$ (the maximum point dose) at 1.2 cm based on the treatment planning system in order to ensure that 20 Gy was given to the tumor.

The primary disease sites included the tonsils (29%), the base of the tongue (21%), the larynx (14%), the maxillary sinus (14%), the retromolar trigone (7%), the nasopharynx (7%), and the parotid gland (7%). The T-stage distribution was as follows: T1 (21%), T2 (21%), T3 (29%), and T4 (29%). Sixty-four percent of the

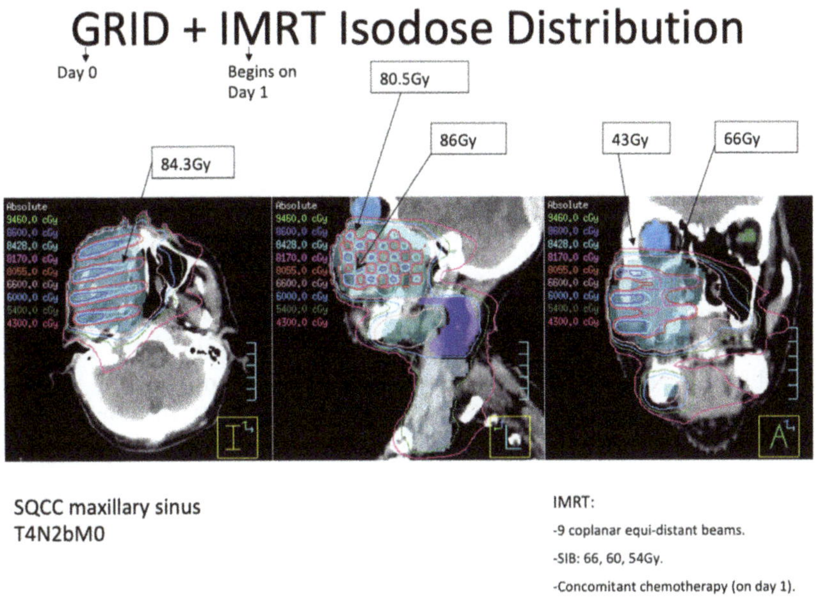


**Figure 6.2.** Combined MLC GRID and IMRT dose distribution administered to T4N2bM0 squamous cell carcinoma of the right maxillary sinus. Adapted from [23] with permission from Elsevier and adapted from [24] with permission of the Journal of the Arkansas Medical Society.

patients had N3 disease, while the rest had N2b/c disease. The GRID therapy was administered to the primary tumor in six patients (four of whom had T4 disease and two of whom had T3 disease) and to the lymph node region in eight patients (all of whom had N3 disease).

The concurrent chemotherapy consisted of carboplatin–docetaxel in 79% (11/14 patients), and the remaining three patients each received carboplatin–paclitaxel, 5-flurouracil–cisplatin, or cisplatin alone. A GRID dose of 20 Gy was given on day zero. The dose levels used for the SIB-IMRT were 66 Gy, 60 Gy, and 54 Gy in 30 fractions for high-, intermediate-, and low-risk patients, respectively; patients were started on concurrent chemotherapy on the next day, i.e. day one.

Ten patients had planned neck dissections or primary tumor biopsies of the GRID area. Eight of out of ten (80%) achieved a pCR. The other two patients had no clinical evidence of disease after radiation, but were found to have one lymph node each containing squamous cell cancer on neck dissection. Four patients did not have any surgery and three of them were without evidence of disease at 18, 19, and 33 months, giving a clinical complete response of 75%. One remaining patient was not compliant and died of recurrent disease at 13 months. The median follow-up was at 19.5 months (2–38 months). Figure 6.2 presents an example of the treatment planning images and dosimetry for GRID therapy in head and neck cancer.

Out of the eight patients with N3 disease treated by GRID, seven had planned neck dissections, and two of these showed residual squamous cells in their specimens. The pCR for N3 disease treated using neck dissection was 71% (5/7). One patient did not have the neck dissection, but was clinically and radiographically disease free at 33 months. Of the seven who had surgery, no wound healing issues occurred, but one died at ten months due to carotid blowout from a skin-to-carotid fistula. This complication was not thought to be related to the radiation but rather the lack of tissue overlying the carotid after surgery.

Figure 6.3 illustrates the complete imaging response in a patient with bulky neck node involvement.

In the six patients treated by GRID at the primary site, three had biopsies that demonstrated a complete pathological response rate. Two of the other three patients had no evidence of disease (NED) at 18 and 19 months. The one patient who died had a recurrence, but this patient had not been compliant with treatment. The median follow-up took place at 11.5 months (2–19 months). The primary sites treated by GRID included the maxillary sinus (two patients), the parotid gland, the base of the tongue, the retromolar trigone, and the tonsils.

No patient had grade 4 toxicities. The mucosal acute toxicity was similar to that due to combined chemoradiation in other case series. Ten of 14 patients lived for more than one year; grade 1 (30%), grade 2 (30%), and grade 3 (10%) skin fibroses were seen in these patients. Two patients became percutaneous endoscopic gastrostomy (PEG)-tube dependent, likely due to trismus seen at presentation.

Overall, among all 14 patients, only three had recurrent disease, resulting in an overall local control rate of 79%. For two of these, residual disease was found during neck dissection despite their apparent clinical response to GRID; they suffered from recurrence and died of their disease. The other patient had not been compliant with treatment. One patient with local control at the GRID site died of distant metastasis at eight months.

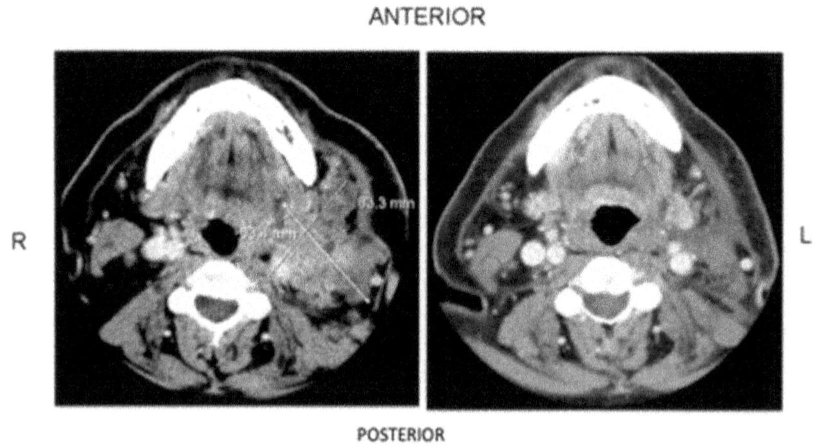


**Figure 6.3.** Pre-GRID (left) and post-treatment axial CT scans of a patient with head and neck cervical lymphadenopathy showing a complete radiographic response; the patient also showed no pathological evidence of disease upon neck dissection. Reproduced from [24] with permission of the Journal of the Arkansas Medical Society.

### 6.3.6 University of Texas at San Antonio

Experience gained at the University of Texas at San Antonio was reported by Choi *et al* in 2019 [25]. Twenty-one patients with large cancers (>5 cm) of the head and neck region were treated definitively between 2007 and 2015. Prior to 2008, most patients were treated with MLC-based GRID. After 2009, they were treated with a commercially available GRID block (.decimal Inc., Sanford, FL). Each hole projected a 1 cm diameter circular field with a 2 cm center-to-center spacing in a hexagonal array at the isocenter (as further detailed in chapter 9). A GRID dose of 15 Gy was delivered at $D_{\max}$ (the depth of the maximum dose) using a source-to-surface distance of 100 cm for 16 patients. In 2010–11, this study used 20 Gy palliatively in one fraction for five patients. GRID was given on day zero, followed by external beam radiation therapy the next day.

Sixteen of the 21 patients had squamous cell cancer, and nine of those 16 were treated definitively with curative intent. These nine patients had a median tumor size of 9 cm (5–13,14 cm), a median Karnofsky Performance Scale (KPS) score of 80, and a median age of 59 years (52–64 years). They all received 15 Gy of GRID therapy alone followed the next day by IMRT at a dose of 69.96–72.08 Gy in 2.12 Gy per fraction. All of these patients received chemotherapy concurrently with the IMRT, not the GRID.

Cisplatin alone was used in four patients, cisplatin and paclitaxel in four patients, and cetuximab in one patient.

Forty-four percent had a complete response to therapy. A partial response (PR) was defined as a greater than 50% reduction in the tumor's maximum diameter. One patient had a partial response. Twenty-two percent had less than a partial response and underwent subsequent neck dissection. Twenty-two percent had no response at all; one of those patients received cetuximab and only one of the 33 fractions of the prescribed IMRT dose. Seven of the nine patients treated definitively were still alive at a median follow-up time of seven months (4–16 months). Two patients died at four and 17 months after treatment. If we exclude the one patient who did not receive the external beam, there was an 87.5% overall response rate seen in patients treated definitively who also received >75% of the IMRT dose, and 50% of these patients achieved a complete clinical response. Conversely, among those with <75% of the IMRT dose, only 25% experienced an improvement in their symptoms.

Among all 21 patients, there were no grade 3 or 4 acute mucosal toxicities. Grade 3 or 4 skin toxicities were seen in five patients, including bleeding in three patients and skin ulceration from tumor regression. The authors noted that given the inherent invasiveness of the head and neck tumors, which compromised the overlying skin and surrounding tissues, the bleeding and ulceration seen with tumor regression may have been the natural course of the tumor response and not a separate side effect of treatment.

### 6.3.7 Summary and discussion of studies

Total tumor volume is a relevant prognostic factor for overall survival and local control, and bulky involvement continues to be a challenge. The local control achieved through the addition of chemotherapy to radiation has been reported to be as high as 80% in early-stage head and neck cancers, but in case series of N2 or N3 disease, the pCR rate is closer to 54%–65%. Chemotherapy and radiation followed by planned neck dissection in N3 disease with complete response to therapy can still result in a neck relapse rate of 28% [26].

In the study by Huhn *et al*, the pCR rate was 85% with a neck control rate of 92% [19]. In the study by Peñagarícano, the pCR rate was 80% and the pathological and clinical complete response rate was 79% [23]. The results of these independent studies are all greatly improved compared to the historical reports of 35%–46% of residual disease at the time of neck dissection in N2/N3 disease treated with conventional chemoradiation [18, 27].

While Huhn *et al*'s study in 2006 was the first to use GRID definitively for head and neck cancer, it used older radiation techniques [19]. It used the GRID block and two-dimensional radiation planning as opposed to IMRT. The GRID therapy was limited to 15 Gy and to nodal regions only and was mainly followed by the use of external beam only (i.e. without chemotherapy).

In comparison, the University of Arkansas series was more uniform: all patients received chemotherapy, were treated with curative intent, received MLC GRID, and received a uniform GRID dose of 20 Gy [23]. It also differed from Huhn *et al*'s series in that GRID therapy was also given at the primary site in some cases and not only to the nodal disease. The use of planned neck dissection or biopsy in the majority of their patients further confirmed Huhn *et al*'s high pCR rate (figure 6.3).

The University of Texas at San Antonio used a Cerrobend GRID block at a dose of 15 Gy; their study contained nine patients treated with curative intent using modern chemotherapy and IMRT planning [25]. They reported a 44% clinical complete response rate, which independently corroborated the positive experience reported by the preceding studies [19, 23].

While slightly different GRID doses and techniques were used, the University of Maryland experience suggests that the use of a Cerrobend or brass block is clinically equivalent to the use of MLC GRID, apart from the longer treatment times and increased monitoring units needed with an MLC [6]. MLC-based and collimator-based GRID techniques are reviewed in more detail in chapter 9. A typical MLC-based GRID pattern is illustrated in figure 6.4. At the University of Arkansas, MLC-based GRID tended to be used to treat tumors 6–8 cm in size. A GRID block was used for lesions larger than 8 cm because MLC-based GRID requires a longer delivery time [24]. The group later transitioned to tomotherapy or volumetric modulated arc therapy (VMAT)-based GRID (source: correspondence with Peñagarícano).

### 6.3.8 Future applications in the developing world

Poh *et al* made a special appeal for the use of GRID treatment in the treatment of nasopharyngeal cancer [28]. Nasopharyngeal carcinoma (NPC) is endemic to

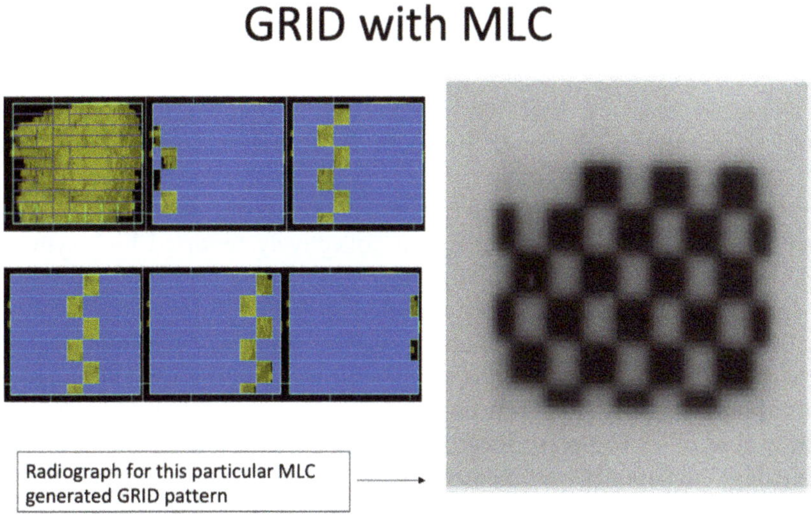


**Figure 6.4.** MLC GRID pattern used by Peñagarícano *et al.* Reprinted from [23], Copyright (2010), with permission from Elsevier.

low-to-middle-income countries. Without access to care, NPC patients often present with locally advanced disease. NPC often presents with large bilateral cervical lymphadenopathy.

GRID therapy allows dose escalation and can be done without complex treatment planning procedures if necessary. A single fraction can therefore provide immediate relief from symptoms, and it may allow a form of 'neoadjuvant' treatment that harnesses immune-activating properties in the patient. Customarily, induction chemotherapy (as commonly practiced in the U.S.) is not often an option for patients in these low-income countries; even if available, it is much more challenging to administer due to lack of sanitation, distance to the treatment facility, and lack of medical and nutritional support. The high observed local response rates, local control, and the unexpectedly low metastasis rate in one of the preceding studies [19] suggest that GRID therapy may generate a bystander effect that may result in immune priming and favorably influence the distant metastasis rate. While robust confirmation of these findings is needed, clinical trials of GRID therapy for head and neck cancer, such as nasopharyngeal cancer, may be particularly useful and impactful in third-world nations without easy access to standard chemotherapy and radiation.

Head and neck cancer may be a good area for a future international trial in a definitive setting. The International Atomic Energy Agency (IAEA) has approved an active clinical trial of SFRT for the palliative treatment of lung and cervical cancer patients [29]. It is aimed at poorer countries without VMAT or IMRT capabilities. The trial will run from April 2020 through September 2025 in Argentina, Azerbaijan, Belarus, Ghana, India, Indonesia, and Kyrgyzstan.

## 6.4 Lung cancer

### 6.4.1 Lung experience gained in the United Kingdom

As in advanced cases of head and neck cancer, bulky advanced lung cancer continues to present a challenge for both local tumor control and metastatic failure [30].

Most GRID experience with lung cancer has been reported in multidisease series of largely palliatively treated patients that collectively reported high symptomatic response but did not separately analyze lung cancer patients [5, 6]. Only one lung-cancer-specific GRID series has been reported to date.

Locally advanced non-small cell lung cancer ⩾6 cm in size has been treated at the Royal Marsden Hospital and Saint George's Hospital in the United Kingdom in a feasibility phase II study [31]. Ten patients were treated using a Cerrobend GRID block at a dose of 15 Gy prescribed at the mid-tumor using 10 MV photons. The following day, the patients were treated with cERT of 36 Gy in 12 fractions over 2½ weeks. Seven patients noted temporary skin erythema in the form of the GRID. Two patients had grade 2 moderate symptomatic lung fibrosis. No grade 3/4 acute toxicities were recorded.

Of the patients who had presented with chest pain, 71.4% attained a complete response and 28.5% achieved a sustained partial response up to the last follow-up. Three patients with Pancoast tumors had presented with severe pain with chest wall numbness that restricted arm abduction. After one month, all three had completely responded. On imaging, 90% of the patients had a partial response in the lung primary site which was sustained until the end of follow-up at a median of four months (range 2–24 months). The authors concluded that the GRID therapy allowed safe dose escalation without any significant acute or late morbidity and that further research was warranted in lung cancer.

### 6.4.2 Dosimetric considerations for lung GRID

Costlow *et al* investigated different types of potential GRID plan that could be clinically used for lung cancer in an attempt to increase the TR [32]. They evaluated six different MLC-based GRID plans using IMRT and electron compensation that had varying hole patterns. They modeled the six plans in five lung patients while assuming a radiosensitive lung cancer cell line. The therapeutic ratios ranged from 4.5 to 132, meaning that the GRID therapy plans could spare 4.5–132 times more normal cells than the open-field therapy could at the same EUD of 4.2 Gy, where equivalent EUDs represent the same cancer cell killing ability. Of the six plans, two attempted a weave pattern that created a dose volume histogram (DVH) with only one medium 10 Gy peak instead of the usual two peaks (3 and 18 Gy) that are seen with the customary GRID block. The presence of two peaks suggests that the tumor is receiving a significant amount of high-dose radiation as well as a significant dose of low-dose radiation, enhancing the therapeutic ratio. This would suggest that the weave-pattern plans are not as clinically useful in lung cancer. One advantage of

MLC/IMRT plans is the lower dose administered to the organs at risk as compared to that of a standard block plan using photons.

## 6.5 Other tumor types

A number of other disease sites including breast and cervical cancer have been treated in primary settings using GRID, but unfortunately, these have not been published as case series in the literature due to their small numbers. The authors have treated these disease sites, as well as rectal cancer, in a palliative setting with good local response effect, as illustrated in figure 6.5.

## 6.6 Breast cancer

Murphy *et al* modeled the use of MLC-based GRID planning in 12 prone breasts [33]. Each GRID plan was made of four fields: two medial and two lateral tangent fields. Each medial tangent was collimated at 90 degrees to the other medial tangent, as were the lateral tangents. This created a series of 1 cm wide striped blocks for each tangent when the MLCs were extended to the opposing collimator jaw. Taken together as four fields, they created a $1 \times 1$ cm grid in the sagittal direction. A dose of 20 Gy was prescribed using 6 MV beams, and the maximum dose was limited to 120%. At least 95% of the breast volume received 5 Gy, the dose covering 50% of the target volume was 50% of the maximum dose, and the maximum rib dose was limited to 20 Gy. The planning target volume (PTV) was the whole left or right breast with a negative 0.5 cm margin in the prone position, and it varied from 354 to 1778 $cm^3$ (average 814.5 $cm^3$). The $\alpha/\beta$ ratio of the breast cancer was taken to be 4 Gy but was modeled using two cell lines of 10 Gy (acute responding) and 3.846 Gy (late responding) using the MLQ model.

When the authors of this paper expanded the aperture size from 1 cm to 2 cm, the peak–valley ratio increased, but this came at the cost of a reduced EUD and a reduced TR. This meant that the high-dose zone increased, but more of the overall dose moved into the lower range. There appears to be more advantage with the 1 cm aperture, as a larger EUD suggests a larger possibility of tumor control, and a larger TR means a larger portion of normal tissue sparing. The 1 cm aperture at 20 Gy

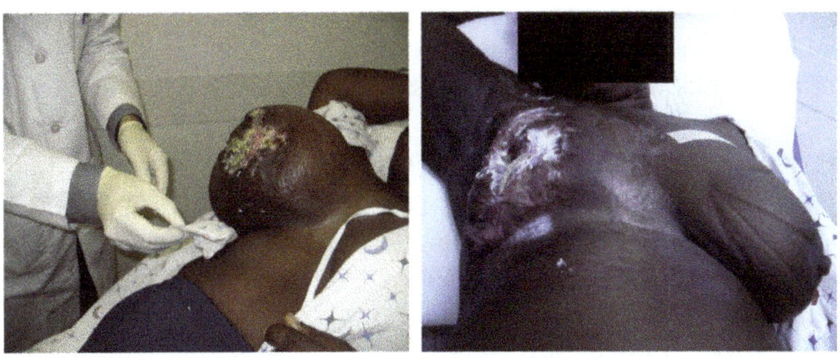

**Figure 6.5.** Clinical images of locally advanced right breast cancer before (left) and after (right) GRID therapy. Reprinted from [6], Copyright (2012), with permission from Elsevier.

seemed to give an EUD of 8–10 Gy and a peak–valley dose ratio (PVDR) from 2.34 to 2.92. The authors also argued that the advantage of using the MLC design over the Cerrobend block may be that at 20 Gy, MLCs allowed a greater EUD of 8.7 vs 4.2 and a TR of 9 vs 2.5 but a smaller peak–valley dose of 2.7 vs 4.9.

The breast is a site that is amenable to GRID therapy, but has customarily received neoadjuvant chemotherapy and/or mastectomy in locally advanced cases. The role of integrated GRID in a definitive setting has not yet been explored in a clinical trial or series. However, the breast is a site that has been treated palliatively with success. In the University of Maryland study, the leading author of this chapter can be seen next to a patient with locally advanced right breast cancer who presented with foul smell, necrotic ulceration, peau d'orange, and axillary lymphadenopathy [6]. The patient was treated with MLC-based GRID at 15 Gy followed by 60 Gy of external beam radiation therapy. Other than some minor debridement and wound care for necrotic tissue, a CT scan performed four months later was reported as 'interval mastectomy with no recurrence in the chestwall,' although no surgery was ever performed.

## 6.7 Cervical cancer

### 6.7.1 Cervical cancer hypofractionated modeling

Zhang *et al* used a Monte Carlo simulation of a Cerrobend GRID block to examine whether there is an advantage to giving a 15 Gy GRID dose in a single fraction as compared to 2 Gy per fraction of conventional radiation to debulk cervical cancers that have different LQ parameters [34]. As in the studies of lung tumors and melanomas that were published later, the researchers found that GRID treatment favors acutely responding tumors ($\alpha/\beta > 6$) inside radiosensitive normal tissues. Theoretical predictions using an LQ model of five cervical cancer cell lines with $\alpha/\beta$ ratios of 5.9, 12.4, 12.6, 19.4, and 20.9 showed that the TR was also dependent on the individual $\alpha$ and $\beta$ values, preferring large values of $\alpha$. Late-responding tumors and radioresistant normal tissues did not benefit from GRID therapy. A 15 Gy GRID dose can increase the normal cell survival ratio by at least 37% compared with open-field debulking radiation. Using EUD, Zhang *et al* calculated that two 15 Gy fractions of GRID would equal 5.26 Gy in a single-fraction open field or two fractions of 3.68 Gy as an open field. This also suggests that multiple fractions of GRID could be given to try and increase tumor control, which may allow more sparing of normal tissues beyond that possible using just GRID collimation.

### 6.7.2 'Internal' GRID mimicking virtual tandem brachytherapy

Cervical cancer often presents as large and bulky disease, designated as 'barrel-shaped.' The outcomes of locally advanced cervical cancer diminish greatly with increasing tumor volume. For small (<40 $cm^3$), intermediate (40–99 $cm^3$), and large (>100 $cm^3$) tumor volumes, the five-year local control rates are 92%, 59%, and 36%. Likewise, the five-year disease-free survival (DFS) rate decreases from 75% to 48% to 18%, respectively, and the five-year overall survival (OS) rate drops precipitously from 40%–51% to 0% [35].

The current paradigm is to initially use chemotherapy and radiation to the pelvis and then low-dose-rate (LDR) or high-dose-rate (HDR) brachytherapy at around week four or five of the pelvic radiation therapy. The hope is that the pelvic radiation will shrink the bulky tumor to a small enough volume to be encompassed by the brachytherapy device's dose cloud, usually via a tandem and ring, tandem and ovoids, or interstitial implant.

Interestingly, the use of tandem-based devices introduces the idea of using high doses of 'internal' radiation administered heterogeneously to the cervix and fundus area. The HDR dose of 6 Gy in five fractions was historically prescribed at Manchester point A, representing a geometrical and anatomical region in relation to the cervical os. As 3D conformal techniques increased with the use of CT and MR planning, there has been a push to prescribe using more volumetric definitions. As seen volumetrically in computer planning systems, the 6 Gy prescription at point A more accurately describes a very heterogeneous, central tandem dose of 200%–300% to the cervix and fundus, with a lower dose of 6 Gy actually reaching the edges of the tumor volume. The point B dose, representing the pelvic sidewall, is usually 25% of the prescribed dose. Moreover, in studies using CT planning, it has been demonstrated that the brachytherapy device very often cannot encompass the entire gross tumor volume (GTV) with the 6 Gy dose cloud, even after pelvic radiation [36]. If cervical treatment had relied on covering the whole GTV with the full dose, one would have expected marginal misses and higher local failure rates than are seen clinically in brachytherapy. Knowing that very large cervical tumors do not respond in time for the brachytherapy by week four or five, the University of Washington St. Louis often introduces HDR brachytherapy in week one. They do so knowing that the HDR dose does not cover the entire GTV, but by giving it early, they can induce a more rapid and pronounced shrinkage by introducing a heterogeneous high dose early in the treatment, even if it is given over a partial volume. In essence, they are delivering a form of 'internal' spatial fractionation through the use of brachytherapy. In fact, the rate of weekly regression may be a more important predictor of outcome than initial tumor size [35].

While the customary GRID therapy mimics lines of interstitial catheters, and lattice therapy mimics individually spaced LDR seed implants, as seen in prostate cancer, there is a role for introducing a form of 'internal' GRID to mimic the high-dose tandem used in cervical cancer. In March 2010, Mohiuddin presented the University of Maryland experience at the International Conference on Radiation Medicine: Clinical Applications and Innovative Approaches, using what he dubbed 'internal GRID' of a stereotactic tandem [37]. This was a form of VMAT-arc-based stereotactic treatment for cervical cancer that prescribed a core of high dose to the center of the bulky cervical cancer. In essence, the GTV of the cervix and fundus was contoured similarly to the approach now used in lattice therapy (further detailed in chapter 7). An 'internal GRID' core volume was then created by subtracting a 2 cm margin from the edges of the tumor. This central core cylinder of the GTV was then prescribed a central point dose of 10–15 Gy (median 12 Gy). The dose was planned using 360-degree arcs, which allowed for very rapid dose fall-off with rings of heterogeneous doses from the center (figure 6.6). Eight to ten Gy reaches most of the internal GRID volume, while the dose ring used at the periphery of the cervix's GTV

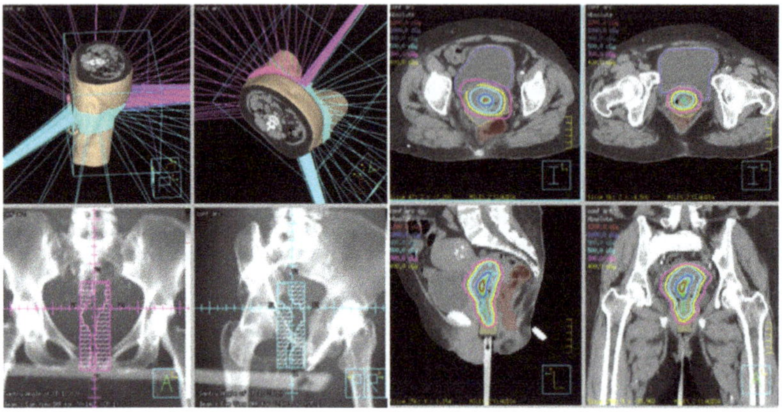

**Figure 6.6.** 'Stereotactic virtual tandem' showing irregular 'internal' GRID dose distribution with vaginal immobilization device and a prescription of 12 Gy (red) given to a cervical GTV (pale orange) via two VMAT arcs [37].

is usually <4 Gy (median 2 Gy), which is tolerable to the organs at risk, such as the bladder and rectum. This dose was repeated three times, once a week during weeks one to three of the pelvic radiation. Replanning was often necessary due to significant shrinkage after week two.

The cervix was immobilized by an internal vaginal cylinder that was mounted on a fixed arm and indexed to the linac couch. Cone-beam CT imaging was performed to ensure reproducibility. The tumor was often so advanced that it was fixed in position in the pelvis. The bulky configuration of the cervix often displaced the bladder and small bowel. The vaginal cylinder immobilization device displaced the rectum posteriorly, much like a vaginal retractor in some tandem and ring brachytherapy kits. Unlike the tandem and ring, which has a fixed pear-shaped distribution, the 'internal' GRID volume could be irregularly shaped in the axial plane and conform to the bend of the cervix and uterus in the sagittal plane, taking on the conformal shape of patient's tumor. The intention of the 'internal GRID' was to induce an early rapid response to allow for subsequent brachytherapy in very large tumors, in which such a response would be unlikely with only 45 Gy of conventional radiation and cisplatin.

In a pilot study, ten patients were treated with stage IB2 bulky, stage III, or stage IV cancers and with tumor sizes >200 cc. The median tumor size was 343 cc (range of 258–556 cc). Most patients had ureteral stents placed and all were treated with 45 Gy of pelvic radiation and 40 mg $m^2$ of cisplatin weekly. The 'internal GRID stereotactic virtual tandem' dose was delivered alone (without the pelvic dose for that day) once a week for the first three weeks of treatment. A parametrial and sidewall boost was given at 60 Gy as needed. The internal tandem GRID dose was excluded from the total prescription dose except as related to bladder and rectum tolerances, and seven patients received interstitial implants at a dose of 75–80 Gy. Three patients refused interstitial implants due to anesthesia concerns and were treated with IMRT as a dose escalation to 75 Gy using the vaginal cylinder immobilizer.

At a median of 18 months (9 to 36 months), all patients were positron emission tomography (PET) negative at the last follow-up. After 23.4 Gy of pelvic radiation, the size of the tumoral regression was 44% (30%–65%) based on cone-beam computed tomography (CBCT), and after 45 Gy of pelvic radiation, it was 83% (68%–91%) based on a replanning CT scan. The residual cervix size (which includes scarring) at the last follow-up was 0–72 cc. All patients had no evidence of disease at the last follow-up. There were no cases of grade 3+ late side effects to the bladder, rectum, ureter, or bowel, though closure of the cervical os and proximal vaginal stenosis was very common (personal correspondence).

This technique may present an alternative to stereotactic radiation in the treatment of unresponsive bulky cervix cancer. Stereotactic boost therapy treats the entire GTV with a high dose of 6–7 Gy per fraction, but cannot mimic the very high central dose of at least 12–18 Gy provided by the tandem. In 2020, a phase II study of stereotactic cervical boost (28 Gy in four fractions) was closed early due to excessive toxicity and suboptimal results, attributed to large tumor sizes at a median of 139 cc (range 51–268 cc) [38]. In contrast, the University of Maryland study had favorable results despite even larger tumor sizes (it only included tumors >200 cc with a median volume of 343 cc). The high observed response rates provide subtle evidence that the high central dose and heterogeneity of brachytherapy provides a radiobiological advantage, and that the proposed 'internal' GRID approach may mimic it.

## 6.8 Rectal cancer

The clinical total response to GRID therapy of colorectal cancer was reported to be 100% by Mohiuddin *et al* [3, 39]. In an early palliative setting, the majority of the Thomas Jefferson University study treated the abdomen/pelvis (64%) without any major side effects. Despite high-dose beamlets traversing organs such as the bladder and bowel, only one patient suffered a small bowel obstruction which was found at laparotomy to be due to a recurrent tumor, not the radiation. That said, GRID has not been used to date in definitive settings for rectal cancer. It may play a role in clinical trials in a neoadjuvant setting for T4 and/or N2/3 disease, especially if the rectal tumor is expected to be removed at the time of surgery.

## 6.9 Conclusions

GRID treatment holds particular promise for the treatment of large primary tumors that do not have good existing conventional treatments. Both block- and MLC-based GRID treatments have been used with near-equal efficacy. Mathematical modeling using the MLQ model with cell lines in melanomas and lung, breast, and cervical cancers has shown the therapeutic ratio advantage of the heterogenous dose pattern of GRID compared to that of open-field radiation. In cases of melanoma, which responds better to hypofractionation, GRID delivers a high dose to a significant portion of the tumor volume, which results in approximately 80% local control. In addition, it may immunologically prime the tumor for an enhanced response to radiation and drugs targeting checkpoint inhibition. In cases of head and neck cancer, there is a relatively higher response rate to GRID as compared to the responses at other tumor sites, and it can be combined with IMRT and concurrent chemotherapy (and salvage surgery if needed) without an increase in toxicity. The pathological response rate is close to 80% when GRID therapy is added, as compared to 45% in locally advanced head and neck cancer patients treated using conventional radiation only. In cases of lung cancer, GRID treatment can provide rapid responses by three months, particularly in Pancoast tumors. In cases of locally advanced breast cancer, GRID therapy shows a good local response effect, but may require wound care if the breast skin is already compromised. In cases of barrel-shaped, bulky unresponsive cervical cancer, SFRT can be safely delivered using an 'internal' GRID via arcs that mimic the high-dose tandem of HDR brachytherapy while restricting the adjacent organs at risk to a low peripheral dose. The dose given to organs at risk can be further clinically reduced using technologies such as protons [40].

In summary, GRID therapy can be safely incorporated into current treatment protocols for a variety of tumors in definitive settings. More prospective studies and controlled clinical trials need to be done to further establish its role.

## References


[1] Billena C and Khan A J 2019 A current review of spatial fractionation: back to the future? *Int. J. Radiat. Oncol. Biol. Phys.* **104** 177–87

[2] Yan W, Khan M K, Wu X, Simone C B, Fan J and Gressen E *et al* 2020 Spatially fractionated radiation therapy: history, present and the future *Clin. Transl. Radiat. Oncol.* **20** 30–8

[3] Mohiuddin M, Curtis D L, Grizos W T and Komarnicky L 1990 Palliative treatment of advanced cancer using multiple nonconfluent pencil beam radiation: a pilot study *Cancer.* **66** 114–8

[4] Mohiuddin M, Stevens J H, Reiff J E, Huq M S and Suntharalingam N 1996 Spatially fractionated (GRID) radiation for palliative treatment of advanced cancer *Radiat. Oncol. Investig.* **4** 41–7

[5] Mohiuddin M, Fujita M, Regine W F, Megooni A S, Ibbott G S and Ahmed M M 1999 High-dose spatially-fractionated radiation (GRID): a new paradigm in the management of advanced cancers *Int. J. Radiat. Oncol. Biol. Phys.* **45** 721–7

[6] Neuner G, Mohiuddin M M, Vander Walde N, Goloubeva O, Ha J and Yu C X *et al* 2012 High-dose spatially fractionated GRID radiation therapy (SFGRT): a comparison of treatment outcomes with Cerrobend vs. MLC SFGRT *Int. J. Radiat. Oncol. Biol. Phys.* **82** 1642–9

[7] Kudrimoti M R, Regine W F, Meigooni A S, Ahmed M and Mohiuddin M 2001 High dose spatially fractionated radiation (GRID): a new paradigm in the management of advanced cancers *Int. J. Radiat. Oncol. Biol. Phys.* **51** 50–1

[8] Ang K K, Peters L J, Weber R S, Morrison W H, Frankenthaler R A and Garden A S *et al* 1994 Postoperative radiotherapy for cutaneous melanoma of the head and neck region *Int. J. Radiat. Oncol. Biol. Phys.* **30** 795–8

[9] Ballo M T, Strom E A, Zagars G K, Bedikian A Y, Prieto V G and Mansfield P F *et al* 2002 Adjuvant irradiation for axillary metastases from malignant melanoma *Int. J. Radiat. Oncol. Biol. Phys.* **52** 964–72

[10] Zhang H, Zhong H, Barth R F, Cao M and Das I J 2014 Impact of dose size in single fraction spatially fractionated (grid) radiotherapy for melanoma: impact of dose size in grid radiotherapy *Med. Phys.* **41** 021727

[11] Kudrimoti M, Regine W F, Huhn J L, Meigooni A S, Ahmed M and Mohiuddin M 2002 Spatially fractionated radiation therapy (SFR) in the palliation of large bulky (>8 cm) melanomas *Int. J. Radiat. Oncol. Biol. Phys.* **54** 342–3

[12] Reits E A, Hodge J W, Herberts C A, Groothuis T A, Chakraborty M and Wansley E K *et al* 2006 Radiation modulates the peptide repertoire, enhances MHC class I expression, and induces successful antitumor immunotherapy *J. Exp. Med.* **203** 1259–71

[13] Formenti S C and Demaria S 2012 Radiation therapy to convert the tumor into an *in situ* vaccine *Int. J. Radiat. Oncol. Biol. Phys.* **84** 879–80

[14] Mohiuddin M, Park H, Hallmeyer S and Richards J 2015 High-dose radiation as a dramatic, immunological primer in locally advanced melanoma *Cureus* **7** e417

[15] Formenti S C and Demaria S 2009 Systemic effects of local radiotherapy *Lancet Oncol.* **10** 718–26

[16] Beitler J J, Zhang Q, Fu K K, Trotti A, Spencer S A and Jones C U *et al* 2014 Final results of local-regional control and late toxicity of RTOG 9003: a randomized trial of altered fractionation radiation for locally advanced head and neck cancer *Int. J. Radiat. Oncol. Biol. Phys.* **89** 13–20

[17] Forastiere A A, Zhang Q, Weber R S, Maor M H, Goepfert H and Pajak T F *et al* 2013 Long-term results of RTOG 91-11: a comparison of three nonsurgical treatment strategies to preserve the larynx in patients with locally advanced larynx cancer *J. Clin. Oncol.* **31** 845–52

[18] Brizel D M, Albers M E, Fisher S R, Scher R L, Richtsmeier W J and Hars V *et al* 1998 Hyperfractionated irradiation with or without concurrent chemotherapy for locally advanced head and neck cancer *N. Engl. J. Med.* **338** 1798–804

[19] Huhn J L, Regine W F, Valentino J P, Meigooni A S, Kudrimoti M and Mohiuddin M 2006 Spatially fractionated GRID radiation treatment of advanced neck disease associated with head and neck cancer *Technol. Cancer Res. Treat.* **5** 607–12

[20] Edwards J M, Shah P H, Huhn J L St., Clair W, Regine W F and Mohiuddin M *et al* 2015 Definitive GRID and fractionated radiation in bulky head and neck cancer associated with low rates of distant metastasis *Int. J. Radiat. Oncol. Biol. Phys.* **93** E334

[21] Vermorken J B, Remenar E, van Herpen C, Gorlia T, Mesia R and Degardin M *et al* 2007 Cisplatin, fluorouracil, and docetaxel in unresectable head and neck cancer *N. Engl. J. Med.* **357** 1695–704

[22] Budach W, Bölke E, Kammers K, Gerber P A, Orth K and Gripp S *et al* 2016 Induction chemotherapy followed by concurrent radio-chemotherapy versus concurrent radio-chemotherapy alone as treatment of locally advanced squamous cell carcinoma of the head and neck (HNSCC): a meta-analysis of randomized trials *Radiother. Oncol.* **118** 238–43

[23] Peñagarícano J A, Moros E G, Ratanatharathorn V, Yan Y and Corry P 2010 Evaluation of spatially fractionated radiotherapy (GRID) and definitive chemoradiotherapy with curative intent for locally advanced squamous cell carcinoma of the head and neck: initial response rates and toxicity *Int. J. Radiat. Oncol. Biol. Phys.* **76** 1369–75

[24] Peñagarícano J A, Griffin R, Corry P, Moros E, Yan Y and Ratanatharathorn V 2009 Spatially fractionated (GRID) therapy for large and bulky tumors *J. Ark. Med. Soc.* **105** 263–5

[25] Choi J I, Daniels J, Cohen D, Li Y, Ha C S and Eng T Y 2019 Clinical outcomes of spatially fractionated GRID radiotherapy in the treatment of bulky tumors of the head and neck *Cureus* **11** e4637

[26] Argiris A, Stenson K M, Brockstein B E, Mittal B B, Pelzer H and Kies M S *et al* 2004 Neck dissection in the combined-modality therapy of patients with locoregionally advanced head and neck cancer *Head Neck* **26** 447–55

[27] Brizel D M, Prosnitz R G, Hunter S, Fisher S R, Clough R L and Downey M A *et al* 2004 Necessity for adjuvant neck dissection in setting of concurrent chemoradiation for advanced head-and-neck cancer *Int. J. Radiat. Oncol. Biol. Phys.* **58** 1418–23

[28] Poh S S, Chua M L K and Wee J T S 2018 Why we should give spatially fractionated radiation therapy (GRID) a second look—especially in nasopharyngeal carcinoma *Ann. Nasopharynx Cancer* **1** 1

[29] IAEA CRP 2020 (https://iaea.org/projects/crp/e33043)

[30] Tam K, Daly M and Kelly K 2017 Treatment of locally advanced non-small cell lung cancer *Hematol./Oncol. Clin. North Am.* **31** 45–57

[31] Somaiah N, Warrington J, Taylor H, Ahmad R, Tait D and Glees J 2008 High dose spatially fractionated radiotherapy (SFR) using a megavoltage GRID in advanced lung tumors: preliminary experience in UK *Int. J. Radiat. Oncol. Biol. Phys.* **72** S490

[32] Costlow H N, Zhang H and Das I J 2014 A treatment planning approach to spatially fractionated megavoltage grid therapy for bulky lung cancer *Med. Dosim.* **39** 218–26

[33] Murphy N L, Philip R, Wozniak M, Lee B H, Donnelly E D and Zhang H 2020 A simple dosimetric approach to spatially fractionated GRID radiation therapy using the multileaf collimator for treatment of breast cancers in the prone position *J. Appl. Clin. Med. Phys.* **21** 105–14

[34] Zhang H, Wang J Z, Mayr N, Kong X, Yuan J and Gupta N *et al* 2008 Fractionated grid therapy in treating cervical cancers: conventional fractionation or hypofractionation? *Int. J. Radiat. Oncol. Biol. Phys.* **70** 280–8

[35] Mayr N A, Taoka T, Yuh W T C, Denning L M, Zhen W K and Paulino A C *et al* 2002 Method and timing of tumor volume measurement for outcome prediction in cervical cancer using magnetic resonance imaging *Int. J. Radiat. Oncol. Biol. Phys.* **52** 14–22

[36] Wahab S H, Malyapa R S, Mutic S, Grigsby P W, Deasy J O and Miller T R *et al* 2004 A treatment planning study comparing HDR and AGIMRT for cervical cancer *Med. Phys.* **31** 734–43

[37] Mohiuddin M 2010 Stereotactic treatment for advanced cervical cancer 2010 Int. Conf. on Radiation Medicine: Clinical Applications and Innovative Approaches *(Riyadh, Saudi Arabia)* (http://radmed.org/scientific_program.php)

[38] Albuquerque K, Tumati V, Lea J, Ahn C, Richardson D and Miller D *et al* 2020 A phase II trial of stereotactic ablative radiation therapy as a boost for locally advanced cervical cancer *Int. J. Radiat. Oncol. Biol. Phys.* **106** 464–71

[39] Gholami S, Nedaie H A, Longo F, Ay M R, Wright S and Meigooni A S 2016 Is grid therapy useful for all tumors and every grid block design? *J. Appl. Clin. Med. Phys.* **17** 206–19

[40] Mohiuddin M, Lynch C, Gao M and Hartsell W 2020 Early clinical results of proton spatially fractionated GRID radiation therapy (SFGRT) *Br. J. Radiol.* **93** 20190572

# Chapter 7

# Lattice Radiotherapy SFRT: definitive radiation therapy in bulky primary tumors

**Beatriz E Amendola, Naipy C Perez, Benhua Xu, Nina A Mayr, Marco A Amendola and Xiaodong Wu**

Lattice Radiotherapy (LRT) is a novel spatially fractionated radiation therapy (SFRT) technique used to deliver inhomogeneous doses of radiation to voluminous tumors. LRT was derived from two-dimensional GRID therapy, the initial SFRT modality, by applying recent technological advances, including intensity-modulated radiation therapy (IMRT) and image-guided radiation therapy (IGRT), to generate a three-dimensional and individualized configuration of the SFRT dose heterogeneity. LRT allows for the delivery of very high ablative radiation doses to individually placed small high-dose spheres within the tumor volume, while limiting the exposure to surrounding normal tissues according to their respective tolerances. Technical approaches and the clinical experience with LRT are presented and discussed in this chapter.

## 7.1 The history, origins, and development of Lattice therapy

LRT is rooted in the original concept and early inception of SFRT, which dates back to Alban Köhler's work of more than 100 years ago [1, 2]. Köhler introduced the original GRID device in 1909, which delivered a heterogeneous radiation dose as further described in chapter 1. This dose heterogeneity enabled a reduction in the skin toxicity when treating large tumors compared to the toxicity caused by whole-field irradiation. In the ortho- and kilovoltage x-ray era, Köhler used doses ten and twenty times higher than usual at that time. It was soon recognized that these doses were tolerable, despite the technical limitations of radiotherapy delivery. Köhler named this form of therapy 'fractionation of the x-ray dosage in space' in the 2D GRID era, a term remarkably similar to today's term 'spatially fractionated radiation therapy,' which describes the range of SFRT technologies and techniques from 2D and 3D GRID therapy to LRT.

doi:10.1088/978-0-7503-4046-5ch7  

Throughout the technological advancement of radiation therapy delivery, the concept of dose heterogeneity in SFRT has remained the same. In common with other SFRT techniques, LRT does not attempt to treat the whole tumor volume, as is done in conventional radiation therapy approaches. Instead, SFRT (including both GRID therapy and LRT) allows for the delivery of high radiation doses to partial tumors using similar doses to those administered to the target volume by stereotactic radiosurgery (SRS) or stereotactic body radiation therapy (SBRT). Delivering partial tumor radiation to bulky tumors reduces the dose and ensuing toxicities to surrounding normal tissues, such as the bowel, bladder, lungs, neural structures, and others.

The original ortho- and kilovoltage GRID therapies were commonly used from the 1930s to the 1950s [3] and fell out of favor after the introduction of megavoltage radiation in the 1960s. However, the limitations of megavoltage therapy in terms of normal tissue sparing were soon recognized, especially for recurrent and therapy refractory tumors. The GRID concept was therefore reintroduced and adapted to megavoltage therapy in the 1980s [4–6].

The recent advances in IMRT, volumetric modulated arc therapy (VMAT), and other advanced delivery techniques have led to a further advance in megavoltage SFRT using multileaf collimator (MLC)-based GRID approaches [7, 8] and the emergence of LRT [9].

Advances in delivery platforms, including IMRT, VMAT, TomoTherapy, and CyberKnife, and increases in dose rate capabilities have been essential for the development of LRT. LRT was first described in 2010 [9] as a way to extend the SFRT dose heterogeneity to an individualized 3D configuration, in which an array of high-dose regions (vertices) could be created within the tumor volume through converging photon beams (figure 7.1). In LRT, the high-dose vertices are separated by a certain distance to give rise to the peak-to-valley dose distributions required to deliver the inhomogeneous dose distributions. The use of LRT has also been

Innovative Cancer Institute (ICI) Experience from 4/2010 to 10/2021

| Pathologic Diagnosis | n |
|---|---|
| Gynecological * (26 cervical ca; 4 uterine sarcomas) | 37 |
| Lung Cancer (one SCLC) | 30 |
| Head and Neck | 11 |
| RCC | 7 |
| Sarcoma | 6 |
| Breast | 5 |
| Colon | 4 |
| Anorectal | 2 |
| Melanoma | 1 |
| Skin | 1 |
| Plasmacytoma | 1 |
| Neuroendocrine | 1 |
| Total | 106 |

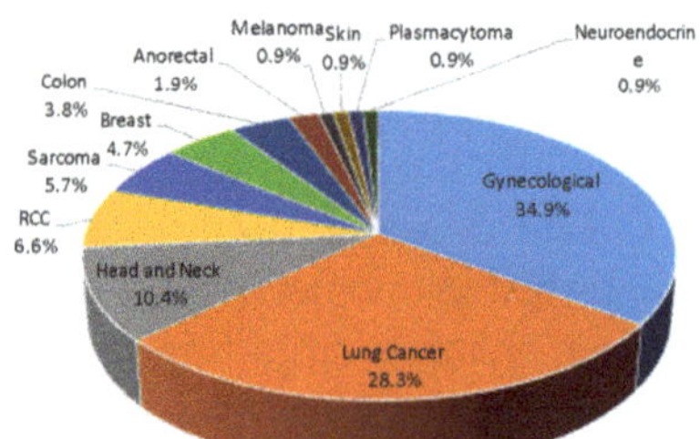


**Figure 7.1.** Patients treated with LRT at the Innovative Cancer Institute between 2010 and 2022. Patients are tabulated by diagnosis and tumor site, number ($n$), and percentages of total.

explored to create high-dose regions, peaks, and valleys using the Bragg peaks of charged particle beams, such as proton therapy [10, 11].

LRT leverages the highly variable placement of high-dose vertices whose configuration can be individualized to cover the tumor bulk but spare nearby normal tissues [12]. While the optimal distribution of the high-dose vertices and low-dose valleys remains to be determined, LRT allows for the individualized reduction of the doses given to adjacent normal structures, such as the bowel, bladder, lungs, neural structures, or other sensitive structures [12–16].

Over the ensuing several decades, the clinical experience with megavoltage GRID therapy has accumulated (see chapters 5 and 6), first in palliative radiation [4–6, 8] and subsequently in selected definitively treated diseases (with curative intent), such as head and neck cancer [17–19], lung cancer [15, 20], and sarcoma [21–23]. Meanwhile, a consensus has been gradually established among the GRID therapy community on treatment delivery treatment planning and reporting [24].

LRT, which is described in more detail in chapter 10. LRT requires more complex dosimetric and physical parameters than conventional megavoltage therapy and GRID therapy. While GRID heterogeneity patterns are largely fixed by the GRID collimator hardware configuration, in the LRT method, the variability of vertex positioning must be closely planned and documented. Specific recommendations have been developed for the vertex geometry [12]. The vertex size generally ranges from 0.5 to 1.5 cm, and the vertex spacing (separation) generally ranges from 2 to 5 cm. This allows variability tailored to the tumor and normal tissue configuration. The volume of the vertices which receive the prescribed high LRT dose generally encompasses 1%–10% of the total gross tumor volume (GTV), resulting in an achievable low peripheral dose of 2–5 Gy [12]. Despite the resulting variability in the SFRT heterogeneity pattern, clinical results [13–16, 20, 25] have been remarkably consistent with those of the GRID therapy outcomes [5, 6, 8, 17, 18, 21, 26–29].

## 7.2 Clinical LRT experience

LRT is a young modality that has only existed for little more than a decade, and clinical outcome results are just emerging.

As in GRID therapy [5, 6, 8, 17, 18, 21, 26–29], current outcome results in LRT are based on single-institution studies. These clinical data have shown overall favorable outcomes in patients with advanced bulky primary tumors and in the use of LRT to treat patients with recurrent or metastatic lesions [14, 15, 20, 30]. The vast majority of the current clinical LRT experience has been gained at the Innovative Cancer Institute (ICI), South Miami [13–16, 25], and additional data are emerging from other institutions. A second small case series focused on lung cancer was recently presented at the 2021 Annual Meeting of the American Society for Radiation Oncology (ASTRO) [20].

From 2010 to the present, more than 100 patients with tumors of multiple histologies and at various tumor sites have been treated using LRT at the ICI. This includes patients with recurrent and metastatic tumors, as well as non-metastatic primary lung cancer; cervical cancer [13, 14]; other gynecologic cancers, including uterine and ovarian cancers [16]; head and neck cancers; and soft-tissue sarcomas. ICI's updated experience is summarized in figure 7.1.

### 7.2.1 LRT in gynecologic cancer

Among primary gynecologic tumors, the most clinical experience has been reported for cervical cancer [14]. In addition, LRT has been used in advanced ovarian cancer [16], and in vulvar cancer (unpublished data).

#### *7.2.1.1 Cervical cancer*

Cervical cancer continues to be a major global public health concern as the fourth most frequently diagnosed cancer and the fourth leading cause of cancer death in women, with an estimated 604 000 new cases and 342 000 deaths worldwide in 2020 [31]. Advanced cervical cancer remains a challenge to the delivery of radiation therapy, particularly in patients who have advanced voluminous tumors and those with severe anatomical distortions that severely challenge or prohibit the use of brachytherapy.

The first case series of SFRT used for the definitive treatment of advanced/bulky cervical cancer was reported in 2020 [14]. In this series patients were treated with LRT. There was no prior reported cohort of cervical cancer patients treated using GRID therapy. This LRT series was preceded by two pilot case reports of LRT in gynecologic cancer: one in a patient with advanced cervical cancer [13] and one in a patient with bulky abdominal recurrence from ovarian carcinosarcoma [16]. Both pilot cases showed a rapid and drastic response and minimal toxicity.

The LRT cervical cancer series included ten patients aged 44–90 years, with very advanced bulky squamous cell carcinomas (seven) and adenocarcinomas (three) at stages IIIB–IVA. The majority of patients (eight out of ten) had lymph node involvement. Tumors were characterized by an excessive tumor bulk of >7 cm and/or severe anatomical distortion deemed to severely interfere with brachytherapy [14]. The patients' pre-therapy tumor volumes ranged from 74.1 to 412.4 $cm^3$ (mean: 200.35 $cm^3$).

LRT was given at a dose of 24 Gy in three fractions and followed by conventionally fractionated external beam radiation therapy (cERT) at doses of 39.6 to 45.0 Gy (mean: 44.28 Gy) in 1.8 Gy fractions. LRT was prescribed for the gross tumor volume, inclusive of organ motion considerations, based on simulations with both, a full and an empty bladder that were used to generate an internal target volume (ITV) with a 3–5 mm expansion. For treatment planning, multiple vertices were evenly placed throughout the GTV and further adjusted to reduce the dose given at the ITV periphery. The ITV peripheral dose was constrained to 9 Gy in three fractions. As a result of the variability in tumor size, the number of vertices ranged from two to eleven (mean: five). An example of vertex placement is shown in figure 7.2. The vertex diameter was most commonly 1 cm, resulting in a total vertex tumor volume (VTV) of 0.80–4.83 $cm^3$.

The three LRT fractions were delivered on consecutive days using the VMAT technique, stereotactic localization, and daily image guidance. The LRT was

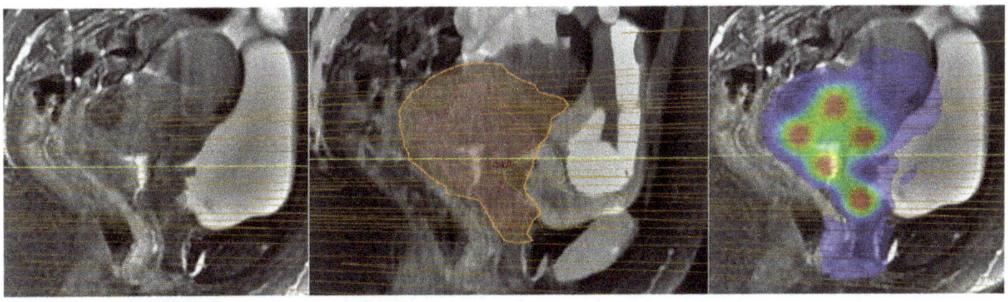

**Figure 7.2.** Example of the distribution of vertices in a patient with a voluminous cervical cancer. The patient had stage IVA cervical cancer with massive extension to the bladder that was confirmed by biopsy. The left image shows the fusion of computed tomography (CT) and magnetic resonance (MR) imaging, depicting the invasion of the bladder by the tumor. The planning target volume (PTV) (middle) and vertex distribution (right image) are shown.

immediately followed by the cERT. All patients received concurrent weekly chemotherapy with cisplatin. Chemotherapy was also given during the SFRT portion of the treatment. No brachytherapy was performed due to infeasibility, generally because of severe anatomic distortion. Four patients had post-radiation hysterectomies. An additional cERT tumor boost was given in two patients.

Tumor response was assessed in three ways: (i) clinically, by serial morphological imaging, including intratreatment cone beam CT (CBCT), (ii) by pre- and post-therapy CT and/or magnetic resonance imaging (MRI), and (iii) by molecular imaging with [18] fluorodeoxyglucose (FDG) positron emission tomography (PET)/CT. This was the first SFRT case series to apply pre- and post-therapy molecular imaging to assess SFRT response and was also the first series to apply intratreatment CBCT and pre- and post-therapy volumetric imaging (CT, MRI) for SFRT response assessment. The serial imaging data produced by this case series provided early insights into the morphologic and metabolic response dynamics of SFRT.

All patients had local pelvic tumor control at a median follow-up of 16 months (1–77) months, including one patient with bladder invasion and para-aortic lymph node involvement. This patient's pre-therapy imaging, post-therapy CT, and metabolic response are illustrated in figure 7.3.

The volumetric tumor response as measured via CBCT on the last day of pelvic radiotherapy was highly variable and frequently rapid, showing tumor regressions of 6%–91% (mean: 54%). Figure 7.4 shows an example of rapid tumor regression at the end of cERT.

The morphologic imaging response as seen on CT and/or MRI was high, with a complete response (per RECIST criteria) in 55% of patients in the early post-therapy phase (at a median 2.2 months after treatment completion) and a partial response in all others. When molecular imaging was included in the response assessment, 67% attained a complete metabolic response within six months post-therapy, and all others had a partial response. The ultimate metabolic response, scored at the last follow-up (at a median of 28.5 months for surviving patients) was high at 89% (eight of nine patients according to PET/CT), and one patient had a partial response. The pathologic response was assessable in four patients who underwent post-radiation

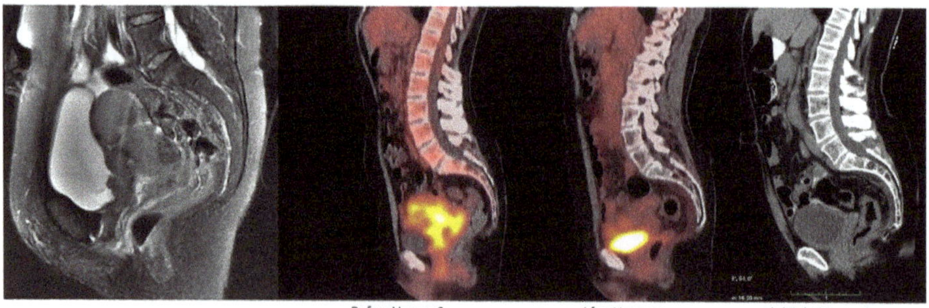


**Figure 7.3.** Metabolic tumor response to LRT in a patient with bulky advanced cervical cancer. Pre-therapy MRI and PET/CT (left two images) show the extensive involvement of stage IV cervical cancer in a 59-year-old woman who presented with vaginal bleeding, renal failure, and a large tumor invading the bladder. PET/CT and CT images obtained nine months after LRT and cERT with concurrent chemotherapy show a complete response. The patient subsequently underwent total abdominal hysterectomy/bilateral salpingo-oophorectomy and had no evidence of disease three months after therapy.

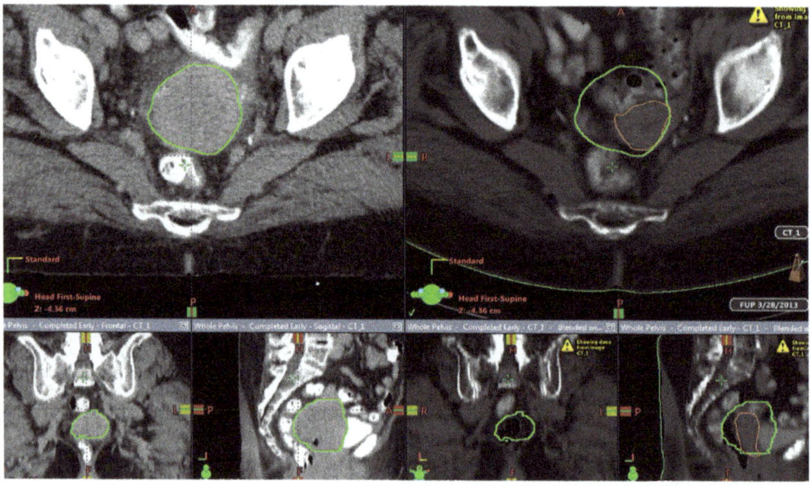

**Figure 7.4.** Tumor response to LRT in advanced cervical cancer. Left images: bulky cervical tumor (green contour) in pre-therapy CT simulation images. Right images: rapid regression (orange contour) is seen in the CT image obtained at the end of LRT and cERT with concurrent chemotherapy.

therapy hysterectomy for severe anatomical distortion (precluding brachytherapy) and/or suspicion of residual disease. Two of the four patients had a pathologic complete response, one had a partial response, and one had extensive residual involvement. Since the publication of this case series, another patient underwent post-therapy hysterectomy and had no residual tumor. This brings the complete pathologic response to three patients out of five.

The two-year disease-specific survival rate for the entire cohort was 53.3%. All cancer deaths were related to metastatic failure in this advanced patient population, and local control was maintained.

The toxicity that occurred during treatment was mild, including grade 1 diarrhea that was easily controlled with symptomatic management and one case of grade 2 bladder cystitis in a patient with bladder involvement. No short-term or long-term treatment-related complications were seen at grades $\geq$3. These early results suggest that LRT is generally well tolerated when applied to the pelvic region and confirm similar observations of low toxicity for palliative GRID therapy in unspecified pelvic tumors [5].

The overall results also suggest high complete response rates without brachytherapy (as shown in the pathologic response data) and high local control in the pelvis with definitive LRT and cERT for advanced cervical cancer. The experience gained from these early results for cervical cancer confirms prior reports of high and often drastic responses and of favorable tumor control in other advanced/bulky malignancies, such as head and neck cancers treated with GRID therapy [17, 18, 28]. However, these encouraging outcomes need confirmation through rigorous studies of larger patient cohorts and controlled clinical trials.

The variable and often rapid volumetric tumor response during therapy seen in this pilot series emphasizes the need for image guidance and close intratreatment response monitoring in LRT, and likely for SFRT in general. This is critical to prevent toxicity caused by tumor and normal tissue shifts and to prevent geographic misses and inconsistency in the LRT delivery, particularly in an anatomic region of significant target and normal tissue mobility and when using an SFRT schedule involving more than one fraction, as was the case in this series. Adaptive replanning was necessary for seven of the ten patients and was needed twice for one patient. The timing of the adaptive replanning tended to be variable. It was required after an average of 16 fractions but had a wide range of 11–23 fractions and was deployed when tumor volumes had regressed by an average of 43% (range: 23%–83%).

*7.2.1.2 Other gynecologic tumors*

Overall, over 37 women with cervical cancer and other bulky gynecological tumors which were unsuitable for conventional treatment have been treated with LRT at the ICI to date. These include patients with advanced/recurrent vulvar cancers, uterine carcinomas and sarcomas, and ovarian cancers. These patients commonly presented with advanced disease, frequent bladder involvement, and lymph node involvement, including para-aortic node involvement. The outcomes of these cases mirror those of the cervical cancer experience, with high local tumor control and minimal toxicity.

### 7.2.2 LRT in lung cancer

Lung cancer constitutes another malignancy that creates a major challenge for the delivery of sufficient radiation doses, which is frequently constrained by dose-limiting nearby critical normal structures. Therefore, local control remains a major challenge in lung cancer [32, 33]. In 2021, 1 898 160 new cancer cases and 608 570 cancer deaths are projected to occur in the United States, despite recent public health achievements in smoking cessation and improved advances in early detection and treatment [34]. Despite this progress, we still see patients with large tumors unfit for conventional management.

The initial ICI lung cancer experience consisted of a case series of ten lung cancer patients with non-small cell lung cancer (NSCLC) [15], which was preceded by an initial case report of a patient with bulky lung cancer treated successfully with LRT [25]. In this case, a 72-year-old male with a stage IIIA, 6 cm left upper lobe NSCLC was treated with an LRT dose of 18 Gy, followed by cERT. The tumor responded rapidly and the patient remained disease-free six years later. He experienced no toxicity except transient mild focal skin erythema.

The subsequent series of ten NSCLC patients [15] constituted the first published cohort of lung cancer patients treated with LRT. Our work builds on the prior experience with lung cancer using GRID therapy that was reported in several multidisease studies [5, 8], although the outcome statistics of the lung cancer patients were not separately reported within the multidisease case series. These GRID therapy case series have nevertheless provided indirect evidence that SFRT is effective in palliative treatment for local control in the treatment of thoracic tumors and in some cases for definitive curative-intent treatment.

In the ICI lung cancer series [15], all patients had a pathologic diagnosis of NSCLC, were not surgical candidates, and had locally advanced or recurrent disease with poor prognosis after failing systemic therapy. Five patients had stage III and five had stage IV lung disease (i.e. with distant metastases). Patients with prior chest radiation were excluded. Nine patients were male, one was female, and their mean age was 71 years (range: 49–87 years).

Tumors were bulky at presentation, ranging from 5 to 14 cm (mean: 8 cm). CT-based volumetric assessment (at the time of simulation) showed pre-radiation therapy tumor volumes ranging from 46 $cm^3$ to 487 $cm^3$ (mean: 195 $cm^3$).

LRT was given first at a dose of 18 Gy in a single fraction to the vertex tumor volume (VTV), and the dose to the peripheral GTV was constrained to 3 Gy using VMAT with 6 MeV photons (figure 7.5). Daily CBCT image guidance was employed. For the LRT fraction, the number of vertices ranged from three to seven, and the median center-to-center vertex separation was 3.6 cm. Image guidance and respiratory motion management with an optical surface management system were used for treatment delivery. LRT was immediately followed with cERT at a definitive dose of 45.0–59.4 Gy, delivered in 1.8–2 Gy fractions. Seven of the ten patients additionally received a boost delivered via IMRT or SBRT to the residual tumor. Adaptive therapy for rapid tumor regression was required in all patients at variable times during the treatment course.

All but one patient had an objective tumor response at the end of radiation therapy (based on pre-therapy planning CT and a CBCT image obtained at the time of the last treatment fraction), with variable tumor volume reduction ranging from 15% to 83% (mean: 52%), corresponding to a mean tumor diameter decrease from 7.7 cm to 5.4 cm in the nine patients who responded. In the non-responder, who had a large cavitary lesion, the tumor progressed.

The imaging follow-up period ranged from one month to 71 months (median six months). Nine of the ten patients had 18FDG PET/CT, which was used as a baseline and for follow-up assessment.

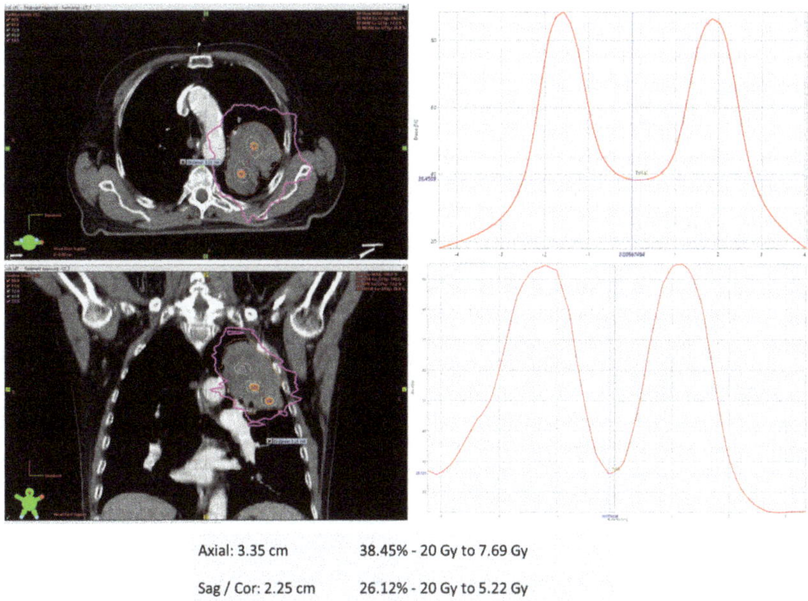


**Figure 7.5.** Dose distribution in LRT for lung cancer. Peak (vertices) and valley distributions are shown in the axial and coronal planes. The same valley dose can be obtained with less separation between the vertices in the coronal plane than in the axial plane. This is due to the position of the leaves with respect to the orientation of the treatment plane in the patient.

Of the ten patients, five were alive 18–86 months after treatment completion, three with sustained metabolic tumor response and two with partial metabolic response and extra-thoracic disease. While PET/CT imaging showed grade 1 pneumonitis, there was no clinical toxicity at grades >1.

The outcome results in this series are consistent with the earlier GRID therapy experience gained in several studies. Neuner *et al* [8] treated a mixed population of 78 patients with predominately head and neck and lung cancer using both collimator- and MLC-based GRID therapy techniques, followed by cERT in 80% of these patients. While the lung cancer population was not analyzed separately, the investigators found overall high symptomatic response and minimal toxicity, and this result agrees with our findings. Somaiah *et al* [35] treated ten patients with locally advanced bulky (>6 cm) NSCLC with 15 Gy using GRID therapy, followed by cERT at 36 Gy in 12 fractions. They reported a complete response in 71% and a partial response to chest pain in 29%, and a partial tumor response based on imaging in 90% of patients. No toxicities were reported at grades >2.

In our LRT lung cancer case series, the median overall survival is 16 months (range: 4–86) months. Five of the ten patients are alive at 18–86 months (median: 25 months) post-therapy. Three of these have a continued complete metabolic response according to PET–CT results, despite having a residual mass in CT imaging (with a 48% average volume decrease). The other two are alive with disease outside the chest and partial metabolic response of the treated tumor. ICI has now treated more than 30 lung cancer patients using LRT, and our results have generally been consistent with this reported series.

A very recent European series presented at the 2021 ASTRO Annual Meeting [20] confirmed our results. Eleven NSCLC patients with bulky unresectable tumors or medical inoperability, who were unfit for systemic neoadjuvant therapy, were treated with LRT of 15 Gy in one fraction. The LRT was delivered using the VMAT technique and IGRT with a minimum of four vertices separated by 2.5–3 cm. The valley dose was <5 Gy. LRT was followed by a more hypofractionated cERT regimen than in Amendola *et al*'s [15] series. A dose of 55 Gy was given in 20 fractions. Concurrent chemotherapy was given to nine of the ten patients.

As in Amendola *et al*'s [15] series, adaptive replanning was commonly needed. It was required in half of the patients within ten days of the LRT fraction. Six of eight evaluable patients had >50% tumor regression, including two patients with complete metabolic response according to PET–CT scans, and two patients had a partial response. Two patients died in the early post-therapy phase, one of infectious pneumonia (six weeks after therapy) and one of hemoptysis (three months after therapy).

These results, obtained using a similar LRT regimen, generally confirm Amendola *et al*'s [15] observations of rapid tumor response, the need for adaptive replanning, high response, and low toxicity.

Based on these observations, ICI currently considers patients with bulky (>5 cm) inoperable stage IIB, IIIA, or IIIB NSCLCs (without prior treatment), patients with recurrent lung cancer after chemo- or immunotherapy failure or prior irradiation, and patients with metastatic lung cancer for palliation eligible for LRT.

In general, ICI uses two regimens: LRT of 18 Gy followed cERT, as previously described above and in our report [15], and LRT SBRT, an extreme hypofractionated technique that delivers five fractions of SBRT at 5 Gy to the periphery of the GTV and 50–60 Gy in five fractions (10–12 Gy per fraction) of SFRT to the vertex volume, as shown in figure 7.6.

## 7.3 Emerging experience with LRT in other tumors and related techniques

Our overall experience has shown that in general, voluminous tumors in almost any location can be debulked using LRT, under the conditions that the low peripheral target dose is maintained and the dose to organs at risk is kept within current recommendations using the abovementioned techniques (see also chapter 10). An example of a bulky liver metastasis that originated from cervical cancer and its rapid metabolic response after LRT are illustrated in figure 7.7.

Based on our initial experience, LRT should be used as the initial treatment and should be immediately followed by cERT and systemic therapy, either chemotherapy or immunotherapy, depending on the tumor type and pathology. The specific tumor types of the 106 patients treated to date with LRT at ICI are presented in figure 7.1.

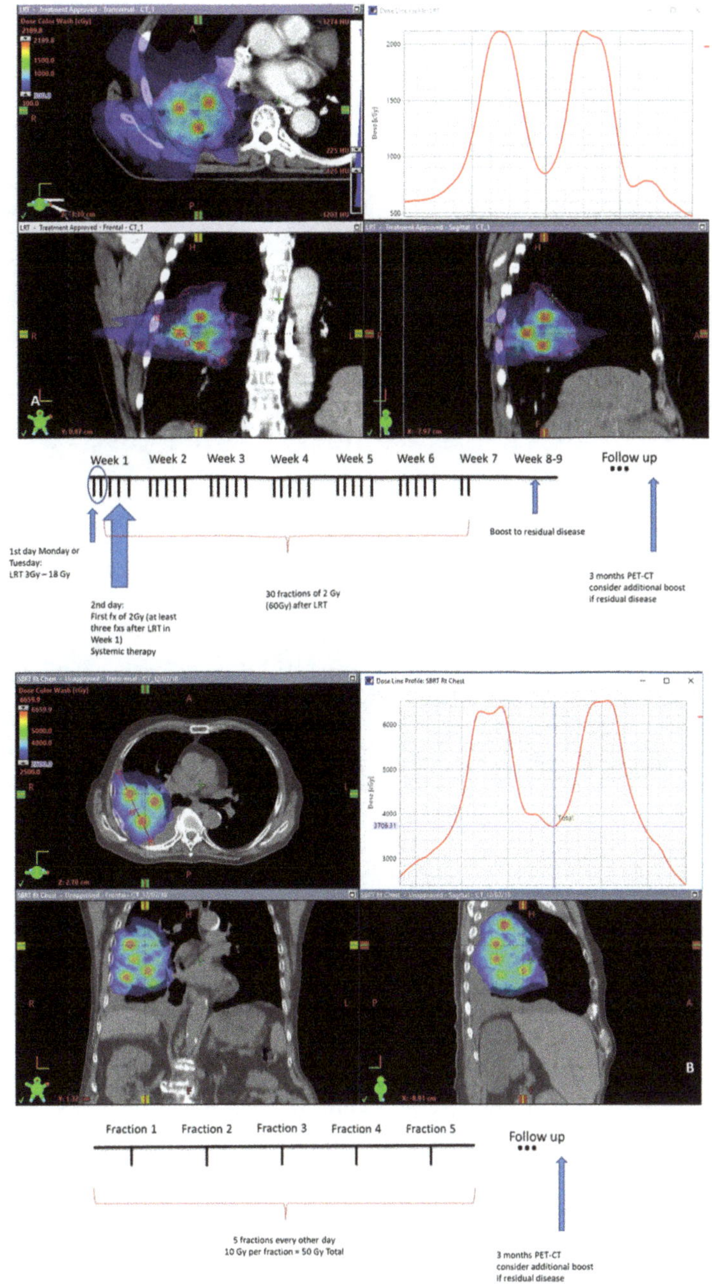


**Figure 7.6.** Comparison of plans developed for classic LRT and LRT SBRT. Left panel: an LRT treatment regimen of 18 Gy given to the vertex tumo in a single fraction together with 3 Gy given to the periphery of the target, followed by conventional IMRT. Right panel: an LRT SBRT extreme hypofractionation regimen, delivering 10–12 Gy to the VTV and 5 Gy to the target periphery every other day. This regimen is used as a palliative tool for dose escalation and does not produce the low valley dose of classic LRT. The respective fractionation schemes are shown below each panel. Adapted from [15], with permission from Cureus.

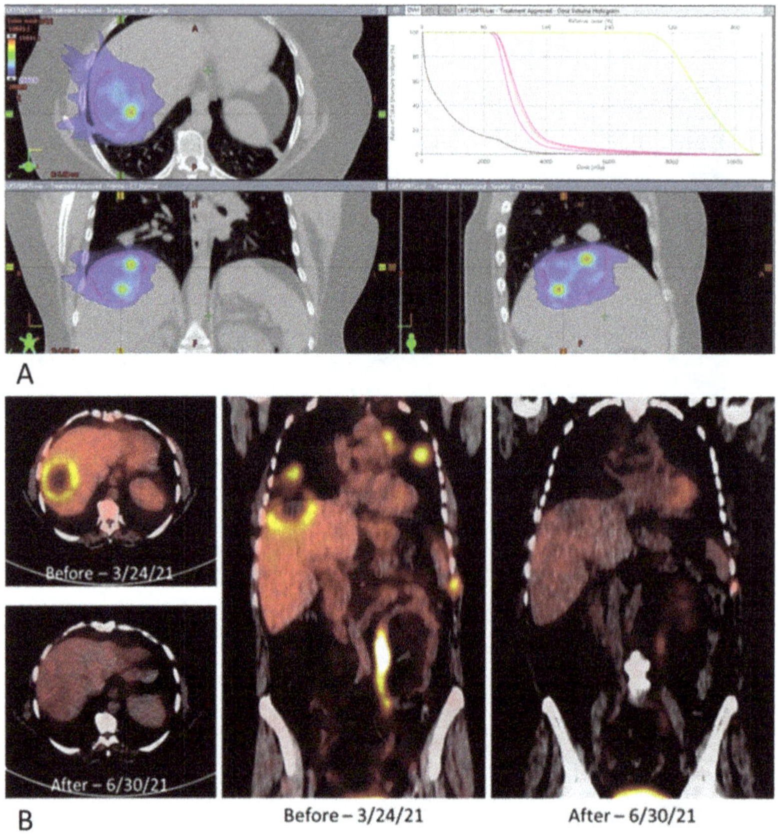


**Figure 7.7.** Bulky single liver metastasis from cervical cancer 50-year-old female with stage IIA HPV-positive endocervical adenocarcinoma, who later developed a bulky liver metastasis. A. The tumor GTV 127.13 cc (~ 6.2 cm diameter). The prescription dose is 15 Gy for 4 fractions to the VTV and 5 Gy to the target periphery (25 Gy total). The 15 Gy to the VTV are given with 4 vertices of 1 cm diameter each. The total dose to the VTV is 75 Gy. The ratio of VTV/GTV is 1.4%. B. At follow-up 3 months after LRT, repeat PET/CT shows complete metabolic response. The patient died of brain metastases and with local control in her liver metastasis.

Our early experience with LRT in locally advanced, voluminous primary *head and neck cancer* suggests that it appears safe and effective when delivered at high vertex doses. Our LRT experience is consistent overall with that reported in several case series of primary head and neck cancer treated using GRID-based SFRT [17–19]. Our experience in *sarcoma* mirrors the high response rates to GRID therapy observed by Mohiuddin *et al* [21, 22] and Snider *et al* [29]. However, the SFRT clinical experience in individual disease sites requires confirmation by prospective clinical trials with consistent and standardized dosimetric parameters, as described in chapter 10 and in the recent white paper on the technical implementation of LRT [12].

Partial tumor irradiation, a concept akin to SFRT, has also been recently investigated. Tubin and colleagues [36, 37] developed an SBRT regimen for partial tumor irradiation targeting the hypoxic regions (SBRT for PArtial Tumor irradiation of unresectable bulky tumors targeting exclusively their HYpoxic segment, 'SBRT PATHY') in bulky tumors, assessed by PET/CT and contrast CT, with the goal of generating intratumoral bystander effects and distant abscopal effects. The hypoxic region received one to three factions of 10–12 Gy each, and the remainder of the tumor, involved lymph nodes, and metastases were not irradiated. Patients with unresectable bulky malignancies located in the chest, the abdomen, or the head and neck area were included. The local response (bystander response) rate was 96%. The response rate in non-irradiated tumor sites (i.e. the abscopal response) was 52%. There was no early (acute) or late toxicity. The tumor volumes regressed by 30%–100% (median: 70%), and 87% of patients remained progression free at a 4–20 (median: 9.4) month follow-up. The investigators are currently conducting a prospective trial of this regimen.

Other concepts related to LRT have since been proposed. Duriseti *et al* [38] reported a dosimetry and quality assurance feasibility study of a variation of LRT using extreme hypofractionation, named Lattice SBRT. In a cohort of CT simulation data sets of 12 large (>10 cm) deep-seated tumors, plans were computed to deliver 20 Gy in five fractions to the entire tumor target with a simultaneous integrated boost of 66.7 Gy to vertices arranged in regular geometric patterns within the target volume. This regimen was characterized by significantly higher valley doses (related to the contribution from the whole-field dose) than the classic LRT described above. No cERT was used. The investigators have since reported 20 patients (22 tumors) treated with this technique in a phase I trial [39]. The tumor volumes decreased by 2.4%–91.7% (median: 24.4%) at a median follow-up imaging interval of 1.8 months. Short-term toxicity was found to be acceptable, but included a grade 4 acute toxicity (urosepsis during the treatment course in a patient with bulky retroperitoneal leiomyosarcoma with ureteral involvement and percutaneous nephrostomies). Since then, an additional acute grade 4 toxicity consisting of tumor lysis syndrome has been reported [40].

Our clinical experience highlights LRT's ability to flexibly adapt the dose heterogeneity pattern to the individual patient. Each LRT treatment plan should be carefully individualized to the tumor geometry and the proximity, type, and radiation tolerance of critical normal tissues. Treatment planning and reporting guidelines have been established [9, 12] (chapter 10) that serve as a helpful guide for building a clinical LRT program. The experience gained from the early clinical outcomes [13–16, 25. 41, 42] has demonstrated the feasibility, safety, and low toxicity of LRT applications for both palliation and up-front tumor boosting/debulking. The unexpectedly high tumor responses seen with LRT are consistent with the observations made since the beginning of the megavoltage SFRT era that are well demonstrated by the GRID experience. In addition, the early LRT experience has established data for the tumor response velocity and molecular response characteristics associated with SFRT. In conjunction with the promising preclinical experimental findings for the use of LRT and GRID (detailed further in chapter 2), current clinical observations with LRT support the notion of bystander and immunomodulatory effects that may contribute to the tumor response seen with heterogenous irradiation in SFRT.

The guidelines, recommendations, and parameters presented in this article are derived from limited clinical LRT experience and are provisional in nature. As pointed out by Drs. Norman Coleman and Mansoor Ahmed in an editorial [43] following the inaugural Radiosurgery Society—NCI Workshop: '… *we emphasize that medical treatments that are technically feasible are not necessarily clinically indicated…*' '*Rigorous clinical studies are imperative to advance the experience from the small SFRT community to systemic proof. Until such time, for each patient to be considered for SFRT, the merits and risks must be strictly, individually justified.*'

## 7.4 Knowledge gaps and future perspectives

Our successful experience with LRT in gynecologic cancer, which has converted patients in our cervical cancer series from a palliative status to operability with a high probability of complete pathologic response and subsequent sustained tumor control [13, 14] may serve as a hypothesis-generating finding. This SFRT experience gained from pelvic tumors is supported by the same high pathologic response findings as those observed for the use of GRID SFRT in head and neck cancer [5, 18, 19] and sarcoma [21, 23], and supports the concept of studying SFRT as a preoperative modality in wider patient populations.

Despite encouraging early clinical results, knowledge gaps abound in the LRT field. The optimal dose heterogeneity pattern and the ideal distribution of valley and peak doses within the tumor target that may generate an optimal tumor response have not been experimentally or clinically determined; these require meticulous study and clinical translation.

While concurrent chemotherapy has been successfully used with both GRID- and LRT-based SFRT [14, 15, 17–19], the role, timing, and types of systemic therapy require further exploration. In particular, experience with combinations of SFRT and immunotherapy is minimal [42], and well-designed prospective studies are needed.

## 7.5 Conclusions

SFRT's concept of covering the whole or partial tumor with an inhomogeneous radiation dose provides a potential new dimension to the field of radiation oncology. While its clinical use to date has been limited to select centers, and it has most commonly been aimed at palliative or recurrent cases, its clinical use is rapidly increasing. SFRT has the potential to treat primary cancers, such as head and neck, lung, gynecologic cancer, and sarcoma definitively with curative intent. LRT may further individualize the SFRT approach and further reduce normal tissue dose. Clinical trials incorporating SFRT as an up-front boost or as the primary radiotherapy component are warranted. The future application of the SFRT concept will depend on the refinement of its implementation and technique together with a fuller understanding of the biological mechanisms underlying the tumoral and normal tissue responses.

## References

[1] Köhler A 1909 Röntgentiefen Therapie mit Massendosen *Münch. Med. Wochenschr.* **56** 2314–16 (in German)

[2] Laissue J A, Blattmann H and Slatkin D N 2012 Alban Köhler (1874–1947): inventor of grid therapy *Z. Med. Phys.* **22** 90–9 (in German)

[3] Marks H 1952 Clinical experience with irradiation through a grid *Radiology* **58** 338–42

[4] Mohiuddin M, Curtis D L and Grizos W T *et al* 1990 Palliative treatment of advanced cancer using multiple nonconfluent pencil beam radiation. A pilot study *Cancer* **66** 114–8

[5] Mohiuddin M, Fujita M and Regine W F *et al* 1999 High-dose spatially-fractionated radiation (GRID): a new paradigm in the management of advanced cancers *Int. J. Radiat. Oncol. Biol. Phys.* **45** 721–7

[6] Mohiuddin M, Stevens J H and Reiff J E *et al* 1996 Spatially fractionated (GRID) radiation for palliative treatment of advanced cancer *Radiat. Oncol. Invest.* **4** 41–7

[7] Ha J K, Zhang G and Naqvi S A *et al* 2006 Feasibility of delivering grid therapy using a multileaf collimator *Med. Phys.* **33** 76–82

[8] Neuner G, Mohiuddin M M and Vander Walde N *et al* 2012 High-dose spatially fractionated GRID radiation therapy (SFGRT): a comparison of treatment outcomes with Cerrobend vs. MLC SFGRT *Int. J. Radiat. Oncol. Biol. Phys.* **82** 1642–9

[9] Wu X, Ahmed M M and Wright J *et al* 2010 On modern technical approaches of three-dimensional high-dose Lattice radiotherapy (LRT *Cureus* **2** e9

[10] Dilmanian F A, Eley J G and Krishnan S 2015 Minibeam therapy with protons and light ions: physical feasibility and potential to reduce radiation side effects and to facilitate hypofractionation *Int. J. Radiat. Oncol. Biol. Phys.* **92** 469–74

[11] Gao M, Mohiuddin M M and Hartsell W F *et al* 2018 Spatially fractionated (GRID) radiation therapy using proton pencil beam scanning (PBS): Feasibility study and clinical implementation *Med. Phys.* **45** 1645–53

[12] Wu X, Perez N and Zheng Y *et al* 2020 The technical and clinical implementation of LATTICE radiation therapy (LRT) *Radiat. Res.* **194** 737–46

[13] Amendola B E, Perez N and Amendola M *et al* 2010 Lattice radiotherapy with RapidArc for treatment of gynecological tumors: dosimetric and early clinical evaluations *Cureus* **2** 1–6

[14] Amendola B E, Perez N C and Mayr N A *et al* 2020 Spatially fractionated radiation therapy using lattice radiation in far-advanced bulky cervical cancer: a clinical and molecular imaging and outcome study *Radiat. Res.* **194** 724–36

[15] Amendola B E, Perez N C and Wu X *et al* 2019 Safety and efficacy of lattice radiotherapy in voluminous non-small cell lung cancer *Cureus* **11** e4263

[16] Blanco Suarez J M, Amendola B E and Perez N *et al* 2015 The use of lattice radiation therapy (LRT) in the treatment of bulky tumors: a case report of a large metastatic mixed mullerian ovarian tumor *Cureus* **7** e389

[17] Choi J I, Daniels J and Cohen D *et al* 2019 Clinical outcomes of spatially fractionated GRID radiotherapy in the treatment of bulky tumors of the head and neck *Cureus* **11** e4637

[18] Huhn J L, Regine W F and Valentino J P *et al* 2006 Spatially fractionated GRID radiation treatment of advanced neck disease associated with head and neck cancer *Technol. Cancer Res. Treat.* **5** 607–12

[19] Penagaricano J A, Moros E G and Ratanatharathorn V *et al* 2010 Evaluation of spatially fractionated radiotherapy (GRID) and definitive chemoradiotherapy with curative intent for locally advanced squamous cell carcinoma of the head and neck: initial response rates and toxicity *Int. J. Radiat. Oncol. Biol. Phys.* **76** 1369–75

[20] Larrea L, Gonzalez V and Antonini P *et al* 2021 Lattice radiotherapy (LRT)-spatially fractionated radiotherapy (SFRT): advanced non-small cell lung cancer (NSCLC): early experience (abst.) *Int. J. Radiat. Oncol. Biol. Phys.* **111** e443

[21] Mohiuddin M, Memon M and Nobah A *et al* 2014 Locally advanced high-grade extremity soft tissue sarcoma: response with novel approach to neoadjuvant chemoradiation using induction spatially fractionated GRID radiotherapy (SFGRT) (abst.) *J. Clin. Oncol.* **32** 10575

[22] Mohiuddin M, Miller T and Ronjon P *et al* 2009 Spatially fractionated grid radiation (SFGRT): a novel approach in the management of recurrent and unresectable soft tissue sarcoma (abstr) *Int. J. Radiat. Oncol. Biol. Phys.* **75** S526

[23] Snider J W, Molitoris J and Shy S *et al* 2019 *Radiat. Res.* **194** 707–14 Spatially fractionated GRID radiotherapy prior to neoadjuvant conventionally fractionated radiotherapy for very high-risk soft tissue and osteo-sarcomas: promising pathologic response with safe dose escalation (abst.) *The Connective Tissue Oncology Society (CTOS) Meeting (Tokyo, Japan, 2019)* https://www.ctos.org/Portals/0/PDF/2019%20CTOS%20Final%20Program.pdf

[24] Zhang H, Wu X and Zhang X *et al* 2020 Photon GRID radiation therapy: a physics and dosimetry white paper from the radiosurgery society (RSS) GRID-lattice-microbeam-FLASH radiotherapy working group *Radiat. Res.* **194** 665–77

[25] Amendola B E, Perez N C and Wu X *et al* 2018 Improved outcome of treating locally advanced lung cancer with the use of Lattice Radiotherapy (LRT): a case report *Clin. Transl. Radiat. Oncol.* **9** 68–71

[26] Kudrimoti M, Regine W F and Huhn J L *et al* 2002 Spatially fractionated radiation therapy (SFR) in the palliation of large bulky (>8 cm) melanomas (abstr) *Int. J. Radiat. Oncol. Biol. Phys.* **54** 342–3

[27] Mohiuddin M, Park H and Hallmeyer S *et al* 2015 High-dose radiation as a dramatic, immunological primer in locally advanced melanoma *Cureus* **7** e417

[28] Penagaricano J A, Griffin R and Corry P *et al* 2009 Spatially fractionated (GRID) therapy for large and bulky tumors *J. Ark. Med. Soc.* **105** 263–5

[29] Snider J W, Molitoris J and Shyu S *et al* 2020 Spatially fractionated radiotherapy (GRID) prior to standard neoadjuvant conventionally fractionated radiotherapy for bulky, high-risk soft tissue and osteosarcomas: feasibility, safety, and promising pathologic response rates *Radiat. Res.* **194** 707–14

[30] Amendola B E, Perez N and Amendola M A *et al* 2020 The use of lattice radiation therapy in patients with voluminous tumors (abstr): *Int. J. Radiat. Oncol. Biol. Phys.* **108** e520

[31] Sung H, Ferlay J and Siegel R L *et al* 2021 Global cancer statistics 2020: GLOBOCAN estimates of incidence and mortality worldwide for 36 cancers in 185 countries *CA Cancer J. Clin.* **71** 209–49

[32] Jegadeesh N, Liu Y and Gillespie T *et al* 2016 Evaluating intensity-modulated radiation therapy in locally advanced non-small-cell lung cancer: results from the national cancer data base *Clin. Lung Cancer* **17** 398–405

[33] Movsas B, Hu C and Sloan J *et al* 2016 Quality of life analysis of a radiation dose-escalation study of patients with non-small-cell lung cancer: a secondary analysis of the radiation therapy oncology group 0617 randomized clinical trial *JAMA Oncol.* **2** 359–67

[34] Siegel R L, Miller K D and Fuchs H E *et al* 2021 Cancer statistics, 2021 *CA Cancer J. Clin.* **71** 7–33

[35] Somaiah N, Warrington J and Taylor H *et al* 2008 High dose spatially fractionated radiotherapy (SFR) using a megavoltage GRID in advanced lung tumors: preliminary experience in UK (abst) *Int. J. Radiat. Oncol. Biol. Phys.* **72** S490

[36] Tubin S, Ashdown M and Jeremic B 2019 Time-synchronized immune-guided SBRT partial bulky tumor irradiation targeting hypoxic segment while sparing the peritumoral immune microenvironment *Radiat. Oncol.* **14** 220

[37] Tubin S, Popper H H and Brcic L 2019 Novel stereotactic body radiation therapy (SBRT)-based partial tumor irradiation targeting hypoxic segment of bulky tumors (SBRT-PATHY): improvement of the radiotherapy outcome by exploiting the bystander and abscopal effects *Radiat. Oncol.* **14** 21

[38] Duriseti S, Kavanaugh J and Goddu S *et al* 2021 Spatially fractionated stereotactic body radiation therapy (Lattice) for large tumors *Adv. Radiat. Oncol.* **6** 100639

[39] Duriseti S, Kavanaugh J A and Szymanski J *et al* 2021 LITE SABR M1: a phase I trial of Lattice stereotactic body radiotherapy for large tumors *Radiother. Oncol.* **167** 317–22

[40] Schiff J P, Spraker M B and Duriseti S *et al* 2022 Tumor lysis syndrome in a patient with metastatic endometrial cancer treated with lattice stereotactic body radiation therapy *Adv. Radiat. Oncol.* **7** 100797

[41] Amendola B E, Perez N and Amendola M A *et al* 2019 Single institution experience in the use of lattice radiosurgery in voluminous tumors (abstr) *Radiosurgery Society Scientific Meeting 2019* (abst.) https://www.cureus.com/channels/therss/meetings/49/abstracts

[42] Jiang L, Li X and Zhang J *et al* 2021 Combined high-dose LATTICE radiation therapy and immune checkpoint blockade for advanced bulky tumors: the concept and a case report *Front. Oncol.* **10** 548132

[43] Coleman C N and Ahmed M M 2019 Implementation of new biology-based radiation therapy technology: when is it ready so 'perfect makes practice?' *Int. J. Radiat. Oncol. Biol. Phys.* **105** 934–37

# Chapter 8

# Proton beam spatially fractionated radiation therapy: clinical data

**Ronald Chow, Minglei Kang and Charles B Simone, II**

There is increasing interest in delivering spatially fractionated radiation therapy (SFRT) due to its unique potential to reduce normal tissue toxicities or even improve tumor control. By combining the potential biological advantages of SFRT with the physical advantages of proton therapy (which allows for a rapid radiation dose falloff beyond the target volume), the delivery of SFRT via proton therapy holds great potential to further reduce toxicities or to allow for safer radiation dose escalation. As yet, the data for proton SFRT are quite limited. This chapter assesses the potential clinical advantages and pitfalls of proton SFRT; details the clinical experience to date using proton therapy to deliver GRID, minibeam radiation therapy, and FLASH radiation therapy; and discusses the clinical trial roadmap for proton FLASH.

## 8.1 Introduction and rationale for delivering spatially fractionated modalities with proton therapy

Traditional photon radiation therapy can cause acute and late toxicities due to the deposition of ionizing radiation in normal tissues surrounding the target volume being treated. As a result, clinical practice often reduces the dose of radiation therapy that is delivered compared to the dose that may most effectively optimize tumor local control, thus hindering the utilization of radiation therapy for curative purposes. The toxicities to normal tissues associated with photon therapy are often further magnified in the setting of today's chemotherapy [1].

Proton therapy may be an effective alternative way to reduce acute and late toxicities compared with traditional photon therapy. On a molecular level, protons are heavier than photons and are charged particles; they therefore have different physical properties than photons or electrons [2]. While photons often experience an exponential attenuation with increased depth after the initial few centimeters of

doi:10.1088/978-0-7503-4046-5ch8

entrance and peak dose and therefore deposit their energy in normal tissues beyond the tumor [3], protons can be delivered with precise energies to a desired depth known as the Bragg peak. Beyond this depth, protons can have no exit dose, thus sparing critical structures distal to the desired target volume from unnecessary irradiation. As a result, reduced toxicities and/or improved clinical outcomes have been observed for proton therapy compared to photon therapy for patients with head and neck cancers [4], esophageal cancers [5], lung cancers [6], liver cancers [7], and pediatric malignancies [8]. Reductions in toxicities and hospitalizations [9] and better preservation of quality of life [10] across multiple solid malignancies have also been reported for patients receiving proton therapy compared with those receiving photon therapy.

## 8.2 Current limitations of proton therapy

To date, proton therapy has not been as widely available as photon therapy, likely due the significant up-front and ongoing expenses associated with this technology. As a result, with only 39 proton centers in operation in the United States as of early 2022, proton therapy has been administered for fewer than 2% of annual external beam radiation therapy treatment courses completed in the United States to date. Currently, developments in accelerator technology are focusing on lower initial investment costs, with an increase in the proliferation of single-room treatment facilities or facilities without a full 360° gantry [11].

Proton therapy is also more sensitive to organ motion or other anatomical changes than photon therapy. As such, there is more limited experience to date using proton therapy for stereotactic body radiation therapy (SBRT) delivery relative to photon therapy, as intrafractional and interfractional variations in organ motion are generally smeared out when delivering more prolonged treatment courses. Furthermore, accounting for and, when necessary, mitigating tumor motion is often critical for proton therapy when delivering shorter courses of treatment [12]. The data supporting proton therapy as an effective treatment option when delivered as stereotactic body radiation therapy in five or fewer fractions have increased over the last few years [13], including a recently reported small, single-institution randomized trial comparison of proton versus photon stereotactic body radiation therapy for early-stage non-small cell lung cancer (NSCLC), which showed favorable outcomes with proton therapy [14]. These lessons with proton therapy homogenously delivered to target volumes in the clinic in five or fewer fractions can be directly applied to SFRT delivered via proton therapy that is often administered in just a single fraction.

## 8.3 Clinical experience with proton GRID therapy

Historically, GRID therapy has been delivered using single-field photon-beam grids irradiated from a single direction. GRID plans are generated to achieve dose distributions with high and low doses, termed peaks and valleys, respectively, in an attempt to better spare normal tissues from radiation-induced toxicities.

The delivery of GRID with protons rather than photons, however, has several potential advantages. With photon-based GRID therapy, select patients may not be amenable to therapy due to the beam entry and exit angles and due to critical organs at risk that might receive significant irradiation doses. Proton-based GRID therapy, in contrast, allows for rapid dose falloff after the Bragg peak, thus better sparing normal tissues beyond the target volume.

Early reports have demonstrated the feasibility of using protons to deliver a single field of spatially fractionated GRID therapy. Investigators from the Northwestern Medicine Proton Center in Chicago, IL performed a feasibility and clinical implementation study of the use of pencil beam scanning (PBS) proton therapy to deliver GRID therapy. Their feasibility study showed that proton GRID therapy can provide a more uniform beamlet dose within the tumor and can better spare normal tissues distal to the tumor compared with photon GRID. They employed their technique to treat four patients using proton GRID, and the treatment was well tolerated [15].

These investigators subsequently reported on ten patients with large and bulky tumors resistant to prior treatments who could benefit from SFRT but were not suitable candidates for photon-based GRID therapy and were instead treated with proton-based GRID therapy. These patients received 15–20 cobalt Gray equivalent using a single-proton GRID field with 7–51 beamlets, followed in eight of the ten patients by adjuvant radiation therapy (range 13.7–63.8 Gy). This treatment was well tolerated, and 80% of the cohort had tumor regression and/or local symptom improvement [16].

Uniquely, protons can offer the opportunity to deliver GRID therapy using interlacing and crossfiring with millimeter-wide proton beams covering the desired target volume [17]. An early proof-of-principle report on the delivery of interlacing–crossfiring geometry for proton GRID therapy was authored by investigators from Sweden, who showed that a nearly homogeneous dose distribution is achievable in a target volume by crossfiring proton-beamlet grids while maintaining the grid pattern of dose distribution at the desired depth [18].

## 8.4 Proton minibeam radiation therapy

Microbeam radiation therapy is another advanced spatially fractionated radiation modality that has the potential to reduce normal tissue toxicities. Microbeam radiation therapy combines the benefits of spatially fractionating the irradiation dose (to reduce normal tissue toxicities) with extremely narrow beams of $\leqslant$100 μm that have also been shown to reduce the expected normal tissue toxicities [19]. Although a significantly improved tolerance to extreme doses of radiation therapy can be achieved when micrometer-scale beams are used, extremely high dose rates are needed to maintain the patterns of peaks and valleys. As a result, such an approach is currently limited to very select centers with synchroton light facilities [20], and, to date, is lacking appreciable clinical implementation.

In contrast, minibeam radiation therapy may also allow for normal tissue toxicity reduction while still being more feasible to deliver clinically. While the field width is still only a fraction of that delivered with conventional radiation therapy, minibeam radiation therapy uses wider field sizes than microbeam radiation therapy, typically 400–700 μm. Investigators from the Orsay Proton Therapy Center recently implemented minibeam radiation therapy delivered with proton beams. Preclinical data show significant normal tissue sparing in the skin and brain [21, 22], perhaps even accompanied by improved tumor killing [23].

With an eye toward clinical treatments using minibeam radiation therapy, the delivery of minibeam radiation therapy through proton therapy may be optimal compared to photon-based minibeam delivery in allowing for a more localized release of the dose. Proton minibeam radiation therapy can be delivered with either passive scattering proton therapy or PBS proton therapy that employs magnetically scanned multiple pencil beams over the target volume while modulating the beam, which can better allow spatial fractionation to be maintained at shallow depths. Clinical data for proton therapy microbeam radiation therapy and minibeam radiation therapy are lacking at this time.

## 8.5 Proton FLASH: rationale, preclinical data, and the first treated patient

Recently, the delivery of ultrahigh-dose-rate radiation therapy to achieve a FLASH effect has been introduced as an option to further reduce toxicities. Whereas linear accelerators and proton accelerators typically deliver 0.06–0.40 Gy $s^{-1}$ and 1.67 Gy $s^{-1}$, respectively, FLASH involves the delivery of radiation therapy at dose rates in excess of 40 Gy $s^{-1}$, as described in more detail in chapters 4 and 22.

Research into FLASH, while rapidly proliferating, is still relatively sparse, but the mechanism by which it spares normal tissues from toxicity is postulated to be multifactorial. FLASH can mimic hypoxia in normal tissues and therefore prevent free radicals from reacting with oxygen, forming damaging peroxyl radicals, and increasing normal tissue radioresistance [24, 25]. In addition, FLASH radiotherapy (RT) may not cause G2 cell cycle arrest as profoundly as conventional-dose-rate radiation therapy, and it thus results in less damage to normal tissues [26]. Furthermore, FLASH may cause fewer double-strand DNA breaks than conventional-dose-rate radiation therapy and may thus lead to a differential inflammatory response [27, 28]. Finally, FLASH may be associated with greater preservation of normal stem cells [29, 30].

The preponderance of preclinical studies to date suggest that FLASH is equally efficacious but can decrease the likelihood of toxicities relative to conventional-dose-rate radiation therapy. In a pivotal study by Favaudon *et al* [31], C57BL/6J mice were irradiated with either conventional-dose-rate or ultrahigh-dose-rate radiation therapy. Significant fibrosis was observed in mice treated with conventional-dose-rate radiation therapy, but no damage was observed in mice treated with FLASH radiation therapy. In another study by Vozenin *et al* [32], cats with locally advanced T2/T3 N0 M0 squamous cell carcinoma of the nasal planum were treated in a dose escalation trial with FLASH RT doses ranging from 25 to 41 Gy in a single fraction. All cats experienced complete responses at three and six months, and all but one cat had sustained a complete response at 16 months. No erythema, moist desquamation, fibronecrosis, hyperkeratosis, inflammatory infiltrates, or dermal remodeling were reported.

In the first human case study, FLASH was similarly reported to be effective and safe. Bourhis *et al* [33] reported on the case of a 75-year-old male with CD30+ T-cell lymphoma with ulcerative and/or painful cutaneous lesions treated with radiotherapy at 110 prior tumor sites. In an attempt to provide equivalent tumor control while limiting skin toxicities in this heavily pretreated patient, the patient was then treated with 15 Gy in a single fraction over 90 ms, or equivalently 167 Gy $s^{-1}$, which was administered to a skin tumor 3.5 cm in diameter. Tumor shrinkage began 10 days after irradiation, and complete response was observed at 36 days. Furthermore, three weeks after irradiation, only grade 1 epithelitis and transient grade 1 edema in soft tissue was observed.

Notably, the aforementioned preclinical studies and human case study employed electron FLASH, which has several inherent limitations relative to proton FLASH. Today, electron FLASH has low penetration and an inability to treat deep-seeded tumor volumes, akin to conventional-dose-rate electron therapy. Furthermore, given its less conformal dose distribution and limited field size, electron FLASH has been limited to the treatment of superficial cancers, namely skin cancers and cutaneous lymphomas [34]. Proton FLASH can overcome these limitations and deliver treatment at much greater depths within the body. Additionally, today's proton accelerators are better and more readily able to deliver FLASH RT compared with photon and electron linear accelerators that currently require significant machine manipulation in order to achieve the ultrahigh dose rates necessary for the induction of a FLASH effect, and the latter are also limited by field-size restrictions [35]. These are the driving factors that explain why the first clinical trial to investigate the FLASH effect in humans using ultrahigh-dose-rate radiation therapy was delivered with protons and not electrons or photons.

## 8.6 Proton FLASH: methods of delivery

At present, the easiest way to deliver FLASH using proton therapy is to intentionally place the Bragg peak outside, or behind, the patient (figure 8.1). This is termed transmission FLASH, and this method eliminates uncertainties associated with the positioning of the Bragg peak that could be significant when delivering ultrahigh dose rates. This approach thus standardizes delivery in order to minimize the risk of underdosing tumors or overdosing normal tissues [36] (figure 8.2).

The most optimal way to deliver proton FLASH, however, is with Bragg peak beams. Early reports have begun to assess the feasibility of delivering Bragg peak beams for which the proton Bragg peak is intentionally placed in the patient, akin to the clinical practice delivery of proton therapy at conventional dose rates, thus uniquely allowing for the complete elimination of the exit dose. This approach stands in contrast to electron FLASH and transmission proton FLASH, therefore allowing a corresponding reduction in the radiation delivered to normal tissues beyond the target volume [37] (figure 8.3). Investigators at the New York Proton

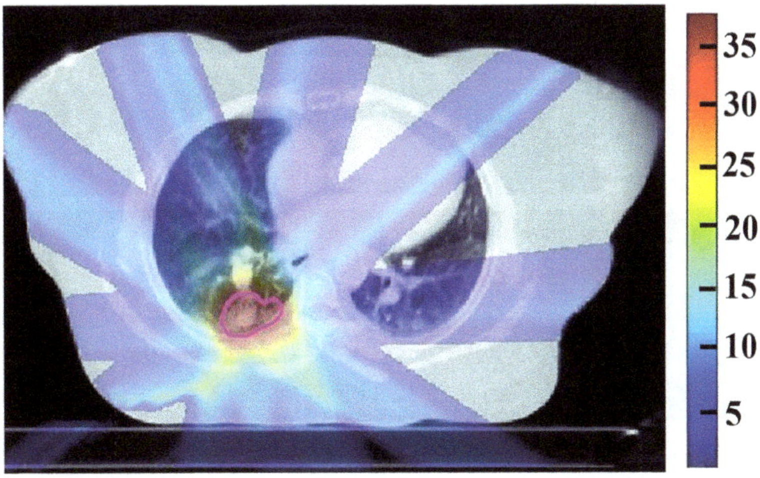


**Figure 8.1.** Lung cancer proton transmission FLASH plan. Five-field proton transmission FLASH plan for a patient with a right-sided early-stage NSCLC.

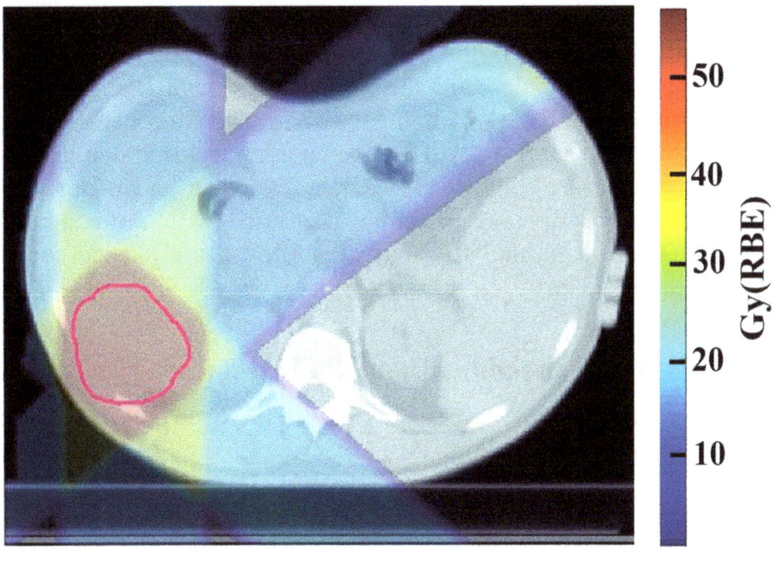


**Figure 8.2.** Liver cancer proton transmission FLASH plan. Three-field proton transmission FLASH plan for a patient with a primary hepatocellular carcinoma.

Center have authored a series of publications demonstrating the feasibility of delivering Bragg peak FLASH [38], the ability of Bragg peak proton FLASH to achieve superior organ-at-risk sparing compared with transmission proton FLASH [39], and quantitative methods for assessing the dose rate for PBS FLASH radiotherapy [40].

Bragg peak planning for proton FLASH therefore optimizes the true physical potential of proton therapy, while still affording the ability to deliver ultrahigh dose

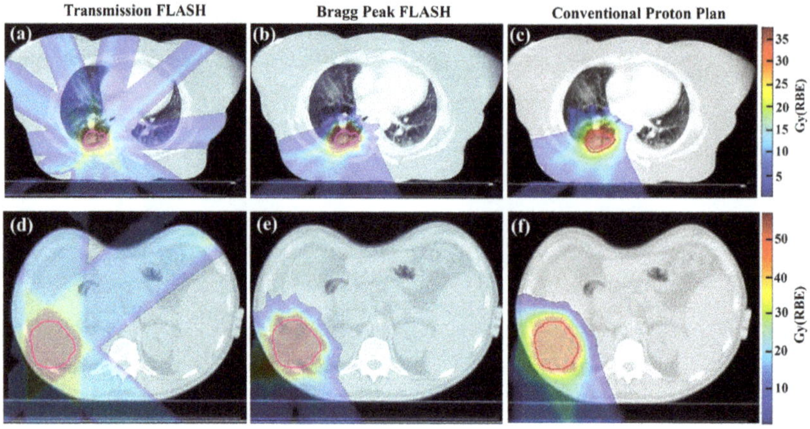


**Figure 8.3.** Comparison of conventional proton, proton transmission FLASH, and proton Bragg peak FLASH plans. Dose distributions for proton PBS FLASH treatment planning using different techniques for lung (a) and (b) and liver (d) and (e) cancers, and the conventional proton PBS technique ((c) for lung, (f) for liver). The left, middle, and right columns represent treatment plans based on proton transmission beams, single-energy Bragg peak beams, and conventional multiple-energy-layer proton PBS beams, respectively.

rates and to treat deep targets in the body offered by transmission proton FLASH planning. This lack of an exit dose and the optimal physical advantages of delivering FLASH using proton Bragg peak planning may be particularly beneficial compared to electron FLASH and proton FLASH delivered using transmission planning when treating patients via dose escalation. The latter is used in an attempt to improve tumor control rates for diseases currently associated with more limited tumor control outcomes due to an inability to escalate doses safely using conventional-dose-rate radiation therapy.

## 8.7 Proton FLASH: preclinical and clinical data

Over the last two years, notable preclinical research has been conducted into the use of proton therapy to deliver ultrahigh-dose-rate radiotherapy and has demonstrated the FLASH effect with normal tissue sparing. Investigators from Denmark demonstrated reduced acute moist desquamation of the skin in irradiated mice that received FLASH radiation therapy with protons relative to conventional-dose-rate radiation therapy [41]. Investigators from University of Pennsylvania demonstrated better preservation of mouse intestinal crypts in a pancreatic tumor model when irradiated with proton FLASH relative to standard-dose-rate proton radiotherapy, without differences in tumor growth responses [42]. Furthermore, investigators from Cincinnati Children's Hospital Medical Center and the University of Cincinnati demonstrated the benefits of FLASH over conventional PBS proton therapy for skin and soft-tissue toxicities [43].

Recognizing the value and potential benefits of proton FLASH in overcoming current limitations of electron and photon FLASH, the first in-human clinical trial assessing the feasibility of FLASH was started in November 2020 using PBS proton therapy. The trial, termed 'Feasibility Study of FLASH Radiotherapy for the Treatment of Symptomatic Bone Metastases (FAST-01),' is an open label, single-arm prospective feasibility study conducted at the Cincinnati Children's Proton Therapy Center; it aimed to enroll ten patients greater than 18 years old who had a life expectancy of at least two months with up to three painful bone metastases in the extremities (ClinicalTrials.gov Identifier NCT04592887). Patients were treated for a durations of <1 s using proton FLASH at dose rates of 40 Gy $s^{-1}$ or greater in a single fraction of up to 8 Gy using a single-transmission proton beam and a predefined treatment field size. Patients were treated to the gross tumor volume with a margin of 0.5 cm or more. The study had prespecified primary endpoints of workflow feasibility and radiation-induced toxicities. The secondary endpoints were pain relief, pain flare, and the use of pain medication. The trial recently completed study accrual, and its results are eagerly awaited.

## 8.8 Proton FLASH: clinical trial roadmap

Further human studies are needed and are being developed to afford greater insight into the efficacy and safety of proton FLASH. As FLASH's flagship benefit is its potential to reduce toxicities, the greatest benefit of this modality may be observed in disease sites with high expected toxicity rates. Suitable targets include locally advanced NSCLC, early-stage NSCLC, thoracic metastases, glioblastoma multiforme, hepatocellular carcinoma, and locally advanced pancreatic cancer. The endpoints of future studies are expected to focus on the reduction of high-grade toxicities that occur between FLASH and conventional-dose-rate radiation therapy treatments in the aforementioned sites.

Locally advanced NSCLC may be a good disease site and presentation for early curative-intent trials of proton FLASH, given the high normal tissue toxicity burden associated with conventional-dose-rate radiation therapy, a five-year survival rate of less than 50% [44–46], and reports that dose escalation can improve local control and thereby improve overall survival when delivered safely [47]. However, treatment may be complicated by tumor motion that occurs during respiration as well as intrafractional motion that is a common concern in conventional-dose-rate radiation therapy. The concerns for the latter, however, may be less significant with FLASH proton therapy, as it is delivered in less than a second per beam and as a single fraction or just a few fractions. The use of a 4D computed tomography (CT) scan to account for motion and methods for mitigating tumor motion, especially if the maximum target excursion is >10 mm (such as abdominal compression or breath-holding strategies [48–50]), may be particularly important in the planning of future FLASH trials involving lung cancer and other thoracic and upper gastrointestinal tumors associated with intrafractional motion due to respiration.

Early-stage NSCLC may also be a good disease site and presentation for human trials of proton FLASH, especially for patients with central or ultracentral tumors that experience high rates of toxicities from stereotactic body radiation therapy, which can induce treatment-induced fistulas, necrosis, major bleeds, and death [51–54]. Given the high incidence rates of NSCLC and the increasing proportion of patients being diagnosed at earlier stages due to the increased utilization of lung cancer screening imaging and the general increase in the use of medical imaging, study accrual would be anticipated to be relatively robust. Treating patients with early-stage NSCLC, who often have the same or even increased tumor motion relative to locally advanced NSCLC patients, will pose similar technological challenges to those encountered in the treatment of patients with locally advanced NSCLC. However, given that there is currently no definitive dose and fractionation of conventional-dose-rate radiation therapy that is thought to be a safe standard of care for the treatment of ultracentral lung tumors, the potential for FLASH to reduce toxicities in this curative population holds great promise.

Patients with thoracic metastases also have a relatively high toxicity rate when radiotherapy is delivered to the chest, especially in patients who are actively managed on or have received several lines of systemic therapy; this cohort may also provide suitable candidates for FLASH trials. Given the large proportion of patients who develop intrathoracic metastases during the course of their malignancy, it is anticipated that there would be ample opportunity to add patients with thoracic metastases to FLASH proton trials. In this population, in the event that FLASH does not provide the desired local control or symptomatic response, patients can be treated with the salvage options of surgery, alternative ablative therapies, the next line of systemic therapy, or other modalities. The challenges raised in treating patients with thoracic metastases, however, are the high heterogeneity of histologies and systemic therapies (including the possibility of concurrent chemotherapy or immunotherapy) that would serve as competing contributors to patient toxicity, in addition to the aforementioned complexities of tumor motion.

It may also be of interest to treat patients with upper gastrointestinal malignancies using FLASH RT [55, 56]. Today, conventional-dose-rate radiation therapy for hepatocellular carcinoma is limited by the radiosensitivity of hepatocytes and the high risk of radiation-induced liver toxicities. Such toxicities could potentially be minimized through the FLASH effect by delivering proton therapy at ultrahigh dose rates. Challenges are present in the planning for FLASH hepatocellular carcinoma and/or liver metastases trials, including heterogeneous systemic therapies the serve as competing contributors to toxicities, the complexities of tumor motion, and also greater difficulty in directly visualizing the tumor within the liver prior to and during treatment. FLASH proton therapy could serve to reduce the risk of duodenal toxicity that is often dose limiting for pancreatic cancer conventional-dose-rate radiation therapy, especially when delivered in the form of stereotactic body radiation therapy. The complexities of delivering FLASH to pancreatic cancers largely mirror those encountered while delivering FLASH to liver tumors; these include the toxic effects of systemic therapies, tumor motion, and difficulties with pretreatment tumor visualization.

Finally, glioblastoma multiforme and soft-tissue sarcoma may be suitable disease sites for early in-human clinical trials of proton FLASH. Glioblastoma multiforme has a failure pattern that is predominantly local, and while prior attempts at dose escalation have not been shown to improve outcomes for this malignancy [57], it is possible that the risk–benefit ratio of dose escalation could be improved by ultrahigh-dose-rate radiation therapy. As soft-tissue sarcoma is often treated with radiation therapy in the neoadjuvant setting prior to a definitive surgical resection, a trial in this patient population tumor might allow for a unique opportunity to study the biological effects of FLASH radiation therapy on tumors and their surrounding normal tissues by assessing post-FLASH irradiated surgical specimens.

For each disease site and condition discussed, several important factors need to be considered and controlled for before clinical trials are conducted using proton FLASH in potentially curative patients. Careful deliberation is needed for the total irradiation per voxel, the number of times a voxel is irradiated, and overlapping beams when employing more than one treatment field. The definition of the FLASH dose rate needs to be standardized, and further research is needed to determine whether there is a differential effect with higher radiation dose rates. FLASH is most typically defined simply as a treatment of 40 Gy $s^{-1}$ or greater, and the terminologies of delivering an ultrahigh dose rate and actually achieving the FLASH effect of normal tissue sparing are often used interchangeably. It is uncertain whether 40 Gy $s^{-1}$ is adequate to optimize normal tissue sparing, or whether dose rates closer to 80–120 Gy $s^{-1}$ may be superior in consistently achieving the FLASH effect and normal tissue sparing. In addition, further technological advancements will likely contribute to the evolution of proton FLASH over time. Further development of Bragg peak delivery for FLASH is expected to optimize dose conformality and to circumvent the current limitation of maximum beam energy that could create challenges for the use of transmission beam methods to treat deep-seated tumors in larger patients. Bragg peak delivery, however, creates additional challenges related to dose-rate measurements and dose deposition verification when treatment is delivered in a fraction of a second.

## 8.9 Conclusions

Proton radiation therapy has physical advantages that may allow for fewer toxicities than photon therapy. SFRT has biological advantages that may allow for fewer toxicities than conventional radiation therapy modalities. The use of proton therapy to deliver SFRT can allow for the optimal combination of biological and physical advantages that can significantly advance our current ability to spare normal tissues from toxicities that are currently dose limiting in conventional radiation therapy. While the use of proton therapy to deliver GRID therapy, minibeam radiation therapy, and FLASH radiation therapy is in its infancy, early preclinical and clinical data have emerged supporting the use of proton therapy as a potentially optimal way to deliver these advanced SFRT modalities. Additional data and clinical trials in potentially curative patients are needed to assess whether modalities such as proton FLASH will prove to be transformational advancements that will significantly change the field of oncology.

## Conflict of interest

CBS reports Varian Medical Systems honoraria.

## Funding

None.


## References


[1] Simone C B 2nd 2017 Thoracic radiation normal tissue injury *Semin. Radiat. Onco.* **27** 370–7

[2] Kaiser A, Eley J G and Onyeuku N E *et al* 2019 Proton therapy delivery and its clinical application in select solid tumor malignancies *J. Vis. Exp.* **144** e58372

[3] Chun S G, Solberg T D and Grosshans D R *et al* 2017 The potential of heavy-ion therapy to improve outcomes for locally advanced non-small cell lung cancer *Front. Oncol.* **7** 201

[4] Patel S H, Wang Z and Wong W W *et al* 2014 Charged particle therapy versus photon therapy for paranasal sinus and nasal cavity malignant diseases: a systematic review and meta-analysis *Lancet Oncol.* **15** 1027–38

[5] Lin S H, Hobbs B P and Verma V *et al* 2020 Randomized phase IIB trial of proton beam therapy versus intensity-modulated radiation therapy for locally advanced esophageal cancer *J. Clin. Oncol.* **38** 1569–79

[6] Higgins K A, O'Connell K and Liu Y *et al* 2017 National cancer database analysis of proton versus photon radiation therapy in non-small cell lung cancer *Int. J. Radiat. Oncol. Biol. Phys.* **97** 128–37

[7] Sanford N N, Pursley J and Noe B *et al* 2019 Protons versus photons for unresectable hepatocellular carcinoma: liver decompensation and overall survival *Int. J. Radiat. Oncol. Biol. Phys.* **105** 64–72

[8] Kahalley L S, Peterson R and Ris M D *et al* 2020 Superior intellectual outcomes after proton radiotherapy compared with photon radiotherapy for pediatric medulloblastoma *J. Clin. Oncol.* **38** 454–61

[9] Baumann B C, Mitra N and Harton J G *et al* 2020 Comparative effectiveness of proton vs photon therapy as part of concurrent chemoradiotherapy for locally advanced cancer *JAMA Oncol.* **6** 237–46

[10] Verma V, Simone C B 2nd and Mishra M V 2018 Quality of life and patient-reported outcomes following proton radiation therapy: a systematic review *J. Natl. Cancer Inst.* **110** 341–53

[11] Paganetti H, Beltran C J and Both S *et al* 2021 Roadmap: proton therapy physics and biology *Phys. Med. Biol.* **66** 05RM01

[12] Chang J Y, Zhang X and Knopf A *et al* 2017 Consensus guidelines for implementing pencil-beam scanning proton therapy for thoracic malignancies on behalf of the ptcog thoracic and lymphoma subcommittee *Int. J. Radiat. Oncol. Biol. Phys.* **99** 41–50

[13] Westover K D, Seco J and Adams J A *et al* 2012 Proton SBRT for medically inoperable stage I NSCLC *J. Thorac. Oncol.* **7** 1021–5

[14] Nantavithya C, Gomez D R and Wei X *et al* 2018 Phase 2 study of stereotactic body radiation therapy and stereotactic body proton therapy for high-risk, medically inoperable, early-stage non-small cell lung cancer *Int. J. Radiat. Oncol. Biol. Phys.* **101** 558–63

[15] Gao M, Mohiuddin M M, Hartsell W F and Pankuch M 2018 Spatially fractionated (GRID) radiation therapy using proton pencil beam scanning (PBS): feasibility study and clinical implementation *Med. Phys.* **45** 1645–53

[16] Mohiuddin M, Lynch C, Gao M and Hartsell W 2020 Early clinical results of proton spatially fractionated GRID radiation therapy (SFGRT) *Br. J. Radiol.* **93** 20190572

[17] Henry T, Ureba A and Valdman A *et al* 2017 Proton grid therapy: a proof-of-concept study *Technol. Cancer Res. Treat.* **16** 749–57

[18] Henry T, Bassler N and Ureba A *et al* 2017 Development of an interlaced-crossfiring geometry for proton grid therapy *Acta Oncol.* **56** 1437–43

[19] Zeman W, Curtis H J and Gebhard E L *et al* 1959 Tolerance of mouse-brain tissue to high-energy deuterons *Science* **130** 1760–1

[20] De Marzi L, Nauraye C and Lansonneur P *et al* 2019 Spatial fractionation of the dose in proton therapy: proton minibeam radiation therapy *Cancer Radiother.* **23** 677–81

[21] Girst S, Greubel C and Reindl J *et al* 2016 Proton minibeam radiation therapy reduces side effects in an *in vivo* mouse ear model *Int. J. Radiat. Oncol. Biol. Phys.* 1 **95** 234–41

[22] Prezado Y, Jouvion G and Hardy D *et al* 2017 Proton minibeam radiation therapy spares normal rat brain: long-term clinical, radiological and histopathological analysis *Sci. Rep.* **7** 14403

[23] Prezado Y, Jouvion G and Guardiola C *et al* 2019 Tumor control in RG2 glioma-bearing rats: a comparison between proton minibeam therapy and standard proton therapy *Int. J. Radiat. Oncol. Biol. Phys.* **104** 266–71

[24] Smyth L M L, Donoghue J F and Ventura J A *et al* 2018 Comparative toxicity of synchrotron and conventional radiation therapy based on total and partial body irradiation in a murine model *Sci. Rep.* **8** 12044

[25] Wilson P, Jones B and Yokoi T *et al* 2012 Revisiting the ultra-high dose rate effect: implications for charged particle radiotherapy using protons and light ions *Br. J. Radiol.* **85** e933–9

[26] Auer S, Hable V and Greubel C *et al* 2011 Survival of tumor cells after proton irradiation with ultra-high dose rates *Radiat. Oncol.* **6** 139

[27] Buonanno M, Grilj V and Brenner D J 2019 Biological effects in normal cells exposed to FLASH dose rate protons *Radiother. Oncol.* **139** 51–5

[28] Kim Y E, Gwak S H and Hong B J *et al* 2021 Effects of ultra-high doserate FLASH irradiation on the tumor microenvironment in lewis lung carcinoma: role of myosin light chain *Int. J. Radiat. Oncol. Biol. Phys.* **109** 1440–53

[29] Chabi S, To T H V and Leavitt R *et al* 2021 Ultra-high-dose-rate FLASH and conventional-dose-rate irradiation differentially affect human acute lymphoblastic leukemia and normal hematopoiesis *Int. J. Radiat. Oncol. Biol. Phys.* **109** 819–29

[30] Diffenderfer E S, Verginadis, I I and Kim M M *et al* 2020 Design, implementation, and *in vivo* validation of a novel proton FLASH radiation therapy system *Int. J. Radiat. Oncol. Biol. Phys.* **106** 440–8

[31] Favaudon V, Caplier L and Monceau V *et al* 2014 Ultrahigh dose-rate FLASH irradiation increases the differential response between normal and tumor tissue in mice *Sci. Transl. Med.* **6** 245ra93

[32] Vozenin M C, De Fornel P and Petersson K *et al* 2019 The advantage of FLASH radiotherapy confirmed in mini-pig and cat-cancer patients *Clin. Cancer Res.* **25** 35–42

[33] Bourhis J, Sozzi W J and Jorge P G *et al* 2019 Treatment of a first patient with FLASH-radiotherapy *Radiother. Oncol.* **139** 18–22

[34] Montay-Gruel P, Meziani L and Yakkala C *et al* 2019 Expanding the therapeutic index of radiation therapy by normal tissue protection *Br. J. Radiol.* **92** 20180008

[35] Chow R, Kang M and Wei S *et al* 2021 FLASH radiation therapy: review of the literature and considerations for future research and proton therapy FLASH trials *Appl. Radiat. Oncol.* **10** 15–21

[36] Zou W, Diffenderfer E S and Cengel K A *et al* 2021 Current delivery limitations of proton PBS for FLASH *Radiother. Oncol.* **155** 212–18
[37] Verhaegen F, Wanders R G, Wolfs C and Eekers D 2021 Considerations for shoot-through FLASH proton therapy *Phys. Med. Biol.* **66** 06nt01
[38] Kang M, Wei S, Choi J I, Lin H and Simone C B 2nd 2022 A universal range shifter and range compensator can enable proton pencil beam scanning single-energy Bragg peak FLASH-RT treatment using current commercially available proton systems *Int. J. Radiat. Oncol. Biol. Phys.* **113** 203–13
[39] Wei S, Lin H, Choi J I, Simone C B 2nd and Kang M 2021 A novel proton pencil beam scanning flash rt delivery method enables optimal OAR sparing and ultra-high dose rate delivery: a comprehensive dosimetry study for lung tumors *Cancers (Basel)* **13** 5790
[40] Kang M, Wei S, Choi J I, Simone C B 2nd and Lin H 2021 Quantitative assessment of 3D dose rate for proton pencil beam scanning FLASH radiotherapy and its application for lung hypofractionation treatment planning *Cancers (Basel)* **13** 3549
[41] Singers Sørensen B, Krzysztof Sitarz M and Ankjærgaard C *et al* 2021 In vivo validation and tissue sparing factor for acute damage of pencil beam scanning proton FLASH *Radiother. Oncol.* **167** 109–15
[42] Kim M M, Verginadis I I and Goia D *et al* 2021 Comparison of FLASH proton entrance and the spread-out bragg peak dose regions in the sparing of mouse intestinal crypts and in a pancreatic tumor model *Cancers (Basel)* **13** 4244
[43] Cunningham S, McCauley S and Vairamani K *et al* 2021 FLASH proton pencil beam scanning irradiation minimizes radiation-induced leg contracture and skin toxicity in mice *Cancers (Basel)* **13** 1012
[44] Verma V, Simone C B 2nd and Werner-Wasik M 2017 Acute and late toxicities of concurrent chemoradiotherapy for locally-advanced non-small cell lung cancer *Cancers (Basel)* **9** 120
[45] Kong F-M S, Zhao J and Wang J *et al* 2014 Radiation dose effect in locally advanced non-small cell lung cancer *J. Thorac. Dis.* **5** 336–47
[46] Vrankar M and Stanic K 2018 Long-term survival of locally advanced stage III non-small cell lung cancer patients treated with chemoradiotherapy and perspectives for the treatment with immunotherapy *Radiol. Oncol.* **52** 281–8
[47] Ma L, Men Y and Feng L *et al* 2019 A current review of dose-escalated radiotherapy in locally advanced non-small cell lung cancer *Radiol. Oncol.* **53** 6–14
[48] Lin L, Souris K and Kang M *et al* 2017 Evaluation of motion mitigation using abdominal compression in the clinical implementation of pencil beam scanning proton therapy of liver tumors *Med. Phys.* **44** 703–12
[49] Molitoris J K, Diwanji T and Snider J W 3rd *et al* 2018 Advances in the use of motion management and image guidance in radiation therapy treatment for lung cancer *J. Thorac. Dis.* **10** S2437–50
[50] Chuong M D, Hallemeier C L and Li H *et al* 2021 Executive summary of clinical and technical guidelines for esophageal cancer proton beam therapy from the particle therapy co-operative group thoracic and gastrointestinal subcommittees *Front. Oncol.* **11** 748331
[51] Postmus P E, Kerr K M and Oudkerk M *et al* 2017 Early and locally advanced non-small-cell lung cancer (NSCLC): ESMO clinical practice guidelines for diagnosis, treatment and follow-up *Ann. Oncol.* **28** iv1–21

[52] Abel S, Hasan S and Horne Z D *et al* 2019 Stereotactic body radiation therapy in early-stage NSCLC: historical review, contemporary evidence and future implications *Lung Cancer Manag.* **8** LMT09
[53] Simone C B 2nd, Wildt B and Haas A R *et al* 2013 Stereotactic body radiation therapy for lung cancer *Chest.* **143** 1784–90
[54] Tekatli H, Haasbeek N and Dahele M *et al* 2016 Outcomes of hypofractionated high-dose radiotherapy in poor-risk patients with 'ultracentral' non-small cell lung cancer *J. Thorac. Oncol.* **11** 1081–9
[55] Byun H K, Kim H J and Im Y R *et al* 2019 Dose escalation by intensity modulated radiotherapy in liver-directed concurrent chemoradiotherapy for locally advanced BCLC stage C hepatocellular carcinoma *Radiother. Oncol.* **133** 1–8
[56] Herrmann E, Naehrig D and Sassowsky M *et al* 2017 External beam radiotherapy for unresectable hepatocellular carcinoma, an international multicenter phase I trial, SAKK 77/07 and SASL 26 *Radiat. Oncol.* **12** 12
[57] Badiyan S N, Markovina S and Simpson J R *et al* 2014 Radiation therapy dose escalation for glioblastoma multiforme in the era of temozolomide *Int. J. Radiat. Oncol. Biol. Phys.* **90** 877–85

# Part II

## Physics of moderate dose rate SFRT

**IOP** Publishing

Spatially Fractionated, Microbeam and FLASH Radiation Therapy
A physics and multi-disciplinary approach
**Hualin Zhang and Nina A Mayr**

# Chapter 9

# GRID-collimator-based and static-field SFRT

**Hualin Zhang**

GRID collimators provided the initial technology for GRID therapy for decades. Commercial GRID collimators, which evolved from the initial Cerrobend GRID block and consist of a hexagonal pattern of circular divergent holes, provided the first standardized and easy-to-use spatially fractionated radiation therapy (SFRT) and the only SFRT accessible to patients well before the development of multileaf collimator (MLC)-based SFRT. Most of the published clinical experience with SFRT has been obtained using GRID collimators.

This chapter describes the dosimetric characteristics of commercially available GRID collimators, MLC-based SFRT techniques, and customer-made static 2D GRID collimating devices. It describes the structure and configuration of both the Cerrobend and brass GRID collimators and the dose profiles at different depths; it also compares the peak and valley dose ratios at various depths of two types of commercial GRID and the percentage depth–dose (PDD) curves for different field sizes. The dose properties of other patterns of 2D GRID fields produced by customer-made GRID shapers and MLC-based techniques, such as checkerboard and fenced fields, are discussed.

Commercial GRID collimators have recently been successfully incorporated into some treatment planning systems (TPSs) by installing a vendor-provided DICOM script, but not all TPSs have this capability. This chapter introduces a TPS-aided GRID collimator dose calculation and provides sample dose–volume histograms and dose calculation accuracy verification methods. Dose metrics recommended by the Radiosurgery Society's GRID/Lattice/Flash Working Group are discussed. GRID therapy planning techniques with and without a TPS are introduced and the necessary quality assurance steps are reviewed.

## 9.1 Introduction/overview

GRID therapy is a form of SFRT that was initially used to overcome the challenges of treating deep-seated tumors in the kilovoltage x-ray era before the 1950s, largely for reducing severe skin reactions [1]. The technology was subsequently adapted to megavoltage beams, and the first clinical study using megavoltage GRID therapy was published in 1990 [2]. Megavoltage x-ray GRID therapy has been used successfully to manage patients with bulky tumors, which are often refractory to conventional radiation therapy and other cancer therapies [2, 3]. GRID therapy initially succeeded in reducing tumor size and inducing high rates of symptomatic response in bulky palliatively treated tumors in patients with metastatic cancer. Over the last 30 years, ample clinical evidence has accumulated for the high symptomatic, objective tumor response and minimal toxicity in both palliatively and definitively treated tumors [2, 4–15]. More recently, SFRT has also been used as a boost or 'priming' therapy to improve the response to definitive or preoperative radiation of bulky, locally advanced curable tumors [2, 9–15], as reviewed in chapters 5 and 6. The mechanisms hypothesized to underpin the observed responses in GRID therapy, such as immunological, bystander, and microvascular effects, continue to be actively investigated [16–18].

Traditional GRID therapy employs an x-ray fluence in a purposely designed spatially fractionated irradiation pattern in the shape of a GRID (GRID pattern). This GRID pattern is created using a physical GRID collimator [19] that contains arrays of apertures within a Cerrobend or brass block. Newer technologies also include GRID pattern generation by a treatment planning system that uses a virtual block and operates entirely by MLC modulation [20].

The purpose of this chapter is to describe the physics, dose properties, and examples of the clinical application of commercial and customer-made GRID collimators and MLC-generated SFRT currently used in radiation oncology clinics.

## 9.2 The geometry of commercially available GRID collimators

Today, most clinics use commercially available GRID collimators from one of two companies: High Dose Radiation GRID, Radiation Products Design, Albertville, MN and Dotdecimal, Sanford, FL. Early GRID therapy used a GRID collimator with a hexagonal array of apertures within a Cerrobend block. Before the development of MLCs on board linac accelerators, the early use of GRID collimators did not benefit from MLC-based field shaping, as the GRID-covered field size was only produced by a pair of jaws; thus, the field shapes were always either square or rectangular. The concept was then further developed into the GRID collimators used today, which allow both the jaws and MLC shaping to be used to conform to the target shape; thus, a two-dimensional conformal GRID pattern of irradiation can be delivered to the target. Two typical GRID collimators are shown in figures 9.1(a) and (b).

### 9.2.1 Cerrobend GRID collimator

The first commercial GRID collimator was manufactured by Radiation Products Design (Albertville, MN). It consisted of a 7.5 cm thick cerrobend block perforated by a hexagonal pattern (figure 9.1(a)) of circular divergent apertures. The GRID collimator was designed to be mounted in the standard linear accelerator accessory

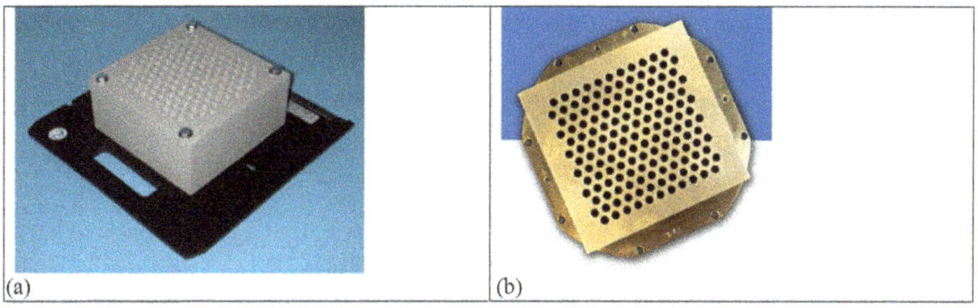

Figure 9.1. (a) Commercially available GRID collimator (High Dose Radiation Grid, Radiation Products Design, Albertville, MN). (b) Commercially available GRID collimator (Dotdecimal, Sanford, FL).

mount, for example, 65.4 cm from the source of a Varian linear accelerator (Varian, Varian Oncology System, Palo Alto, CA). Radiation Products Design also made GRID collimators for other manufacturers' linear accelerator machines. Various linear accelerators have different source-to-accessory mount distances; therefore, different GRID collimators have been designed according to the linacs' different divergences. The weight of a Cerrobend GRID is approximately 22 kg. The hole diameter is 0.60 cm on the top surface and 0.85 cm on the lower surface, and the center-to-center separation of the holes on the block is 1.15 cm on the lower surface. With this GRID collimator design, approximately 50% of the tissues in the collimated areas are irradiated by the collimated primary beam; the remainder are shielded by the Cerrobend block. All holes in the GRID are divergent and roughly concordant with the beam tilt.

### 9.2.2 Brass GRID collimator

The GRID collimator configuration recently advanced to a new design using brass as a construction material (Dotdecimal™, Sanford, FL). The new design of the GRID collimator by Dotdecimal™ is similar in its dimensional configuration and resulting GRID pattern. The thickness of the brass GRID block is also 7.5 cm. At approximately 18 kg, the brass GRID is 4 kg lighter than the Cerrobend GRID, although it is still bulky and heavy. The hole diameter is 0.80 cm on the top surface and 1.00 cm on the lower surface, and the center-to-center separation of the holes on the block is 1.40 cm on the lower surface. All holes in the GRID are divergent and are designed to be concordant with the beam tilt. With this classical GRID design, it is considered that approximately one half of the tissues in the treated areas are irradiated by the collimated primary beam; the remaining zones are shielded by the brass block.

## 9.3 GRID collimation performed by MLC or customer-made GRID formers

In addition, the further development of MLCs has allowed linac machines to form a GRID pattern of irradiation using multileaf collimation alone since 2006 [20–22]. This is also referred to as a virtual GRID block. Although the projected beamlet spot of MLC-generated GRID radiation is square instead of circular, its dosimetric properties can be made very similar to those of the bulky, heavy, and labor-intensive physical GRID collimators; thus, it can greatly facilitate the use of SFRT in the clinic. The MLC-based GRID collimator has numerous advantages over the GRID block: (a) the GRID field can be obtained easily and quickly by simply programming the leaf positions of the collimator; (b) MLCs are readily available in most linear accelerators and may therefore provide the possibility for institutions to start GRID therapy with minimum effort; (c) MLC-based GRID therapy eliminates the inconvenience and injury risk of mounting and/or dismounting a heavy GRID collimator; (d) when MLC-based GRID collimators are used, the dose–volume histograms of the target volume and any nearby organs at risk (OARs) can be calculated and evaluated; thus, any required adjustments to the treatment plan can be made; (e) MLC does not require a physical collimator and is therefore more cost-effective.

### 9.3.1 MLC-formed GRID fields

GRID fields formed by MLCs have been explored by different investigators. One example, presented in a study by Ha *et al* [20], used a Varian clinical linear accelerator equipped with an MLC, which was placed below two sets of rectangular collimator jaws as a tertiary collimator device. The MLC contained 60 pairs of opposing leaves (different machine models may have different numbers of multileaf pairs) capable of shaping a maximum field size of 40 cm × 40 cm on a plane 100 cm from the x-ray source (source-to-surface distance = 100 cm). The central 20 cm was shaped by 80 leaves (40 leaf pairs), each of which had a projected width of 0.5 cm. The outer 20 cm was shaped by the remaining 40 leaves, which had a projected width of 1 cm. Each leaf had a rounded edge to minimize the variation in the transmission penumbra with the leaf position; it also had a tongue on one side and a groove on the other to minimize interleaf leakage. Although the Varian system can deliver multiple segments, it would not permit the collimator jaw positions to change during the delivery of all the segments. For this reason, a multiple beam was used (as opposed to a multiple segment plan). Although the delivery time was slightly longer, the advantage of this approach was that the collimator jaws could be utilized to reduce MLC leakage by tracking the leaf positions with the aim of placing the jaw's end 0.2 cm away from the rounded end of the leaf, subject to the constraint that each collimator jaw could not travel more than 2 cm across the central axis of the collimator head. More specifically, five separate MLC-shaped beams were used, and each was defined by two columns of grid openings. This is a convenient GRID design which is used clinically with the MLC technique (see figure 9.2).

### 9.3.2 GRID collimation performed by customer-made GRID shapers

While most institutions in the U.S. use commercially available GRID collimators, some radiation oncology departments still prefer to design their own GRID collimator. A contemporary example of a such a customer-made GRID collimator is given here, in which Almendral *et al* [23] created a customer-made GRID collimator. A two-dimensional array of beamlets was created by combining two

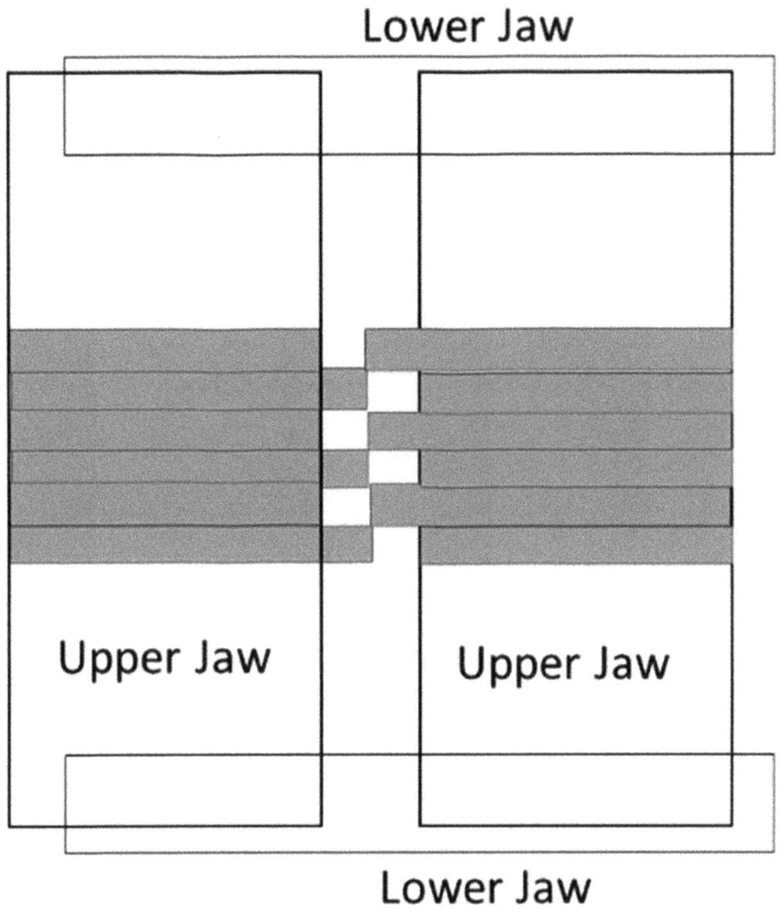


**Figure 9.2.** MLC-formed GRID technique and GRID fields. This schematic diagram illustrates the MLC leaf positions used to deliver one of the beams of a GRID field.

collimators, one of which projected a pattern of equally spaced stripes parallel to the $x$-axis (crossline) and the other of which projected a similar pattern parallel to the $y$-axis (inline). The first collimation was performed by the linac's MLC, which alternated fully closed pairs of leaves with opened pairs, while the second collimation was performed by a tertiary collimator with 14 sheets made from a low-melting-point alloy commonly used for beam shaping (MCP-96, Mining & Chemical Products, Wellingborough, UK). The sheets were individually cast by pouring the melted alloy into an acrylic mold; each one had a height of 7.2 cm and a physical width of 5 mm (about 1 cm projected at the isocenter); they were arranged in a divergent fashion to mimic the dose pattern produced by the MLC, although, since the shape of the sheets was nondivergent, only their central plane and not their sides could exactly match the beam divergence. To maintain the sheets in the correct position, their ends were inserted into the slots of two opposing pieces of acrylic, which were designed using software (QCAD, Ribbon Soft, Switzerland) and cut in

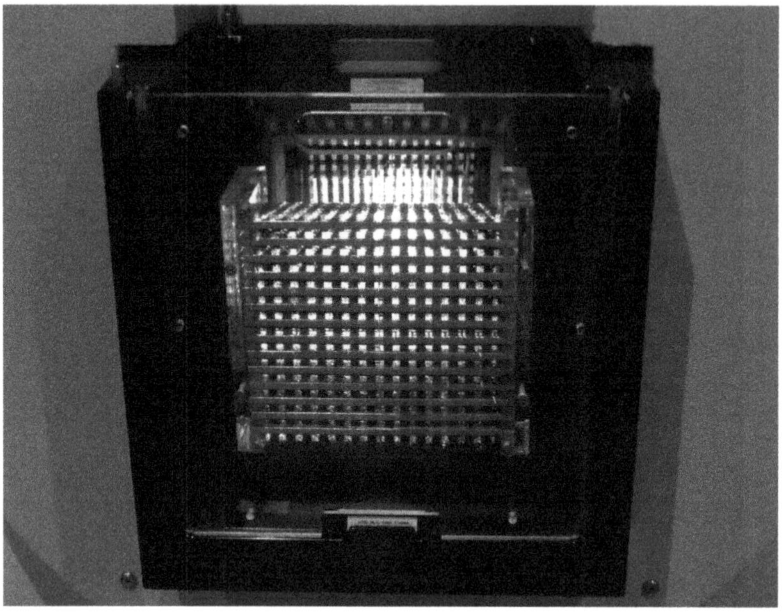

**Figure 9.3.** Customer-made tertiary GRID collimator. Image: Courtesy of Pedro Almendral Manzano, Servicio de Protección Radiológica y Radiofísica Hospitalaria, Hospital Universitario de Badajoz, 06080 Badajoz, Spain.

an external workshop by a computer-controlled cutting machine. These pieces were subsequently assembled with a 1 cm thick acrylic block tray to mount the collimator at the accessory mounting slot (figure 9.3). The combination of the tertiary collimation with the alternating leaf pattern in the MLC projected a GRID pattern of square beamlets (1 cm on each side) aligned in rows and columns separated by 1 cm wide blocked bands at the isocenter distance. This design provided a similar dose heterogeneity to that produced by commercial GRID collimators.

### 9.3.3 GRID fields produced by MLC pairs and the crossfire technique

GRID fields can be formed by two pairs of MLCs. Users can make a fenced field by moving MLC pairs together; the width of fence determines the size of the GRID beamlet. The GRID is formed using two fenced fields. Every other MLC is extended to the opposing collimator jaw in order to create a series of striped blocks that are 1cm wide. The field is copied, and the collimator is then rotated by 90°. The combination of the two fields per gantry angle creates a 1 cm by 1 cm GRID in the direction perpendicular to the beam. The target receives three dose levels: the peak dose, the half-peak dose, and the shielded-zone dose (figure 9.4).

This simple technique based on MLCs has been explored by Pokhrel *et al* in a study of multisite deep-seated tumors [24], and by Murphy *et al* in a breast cancer SFRT study [25]. In Murphy *et al*'s study [25], the GRID was formed by using two fields for both sets of tangents, i.e. a total of four fields. Every other MLC was extended to the opposing collimator jaw to create a series of striped blocks 1 cm

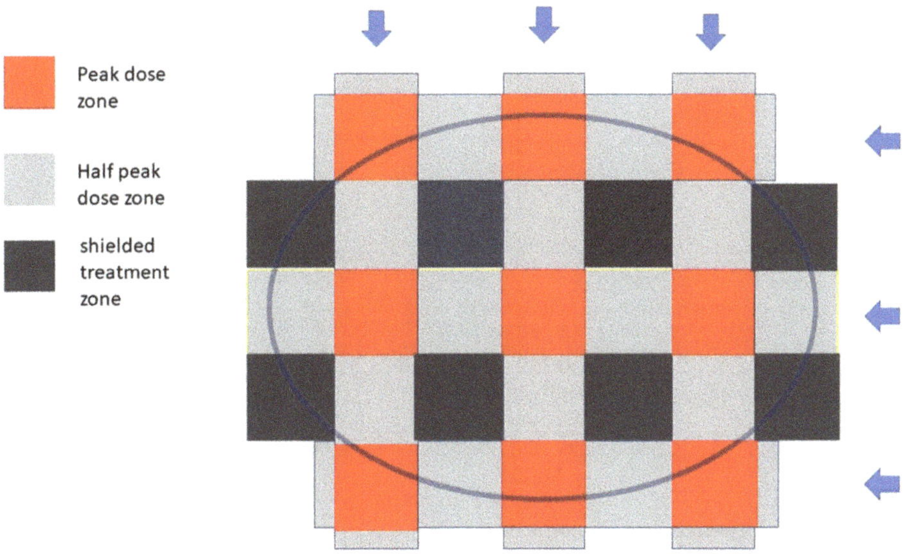


**Figure 9.4.** Schematic diagram of a GRID field formed by a pair of moving MLCs. The three vertical arrows indicate three vertical fence apertures, and three horizontal arrows indicate three horizontal fence apertures. After the crossfire process is complete, they form a GRID field. The GRID field created using this technique has three levels of dose zone: the peak dose zones, the half-peak-dose zones, and the shielded zones.

wide. The field was copied, and the collimator was then rotated by 90°. This process was repeated on the opposing tangent fields. The combination of two fields per tangent created a 1 cm by 1 cm GRID in the sagittal direction. The fields were equally weighted or slightly modified to produce a homogenous peak-pattern distribution. Collimator rotations of 0°–20° were used and designed using the patient's anatomy to minimize MLC leakage into the heart and lung. The GRID therapy plans generated for MLCs by a TPS for a breast in the prone position with this fenced beam crossfire technique showed a strong advantage in accommodating targets, maximally sparing nearby normal structures, and yielding consistent dosimetric quality results, regardless of the shape of the target and its volume [25].

## 9.4 Dosimetric properties of GRID fields

### 9.4.1 Percentage depth–dose and dose profiles of GRID fields produced by commercial GRIDs

The PDD curves and dose profiles of GRID fields produced by commercially available GRID collimators have been published by multiple researchers [13, 14, 19, 26]. Because users started using the Cerrobend GRID collimators much earlier than brass GRID collimators, most of the dosimetric data seen in the literature are for the Cerrobend GRID collimator. Figure 9.5 shows the PDD curves and dose profiles of two commercial GRID collimators. The PDDs and profiles of these two types of GRID collimator are very similar.

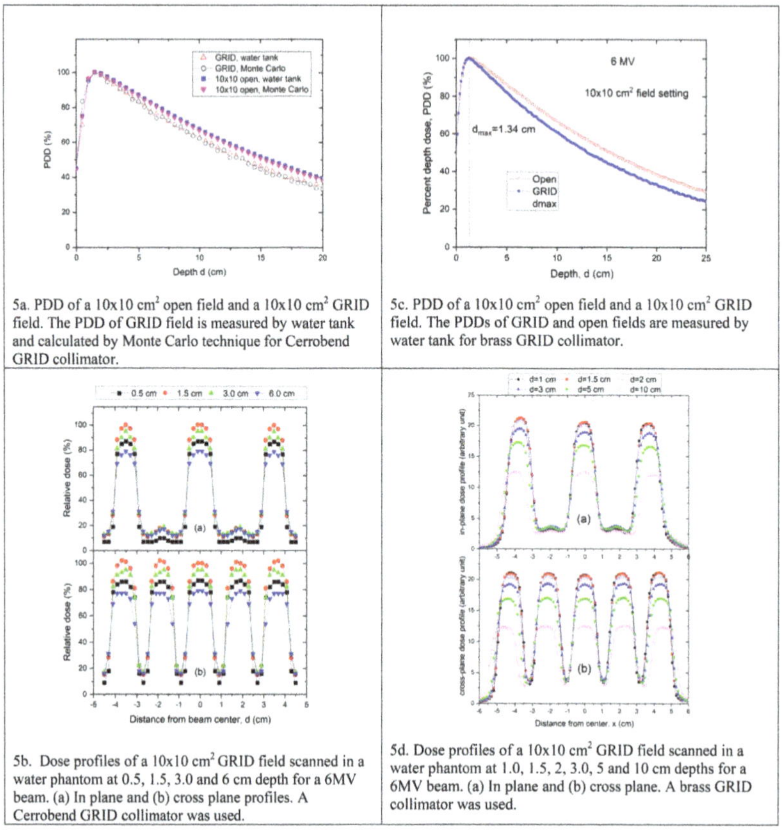


5a. PDD of a 10x10 cm² open field and a 10x10 cm² GRID field. The PDD of GRID field is measured by water tank and calculated by Monte Carlo technique for Cerrobend GRID collimator.

5c. PDD of a 10x10 cm² open field and a 10x10 cm² GRID field. The PDDs of GRID and open fields are measured by water tank for brass GRID collimator.

5b. Dose profiles of a 10x10 cm² GRID field scanned in a water phantom at 0.5, 1.5, 3.0 and 6 cm depth for a 6MV beam. (a) In plane and (b) cross plane profiles. A Cerrobend GRID collimator was used.

5d. Dose profiles of a 10x10 cm² GRID field scanned in a water phantom at 1.0, 1.5, 2, 3.0, 5 and 10 cm depths for a 6MV beam. (a) In plane and (b) cross plane. A brass GRID collimator was used.

**Figure 9.5.** PDD curves and dose profiles of two commercially available GRID collimators. Panels (5a) and (5b) show the curves and profiles of Cerrobend collimators; panels (5c) and (5d) show those of brass GRID collimators.

Figure 9.6 compares the peak/valley dose ratios (PVDR) of two types of GRID collimator. The data for the DotDecimal™ GRID collimator were obtained from a recent water tank scan. The Cerrobend GRID collimator data were derived from a published article [19]. The Cerrobend GRID collimator has a greater PVDR value than the brass GRID collimator at the same depth, because Cerrobend has a greater beam attenuation capability than brass.

### 9.4.2 Dosimetric properties of customer-made GRID fields

The PDD and dose profiles of GRID fields produced by customer-made GRID collimators are different from those produced by commercially available GRID collimators because they are made in different patterns and with different materials. The MLC-based GRID collimator shown in figure 9.2 produces similar dose profiles to those of the Cerrobend and brass GRID collimators [20]. Figure 9.7 shows the dose properties of a similar customer-made tertiary GRID collimator first reported by Almendral *et al* [23], as described in section 9.3.2. With the new aperture

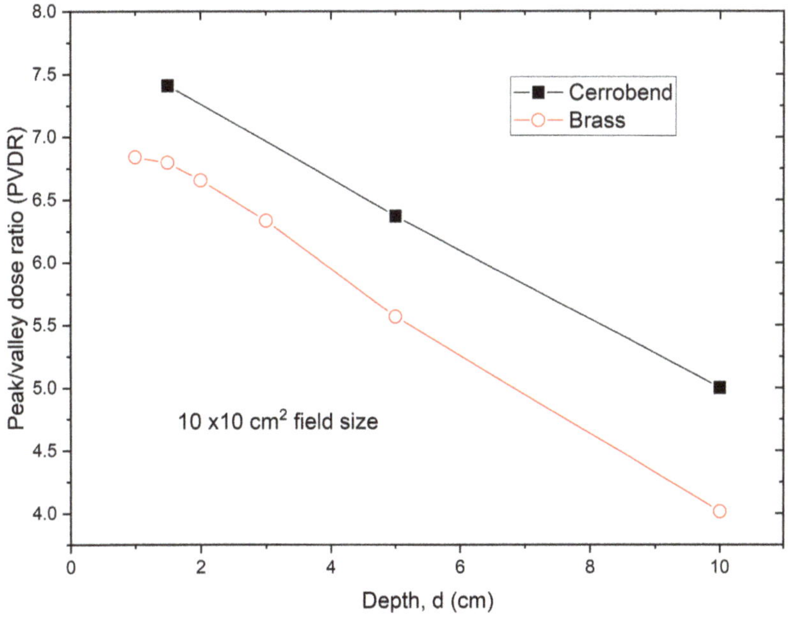


**Figure 9.6.** A comparison between the PVDRs of brass and Cerrobend GRID collimators at a 10 × 10 $cm^2$ field jaw setting. The data for the Cerrobend GRID collimator made by Radiation Products Design Inc. were derived from Meigooni's study [19], while the data for the brass GRID collimator made by Dotdecimal were taken from a recent water tank scan. (The technique involved can be seen in chapter 15).

arrangements, the peak-to-peak distances produced by the inline and the crossline are the same.

### 9.4.3 The use of treatment planning systems to perform GRID therapy dose calculations

The Eclipse system (Varian Oncology System, Palo Alto, CA, USA) is one of the few TPSs that can perform dose computations for commercial GRID collimators. In order to do this, a DICOM file containing the specific geometric features of the GRID collimator and generated by the GRID collimator vendor must be installed in the TPS using the vendor's specific instructions (figure 9.8).

Following the installation of a GRID collimator into the TPS, its calculation accuracy is verified. For this verification, water tank scans of the PDD curves and dose profiles are performed at different depths for various field settings and compared with their TPS-generated counterparts. A calibrated ion chamber suitable for small-field dosimetry or film is used to verify the absolute dose delivered via the GRID field, and a ⩽3% difference, which is generally considered acceptable for radiation therapy plan point dose measurement, is set as a tolerance limit. Figure 9.9 presents an example of a dose profile comparison between the TPS dose projection and values obtained via film measurement for a 10 × 10 $cm^2$ field size performed in our clinic. A comprehensive dose calculation accuracy check is presented in chapter 15. After the GRID dose calculation accuracy has been

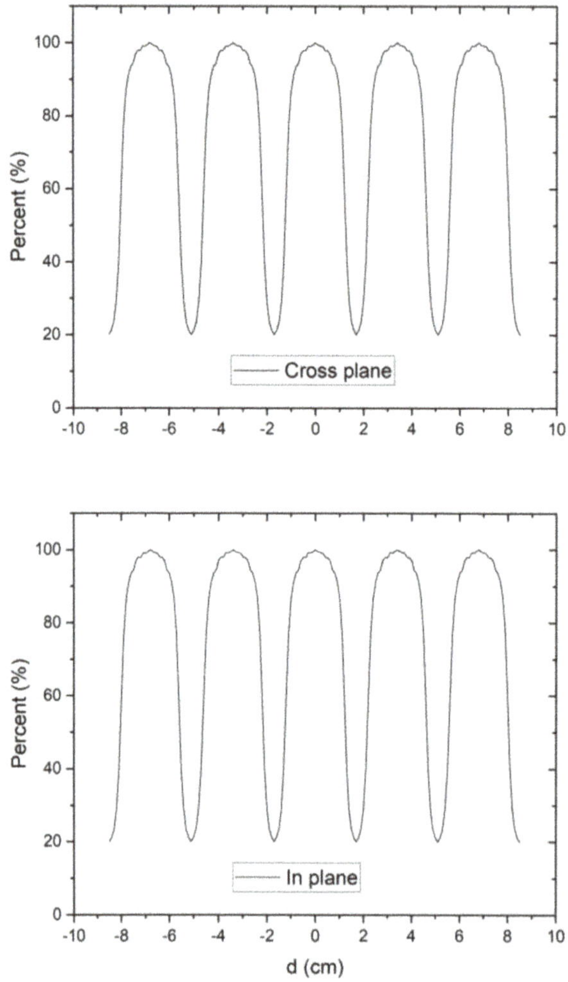


**Figure 9.7.** Schematic dose profiles of the customer-made tertiary GRID collimator shown in figure 9.3.

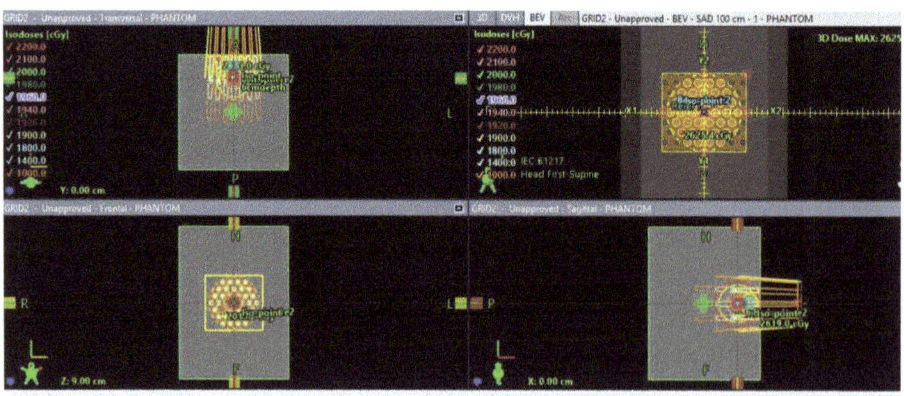

**Figure 9.8.** Schematic diagram of a GRID collimator and its dose projection in a TPS.

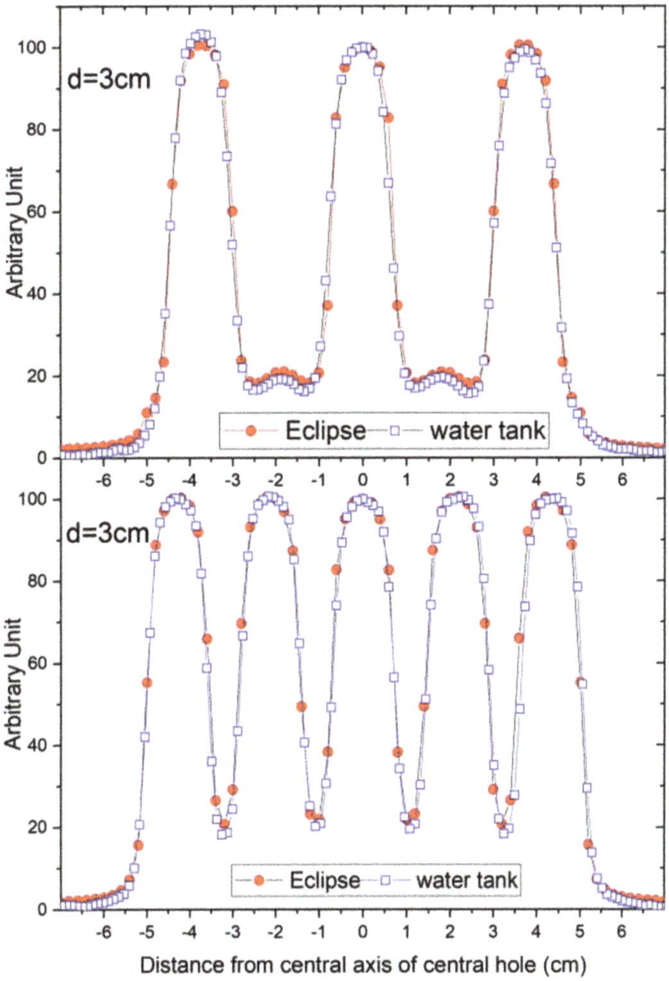


**Figure 9.9.** Dose profile comparison between a TPS dose projection and values obtained via water tank scanning for a Dotdecimal™ GRID collimator.

confirmed, the TPS can be used to create patient treatment plans that use the GRID collimator.

As in the practice of intensity-modulated radiation therapy (IMRT), patient-specific treatment plan QA should be performed to verify the delivered dose for quality assurance and patient safety.

### 9.4.4 Dose–volume histograms for GRID therapy

Because the dose–volume histogram (DVH) contains extensive information about the SFRT dose distribution, the DVHs of the planning target of a GRID therapy plan should be provided when possible, so that the treatment outcomes can potentially be correlated with the relevant dose parameters in the future.

Figure 9.10 shows the differential and cumulative dose–volume histograms (d-DVH and c-DVH) of an ellipsoidal tumor 16 cm in diameter (the height is 6 cm in the beam axis direction) located at depths of 3, 6, and 10 cm. The prescription dose is 20 Gy at the tumor center. The comparisons show that the DVH curves are very similar. When the tumor is located deeper, the curves shift slightly toward the higher dose zone. Another calculation indicates that the equivalent uniform dose (EUD)

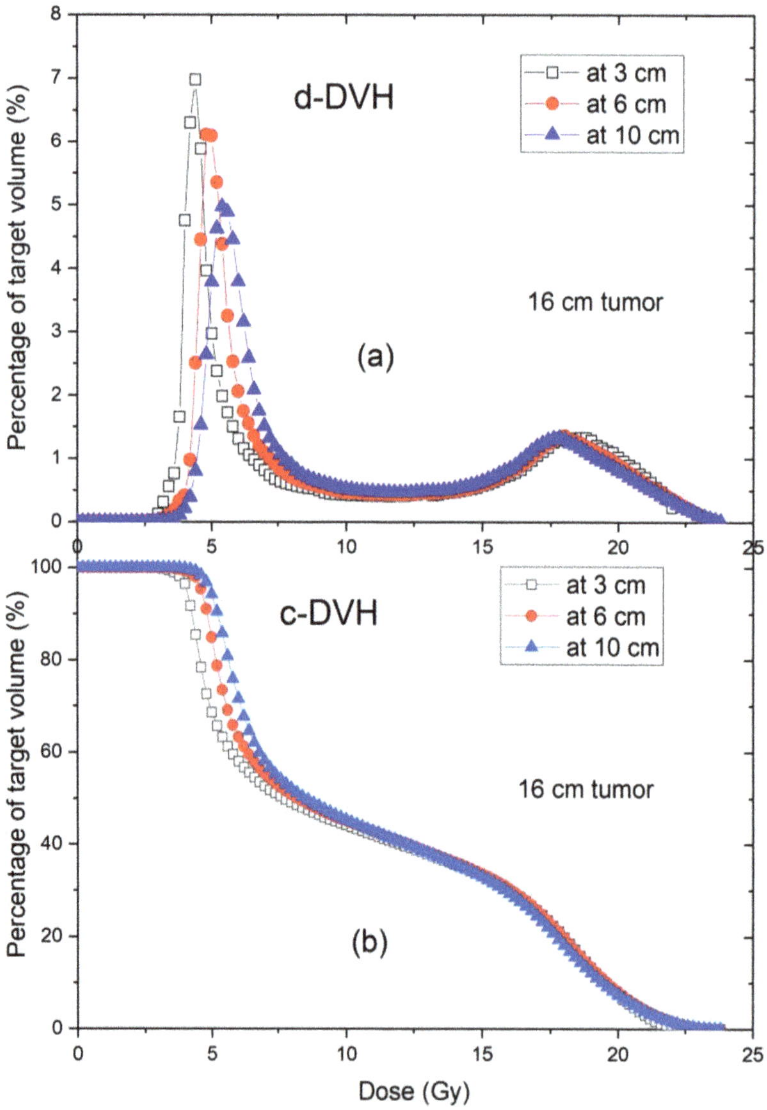


**Figure 9.10.** Differential (a) and cumulative (b) dose–volume histograms of a 16 cm spheroidal tumor located at depths of 3, 6, and 10 cm, respectively. The tumor height (in the beam direction) is 6 cm; on the plane perpendicular to the beam direction at the tumor center, the diameter of the tumor is 16 cm.

increases by less than 1 Gy in a tumor located at a depth of 10 cm compared to a tumor of the same size located at a depth of 3 cm for a prescription dose of 20 Gy.

## 9.5 Dose metrics needed to document GRID therapy

GRID therapy planning is a complex process, and it is a significant departure from traditional radiation therapy practice. The heterogeneous dose distributions can vary significantly from one practitioner to another if MLC-based techniques are involved. It is currently unknown which specific dosimetric parameters within the heterogeneous dose distribution of SFRT play a more important role than others in terms of the radiation response. Thus, the potential correlations between the observed clinical benefit and the dosimetric heterogeneity properties will only be determined through rigorous clinical practice and biological studies. Therefore, a well-defined set of dosimetric metrics that is as comprehensive as possible and standardized based on consensus must be computed for each GRID therapy plan. Such rigorous standardization of reporting may help to elucidate any relationships between the clinical tumor response and heterogenous field properties. The Radiosurgery Society (RSS) GRID, Lattice, Microbeam and FLASH Radiation Therapy Working Group's white paper suggests that the parameters presented in table 9.1 should be documented in each plan [28]. A recent article has validated those parameters in a GRID therapy study [29].

## 9.6 Dosimetric parameters used when creating a GRID therapy plan

For a GRID therapy plan, the prescription dose is the first important plan parameter; it is usually given at the central axis of the central hole at the tumor's

**Table 9.1.** Summary of the recommended GRID plan dosimetric metrics.

| |
|---|
| Prescription dose ($D_p$, in Gy) |
| Equivalent uniform doses (EUDs, in Gy) for tumor and normal tissues |
| Output factor ($OUT_d$) at the prescription depth ($d$) (in Gy/MU), |
| Dose covering 90% of the target (D90, in Gy) |
| Dose covering 50% of the target (D50, in Gy) |
| Dose covering 20% of the target (D20, in Gy) |
| Dose covering 10% of the target (D10, in Gy) |
| Dose covering 5% of the target (D5, in Gy) |
| Valley/peak dose ratio (VPDR) |
| D90/D10 VPDR |
| Peak width (defined at 50% of the max peak dose) |
| Peak-to-peak distance |
| Peak dose |
| Valley dose |

central depth or $d_{max}$. If the central hole does not pass through tumor center, the prescription point should be at a hole-passing tumor geometry and located at or near the tumor center.

In a scenario in which the GRID collimator cannot be implemented within the TPS for dose calculation, the monitor units (MUs) needed to deliver the prescribed peak dose (i.e. 15 or 20 Gy) are calculated based on the measured output factor of the central hole (usually near or passing through the beam's central axis) and are verified by an experimental measurement using either film or an ion chamber in a phantom. The approach is the same for MLC-formed GRID treatments, in which an experimental measurement is performed to determine the output factor used to deliver the prescribed peak dose at the tumor's prescription depth, because the accuracy of TPS-calculated MUs may be affected by field shape and the secondary collimator (or jaws).

In a patient treatment, the jaws and/or MLC can be used to reduce the field size to create a conformal field adapted to the tumor's size and shape. Because the output factor of the GRID field in the central hole at $d_{max}$ ($OUT_{dmax}$) varies with the field size, it needs to be measured. If the prescription dose $D_p$ is prescribed at a depth of $d_{max}$, the MU is calculated according to:

$$\mathrm{MU} = \frac{D_{\mathrm{p(Gy)}}}{\mathrm{OUT}_{\mathrm{dmax}}\left(\frac{\mathrm{Gy}}{\mathrm{MU}}\right)}. \tag{9.1}$$

However, the depth of the tumor's center may be variable because of an irregular tumor shape, and/or the treating physician may decide to prescribe the dose at a depth ($d$) other than $d_{max}$. In addition, if two opposed GRID fields are used [30] then the combined PDD curves are entirely different. If this is the case, then the physicist needs to measure the GRID field output factor at the depth $d$. If the output factor of the GRID field at the depth $d$ is $OUT_d$, then

$$\mathrm{MU} = \frac{D_{\mathrm{p(Gy)}}}{\mathrm{OUT}_{\mathrm{d}}\left(\frac{\mathrm{Gy}}{\mathrm{MU}}\right)}. \tag{9.2}$$

It is worth noting that, because of the dosimetric characteristics of megavoltage x-ray beams, if the dose prescription depth is greater than $d_{max}$, the maximum dose delivered is greater than the prescription dose (the deeper the prescription depth, the greater the maximum dose delivered). The physician needs to decide the prescription point and depth for each patient.

In addition to the prescription dose $D_p$, the depth $d$, and the total MU, the treatment time $T$ also must be documented as a planning parameter. $T$ is calculated by taking the total MU divided by the machine's treatment dose rate. Some physicians also request documentation showing how many holes cover the tumor's maximum cross section at the prescription depth. In addition to the parameters listed in table 9.1, other planning parameters, such as the beam energy, gantry angle, jaw size, and field shape should be documented along with the treatment plan.

## 9.7 Knowledge gaps and future perspectives

Today's commercially available GRID collimators provide a convenient, effective, and dosimetrically consistent SFRT choice for many clinics [29]. However, the initial empirically developed GRID hexagonal pattern of these two GRID collimators, which provide very similar dose modulation, is just one of many potential designs. At present, there are no other available commercial GRID designs, and there are no studies indicating whether the hexagonal pattern is superior or might be improved by alternative designs.

In addition, all commercial GRID devices are tailored to photon beams, and no standard electron-beam GRID collimator is available. The unavailability of GRID dosimetry computations in many TPSs remains an obstacle to the implementation of GRID therapy for clinical use. These are important open questions and gaps that should be investigated and solved in order to advance our understanding of SFRT and further facilitate the clinic use of GRID therapy for patients.

## 9.8 Conclusions

GRID therapy which is based on either a commercially available GRID collimator, an onboard MLC-based method, or a customer-made GRID field shaper, is a convenient and cost-effective way to practice clinical SFRT. Both the Cerrobend and brass GRID collimators can provide similar and consistent GRID field heterogeneity patterns, but the cerrobend GRID collimator provides a greater peak/valley dose ratio than the brass collimator at the same energy and depth. When the GRID collimator is installed in a TPS, more detailed dosimetric information can be derived and the planning accuracy of the GRID therapy can be improved; practitioners are encouraged to take this approach whenever feasible.

## References and additional reading


[1] Marks H 1950 A new approach to the roentgen therapy of cancer with the use of a grid *J. Mt. Sinai Hosp. N. Y.* **17** 46–8

[2] Mohiuddin M, Curtis D L, Grizos W T and Komarnicky L 1990 Palliative treatment of advanced cancer using multiple nonconfluent pencil beam radiation. A pilot study *Cancer* **66** 114–8

[3] Yan W, Khan M K, Wu X, Simone C B 2nd, Fan J and Gressen E *et al* 2020 Spatially fractionated radiation therapy: history, present and the future *Clin. Transl. Radiat. Oncol.* 20 30–8

[4] Liberson F 1933 The value of a multi-perforated screen in deep X-ray therapy *Radiology* **20** 10

[5] Marks H 1950 A new approach to the roentgen therapy of cancer with the use of a grid *J. Mt. Sinai Hosp. N. Y.* **17** 3

[6] Puri D R, Chou W and Lee N 2005 Intensity-modulated radiation therapy in head and neck cancers: dosimetric advantages and update of clinical results *Am. J. Clin. Oncol.* **28** 415–23

[7] Marks H 1952 Clinical experience with irradiation through a grid *Radiology* **58** 338–42

[8] Miller R C, Wilson K G, Feola J M, Urano M, Yaes R J and McLaughlin P *et al* 1992 Megavoltage grid total body irradiation of C3Hf/SED mice *Strahlenther. Onkol.* **168** 423–6

[9] Mohiuddin M, Fujita M, Regine W F, Megooni A S, Ibbott G S and Ahmed M M 1999 High-dose spatially-fractionated radiation (GRID): a new paradigm in the management of advanced cancers *Int. J. Radiat. Oncol., Biol., Phys.* **45** 721–7

[10] Sathishkumar S, Dey S, Meigooni A S, Regine W F, Kudrimoti M S and Ahmed M M *et al* 2002 The impact of TNF-alpha induction on therapeutic efficacy following high dose spatially fractionated (GRID) radiation *Technol. Cancer Res. Treat.* **1** 141–7

[11] Sathishkumar S, Boyanovsky B, Karakashian A A, Rozenova K, Giltiay N V and Kudrimoti M *et al* 2005 Elevated sphingomyelinase activity and ceramide concentration in serum of patients undergoing high dose spatially fractionated radiation treatment: implications for endothelial apoptosis *Cancer Biol. Ther.* **4** 979–86

[12] Huhn J L, Regine W F, Valentino J P, Meigooni A S, Kudrimoti M and Mohiuddin M 2006 Spatially fractionated GRID radiation treatment of advanced neck disease associated with head and neck cancer *Technol. Cancer Res. Treat.* **5** 607–12

[13] Reiff J E, Huq M S, Mohiuddin M and Suntharalingam N 1995 Dosimetric properties of megavoltage grid therapy *Int. J. Radiat. Oncol. Biol. Phys.* **33** 937–42

[14] Trapp J V, Warrington A P, Partridge M, Philps A, Glees J and Tait D *et al* 2004 Measurement of the three-dimensional distribution of radiation dose in grid therapy *Phys. Med. Biol.* **49** N317–23

[15] Penagaricano J A, Moros E G, Ratanatharathorn V, Yan Y and Corry P 2010 Evaluation of spatially fractionated radiotherapy (GRID) and definitive chemoradiotherapy with curative intent for locally advanced squamous cell carcinoma of the head and neck: initial response rates and toxicity *Int. J. Radiat. Oncol. Biol. Phys.* **76** 1369–75

[16] Mackonis E C, Suchowerska N, Zhang M, Ebert M, McKenzie D R and Jackson M 2007 Cellular response to modulated radiation fields *Phys. Med. Biol.* **52** 5469–82

[17] Asur R S, Sharma S, Chang C W, Penagaricano J, Kommuru I M and Moros E G *et al* 2012 Spatially fractionated radiation induces cytotoxicity and changes in gene expression in bystander and radiation adjacent murine carcinoma cells *Radiat. Res.* **177** 751–65

[18] Asur R, Butterworth K T, Penagaricano J A, Prise K M and Griffin R J 2015 High dose bystander effects in spatially fractionated radiation therapy *Cancer Lett.* **356** 52–7

[19] Meigooni A S, Dou K, Meigooni N J, Gnaster M, Awan S and Dini S *et al* 2006 Dosimetric characteristics of a newly designed grid block for megavoltage photon radiation and its therapeutic advantage using a linear quadratic model *Med. Phys.* **33** 3165–73

[20] Ha J K, Zhang G, Naqvi S A, Regine W F and Yu C X 2006 Feasibility of delivering grid therapy using a multileaf collimator *Med. Phys.* **33** 76–82

[21] Costlow H N, Zhang H and Das I J 2014 A treatment planning approach to spatially fractionated megavoltage grid therapy for bulky lung cancer *Med. Dosim.* **39** 218–26

[22] Stathakis S, Esquivel C, Gutierrez A N, Shi C and Papanikolaou N 2009 Dosimetric evaluation of multi-pattern spatially fractionated radiation therapy using a multi-leaf collimator and collapsed cone convolution superposition dose calculation algorithm *Appl. Radiat. Isot.* **67** 1939–44

[23] Almendral P, Mancha P J and Roberto D 2013 Feasibility of a simple method of hybrid collimation for megavoltage grid therapy *Med. Phys.* **40** 051712

[24] Pokhrel D, Halfman M, Sanford L, Chen Q and Kudrimoti M 2020 A novel, yet simple MLC-based 3D-crossfire technique for spatially fractionated GRID therapy treatment of deep-seated bulky tumors *J. Appl. Clin. Med. Phys.* **21** 68–74

[25] Murphy N L, Philip R, Wozniak M, Lee B H, Donnelly E D and Zhang H 2020 A simple dosimetric approach to spatially fractionated GRID radiation therapy using the multileaf collimator for treatment of breast cancers in the prone position *J. Appl. Clin. Med. Phys.* **21** 105–14

[26] Zhang H, Johnson E L and Zwicker R D 2006 Dosimetric validation of the MCNPX Monte Carlo simulation for radiobiologic studies of megavoltage grid radiotherapy *Int. J. Radiat. Oncol. Biol. Phys.* **66** 1576–83

[27] Zhang H, Zhong H, Barth R F, Cao M and Das I J 2014 Impact of dose size in single fraction spatially fractionated (grid) radiotherapy for melanoma *Med. Phys.* **41** 021727

[28] Zhang H, Wu X, Zhang X, Chang S X, Megooni A and Donnelly E D *et al* 2020 Photon GRID radiation therapy: a physics and dosimetry white paper from the radiosurgery society (RSS) GRID/LATTICE, microbeam and FLASH radiotherapy working group *Radiat. Res.* **194** 665–77

[29] Zhang H, Grams M P, Foy J J and Mayr N A 2022 A dosimetric parameter reference look-up table for GRID collimator-based spatially fractionated radiation therapy *Cancers (Basel)* **14** 1037

[30] Meigooni A S, Gnaster M, Dou K, Johnson E L, Meigooni N J and Kudrimoti M 2007 Dosimetric evaluation of parallel opposed spatially fractionated radiation therapy of deep-seated bulky tumors *Med. Phys.* **34** 599–603

# Chapter 10

# The technical aspects of 3D lattice radiation therapy (LRT)

**Xiaodong Wu, Naipy C Perez, Xiaobo Li, Beatriz E Amendola, Georges F Hatoum and Benhua Xu**

The concept of lattice radiation therapy (LRT) was proposed in March 2010. It extends 2D GRID therapy to a 3D configuration that uses converging x-ray beams or charged particle beams. The first clinical case that used LRT in the treatment of a large gynecologic tumor was reported in September 2010. Since then, more than 1000 patients have been treated with LRT worldwide. As in GRID therapy, the key dosimetric characteristic of LRT is the peak–valley dose distribution, but LRT uniquely confines the high-dose islands (peaks or vertices) within the target volume, thus reducing the dose outside the target and decreasing the toxicity risk for surrounding normal structures. The essence of spatially fractionated radiation therapy (SFRT) is its extreme dose heterogeneity. The specific geometric configurations (or shapes) of the heterogeneous dose distribution may or may not be crucially important, depending on the treatment's intent. In this chapter, we focus on presenting the clinical planning and delivery techniques of LRT based on the clinical experience accumulated to date, with the aim of providing guiding principles and practical approaches for clinical implementation.

## 10.1 Introduction

The early inception of GRID radiation therapy was motivated by a desire to spare skin while delivering therapeutic high doses to large, deep-seated tumors [1–5] and was adapted to megavoltage GRID therapy in the 1980s, initially using a 2D GRID-block approach, as further reviewed in chapter 1. Although MV x-rays can generally spare the skin, in cases involving deep-seated tumors, normal tissues and critical organs surrounding the target volume can still receive a relatively high dose when a 2D GRID is employed because it delivers high-dose stripes beyond the anterior/posterior boundaries of the target. The use of modern advanced MV linear

doi:10.1088/978-0-7503-4046-5ch10

accelerators together with parallel advances in radiation oncology physics and the planning capabilities of these new technologies have made it feasible to reconfigure the GRID concept into a 3D form. This 3D GRID can generate arrays of individually distributed high-dose 'islands' or spheres (vertices) at specific separations that form lattice-like peak–valley dose distributions. As the vertices are all confined *within* the tumor volume, unnecessary high-dose exposure to the surrounding normal tissues is eliminated. This three-dimensional SFRT approach was given the name LRT [6] and has been successfully used in clinical studies, as further described in chapter 7.

There have been several steps and evolutions in the logical deliberations involved in transitioning from 2D GRID to 3D LRT. We remind the reader that the fundamental objective of the original GRID approach was not to create heterogeneous peak–valley dose distributions, but to spare the skin to enable the treatment of deep-seated tumors in the orthovoltage era, mostly with short-term palliative intent. Dose heterogeneity was a necessary condition for achieving this initial goal, and the observed clinical tumor response validated this technique until the arrival of megavoltage beams.

Since the megavoltage x-rays produced by modern delivery techniques such as intensity-modulated radiation therapy (IMRT), volumetric modulated arc therapy (VMAT), and charged particle systems can readily spare the skin and other normal tissues, what is the rationale for GRID therapy or even SFRT in general? While SFRT has been adapted to megavoltage therapy to overcome the even greater challenges of inducing a response in advanced voluminous, recurrent, and refractory tumors, the answers to this paradox have begun to emerge. These answers lie in the postulated unconventional biological advantages of highly heterogeneous dose distributions over traditional 'uniform' dose distributions in conjunction with those of the established advantages of single- or hypo-fractionated ablative doses over conventionally fractionated doses.

The unconventional biological effects are thought to result from the highly heterogeneous dose distributions and are often referred to as bystander effects and abscopal effects; the most intriguing underlying mechanisms include radioimmune modulation, radiation-induced reperfusion, and sensitization of tumors to chemotherapy or conventional radiation therapy. Much basic research and some preclinical studies have been carried out [7–12] and are reviewed in the biology sections of this book's chapters 1–3.

These biological considerations may be impacted by the geometric configuration of the dose heterogeneity pattern, and this may be particularly important for LRT-generated dose heterogeneity, which allows much greater variability than those of GRID-based SFRT technologies. Therefore, rigorous guidance on the optimal geometric configuration of SFRT that may correlate with the best tumor response, provided by biologists, and based on preclinical investigations and response models are critically important to physicists, so that dose heterogeneity patterns can be leveraged for better clinical outcomes. Such rigorous biological insights are still evolving in the preclinical research domain and are not yet robustly available to practitioners in clinical settings. Therefore, as in the case of GRID therapy, the principles and methodologies that guide the practice of LRT have largely been heuristic in nature, based on clinical experience accumulated collectively.

LRT dose distributions can be achieved through a number of techniques [6, 13–18]. With x-rays, highly focused irradiation is the overall guiding principle; this depends on specific delivery technology and instrumentation. It can be accomplished by 3D beam focusing, coplanar or non-coplanar IMRT, or static or arc-based approaches, such as VMAT. In the cases of proton and heavier ion beams, the proposed approach has been multiple spaced-out pencil beams with different energies that deliver arrays of singular Bragg peaks [6, 13, 19], but no clinical patient has been treated in this way to date. Photon-based LRT will be the main focus of this chapter.

## 10.2 Clinical intent and LRT configuration

The clinical intent of LRT is generally divided into three categories: partial volume boost or debulking; the induction of bystander/abscopal effects; and the combination of the two.

### 10.2.1 Partial tumor boost or debulking

The purpose of partial tumor boost or debulking is simply to deliver the largest possible radiation dose to the tumor in the safest possible way. With this intent, the major focus is to cover the largest possible portion of the tumor with a high dose, delivered either throughout the course of radiation treatment using the dose-painting (field within field) technique or as standalone LRT boost fraction(s). In this setting, the peak dose can have a wide range, for example 5–20 Gy, and the value of the valley dose is not crucial as long as the normal tissue dose can be adequately reduced.

The 'field within field' approach was first reported by Amendola *et al* in 2012. It was used to treat an inoperable large cervical tumor amounting to 250 cc [20]. A VMAT technique using two complete 6 MV arcs was employed to deliver the LRT plan prescribed as follows: PTV received 1.8 Gy × 20 fractions to the total of 36 Gy, while 15 vertices of 1 cm spheres receiving 2.4 Gy × 20 fractions to the total of 48 Gy to. Only 3% of the planning target volume (PTV) received the escalated (LRT) dose. At the completion of radiation therapy, the patient achieved a 70% tumor volume reduction and subsequently underwent total abdominal hysterectomy and bilateral salpingo-oophorectomy six weeks after the completion of radiation therapy, showing a complete pathological response (no residual tumor in the specimen). Spraker *et al* recently described 'lattice stereotactic body radiation therapy (SBRT),' a dose-painting technique used for the palliative treatment of large tumors, in which the doses administered to the vertices by the SBRT dose vary [21].

The standalone LRT boost approach has been used in most of the reported cases [13, 20, 22–25]. The LRT dose and fractions have varied and have been commonly given prior to conventional (non-heterogeneous) radiation therapy (cERT) or in between doses of cERT, for example, by delivering LRT once a week. Because of the dosimetric properties of LRT, it is easy to keep to conventional dose/fractionation levels (2–3 Gy per fraction) at the tumor periphery. Therefore, the addition of LRT with a high vertex dose (>10 Gy per fraction) to cERT does not generally result in higher toxicity. The main objective of the LRT boost is dose escalation for better local tumor control. In the setting of preoperative radiation for sarcoma, for example, a high incidence of therapy-induced necrosis (known to be a major prognostic factor) has been observed [26–28].

### 10.2.2 Induction of bystander and abscopal effects

For the induction of bystander and abscopal effects, the guidelines of the heuristic principle are that the peak dose should be sufficiently high to induce bystander and distant cell killings through cytokine/chemokine pathways and/or by the tumor immunogenic response due to the mechanism of radiation-based in-situ vaccination [29–45]; the valley dose should be low enough (<5 Gy) to preserve tumor microvasculature and perfusion, thereby allowing the circulation of cytokines, chemokines, and/or immunogenic factors [46–51]. Based on theoretical principles and early observations in tumor biology studies, the recommended peak dose is 15–25 Gy (or higher), and the valley dose is less than 5 Gy (or as low as reasonably achievable). Clinical data in this area are limited. However, increasing evidence from basic research (described in more detail in chapters 2 and 3) has inspired a high level of interest in investigating the potential of harnessing the bystander and abscopal effects of SFRT.

### 10.2.3 LRT configuration and treatment planning

The principle of LRT is to create an array of high-dose islands or vertices, which receive peak doses; these have a certain separation that allows for lower doses (valley doses) in between. The dimensions or scale of such a geometric configuration is generally based on that of the historical GRID experience (described in detail in chapter 9). Given the clinical objective of dose heterogeneity, symmetry is not a rigorous requirement. Therefore, the size and shape of the vertices and the separation between them may vary from case to case or even within the same LRT plan. The characteristics of radiation delivery technologies (linacs and linac specifications, such as multileaf collimator (MLC) size, TomoTherapy, Gamma Knife, CyberKnife and others) are also significant factors that influence the LRT configuration used to achieve certain dose objectives.

To demonstrate the general process of creating an LRT plan, we take a liposarcoma of 2933 cc in the left thigh as an example. Referring to figure 10.1, the following procedures can serve as general guides:

i. *Creating an LRT volume* ($V_L$). Restricting the tumor periphery to a low dose is an important principle in LRT dosimetric planning. For this purpose, an LRT volume ($V_L$) is created by contracting the gross tumor volume (GTV) inward by a certain margin, generally approximately 5 mm (which does not need to be uniform). The purpose of $V_L$ is to prevent high-dose vertices from being placed too close to the edge of the GTV, which might abut critical normal structures.

ii. *Creating vertices within the $V_L$ of certain shapes and sizes at certain separations.* This can commonly be done by creating a number of spheres

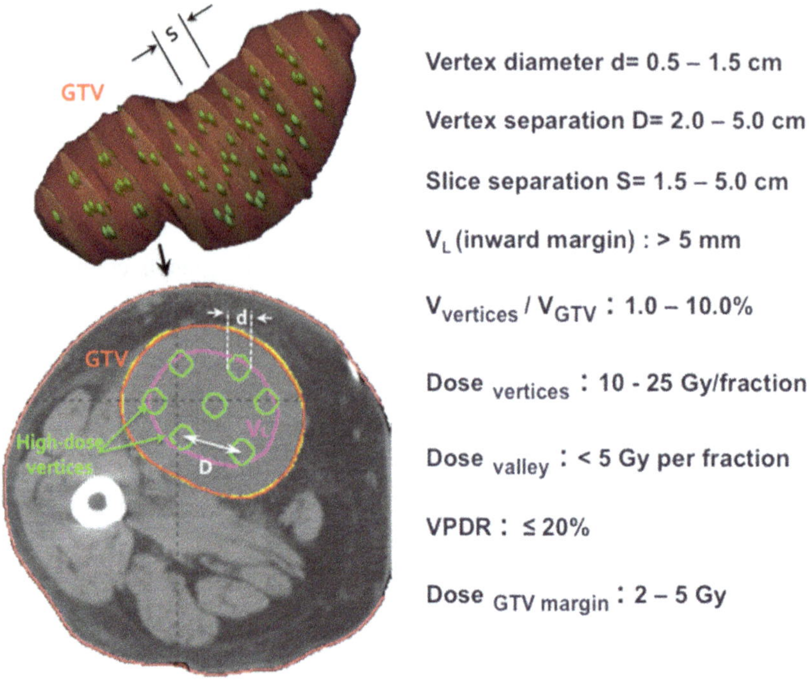


**Figure 10.1.** LRT vertex configuration and planning parameters.

with diameter $d$ (0.5–1.5 cm) within an axial CT slice, separated (center-to-center) by a certain distance $D$ (2–5 cm), and repeating the same in other axial slices with a certain separation between slices $S$ (1.5–5 cm). Placing vertices on critical structures, such as large vessels or nerves within the target volume, or in a location close to critical organs adjacent to the GTV is to be avoided.

For IMRT or VMAT, which have a gantry rotational plane parallel to the slices where the vertices are generated, it is relatively easy to achieve lower valley doses (less than 5 Gy per fraction or less than 20% of the prescribed peak dose) in between slices. Therefore, the separation between slices $S$ can generally be smaller than the vertex separation $D$ within a slice.

iii. *Placing beams with the appropriate parameters (collimator rotation, couch rotation, gantry position, or arc range) and specifying optimization criteria.* Additional structures can be created to assist optimization control, in particular to lower the dose between vertices. The following optimization parameters can be used as a reference:
   a. The LRT prescription dose $D_{\mathrm{p}}$, specified as the high dose delivered to the vertices, should cover 1.0%–10.0% of the GTV.
   b. The lowest 5% of $V_{\mathrm{L}}$ should have a mean dose $D_{\mathrm{mean}}$ (100%–95%) of less than 5 Gy per fraction or less than 20% of the $D_{\mathrm{p}}$, which is defined as the valley-to-peak dose ratio ($VPDR$) for LRT:
      $VPDR = D_{mean}(100\% - 95\%)/D_p$

**Table 10.1.** LRT prescription table.

LRT Prescription: Dp(total Gy): 48.0 Fractions: 4 Photon Energy: 10 MV Technique: VMAT

Vertices

| Number of vertices used | Equiv. dia (cm) per vertex | Effective cc per vertec | Average Distance between vertices center-center (cm) | Dmax (Gy) | Total V(Dp) cc | V(Dp)/GTV |
|---|---|---|---|---|---|---|
| 15 | 1.9 | 3.7 | 4.75 | 73.1 | 55.7 | 0.019 |

Lattice Volume

| $V_L$ (cc) | Dminimum (Gy) | Dmean (100%–95%) Gy | V(≤5 Gy/fx)% | VPDR Dmean(100–95)/Dp |
|---|---|---|---|---|
| 1370 | 7.1 | 9.5 | 70.1 | 0.198 |

GTV

| GTV (cc) | Dminimum (Gy) | Dmean (100%–95%) Gy | V(≤5 Gy/fx)% | VPDR Dmean(100–95)/Dp |
|---|---|---|---|---|
| 2933 | 5.8 | 8.0 | 80.4 | 0.167 |

c. Set the critical structures to receive less than their tolerance doses as per clinical guidelines, considering the SFRT fraction size and the additional cERT dose contribution to critical structures.

iv. It may take several iterations to adjust these parameters; the vertex size *d*, the separations *D* and *S*, the number of beams/arcs, and the couch angles are primarily used to optimally achieve the plan objectives.

v. Record the final plan parameters and dose–volume statistics according to the LRT prescription table (table 10.1).

### 10.2.4 LRT plan review, approval, and reporting

Using the aforementioned general principles, the example plan for this liposarcoma case intended to give preoperative radiotherapy using VMAT to deliver a dose of 50 Gy in 25 fractions, combining four fractions of LRT (12 Gy per fraction to the vertices) with 21 fractions of standard VAMT (2 Gy per fraction to the PTV).

After taking into consideration all the clinical findings, 15 vertices of 1.5 cm diameters ($d$) each were distributed within the LRT volume $V_L$ of 1370 cc with average vertex separations of 4.75 cm ($D$) within slices and 4.0 cm ($S$) between slices. Four coplanar VMAT arcs were used. In the resulting optimized plan, the prescribed LRT dose of 12 Gy in four fractions was distributed to and around the 15 vertices, covering a total volume of 55.7 cc, which was 1.9% of the GTV volume. For $V_L$, the $D_{mean}$ (100%–95%) and *VPDR* were 2.4 Gy per fraction and 19.7% respectively, and for the GTV, they were 2.0 Gy per fraction and 16.7% respectively. The maximum dose delivered to the vertices was 73.1 Gy (figure 10.2).

Note that the layout of the vertices primarily served as a guide to direct the distribution of high-dose islands. Depending on the progression of optimization and the objectives, the final evaluation of an LRT plan rests upon the total volume of the high dose islands and the 'cold' regions surrounding them. In this example, the LRT prescription dose of 12 Gy in four fractions covered each of the 15 predefined vertices with an average volume of 3.7 cm$^3$, equivalent to a sphere with a diameter of 1.9 cm (larger than the predefined vertex size). This resulted in the LRT dose of 12 Gy in four fractions covering a total of 55.7 cm$^3$, or 1.9% of the GTV, in accordance with the guideline that the LRT prescription dose $D_p$ should cover 1.0%–10.0% of the GTV as described in 10.2.3.i.

The dosimetric report of an LRT plan should typically include the parameters listed in table 10.1 (which summarizes the above case example) and the dose–volume histograms (DVHs) of the GTV, $V_L$ (figure 10.3), and the critical normal structures.

The accuracy and reliability with which LRT is delivered are generally secured using the well-established techniques of stereotactic radiosurgery (SRS) or SBRT and IMRT/VMAT delivery. Today's QA technologies can readily be applied to the clinical implementation of LRT. Image guidance and respiratory motion management are essential to assure delivery accuracy.

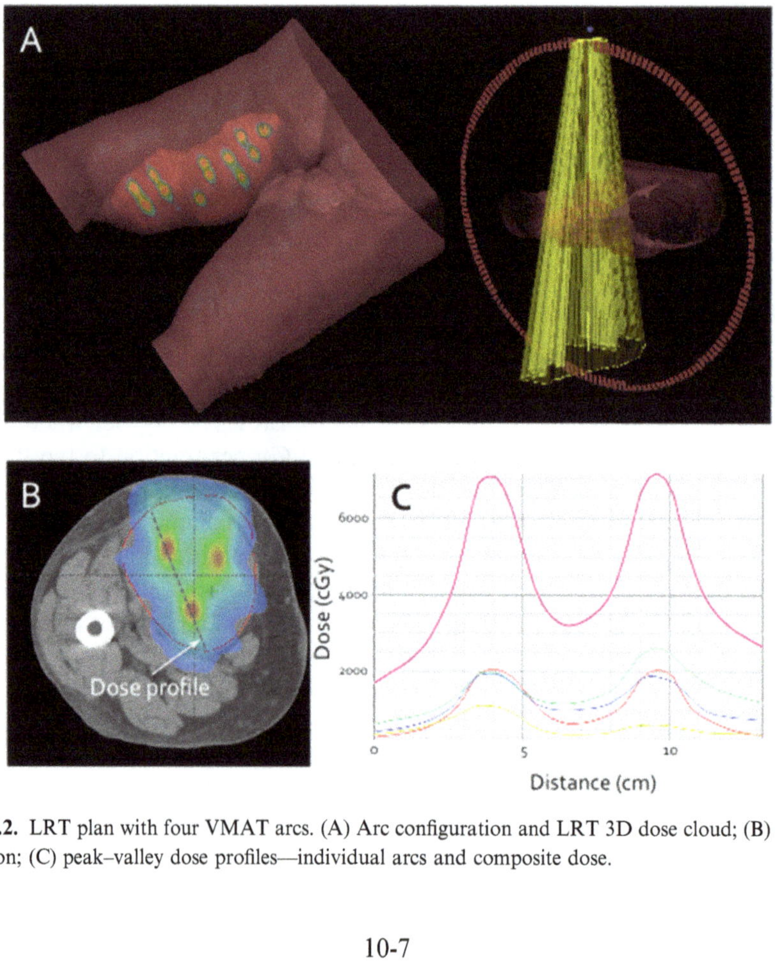


**Figure 10.2.** LRT plan with four VMAT arcs. (A) Arc configuration and LRT 3D dose cloud; (B) axial dose distribution; (C) peak–valley dose profiles—individual arcs and composite dose.

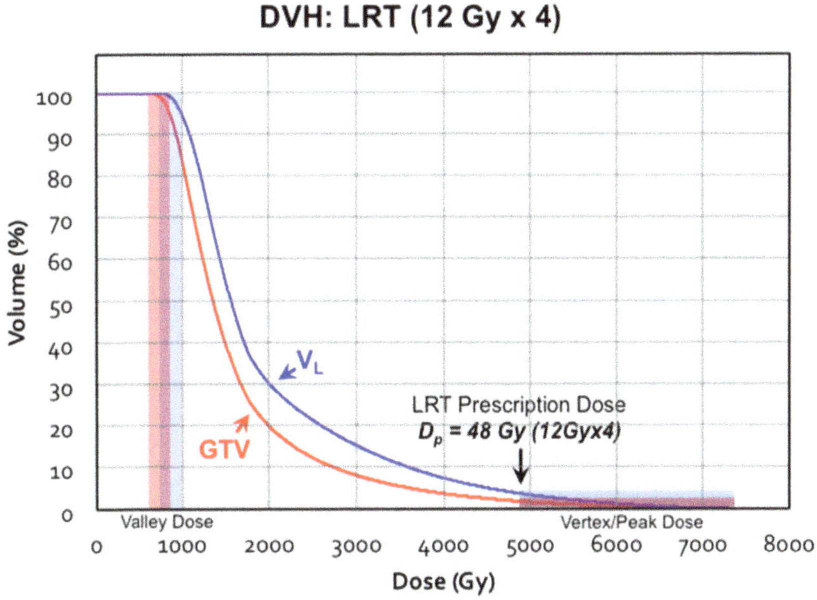


**Figure 10.3.** LRT DVHs of GTV and $V_L$.

## 10.3 Knowledge gaps and future perspectives

The hallmark of SFRT has been its highly heterogeneous dose distribution. Although the clinical data may suggest that it is effective, a range of factors that may impact the treatment outcomes of SFRT has been increasingly observed, yet they lack quantitative correlation. The delivery of an ablative dose to partial tumor volumes is the general objective of SFRT; it may assume various approaches to determine the regions and geometries of the high-dose regions [52–56].

It is evident that a biological basis that can be used to optimize LRT parameters has yet to be rigorously established. Nevertheless, the early clinical data has inspired several systemic clinical studies recently initiated by a number of institutions. With the advent of modern biological science and new clinical data, we may anticipate renewed contributions of the century-old SFRT to cancer treatments.

Advances in radiotherapy instrumentation have also opened new venues for the application of SFRT. Most modern linacs with high-definition MLCs, interactive couch/gantry/collimator motion control, and image guidance are well suited for delivering LRT. The existing treatment planning systems are generally capable of generating LRT plans with or without other assistive software, although a tailored planning module specific to LRT would be highly favorable. Particle systems (proton or heavier ions) could be used to effectively deliver LRT, reaping the additional advantage of Bragg peaks [6, 13]. One of the proposed approaches involves the use of non-intersecting pencil beams from multiple gantry angles at various energies to fill the target volume with high-dose vertices (figure 10.4) [19].

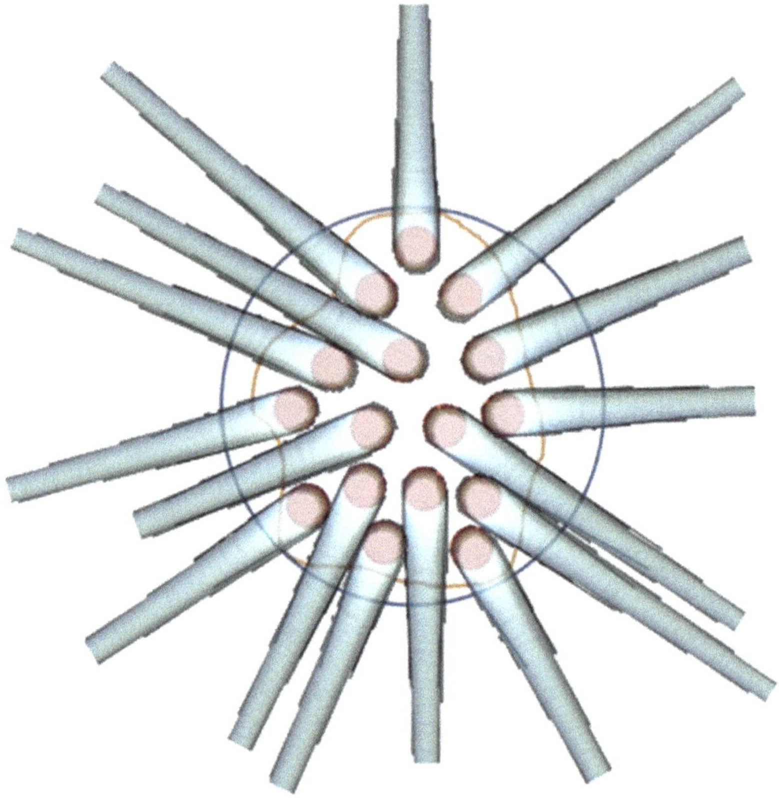

**Figure 10.4.** Bragg-peak vertices generated by non-intersecting proton pencil beams.

## 10.4 Conclusions

Following many decades of the clinical application of GRID therapy, 3D LRT has made its cautious entry into the clinic over the last decade. Over 1000 patients have been treated worldwide with proven safety. LRT can be implemented with relative ease using modern high-energy photon systems. This chapter has focused on providing a general framework for the technical procedures used to plan and deliver IMRT/VMAT-based LRT that may be useful in the initiation of LRT programs, while recognizing that much research will be needed to refine current approaches.

## References


[1] Liberson F 1933 The value of a multi-perforated screen in deep x-ray therapy *Radiology* **30** 186–95

[2] Marks H 1950 A new approach to the roentgen therapy of cancer with the use of a grid *J. Mt. Sinai. Hosp. N. Y.* **17** 46–8

[3] Marks H 1952 Clinical experience with irradiation through a grid *Radiology* **58** 338–42

[4] Laissue J A, Blattmann H and Slatkin D N 2012 [Alban Köhler (1874–1947): inventor of grid therapy] *Z. Med. Phys.* **22** 90–9

[5] Freid J R, Lipman A and Jacobson L E 1953 Roentgen therapy through a grid for advanced carcinoma *Am. J. Roentgenol. Radium. Ther. Nucl. Med.* **70** 460–76
[6] Wu X, Ahmed M M, Wright J, Gupta S and Pollack A 2010 On modern technical approaches of three-dimensional high-dose lattice radiotherapy (LRT) *Cureus.* **2** e9
[7] Sathishkumar S, Dey S, Meigooni A S, Regine W F, Kudrimoti M S and Ahmed M M *et al* 2002 The impact of TNF-alpha induction on therapeutic efficacy following high dose spatially fractionated (GRID) radiation *Technol. Cancer Res. Treat.* **1** 141–7
[8] Sathishkumar S, Boyanovsky B, Karakashian A A, Rozenova K, Giltiay N V and Kudrimoti M *et al* 2005 Elevated sphingomyelinase activity and ceramide concentration in serum of patients undergoing high dose spatially fractionated radiation treatment: implications for endothelial apoptosis *Cancer Biol. Ther.* **4** 979–86
[9] Peters M E, Shareef M M, Gupta S, Zagurovskaya-Sultanov M, Kadhim M and Mohiuddin M *et al* 2007 Potential utilization of bystander/abscopal-mediated signal transduction events in the treatment of solid tumors *Curr. Signal Transduct. Ther.* **2** 129–43
[10] Shareef M M, Cui N, Burikhanov R, Gupta S, Satishkumar S and Shajahan S *et al* 2007 Role of tumor necrosis factor-alpha and TRAIL in high-dose radiation-induced bystander signaling in lung adenocarcinoma *Cancer Res.* **67** 11811–20
[11] Kanagavelu S, Gupta S, Wu X, Philip S, Wattenberg M M and Hodge J W *et al* 2014 In vivo effects of lattice radiation therapy on local and distant lung cancer: potential role of immunomodulation *Radiat. Res.* **182** 149–62
[12] Asur R, Butterworth K T, Penagaricano J A, Prise K M and Griffin R J 2015 High dose bystander effects in spatially fractionated radiation therapy *Cancer Lett.* **356** 52–7
[13] Wu X, Perez N C, Zheng Y, Li X, Jiang L, Amendola B E and Xu B *et al* 2020 The technical and clinical implementation of LATTICE radiation therapy (LRT) *Radiat. Res.* **194** 737–46
[14] Kopchick B, Xu H, Niu Y, Becker S, Qiu X and Yu C 2020 Technical note: dosimetric feasibility of lattice radiotherapy for breast cancer using GammaPod *Med. Phys.* **47** 3928–34
[15] Pokhrel D, Halfman M, Sanford L, Chen Q and Kudrimoti M 2020 A novel, yet simple MLC-based 3D-crossfire technique for spatially fractionated GRID therapy treatment of deep-seated bulky tumors *J. Appl. Clin. Med. Phys.* **21** 68–74
[16] Yan W *et al* 2019 Spatially fractionated radiation therapy: history, present and the future *Clin. Transl. Radiat. Oncol.* **20** 30–8
[17] Zhang X, Penagaricano J, Yan Y, Sharma S, Griffin R J, Hardee M, Han E Y and Ratanatharathom V 2016 Application of spatially fractionated radiation (GRID) to helical tomotherapy using a novel TOMOGRID template *Technol. Cancer Res. Treat.* **15** 91–100
[18] Jin J Y, Zhao B, Kaminski J M, Wen N, Huang Y, Vender J, Chetty I J and Kong F M 2015 A MLC-based inversely optimized 3D spatially fractionated grid radiotherapy technique *Radiother. Oncol.* **117** 483–6
[19] Zhou Y 2020 A prototype of automated lattice particle treatment (LPT) planning system *PhD Thesis* University of Miami https://scholarship.miami.edu/esploro/outputs/991031498089802976
[20] Amendola B E, Perez N, Amendola M, Wu X, Ahmed M M and Iglesias A J *et al* 2010 Lattice radiotherapy with RapidArc for treatment of gynecological tumors: dosimetric and early clinical evaluations *Cureus* **2** 1–6
[21] Duriseti S, Kavanaugh J, Goddu S, Price A, Knutson N, Reynoso F, Michalski J, Mutic S, Robinson C and Spraker M B 2021 Spatially fractionated stereotactic body radiation therapy (Lattice) for large tumors *Adv. Radiat. Oncol.* **6** 100639

[22] Blanco Suarez J M, Amendola B E, Perez N C, Amendola M and Wu X 2015 The use of lattice radiation therapy (LRT) in the treatment of bulky tumors: a case report of a large metastatic mixed mullerian ovarian tumor *Cureus.* **7** e389

[23] Amendola B E, Perez N C, Wu X, Blanco Suarez J M, Lu J J and Amendola M 2018 Improved outcome of treating locally advanced lung cancer with the use of lattice radiotherapy (LRT): a case report. *Clin. Transl. Radiat. Oncol.* **9** 68–71

[24] Amendola B E, Perez N C, Wu X, Amendola M A and Qureshi I Z 2019 Safety and efficacy of lattice radiotherapy in voluminous non-small cell lung cancer *Cureus.* **11** e4263

[25] Amendola B E, Perez N C, Mayr N A, Wu X and Amendola M 2020 Spatially fractionated radiation therapy using lattice radiation in far-advanced bulky cervical cancer: a clinical and molecular imaging and outcome study *Radiat. Res.* **194** 724–36

[26] MacDermed D M, Miller L L and Peabody T D *et al* 2010 Primary tumor necrosis predicts distant control in locally advanced soft tissue sarcomas following preoperative concurrent chemoradiotherapy *Int. J. Radiat. Oncol. Biol. Phys.* **76** 1147–53

[27] Koshy M, Rich S E and Mohiuddin M M 2010 Improved survival with radiation therapy in high-grade soft tissue sarcomas of the extremities: a SEER analysis *Int. J. Radiat. Oncol. Biol. Phys.* **77** 203–9

[28] Snider J W, Molitoris J, Shyu S, Diwanji T, Rice S and Kowalski E *et al* 2020 spatially fractionated radiotherapy (GRID) prior to standard neoadjuvant conventionally fractionated radiotherapy for bulky, high-risk soft tissue and osteosarcomas: feasibility, safety, and promising pathologic response rates *Radiat. Res.* **194** 707–14

[29] Jiang L, Li X, Zhang J, Li W, Dong F, Chen C, Lin Q, Zhang C, Zheng F and Yan W *et al* 2021 Combined high-dose LATTICE radiation therapy and immune checkpoint blockade for advanced bulky tumors: the concept and a case report *Front. Oncol.* **10** 548132

[30] Markovsky E, Budhu S, Samstein R M, Li H, Russell J and Zhang Z *et al* 2019 An antitumor immune response is evoked by partial-volume single-dose radiation in 2 murine models *Int. J. Radiat. Oncol. Biol. Phys.* **103** 697–708

[31] Filatenkov A, Baker J, Mueller A M, Kenkel J, Ahn G O and Dutt S *et al* 2015 Ablative tumor radiation can change the tumor immune cell microenvironment to induce durable complete remissions *Clin. Cancer Res.* **21** 3727–39

[32] Formenti S C and Demaria S 2009 Systemic effects of local radiotherapy *Lancet Oncol.* **10** 718–26

[33] Wennerberg E, Lhuillier C, Vanpouille-Box C, Pilones K A, Garcia-Martinez E and Rudqvist N P *et al* 2017 Barriers to radiation-induced *in situ* tumor vaccination *Front. Immunol.* **8** 229

[34] Chakravarty P K, Alfieri A, Thomas E K, Beri V, Tanaka K E and Vikram B *et al* 1999 Flt3-ligand administration after radiation therapy prolongs survival in a murine model of metastatic lung cancer *Cancer Res.* **59** 6028–32

[35] Ahmed M M, Hodge J W, Guha C, Bernhard E J, Vikram B and Coleman C N 2013 Harnessing the potential of radiation-induced immune modulation for cancer therapy *Cancer Immunol. Res.* **1** 280–4

[36] Buchwald Z S, Wynne J, Nasti T H, Zhu S, Mourad W F and Yan W *et al* 2018 Radiation, immune checkpoint blockade and the abscopal effect: a critical review on timing, dose and fractionation *Front. Oncol.* **8** 612

[37] Rodriguez-Ruiz M E, Vanpouille-Box C, Melero I, Formenti S C and Demaria S 2018 Immunological mechanisms responsible for radiation-induced abscopal effect *Trends Immunol.* **39** 644–55

[38] Demaria S, Ng B, Devitt M L, Babb J S, Kawashima N and Liebes L *et al* 2004 Ionizing radiation inhibition of distant untreated tumors (abscopal effect) is immune mediated *Int. J. Radiat. Oncol.* **58** 862–70

[39] Demaria S, Kawashima N, Yang A M, Devitt M L, Babb J S and Allison J P *et al* 2005 Immune-mediated inhibition of metastases after treatment with local radiation and CTLA-4 blockade in a mouse model of breast cancer *Clin. Cancer Res.* **11** 728–34

[40] Hiniker S M, Chen D S and Knox S J 2012 Abscopal effect in a patient with melanoma *New Engl. J. Med.* **366** 2035

[41] Postow M A, Callahan M K, Barker C A, Yamada Y, Yuan J D and Kitano S *et al* 2012 Immunologic correlates of the abscopal effect in a patient with melanoma *New Engl. J. Med.* **366** 925–31

[42] Yamada Y, Bilsky M H, Lovelock D M, Venkatraman E S, Toner S and Johnson J *et al* 2008 High-dose, single-fraction image-guided intensity-modulated radiotherapy for metastatic spinal lesions *Int. J. Radiat. Oncol. Biol. Phys.* **71** 484–90

[43] Greco C, Zelefsky M J, Lovelock M, Fuks Z, Hunt M and Rosenzweig K *et al* 2011 Predictors of local control after single-dose stereotactic image-guided intensity modulated radiotherapy for extracranial metastases *Int. J. Radiat. Oncol. Biol. Phys.* **79** 1151–7

[44] Savage T and Guha C 2019 Radio-immunology of ablative radiation *Stereotactic Radiosurgery and Stereotactic Body Radiation Therapy* ed D Trifiletti, S Chao, A Sahgal and J Sheehan (Cham: Springer) pp 15–29

[45] Mohiuddin M, Park H, Hallmeyer S and Richards J 2015 High-dose radiation as a dramatic, immunological primer in locally advanced melanoma *Cureus* **7** e417

[46] Potiron V A, Abderrahmani R, Clément-Colmou K, Marionneau- Lambot S, Oullier T and Paris F *et al* 2013 Improved functionality of the vasculature during conventionally fractionated radiation therapy of prostate cancer *PLoS One* **8** e84076

[47] Ministro A, de Oliveira P, Nunes R J, dos Santos Rocha A, Correia A and Carvalho T *et al* 2017 Low-dose ionizing radiation induces therapeutic neovascularization in a pre-clinical model of hindlimb ischemia *Cardiovasc. Res.* **113** 783–94

[48] Mendonca M S, Chin-Sinex H, Dhaemers R, Mead L E, Yoder M C and Ingram D A 2011 Differential mechanisms of x-ray-induced cell death in human endothelial progenitor cells isolated from cord blood and adults *Radiat. Res.* **176** 208–16

[49] Park H J, Griffin R J, Hui S, Levitt S H and Song C W 2012 Radiation-induced vascular damage in tumors: implications of vascular damage in ablative hypofractionated radiotherapy (SBRT and SRS) *Radiat. Res.* **177** 311–27

[50] Klug F, Prakash H, Huber P E, Seibel T, Bender N and Halama N *et al* 2013 Low-dose irradiation programs macrophage differentiation to an iNOS(+)/M1 phenotype that orchestrates effective T cell immunotherapy *Cancer Cell* **24** 589–602

[51] Hellevik T and Martinez-Zubiaurre I 2014 Radiotherapy and the tumor stroma: the importance of dose and fractionation *Front. Oncol.* **4** 1

[52] Tubin S, Khan M K, Salerno G, Mourad W F, Yan W and Jeremic B 2019 Mono-institutional phase 2 study of innovative Stereotactic Body RadioTherapy targeting PArtial Tumor HYpoxic (SBRT-PATHY) clonogenic cells in unresectable bulky non-small cell lung cancer: profound non-targeted effects by sparing peri-tumoral immune microenvironment *Radiat. Oncol.* **14** 212

[53] Pollack A, Chinea F M, Bossart E, Kwon D, Abramowitz M C and Lynne C *et al* 2020 Phase I trial of MRI-guided prostate cancer lattice extreme ablative dose (LEAD) boost radiation therapy *Int. J. Radiat. Oncol. Biol. Phys.* **107** 305–15

[54] Bodo S, Campagne C, Thin T H, Higginson D S, Vargas H A and Hua G *et al* 2019 Single-dose radiotherapy disables tumor cell homologous recombination via ischemia/reperfusion injury *J. Clin. Invest.* **129** 786–801

[55] Greco C, Kolesnick R and Fuks Z 2021 Conformal avoidance of normal organs at risk by perfusion-modulated dose sculpting in tumor single-dose radiation therapy *Int. J. Radiat. Oncol. Biol. Phys.* **S0360-3016** 34105–5

[56] Ferini G, Valenti V, Tripoli A, Illari S I, Molino L, Parisi S, Cacciola A, Lillo S, Giuffrida D and Pergolizzi S 2021 Lattice or oxygen-guided radiotherapy: what if they converge? Possible future directions in the era of immunotherapy *Cancers* **13** 3290

# Chapter 11

## Rotational arc SFRT

**Xin Zhang, José Peñagaricano and Eduardo G Moros**

Spatially fractionated radiation therapy (SFRT) based on GRID technology is usually delivered via an multileaf collimator (MLC) step and shoot approach or through a commercially available alloy GRID block. In either case, a single-portal GRID field is usually delivered for treatment. The dose to the target decreases rapidly with depth; the maximum dose can be located at a shallow depth and possibly outside the target volume. Thus, the spatially fractionated dose distribution may under- or over-treat parts of the target volume. To avoid these shortcomings, rotational arc SFRT using helical tomotherapy or volumetric modulated arc therapy has been developed. These newer SFRT techniques offer a number of advantages, such as providing a patient-specific GRID pattern or a virtual GRID block by customizing the number of openings and the center-to-center distance between openings and by changing the diameters of the openings to accommodate the target border and shapes and offering better skin sparing through the use of multiple gantry angles. This arc therapy SFRT approach allows for better sparing of organs at risk (OARs) by preventing high-dose spill outside the target, while maintaining an SFRT pattern at a similar equivalent uniform dose within the target volume that has been shown to offer a theoretical therapeutic gain in terms of normal-tissue sparing compared to open-field debulking radiation therapy.

### 11.1 Introduction/overview

SFRT has been used to treat bulky tumors for decades. The clinical outcomes have shown that SFRT can effectively debulk large tumor volumes with low toxicity [1, 2]. SFRT usually delivers a single fraction-dose using a single field using a GRID alloy block collimator or an multileaf collimator (MLC) to deliver a highly inhomogeneous dose distribution within the target volume [3, 4].

When either a GRID alloy block or an MLC is used, the maximum dose can be located at a shallow depth or outside the target volume (if the tumor is deep and the shallow region consists of normal tissue). Thus, it can be difficult to spare adjacent

doi:10.1088/978-0-7503-4046-5ch11

OARs. This problem becomes more significant for deep-seated bulky tumors, because the beam's high-dose regions may penetrate any organs in its path. Modern SFRT methods aim to use new and advanced rotational arc radiation therapy delivery techniques, such as helical tomotherapy (HT) and volumetric modulated arc therapy (VMAT) to develop improved, more conformal, and patient-specific SFRT treatment plans [5, 6].

These modalities offer personalized optimization of the GRID pattern, and their main advantage is in treating bulky deep-seated tumors for which a commercial GRID collimator may not deliver the same treatment quality at various depths. In addition, VMAT flattening filter-free (FFF) beams can potentially be used to shorten treatment times, if the treatment time required for VMAT is significantly longer than that using a GRID collimator.

This chapter will focus on the rotational arc SFRT method, including the characteristics of the virtual GRID block (or GRID pattern) generated by software, the design of the virtual GRID block, rotational arc SFRT treatment plan considerations, the treatment plan dosimetric characteristics, as well the treatment plan evaluation methods.

## 11.2 MLC-based SFRT block and beam characteristics

Initially, SFRT was delivered by inserting an alloy block GRID collimator into the linear accelerator accessory mount, as described in more detail in chapter 9, which discusses GRID therapy methods. The GRID collimator could be made in-house or acquired commercially. Others have used MLCs to mimic the dose distribution of SFRT (MLC-based GRID therapy). This was done by defining many beamlets with multiple segments in a step and shoot fashion. Utilizing software, a virtual GRID block (or GRID pattern) could be defined and 'inserted' into the planning system. This virtual GRID block could be modeled to fit the patient's anatomy, tumor volume, and shape.

### 11.2.1 Virtual grid block

The concept of the virtual GRID block is still being developed, and various applications and techniques for generating virtual GRID distributions have been developed and continue to evolve (as also described in chapters 9 and 10). These are in principle applicable to multiple delivery technologies and can be tailored to linear accelerators using IMRT or VMAT as well as to helical tomotherapy. This wide applicability of the virtual GRID block concept broadens the overall access to SFRT as a modality.

The virtual GRID block design created by software also consists of open and blocked areas that are similar to those of commercially available GRID blocks. The open and blocked areas of the virtual GRID block are divided into the GRID target, which represents the open areas, and the areas of GRID avoidance, which represent the closed or blocked areas. The user has the ability to define the GRID target's open diameter and center-to-center distance. A similar concept was used in another GRID therapy study, in which structures known as 'cold tube' and 'hot tube' were used for dose optimization [7]. The prescription specifies the dose to be delivered to the GRID target. The interval between the open areas or blocked areas (devoid of open structures), also known as GRID avoidance, is used in the planning process as an avoidance structure to create the low-dose or valleys within the target volume (figure 11.1). The software can either be coded in-house or purchased commercially (one of the commercially available software products is DICOMANTX) [8]. The two new structures (the GRID target and the GRID avoidance) are then transferred to the treatment planning system (TPS) for dose optimization. This approach seeks to create cylindrical volumes of high dosage (peaks) within the gross tumor volume (GTV) surrounded by low-dose volumes (valleys). The longitudinal axes of the cylinders are perpendicular to the rotational plane of the gantry. Alternatively, one can create the virtual block structures directly from the TPS [7].

### 11.2.2 Design of the alloy block and the optimized virtual GRID block

The potential influence of the GRID block design on the therapeutic ratio has been evaluated in previous studies. Among them, Gholami *et al* (2016) [9] performed Monte Carlo simulations for 25 different patterns of GRID block. They reported that the optimal range of open-field diameters should be between 1.00 and 1.25 cm with an open-field spacing of 1.7 or 1.8 cm and that an appropriate design for the open-field diameter and open-field spacing may lead to a 40% improvement in therapeutic ratio (the authors calculated the results for open-field diameters ranging from 0.5 to 1.5 cm). They also reported that GRID blocks with open-field diameters of 1.0 and 1.25 cm may lead to about a 19% higher therapeutic ratio compared to those of GRID patterns with open-field diameters smaller than 1.0 cm or larger than 1.25 cm.

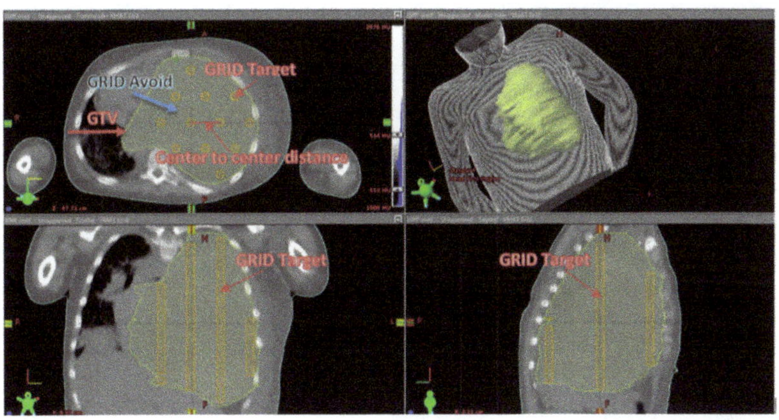


**Figure 11.1.** Example of a virtual GRID block created by the commercially available software DICOMANTX. The user defined the diameters of the GRID target openings and the center-to-center distance. The difference between this approach and lattice therapy (chapter 10) is that rotational arc SFRT creates an array of cylindrical high-dose regions that is more consistent with the heterogeneity dose distribution of classic GRID collimators.

Zhang *et al* [10] investigated the use of a virtual GRID block for VMAT-based SFRT in a study of 25 patients with tumor volumes ranging from 71.6 to 4683 $cm^3$. The virtual GRID block design was optimized by modifying the open area's diameter and the center-to-center spacing to meet the planning goals. The diameter of the average open area was 0.9 cm with a range of 0.8–1.4 cm, and the average center-to-center spacing was 2.7 cm with a range of 2.0–4.6 cm. This study indicated that these parameters can be used as a starting point to design an optimized virtual grid block in the VMAT-based SFRT optimization process.

### 11.2.3 Beam characteristics

Figure 11.2 shows the SFRT dose profile distributions of the alternating peak and valley doses produced by conventional (physical) and virtual GRID blocks.

Figure 11.2 shows that the valley and peak dose distribution is remarkably consistent across the axial plane for the GRID collimator-based SFRT. Ideally, we expect an identical valley–peak dose distribution across the axial plan for rotational SFRT using the virtual GRID block to that produced by the GRID block collimator; however, in the following two cases, the valley–peak dose distributions are variable (figure 11.3).

Figure 11.3 (bottom figure) shows that the valley–peak dose ratio changes across the axial plane for a chest VMAT-SFRT plan. This variability in the magnitudes of the valley and peak doses can be explained as follows: first, the dose under the

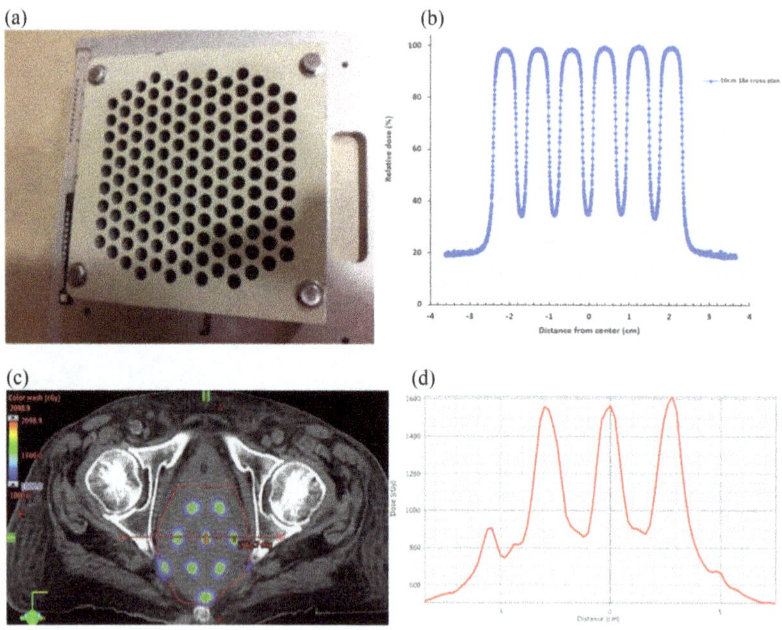


**Figure 11.2.** (a) Conventional alloy GRID block made by Radiation Products Design (Albertville, MN, USA) and the corresponding (b) valley–peak dose distribution; (c) a virtual GRID block and its corresponding (d) valley–peak dose distribution.

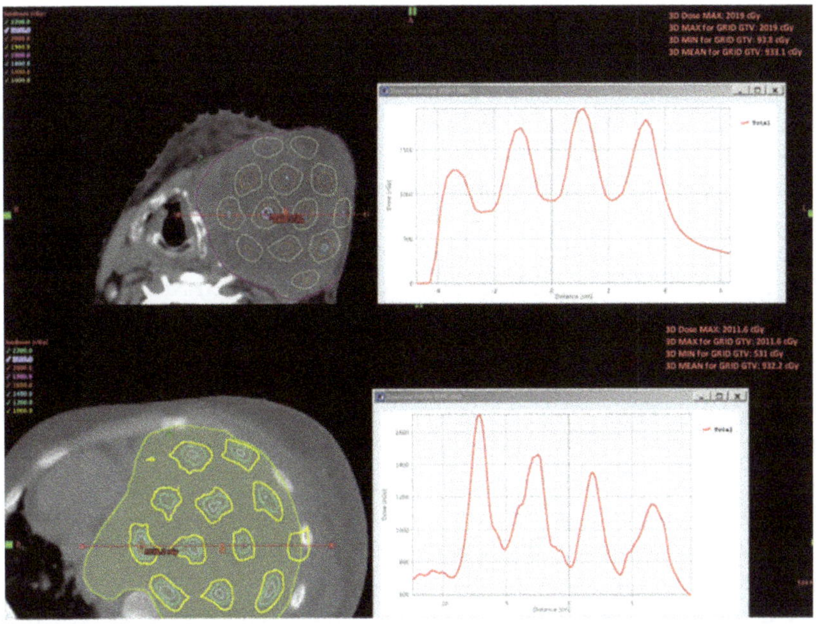

**Figure 11.3.** Variable valley–peak dose distributions for two patients treated with VMAT-SFRT (head and neck (top figure) and chest (bottom figure)).

blocked field consists of beam penetration directly through the virtually blocked areas, the dose fall-off and scatter from the adjacent open area, and the dose leakage from the MLC. Second, the virtual GRID block is patient-specific; if it has a larger open area and a smaller adjacent center-to-center spacing, the dose under the blocked area increases compared to that of a smaller open area with a larger nearby center-to-center spacing due to increased internal scattering. Moreover, the patient with the chest tumor in figure 11.3 (bottom figure) had a large tumor volume (4683.9 $cm^3$) and an irregular tumor shape.

Because of the variable beam profile obtained by defining and using the virtual GRID block, the beam characteristics indicate that a single-point or single-depth valley–peak dose ratio may not represent the target dose inhomogeneity within the SFRT treatment volume. A photon SFRT physics and dosimetry white paper was recently published by the Radiosurgery Society's (RSS's) GRID, Lattice Microbeam and FLASH Radiation Therapy Working Group [11]. The authors recommended that the dosimetric metrics should be reported in SFRT treatment plans. The valley–peak dose ratio (VPDR) at the tumor's central depth was listed as a requirement, but the ratio of D90/D10 of the whole target volume was preferred as a metric with which to characterize the dose inhomogeneity of SFRT. Because clinical situations may vary significantly, the recommendations did not suggest any ranges for these metrics. Zhang *et al* [10] showed that rotational GRID therapy with a virtual block generally has a higher VPDR than SFRT with a physical GRID collimator due to the higher dose given to the GRID blocked area by the scattering of radiation that occurs in the use of VMAT. More studies are needed to evaluate the beam characteristics of modern rotational arc SFRT, so that more flexible and personalized SFRT approaches can be made available for diverse clinical situations. In addition, although there are differences between the dose profiles of GRID collimator-based SFRT and virtual block-based SFRT, Narayanasamy [13] showed that a virtually generated GRID block delivered with a helical tomotherapy unit can produce SFRT patterns that have the same advantage for tumor cell killing (compared to the uniform dose produced by open-field irradiation) as those shown for other types of SFRT, including GRID collimator-based SFRT [9].

## 11.3 Treatment planning considerations

The rotational arc HT or VMAT techniques coupled with the use of a GRID block can address the inability of GRID collimator-based SFRT to optimize the treatment plan to suit a set of dosimetric objectives, particularly the extra-target dose. With SFRT based on rotational arc HT or VMAT, individualized plans can be designed that have improved conformality and reduce the doses given to OARs.

The primary planning goal for rotational arc SFRT using a virtual GRID block is to set the dose constraints for the GRID target, the GRID avoidance structures, and the OARs. By restricting the dose delivered to the GRID avoidance structures, a heterogenous dose distribution is created that shows alternating peak and valley doses.

In order to obtain a maximum dose in the plan that is no larger than the prescription, the dose is prescribed at the maximum point dose of the GTV. The target mean dose is set to fall within the range of 8–10 Gy. In addition, the maximum dose is optimized to be within the GRID target prescription dose. OAR doses are optimized to assure a rapid dose drop-off in the normal-tissue area immediately adjacent to the target. An example of a dose prescription and dose constraint used for planning optimization is as follows: the prescription is set to 20 Gy at the maximum point of the GTV in a single fraction. The plan is optimized with the VMAT technique using two to four arcs with collimator angles of 90° and 270°, and 6 MV FFF beams with a 1400 MU $min^{-1}$ dose rate. Regarding GTV dose constraints, the maximum dose constraint of the GRID target, corresponding to the open area on the virtual GRID block, is set to 20 Gy and the GTV mean dose is set to fall between 8 and 10 Gy.

The normal tissue doses immediately adjacent to the target are optimized to receive a rapid dose fall-off. Two planning structures (ring1, ring2), representing two different normal-tissue areas close to the target, are generated to obtain a rapid dose drop-off from the target surface. Ring1 represents the area that is 5 mm away from the GTV surface and extends outward by 5 mm; ring2 is the area that extends outward by 1 cm from the outer circumference of ring1. The dose constraints for the optimization are 4.5 and 3 Gy for ring1 and ring2, respectively.

Rotational arc beams with collimator angles of 90° and 270° are needed for the virtual block-based GRID therapy to create cylindrical volumes of high dose inside the GTV. Finally, 6 MV FFF beams with 1400 MU $min^{-1}$ or 10 MV FFF beams with 2400 MU $min^{-1}$ dose rates can be used, which can reduce the treatment's beam-on time and reduce patient-motion-related uncertainties.

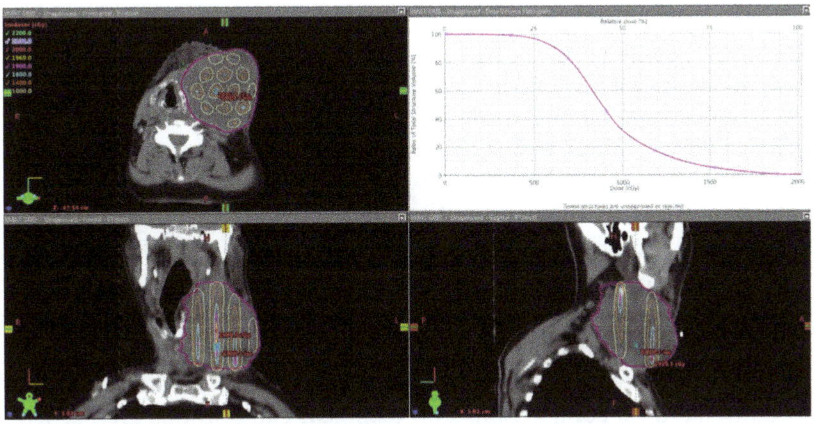

**Figure 11.4.** Example of a DVH of the SFRT in a head and neck cancer patient (the prescription is 20 Gy at the maximum dose point of the GTV); GTV Dmean = 9.33 Gy, GTV EUD = 6.02 Gy, the global maximum dose = 20.2 Gy, and it is located inside the GRID target. The valley–peak ratio = 0.0465, D90/D10 = 0.35, and the virtual GRID block design is as follows: the diameter of the open area = 9 mm and the center-to-center distance = 23 mm.

## 11.4 Treatment plan evaluation

To evaluate a rotational arc SFRT treatment plan, it is recommended to follow the published reporting guidelines as shown in the physics and dosimetry white paper for photon SFRT [11]. The guidelines include parameters such as the GTV mean dose, the GTV equivalent uniform dose (EUD), the GTV inhomogeneity including the VPDR ($D_{min}/D_{max}$), and the ratio of D90/D10. In addition, the location of the global maximum dose is recommended to be located inside the GTV; ideally, the maximum dose should be inside the open areas within the GTV. Figure 11.4 is an example of the dose–volume histogram (DVH) and SFRT isodose distribution for a head and neck cancer patient.

## 11.5 Conclusions and future work

Rotational arc SFRT is a logical progression from physical GRID collimator- or MLC-based SFRT. Rotational arc SFRT not only delivers heterogeneous dose distributions but also exhibits similar peak and valley doses and SFRT patterns consistent with a similar therapeutic ratio advantage to that shown by its predecessor GRID technologies. In addition, this new SFRT approach offers the ability to customize the GRID pattern to suit the patient's individual target volume, while improving OAR sparing with the potential to further decrease the toxicity experienced by normal tissues.

Although SFRT has a long clinical track record in favorably treating large and bulky tumors, there are still many knowledge gaps to be filled. Among these are:

(1) Dosimetric reporting: there is heterogeneity in clinical practice about the dosimetric parameters that are reported in a clinically approved plan. A step forward in working toward a consensus for dosimetric parameter reporting

is the white paper authored by Zhang *et al* [11]. A critical aspect of dosimetric reporting is the prescription dose. In rotational arc SFRT, contrary to routine radiotherapy, the prescription dose has not been correlated with outcomes, and this requires rigorous study.

(2) In rotational arc SFRT, optimization of the planning approach (e.g. the number of arc angle spans) that will provide the best-quality SFRT plans for different target sites remains to be explored. As in the case of the International Consensus [12] on the clinical design of prospective clinical–translational trials in SFRT, a comprehensive physical consensus effort for VMAT-SFRT will provide physical guidelines. A group of experts will establish the guidelines for clinical trials and routine practice in rotational arc SFRT.

(3) Finally, while early studies of rotational arc SFRT have shown promise, additional dose comparisons and technical explorations are needed.

## References

[1] Mohiuddin M S J H, Reiff J E, Huq M S and Suntharalingam N 1996 Spatially fractionated (GRID) radiation for palliative treatment of advanced cancer *Radiat. Oncol. Invest* **4** 41–7

[2] Snider J W, Molitoris J, Shyu S, Diwanji T, Rice S and Kowalski E *et al* 2020 Spatially fractionated radiotherapy (GRID) prior to standard neoadjuvant conventionally fractionated radiotherapy for bulky, high-risk soft tissue and osteosarcomas: feasibility, safety, and promising pathologic response rates *Radiat. Res.* **194** 707–14

[3] Zhang H, Wang J Z, Mayr N, Kong X, Yuan J and Gupta N *et al* 2008 Fractionated grid therapy in treating cervical cancers: conventional fractionation or hypofractionation? *Int. J. Radiat. Oncol. Biol. Phys.* **70** 280–8

[4] Buckey C, Stathakis S, Cashon K, Gutierrez A, Esquivel C and Shi C *et al* 2010 Evaluation of a commercially-available block for spatially fractionated radiation therapy *J. Appl. Clin. Med. Phys.* **11** 3163

[5] Zhang X, Penagaricano J, Yan Y, Sharma S, Griffin R J and Hardee M *et al* 2016 Application of spatially fractionated radiation (GRID) to helical tomotherapy using a novel TOMOGRID template *Technol. Cancer Res. Treat.* **15** 91–100

[6] Zhang X, Penagaricano J, Yan Y, Liang X, Morrill S and Griffin R J *et al* 2016 Spatially fractionated radiotherapy (GRID) using helical tomotherapy *J. Appl. Clin. Med. Phys.* **17** 396–407

[7] Costlow H N, Zhang H and Das I J 2014 A treatment planning approach to spatially fractionated megavoltage grid therapy for bulky lung cancer *Med. Dosim.* **39** 218–26

[8] Yan Y, Penagaricano J and Corry P *et al* 2011 Spatially fractionated radiation therapy (GRID) using a TomoTherapy unit [abstract] *Med. Phys.* **38** 3369

[9] Gholami S, Nedaie H A, Longo F, Ay M R, Wright S and Meigooni A S 2016 Is grid therapy useful for all tumors and every grid block design? *J. Appl. Clin. Med. Phys.* **17** 206–19

[10] Zhang X, Griffin R, Edvaldo P G and Penagaricano J 2021 Feasibility study of 3D-VMAT based GRID therapy *Technol. Cancer Res. Treat.* **21** 15330338221086420

[11] Zhang H, Wu X, Zhang X, Chang S X, Megooni A and Donnelly E D *et al* 2020 Photon GRID radiation therapy: a physics and dosimetry white paper from the radiosurgery society

(RSS) GRID/LATTICE, microbeam and FLASH Radiotherapy Working Group *Radiat. Res.* **194** 665–77

[12] Mayr N A, Snider J W, Regine W F, Mohiuddin M, Hippe D S and Peñagarícano J *et al* 2022 An International Consensus on the Design of Prospective Clinical–Translational Trials in Spatially Fractionated Radiation Therapy *Advances in Radiation Oncology* **7** 100866

[13] Narayanasamy G, Zhang X, Meigooni A, Paudel N, Morrill S, Maraboyina S, Peacock L and Penagaricano J *et al* 2017 Therapeutic benefits in grid irradiation on tomotherapy for bulky, radiation-resistant tumors *Acta Oncol.* **56** 1043–7

# Chapter 12

# Electron beam SFRT

**Hajime Monzen and Mikoto Tamura**

Electron beam spatially fractionated radiation therapy (SFRT) has different dosimetric characteristics from those of megavoltage photon-beam-based SFRT. Its limited penetration capability is mainly used to treat shallowly seated bulky tumors. SFRT fields can be created by either a metal alloy cutout, recently developed tungsten functional paper (TFP), or tungsten-containing-rubber (TCR). The design of the GRID collimator, such as the hole size, the center-to-center spacing of the holes, and its thickness, must be experimentally determined for each patient to cover the target, which includes the therapeutic region as determined by the depth–dose profile, and must produce an adequate peak-to-valley dose ratio (PVDR) from the lateral dose profile. The dosimetric characteristics must be verified to determine the output factor and monitor unit (MU) values based on measurements before any clinical use takes place. In cases in which the GRID collimator can be placed on the patient's skin surface, this is very useful to shape the irradiation field and adapt the radiation volume to the patient's motion. In the future of FLASH radiotherapy, electron beam SFRT FLASH will also be able to fulfill this important role not only for superficial tumors but also for deep-seated tumors with very high energy and ultrahigh dose rate (UHDR) electrons.

## 12.1 Introduction

SFRT was first reported for use in high-dose radiotherapy in the orthovoltage era to increase the skin tolerance by allowing skin regrowth in the areas shielded by the GRID and reducing the dose given to other normal tissues [1, 2]. As the use of the original SFRT decreased with the advent of megavoltage radiotherapy, SFRT was adapted to megavoltage beams to control bulky and refractory tumors that require large doses which exceed the normal tissue tolerance limits achievable with megavoltage beams. SFRT is designed to deliver a large dose with a heterogeneous dose distribution in a single fraction, generally 15 Gy per fraction, to reduce tumor size. The dose pattern of peaks and valleys can deliver this large dose in a single

doi:10.1088/978-0-7503-4046-5ch12  

fraction without increasing the toxicity of the radiation. Low valley doses and large differences in dose between the peaks and valleys are needed to spare normal tissues [3], while the bystander effect is thought to lead to enhanced cell killing in regions adjacent to directly irradiated areas [4, 5]. Utilizing these advantages, the efficacy and safety of SFRT based on photon beams for bulky tumors have been demonstrated in many clinical situations [6–9], as further described in chapters 5–7. However, the use of photon beam SFRT to treat bulky superficial tumors is limited when critical radiosensitive structures are located close behind the malignant neoplasm [10], because photon beams are known to deliver an exit dose beyond these structures.

Electron beam SFRT has the potential to overcome this disadvantage of photon beam SFRT [10, 11]. The electron beam's dosimetric characteristics of a sharp dropoff in dose beyond the tumor [12] provides the rationale for the argument that shallowly seated bulky tumors can benefit from electron SFRT. In this chapter, we focus on: (1) designs of GRID collimators for electron beam SFRT and their dosimetric characteristics; (2) dose calibrations for the accurate and safe delivery of electron beam SFRT; (3) knowledge gaps and the future development of electron beam SFRT.

## 12.2 GRID collimator designs and their dosimetric characteristics for electron beam SFRT

### 12.2.1 Electron beam SFRT based on the metal or alloy cutout method

An optimal design for a low-melting-point alloy (Cerrobend) GRID block was introduced by Meigooni *et al* [10] in 2002, and the design was subsequently tested for 6–20 MeV electron beam SFRT. The thickness of the Cerrobend GRID block was 1.4 cm and its was fabricated to fit the $20.0 \times 20.0\ \text{cm}^2$ electron collimator of a linear accelerator (linac). This initial block was designed for GRID holes with 0.9 cm diameters spaced at 1.5 cm intervals. The percentage depth–dose (PDD) curves for this GRID block are shown in figure 12.1; they indicate that this GRID block could effectively treat a tumor seated at a depth of only 2.0 cm with an 80% isodose line using a 20 MeV electron beam. The optimal GRID hole diameter was then determined using the characteristics of the PDD curve; the objective being to treat to a reasonable depth while maintaining the efficacy of SFRT in terms of the lateral dose profile with the peak and valley doses. Meigooni *et al* [10] defined the optimal diameter as the size which would provide a therapeutic region (e.g. the 80% or 90% isodose lines) to a depth of approximately 50% of the therapeutic region for an open-field electron beam range. For electron beam SFRT with GRID hole diameters of less than 2.5 cm, the penetration characteristics obtained from the PDD curves were clinically suboptimal (figure 12.2), while diameters of more than 2.5 cm limited the number of holes in the radiation field, indicating the loss of SFRT benefits. Therefore, a 2.5 cm diameter was set as an optimal hole size for all electron energies from 6 to 20 MeV. A $5 \times 5$ hole matrix with 2.5 cm diameter holes with a center-to-center hole spacing of 3.0 cm was found to be an optimal Cerrobend GRID block to fit a $20.0 \times 20.0\ \text{cm}^2$ electron applicator, as shown in figure 12.3. When the

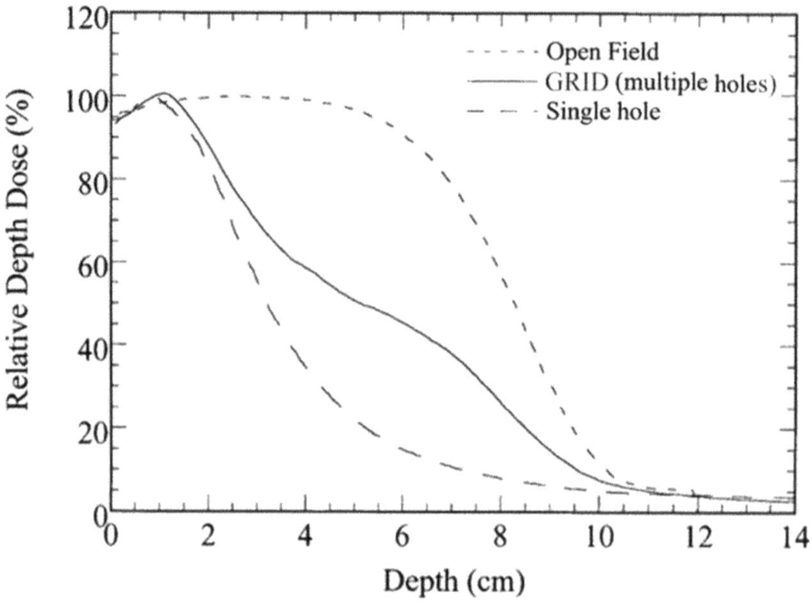


**Figure 12.1.** PDD curves for an open field, a single GRID hole, and multiple GRID hole fields with a 20 MeV electron beam. The hole diameter is 0.9 cm. Reprinted from [10], Copyright (2002), with permission from Elsevier.

irradiation field was 14.5 × 14.5 $cm^2$, the blocked area was approximately about 40%.

In the next step, the lateral dose profile must be verified because the characteristics of the peak and valley doses are important factors for the sparing of normal tissues. Figure 12.4 shows the lateral dose profiles at the maximum dose depth (14 mm), 20, 30, and 40 mm for a 12 MeV electron GRID beam with a Cerrobend GRID collimator. The valley doses are approximately 40%–50% of the peak doses at the maximum dose depth, which indicates that the PVDR is approximately 2.0–2.5. Thus, Meigooni *et al* [10] employed a GRID block with holes 2.5 cm in diameter to carry out electron beam SFRT measurements with the energies from 6 to 20 MeV, although a biological study is needed to verify whether this GRID design can provide favorable electron SFRT treatments in terms of tumor response [10]. It should be noted that there is a drawback in this electron SFRT design: the rigid Cerrobend GRID collimator cannot flexibly change the radiation fields to accommodate different tumor shapes and configurations in different patients. We used premade hole plugs to block some peripheral holes to obtain a preliminary conformal GRID field.

### 12.2.2 Electron SFRT with tungsten functional paper and tungsten-containing rubber

Recent studies have indicated that the nontoxic radiation shielding materials such as TFP and TCR (figure 12.5) can overcome the above-mentioned disadvantages of Cerrobend GRID collimators, such as poor conformality and a time-consuming

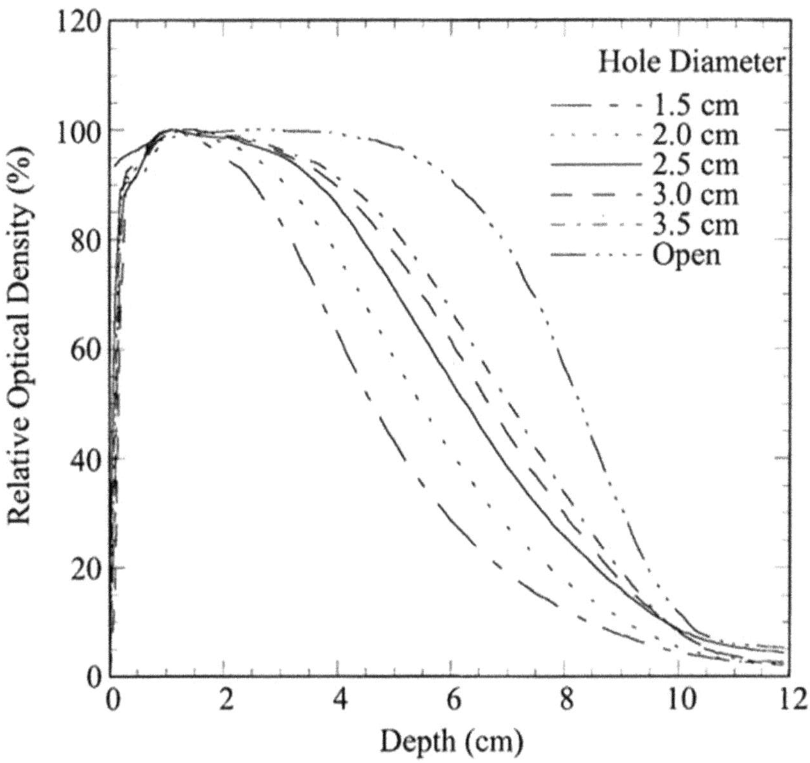


**Figure 12.2.** Comparison of the PDD curves for GRID fields with various GRID hole diameters and a $20 \times 20$ cm$^2$ open field. Reprinted from [10], Copyright (2002), with permission from Elsevier.

manufacturing process [13, 15]. These new flexible materials allow the radiation field to be deformed to fit individual tumor shapes, and the GRID beam can be created with the use of a TFP collimator placed directly on the patient's skin due to its nontoxic features (figure 12.6). We tested the use of TFP for a GRID collimator to create an electron beam SFRT. The study was performed using a Monte Carlo simulation [16]. The TFP (Toppan Printing Co., Ltd, Tokyo, Japan) sheet used in the electron SFRT study was 0.3 mm thick and contained tungsten powder at about 80% of the mass [13]. Multiple TFP sheets could be used together to provide adequate shielding if needed.

As a first step, we investigated whether the TFP GRID collimator could offer the same PDD characteristics as those of the respective Cerrobend GRID collimator [10] for a 9 MeV electron beam [16]. A square radiation field of $14.5 \times 14.5$ cm$^2$ was shaped upstream from a phantom. Similar electron GRID therapy beams to that used with the Cerrobend GRID collimator [10] were shaped by the various thicknesses of TFP placed on a phantom at a source-to-surface distance (SSD) of 100 cm. To determine the dosimetric parameters of the Cerrobend and TFP electron GRID beams, such as the $d_{max}$, $d_{90}$, and $d_{80}$ values, the PDD curves were carefully evaluated. As a second step, we investigated the thickness of the TFP GRID

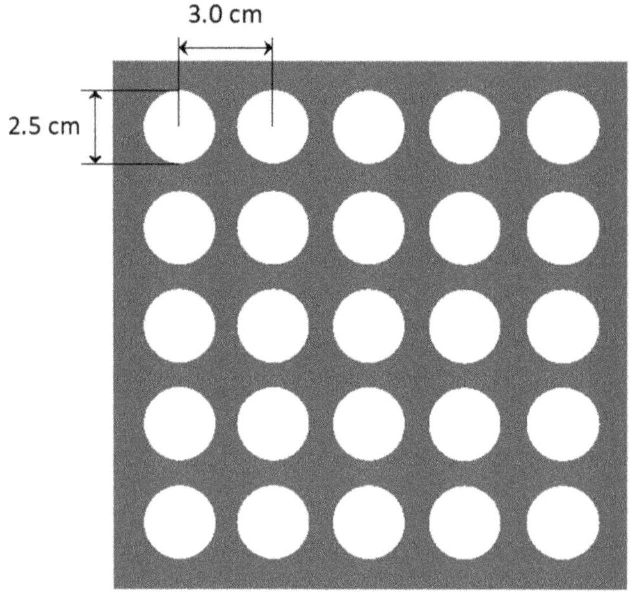


**Figure 12.3.** Schematic diagram of a Cerrobend GRID block design with a 5 × 5 matrix of 2.5 cm diameter holes with a center-to-center hole spacing of 3.0 cm suitable to fit a 20.0 × 20.0 $cm^2$ electron applicator. Reprinted from [10], Copyright (2002), with permission from Elsevier.

collimator required in order to obtain the same PVDR at $d_{max}$, $d_{90}$, and $d_{80}$ as those of the selected Cerrobend GRID block. Based on these values and the dose distributions, we determined the equivalent TFP thickness required to provide similar dosimetric features to those of the Cerrobend electron GRID collimator for an electron beam of the same energy. Figure 12.7 shows the PDDs (a) and lateral dose profiles at $d_{max}$ (b), $d_{90}$ (c), and $d_{80}$ (d) for the Cerrobend electron GRID beams and TFP electron GRID beams at various thicknesses (0.15, 0.6, and 1.2 cm). It can be seen in figure 12.7 that $d_{max}$, $d_{90}$, and $d_{80}$ decreased with increasing TFP thickness, but the PVDR increased with increasing TFP thickness. The relationship between the penetration of the electron beams and the PVDR was shown to be a tradeoff. The PVDR is considered to be an important dosimetric parameter for the heterogeneity of SFRT, although its true role in SFRT remains incompletely understood or quantified to date. According to radiobiological hypotheses, because a higher PVDR has a larger difference between the peak and valley doses within the spatial dose modulation, SFRT might be able to spare the interspersed normal tissues better in its low-dose zones [17]. The equivalent thickness of TFP required was determined to be 0.52 cm based on the dosimetric characteristics of the PDD and the lateral dose profile. At this equivalent thickness, the PVDR of the TFP electron GRID beam is equivalent to that of the Cerrobend electron GRID beam. Our finding that the radiation fields generated by the TFP GRID collimator have almost the same dosimetric characteristics as those generated by the Cerrobend GRID collimator suggests that TFP can be beneficial in electron beam SFRT for

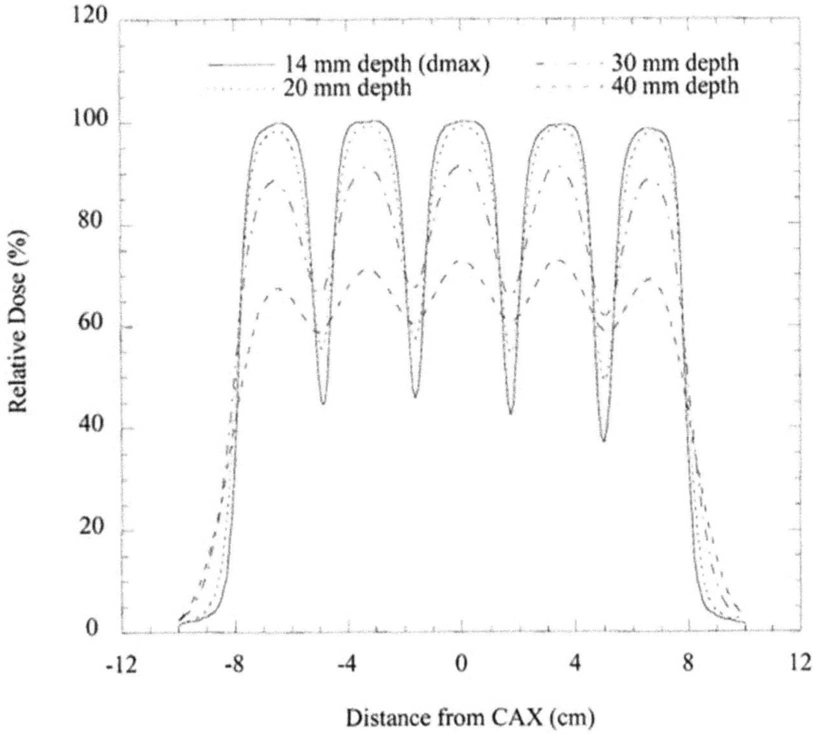


**Figure 12.4.** Lateral dose profiles at the maximum dose depth (14 mm), 20, 30, and 40 mm for a 12 MeV electron GRID beam used with a Cerrobend GRID collimator with a 2.5 cm hole diameter as shown in figure 12.3. Reprinted from [10], Copyright (2002), with permission from Elsevier.

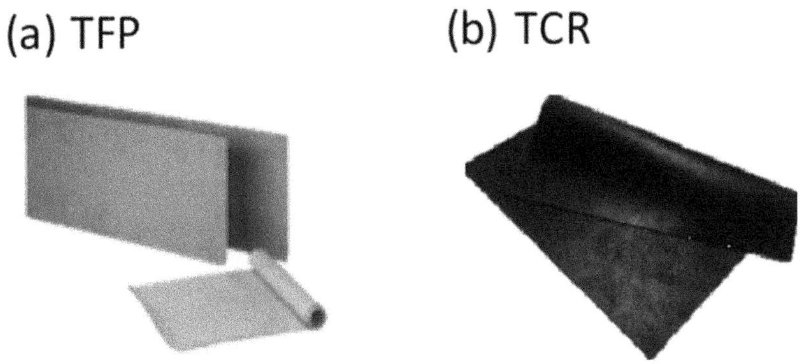


**Figure 12.5.** Nontoxic radiation shielding materials: (a) TFP and (b) TCR. These materials provide adequate shielding for electron beams, as shown in the research literature [13, 15].

bulky superficial tumors, and advantageous due to its increased flexibility and convenience of use in clinic. In the clinical setting, the shapes and depths of tumors differ among patients; when TFP is used for electron beam SFRT, the therapeutic region (surface to $d_{90}$ or $d_{80}$) can be adjusted by using different electron energies

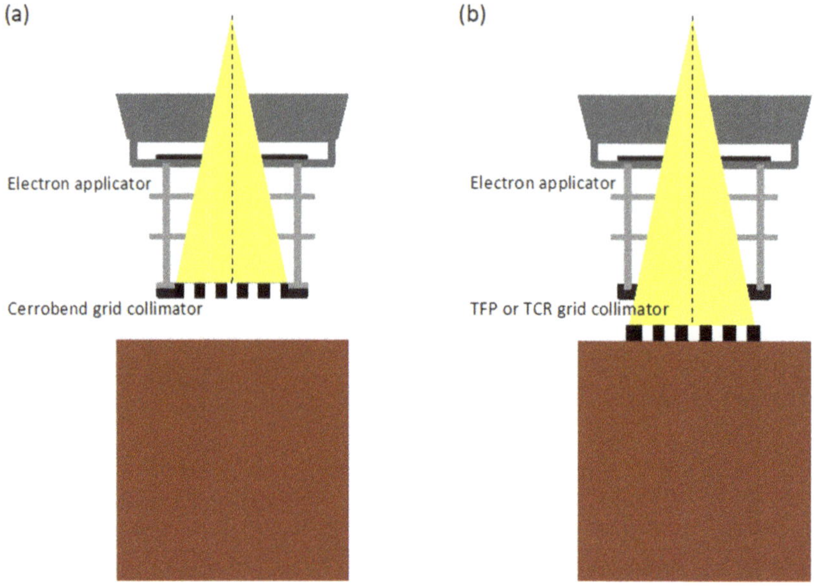


**Figure 12.6.** Schematic diagrams of two types of electron beam SFRT. (a) Irradiation with a conventional Cerrobend GRID collimator attached to the electron applicator. (b) Irradiation provided via a GRID collimator attached to the patient's skin.

and/or different depths of bolus to meet the individual profile of each patient's tumor size and depth [16]. In addition, the tumor motion due to respiration and patient movement may cause blurring of the peak and valley dose distribution [18]. A GRID collimator that is directly placed on the patient's skin surface is useful in adapting to the respiration and motion of the patient, thereby mitigating their potential effects of the delivery of the heterogeneous dose distribution.

## 12.3 Electron beam SFRT dose calibration for clinical safe delivery

In clinical practice, the dosimetric characteristics of the PDD and the lateral dose profile must be verified by the measurements of electron GRID beams that have a variety of energies, radiation field sizes, shapes, and GRID designs. The MU value needed to deliver the prescription dose should be determined using these measurements. First, the output factor, $S_e$ (cGy/MU), as defined by the American Association of Physicists in Medicine (AAPM) Task Group 70 [19], for each treatment situation at the SSD and at $d_{max}$ on the central beam axis is calculated as follows:

$$S_e(r_a, \text{SSD}) = \frac{\text{DMU}\,(d_{max}(r_a),\ r_a,\ \text{SSD})}{\text{DMU}\,(d_{max}(r_0),\ r_0,\ \text{SSD}_0)} \tag{12.1}$$

where DMU is the dose per MU, $d_{max}(r_a)$ is the depth of the maximum dose for the irradiation field size, $r_a$, for the GRID beam, and $d_{max}(r_0)$ is the depth of the maximum dose for the reference field size, $r_0$, for a conventional open field [20].

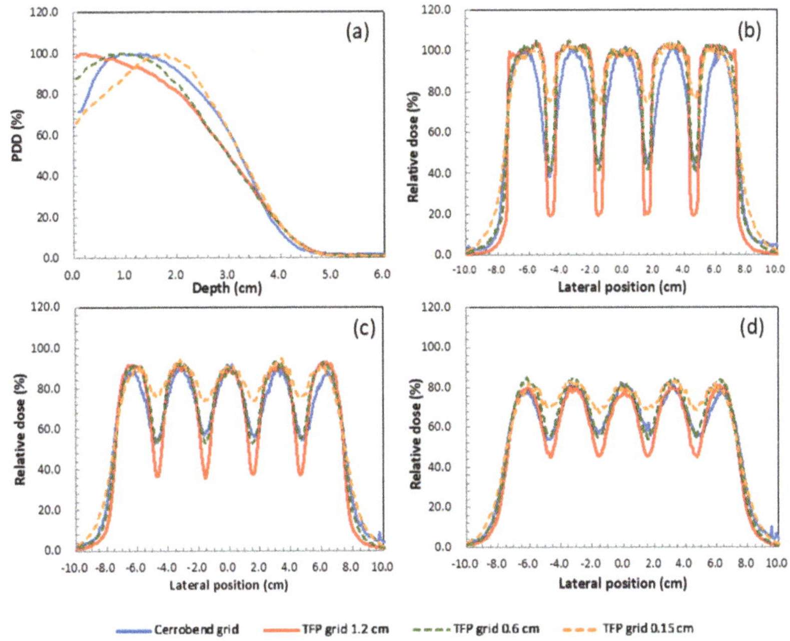


**Figure 12.7.** Comparison of the PDD curves (a) and lateral dose profiles at $d_{max}$, (b) $d_{90}$, (c) and (d) $d_{80}$ for the Cerrobend electron GRID beam and TFP electron GRID beams at various TFP collimator thicknesses (0.15, 0.6, and 1.2 cm). Reproduced from [16]. 

**Table 12.1.** An example of the output factor (cGy/MU) of electron beam SFRT with the optimal Cerrobend GRID collimator at the maximum dose depth on the central beam axis for a 20.0 × 20.0 $cm^2$ electron applicator [10].

| | Output factor (cGy/MU) | |
|---|---|---|
| Electron beam energy (MeV) | GRID field | Open field |
| 6 | 0.817 | 1.000 |
| 9 | 0.936 | 1.000 |
| 12 | 0.951 | 1.000 |
| 16 | 1.011 | 1.000 |
| 20 | 1.065 | 1.000 |



Meigooni *et al* measured and summarized the output factors for each electron energy as shown in table 12.1 [10]. The MU is then calculated as follows:

$$MU = \frac{D}{DMU\,(d_{max}(r_0),\ r_0,\ SSD_0)\ \cdot\ PDD\,(d,\ r_a,\ SSD)\ \cdot\ S_e\,(r_a,\ SSD)} \quad (12.2)$$

where $D$ is the absolute prescribed dose at the point of interest. The PDD term is the value of the GRID field at a depth $d$, at which the prescribed dose is given at a point along the central axis.

## 12.4 Discussion of electron GRID collimators and strategies for clinical use

Although electron beam SFRT using Cerrobend, TFP, and TCR GRID collimators can equally irradiate bulky shallow tumors, Cerrobend GRID collimator-based electron beam SFRT may not be as convenient as the other two options because of its longer manufacturing process and lack of flexibility. In contrast, TCR and TFP electron GRID devices have several clinical advantages. If these collimators can be placed directly on the patient's body, the irradiation field can cover the individual patient's tumor. The treatment can be further individualized by adjusting the hole sizes and center-to-center spacing of the holes to maximize dose heterogeneity and the therapeutic region. In cases in which the patient's surface is rounded or irregular, a GRID collimator made of TCR is more useful; it provides a better fit to the surface because the rubber is flexible (figure 12.5) [21]. GRID collimation can also be achieved with thin layers of TCR. It was found that a TCR GRID collimator only 0.2 cm thick can provide an equivalent quality of spatial dose modulation to that seen in conventional Cerrobend (1.4 cm) and TFP (0.52 cm) GRID collimators in electron beam SFRT [21]. The TFP and TCR collimators are biocompatible, thus they can be placed on the patient's body surface without raising any hazard concerns. If the fitting between the GRID collimator and the patient's skin is poor, the Cerrobend GRID collimator would be preferentially considered, since the dosimetric characteristics of TFP and TCR GRID collimators, such as the dose distribution and PVDR, may be different from those made using a phantom.

The design of a clinical GRID collimator, including parameters such as the hole size and the center-to-center hole spacing, should be determined based on the depth of the tumor, the PDD, and the transverse dose profile, so that it provides an adequate therapeutic region (i.e. a depth of 80% or 90% dose coverage) (figures 12.1 and 12.7(a)) for a given tumor. When a GRID collimator is placed on the patient, it should be noted that the thickness of the collimator also affects the depth–dose profile and the PVDR, as shown in figure 12.7. Therefore, careful experimental evaluation is recommended for each patient. To address the variations of tumor size and location (in terms of depth), the reference look-up table based on the dosimetric parameters reported by Zhang *et al* is also useful to determine the design of the GRID collimator in electron beam SFRT [22]. Because the final dose distribution is affected by many factors, it is recommended that the dosimetric characteristics must be measured and verified after all GRID parameters are set and prior to any clinical use.

## 12.5 Knowledge gaps and future perspectives

The data reviewed in this chapter suggest and it is postulated that electron beam SFRT can be beneficial for patients with bulky superficial tumors; flexible GRID technologies can further help to individualize electron beam SFRT. Further study is needed, both in clinical patients and to investigate the biological effects of electron beam SFRT. It is further speculated that electron beam SFRT FLASH will also fulfill an important role in the future of FLASH radiotherapy, not only in the treatment of superficial tumors but also in the treatment of deep-seated tumors using very high energy and UHDR electrons [23], since current linacs allow UHDR electron beams to be more easily obtained than UHDR photon beams [24].

The design of the electron GRID collimator, including the hole size, the center-to-center spacing of the holes, and thickness (in the case of TFP and TCR GRID collimators) must be experimentally determined for each patient to cover the target by the therapeutic region (e.g. it provides approximately 50% of an open-field electron beam based on a depth–dose profile such as that shown in figure 12.2) and maintain an adequate PVDR ratio (e.g. approximately 2.0–2.5 at $d_{max}$) [2]. The dosimetric metrics must be verified, i.e. users must determine the output factor and MU values using phantom measurements before each SFRT field is clinically used for patients.

## 12.6 Summary

In summary, the SFRT concept can be extended from megavoltage photon beams to electron beam therapy, which requires further evaluation in clinical patients. Electron beam SFRT can be realized using Cerrobend, TFP, and TCR GRID collimators, which can provide SFRT treatment for shallow bulky tumors at same quality as megavoltage SFRT. Electron beam SFRT can further advance the flexibility of SFRT by adapting biocompatible nontoxic GRID collimators to the patient's body surface and contours for highly individualized conformal coverage that may mitigate the effects of patient respiration and motion.

There is a need to broaden the radiation therapy options for bulky, recurrent, or refractory skin and other superficial tumors that are otherwise treatable with electron beams. While there are no reports of the use of electron beam SFRT with clinical patients to date, clinical results with megavoltage beam GRID therapy in skin cancer have been encouraging. A report of favorable symptomatic response (complete and partial responses of 29% and 66%, respectively) by Mohiuddin *et al* [7] included a substantial proportion of skin squamous cell carcinoma and melanoma patients. Kudrimoti *et al* [25] reported a local control rate of 80% with photon GRID therapy for bulky advanced recurrent malignant melanoma, a cancer with rapidly increasing incidence. The treatment of these tumors with electron beam SFRT may take advantage of not only the dose heterogeneity of SFRT but also the well-known shallow dose properties of electron beams that protect deeper-seated sensitive normal tissues.

This chapter provides a strategy for bringing electron beam SFRT into clinical practice. Careful device commissioning, design of the SFRT, treatment planning, individualized adaptation of the dose heterogeneity pattern to the patient's specific condition, and quality assurance, as described, are critically important. Heterogeneity properties, as defined by PVDR and other metrics that may still evolve, will need to be rigorously studied in patients, and their biological correlations require rigorous investigation.

## References

[1] Jolles B 1949 The study of connective tissue reaction to radiation: the sieve or chess methods *Br. J. Cancer* **3** 27–31

[2] Marks H 1952 Clinical experience with irradiation through a grid *Radiology* **58** 338–42

[3] Martinez-Rovira I, Fois G and Prezado Y 2015 Dosimetric evaluation of new approaches in GRID therapy using nonconventional radiation sources *Med. Phys.* **42** 685–93

[4] Zwicker R D, Meigooni A and Mohiuddin M 2004 Therapeutic advantage of grid irradiation for large single fractions *Int. J. Radiat. Oncol. Biol. Phys.* **58** 1309–15

[5] Asur R, Butterworth K T, Penagaricano J A, Prise K M and Griffin R J 2015 High dose bystander effects in spatially fractionated radiation therapy *Cancer Lett.* **356** 52–7

[6] Mohiuddin M, Curtis D L, Grizos W T and Komarnicky L 1990 Palliative treatment of advanced cancer using multiple nonconfluent pencil beam radiation *A pilot study Cancer* **66** 114–8

[7] Mohiuddin M, Fujita M, Regine W F, Megooni A S, Ibbott G S and Ahmed M M 1999 High-dose spatially-fractionated radiation (GRID): a new paradigm in the management of advanced cancers *Int. J. Radiat. Oncol. Biol. Phys.* **45** 721–7

[8] Penagaricano J A, Moros E G, Ratanatharathorn V, Yan Y and Corry P 2010 Evaluation of spatially fractionated radiotherapy (GRID) and definitive chemoradiotherapy with curative intent for locally advanced squamous cell carcinoma of the head and neck: initial response rates and toxicity *Int. J. Radiat. Oncol. Biol. Phys.* **76** 1369–75

[9] Neuner G, Mohiuddin M M, Vander Walde N, Goloubeva O, Ha J and Yu C X *et al* 2012 High-dose spatially fractionated GRID radiation therapy (SFGRT): a comparison of treatment outcomes with cerrobend vs. MLC SFGRT *Int. J. Radiat. Oncol. Biol. Phys.* **82** 1642–9

[10] Meigooni A S, Parker S A, Zheng J, Kalbaugh K J, Regine W F and Mohiuddin M 2002 Dosimetric characteristics with spatial fractionation using electron grid therapy *Med. Dosim.* **27** 37–42

[11] Lin K H, Huang C Y, Lin J P and Chu T C 2002 Surface dose with grids in electron beam radiation therapy *Appl. Radiat. Isot.* **56** 477–84

[12] Khan F M 2009 *The Physics of Radiation Therapy Book* 4th edn (Philadelphia, PA: Lippincott Williams & Wilkins Publishing)

[13] Monzen H, Kanno I, Fujimoto T and Hiraoka M 2017 Estimation of the shielding ability of a tungsten functional paper for diagnostic x-rays and gamma rays *J. Appl. Clin. Med. Phys.* **18** 325–9

[14] Fujimoto T, Monzen H, Nakata M, Okada T, Yano S and Takakura T *et al* 2014 Dosimetric shield evaluation with tungsten sheet in 4, 6, and 9MeV electron beams *Phys. Med.* **30** 838–42

[15] Kijima K, Monzen H, Matsumoto K, Tamura M and Nishimura Y 2018 The shielding ability of novel tungsten rubber against the electron beam for clinical use in radiation therapy *Anticancer Res.* **38** 3919–27

[16] Tamura M, Monzen H, Kubo K, Hirata M and Nishimura Y 2017 Feasibility of tungsten functional paper in electron grid therapy: a Monte Carlo study *Phys. Med. Biol.* **62** 878–89

[17] Zhang H, Wang J Z, Mayr N, Kong X, Yuan J and Gupta N *et al* 2008 Fractionated grid therapy in treating cervical cancers: conventional fractionation or hypofractionation? *Int. J. Radiat. Oncol. Biol. Phys.* **70** 280–8

[18] Naqvi S A, Mohiuddin M M, Ha J K and Regine W F 2008 Effects of tumor motion in GRID therapy *Med. Phys.* **35** 4435–42
[19] Gerbi B J, Antolak J A, Deibel F C, Followill D S, Herman M G and Higgins P D *et al* 2009 Recommendations for clinical electron beam dosimetry: supplement to the recommendations of Task Group 25 *Med. Phys.* **36** 3239–79
[20] Gibbons J P, Antolak J A, Followill D S, Huq M S, Klein E E and Lam K L *et al* 2014 Monitor unit calculations for external photon and electron beams: report of the AAPM Therapy Physics Committee Task Group No. 71 *Med. Phys.* **41** 031501
[21] Kijima K, Krisanachinda A, Tamura M, Nishimura Y and Monzen H 2019 Feasibility of a tungsten rubber grid collimator for electron grid therapy *Anticancer Res.* **39** 2799–804
[22] Zhang H, Grams M P, Foy J J and Mayr N A 2022 A dosimetric parameter reference look-up table for GRID collimator-based spatially fractionated radiation therapy *Cancers* **14** 1037
[23] Esplen N, Mendonca M S and Bazalova-Carter M 2020 Physics and biology of ultrahigh dose-rate (FLASH) radiotherapy: a topical review *Phys. Med. Biol.* **65** 23TR03
[24] Montay-Gruel P, Corde S, Laissue J A and Bazalova-Carter M 2021 FLASH radiotherapy with photon beams *Med. Phys.* **49** 2055–67
[25] Kudrimoti M R W, Huhn J L, Meigooni A S, Ahmed M and Mohiuddin M 2002 Spatially fractionated radiation therapy (SFR) in the palliation of large bulky (>8 cm) melanomas *Int. J. Radiat. Oncol. Biol. Phys.* **54** 342–3

**IOP** Publishing

Spatially Fractionated, Microbeam and FLASH Radiation Therapy
A physics and multi-disciplinary approach
**Hualin Zhang and Nina A Mayr**

# Chapter 13

# Proton beam spatially fractionated radiotherapy

**Mingcheng Gao and Mark Pankuch**

Spatially fractionated radiotherapy (SFRT) is an effective treatment for various bulky tumors. Linac-produced photon beams collimated through GRID collimators or multileaf collimators (MLCs) are the most common methods of SFRT delivery. Taking advantage of the Bragg peak in deep doses, proton beam SFRT may further increase the clinical application of SFRT. Dose inhomogeneity in proton beam SFRT can be achieved using pencil beam scanning (PBS) technology. In this chapter, we discuss the physics aspects of proton beam SFRT. Although the details may vary from one treatment planning system to another, the treatment planning process consists of the placement of pencil beam spots and the use of proper optimization techniques. To achieve a spatially fractionated dose distribution, as in conventional photon GRID therapy, each energy layer of the proton delivery must have an identical diverging spot pattern. PBS spots that have the same diverging trajectories but originate from different energy layers deposit doses at different depths, creating a beamlet that is analogous to the radiation delivered through the hole of a photon GRID collimator or MLC pattern. Proton GRID therapy has been implemented clinically. Compared with GRID based on megavoltage photon beams, proton GRID is dosimetrically advantageous in terms of distal organ sparing, tumor dose, and treatment of deep-seated tumors. The planning techniques presented in this chapter can be readily implemented in most proton centers. Unconventional SFRT dose distributions can be achieved using customized spot patterns or multiple proton beams.

## 13.1 Introduction

The goal of radiation therapy is to treat tumors with a sufficient dose to control disease while limiting the probability of toxicities. The treatment of large tumors always represents a challenge in radiation therapy and typical uniform tumor dose delivery methods may be less effective or even unable to achieve an adequate tumor dose because of their unacceptable toxicity to normal tissues. SFRT aims to deliver

doi:10.1088/978-0-7503-4046-5ch13

an inhomogeneous dose to the tumor using alternating high-dose and low-dose regions and has been shown to be an effective treatment for bulky tumors [1, 2].

Most clinical experience with SFRT is based on megavoltage photon beams; in this approach, a single *en face* field with a distinctive honeycomb-shaped transmission pattern is achieved through photon beam collimation applied to a linac. This type of SFRT is historically referred to as GRID therapy, in reference to the grid-type pattern of the high-dose regions. Photon GRID therapy uses a commercially available Cerrobend block or a brass block mounted on a linac. A typical block has holes approximately 1 cm in diameter that are spaced approximately 2 cm apart when projected at the linac's isocenter [3, 4]. The holes are arranged in a hexagonal pattern and along the beam divergence angle to maintain the most consistent spacing between adjacent holes.

MLCs pre-equipped on linacs can also be used to deliver GRID-type treatments, as demonstrated by Ha *et al* and Stathakis *et al* [5, 6]. The flexibility provided by the design of MLC shapes allows both hexagonal grid patterns and square grid patterns to be achieved. MLC-based GRID has produced clinical results comparable to those of block-based GRID treatments [7]. In addition to single-field GRID treatment, multiple-field 3D conformal radiotherapy (3D-CRT), volumetric modulated arc therapy (VMAT), and helical tomotherapy have been reported to produce traditional GRID-like SFRT dose distributions [8–10], as further described in chapters 9 and 11.

The dosimetry of all these linac-based GRID techniques, however, is bound to the physical laws of a megavoltage photon beam, which deposits its maximal dose at a shallow depth and continues to deliver a significant dose after passing through the tumor. It is therefore challenging to treat deep-seated tumors or tumors that have downstream critical organs. In contrast, due to the Bragg peak phenomenon, a proton beam deposits its maximal dose inside the tumor and exhibits no exit dose [11]. Naturally, combining GRID-type distributions with proton therapy has the potential to further improve the dose gradients between peak and valley doses within the heterogeneity dose patterns of SFRT as well as to lower the normal tissue dose, which may further benefit patients for whom photon-based SFRT cannot sufficiently reduce toxicity.

The vast majority of clinical proton therapy started with the use of passive scattering and uniform scanning technology [12] to spread the proton beam over the target region. Dose-shaping devices must be used to conform the dose to the tumor, for example by using apertures in the direction perpendicular to the beam and compensators for the distal end of the tumor. Although in theory a block similar to the one used in photon GRID might be used with these technologies to achieve a spatially fractionated dose distribution using a proton beam, the ultrasmall beam size calls for more a accurate dose calculation algorithm and differently optimized spread-out Bragg peak (SOBP) layer weights. This has prohibited the clinical application of SFRT using these aperture- and compensator-based delivery methods for proton beams. In addition, the increased neutron dose due to the presence of an additional physical collimator in the proton beam path is another concern which cannot be overcome [13].

In contrast, PBS technology allows proton-based SFRT to be used. PBS is the most advanced proton therapy technology [14]. In the last decade, more and more proton centers have either upgraded to or started to use this delivery method. In PBS, radiation is delivered spot by spot; each magnetically focused 'spot' deposits a highly localized dose through its associated Bragg peak. Through a process called inverse planning, the position, depth, and intensity of each spot can be optimized and a specific objective-driven 3D dose distribution can be achieved by the integrated contributions of all the spots. In a dosimetry study, Gao *et al* [15] demonstrated that a spatially fractionated dose distribution comparable to that of photon GRID can be achieved with PBS technology. Fair [16] delivered a single-energy PBS field with a spot pattern mimicking that of photon GRID therapy to a phantom and found good agreement between the measured dose and the planned dose. Other proton GRID approaches using multiple fields have also been investigated [17]. Today, GRID therapy using proton beams has already been implemented clinically [18]. More than 20 patients have been treated with proton GRID, and the initial clinical experience has been reported [19].

We wish to point out that the proton beam SFRT reviewed in his chapter uses available technologies that can readily be clinically applied in most proton facilities. The goal is to deliver a dose distribution similar to that of conventional photon GRID therapy. This approach is different from SFRT based on proton minibeams, another area of active research. The spot size of current commercial PBS systems is on the order of a few millimeters (4–9 mm sigma). But in proton minibeam radiation therapy, beams of submillimeter width (0.3–0.7 mm full width at half maximum (FWHM)) are proposed; their goal is to deliver a quasi-uniform dose inside the tumor [20–22]. These studies are still in the proof-of-concept, experimental, or preclinical phase, although they have shown promising dosimetry and tumor cell responses. Proton minibeams and proton microbeams are discussed in chapter 21.

## 13.2 Treatment planning

All PBS proton plans consist of multiple discrete energy depositions, called 'layers.' Spots of the highest energy layer deposit their doses at the most distal end of the target and spots of the lowest energy layer deposit their doses at the proximal end. Spots of a single energy layer form a two-dimensional pattern that covers the lateral extent of the target. Spot intensities are determined through an iterative optimization process.

In order to achieve a spatially fractionated dose distribution consistent with that of photon GRID therapy, each layer must have an identical spot pattern with the same diverging spot coordinates from the beam's eye view (figure 13.1(a)). Spots that have the same coordinates but belong to different layers deposit their doses at different depths following the diverging ray from the proton source. This creates a 'beamlet' at that specific spot position that is similar to the radiation that passes through the hole of a photon GRID block (figure 13.1(c)). High-dose regions occur at the beamlet locations and low-dose regions occur between beamlets (figure 13.1(b)). The peak-to-valley dose ratio (PVDR) is an important parameter

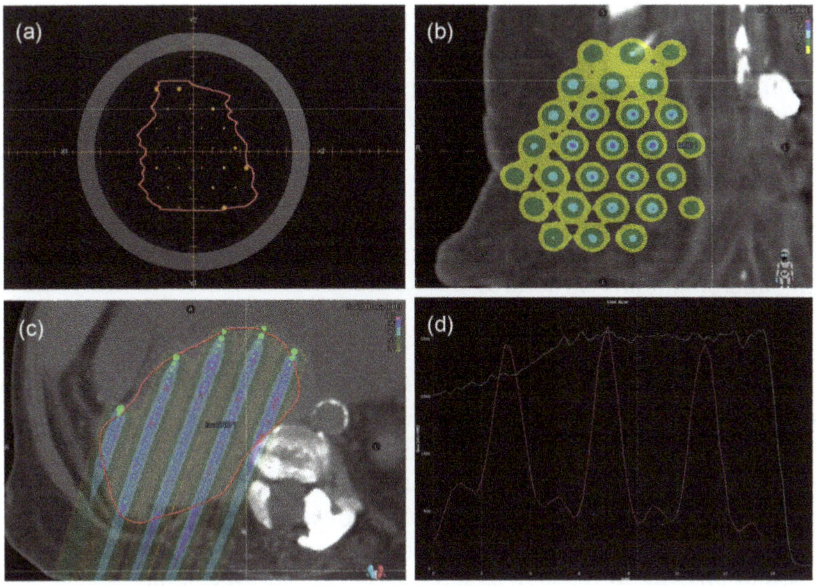


**Figure 13.1.** Proton GRID treatment plan with PBS. (a) Spots of one layer in the beam's eye view. The size of the spot represents its intensity. The spots of the other layers have the same pattern and coordinates. (b) Dose distribution in coronal view at a depth midway between the skin and the target. (c) Dose distribution in axial view. The green crosses represent the locations of the spots. The size of each green dot represents the spot's intensity. (d) The depth–dose curve along a beamlet and the transverse profile in the superior-to-inferior direction. The PVDR is about four.

of GRID therapy and is defined as the ratio of the dose at the center of a beamlet (called a 'peak') to the lowest dose between beamlets (called a 'valley') (figure 13.1(d)).

The two major tasks in proton GRID treatment planning are the lateral placement of spots to form beamlets that give the desired PVDR and the use of appropriate optimization techniques to maximize the tumor mean dose.

### 13.2.1 Placement of spots

The process of setting up spots for proton GRID depends on the treatment planning system (TPS). Alshaikhi *et al* [23] compared the planning parameters of four commercial PBS treatment planning systems: Eclipse (Varian Medical Systems, Palo Alto, CA) version 13.5.35; Pinnacle (Philips Radiation Oncology Systems, Fitchburg, WI) version 16.0; RayStation (RaySearch Laboratories, Stockholm, Sweden) version 4.7.0.15; and Xio (Elekta CMS Software, Maryland Heights, MO) version 4.80.00. Regardless of the system used, the following parameters must be properly set before optimization takes place.

#### *13.2.1.1 GRID pattern*

Proton treatment planning systems typically have a preset grid pattern which is used to arrange spots in an energy layer. Xio and Pinnacle only arrange spots in a square pattern. Eclipse allows a rectangular pattern, but the square arrangement is most appropriate to mimic photon MLC-based patterns. A square spatial fractionation pattern, like those of MLC-based GRID therapy [6], is expected when using these three systems for treatment planning. With RayStation, one can choose either a square or a hexagonal pattern for spot placement. This permits one to mimic the hexagonal spatial fractionation pattern of block-based GRID therapy. It is possible, although considerably more complex, to achieve nearly any pattern desired using any treatment planning system; this requires strategies such as manual editing, scripting, and/or dummy structures.

#### *13.2.1.2 Layer spacing*

Layer spacing is defined as the gap in energy between two adjacent layers. A proper layer spacing is important in reducing dose ripple along the depth axis. All treatment planning systems account for changes in the pristine Bragg peak width as a function of depth. A gap slightly smaller than the standard layer spacing of typical PBS plans is recommended for GRID plans in order to reduce the ripple along a beamlet. This is necessary for proton GRID planning because neighboring beamlets in GRID are much further apart than the spot separation in typical PBS plans. Hence the scatter and dose spill off from other beamlets contribute much less in the optimization to achieve minimal ripple in the depth direction.

#### *13.2.1.3 Spot spacing*

Spot spacing defines the separation between spots within an energy layer. Typical PBS treatment plans require a spot spacing in the order of a few millimeters to achieve a robust, uniform dose within the treated volume. In GRID therapy, the spot spacing is much larger, and the most critical goal is to ensure that the same spot locations are used for all layers in the beam's eye view. Eclipse and Pinnacle use a fixed spot spacing for all layers. All layers can use either a variable value or a fixed value in the RayStation and XiO systems. However, for GRID planning, only fixed spot spacing should be used for these two systems. All treatment planning systems allow the spot spacing to be manually entered. Using a large constant spot spacing results in the formation of beamlets in all treatment planning systems except for Pinnacle. As demonstrated by Alshaikhi *et al* [23], spot placement in the other three systems is based on one 3D grid diverging through the isocenter. In these systems, the spot spacing is defined as the spacing at the isocenter for all depths. In the Pinnacle system, the spot locations are defined by 2D non-divergent square grids for each energy layer, and the spot patterns of different layers are no longer overlaid in the beam's eye view.

The spot spacing directly affects the PVDR in proton GRID treatments. The selection of this parameter depends not only on the treatment depth but also on the type and model of the PBS delivery system, as discussed further in section 13.2.3.

#### *13.2.1.4 Margin*

The lateral, distal, and proximal margins determine how many spots are placed outside the target volume in these respective directions. The margins are handled differently in each treatment planning system. Most systems have a default auto margin. The plans produced by the Eclipse, Pinnacle, and RayStation systems can be made with or without margins [23]. In the XiO system, margins are automatically applied and there are no tools to add or edit these margins.

In regular PBS planning, margins are necessary to ensure dose coverage at the periphery of the target volume. Because GRID therapy is used for debulking or as a boost, absolute tumor coverage is unnecessary and is less critical than normal tissue sparing. For these reasons, zero margins are generally recommended in GRID treatment planning (as further described in chapter 16). If manual spot editing is possible, it is recommended to carefully review the placement of spots and remove any spots that reside outside the target volume. This is routinely practiced in the clinic where the most proton GRID patients have been treated so far [19]. For very shallow tumors, since protons lack the skin sparing property of megavoltage photon beams, it is beneficial to avoid placing spots on subcutaneous tissue to reduce skin toxicity.

### 13.2.2 Plan optimization

During the optimization process, the intensities of spots along each beamlet are optimized to produce a SOBP along the depth of the tumor. Unlike a photon GRID plan, in which the depth–dose profile continuously decreases with depth, in a proton GRID plan, the depth–dose profile along the central axis of a beamlet can be optimized to become quite flat. In a phantom study, it was shown that a variation of less than 5% within the target could be achieved [18]. Ideally, the optimized SOBP along a beamlet is uniform with depth, it has a width that equals the longitudinal extent of the target, and it has an amplitude that equals the prescription dose. If one considers the tradition of prescribing SFRT at the maximum dose point ($D_{\max}$), the use of a constant SOBP dose results in a greater tumor volume receiving the full prescription dose.

The optimization algorithm and functionality vary significantly from one treatment planning system to the other. To achieve the ideal optimization, customized objective functions specific to the treatment planning system should be developed. Dummy or optimization structures are often required to guide the optimizer. For example, a group of thin cylindrical structures can be placed within the target; these represent the central axes of the beamlets and are used for optimization.

As an optimization process example, the proton GRID treatment shown in figure 13.1 was planned with RayStation version 11.0.1.29. The Monte Carlo algorithm was used for dose calculation. The prescription dose is 20 Gy in one fraction. The following objective functions were used:

- Tissue outside GTV: maximum dose < 20 Gy (weight = 100 000)
- 'GTV+5mm' minus GTV: mean dose < 10 Gy (weight = 100 000)
- GTV: maximum dose < 20.6 Gy (weight = 100 000)
- GTV: minimum dose > 20 Gy (weight = 100)

The first objective is to limit the maximum dose given to normal tissues to be no more than the prescription dose. This is consistent with the tradition of SFRT in which $D_{max}$ is used for dose normalization, even though $D_{max}$ may not be inside the target volume. The second objective uses a ring structure to force a rapid dose falloff outside the target. The third objective is to control the hot spot inside the target. The hot spot dose within the target may be slightly higher than the prescription dose, since it is inside the tumor, as long as the volumes and magnitudes of any hot spots are considered acceptable. Due to the nature of GRID therapy, the forth objective cannot be reached. However, since it was assigned a much lower weight than the others, the optimizer tries to increase target coverage as much as possible without violating the other maximum dose controls. As discussed previously, the global optimum was achieved with a uniform SOBP at the prescription dose level, as shown by the line dose along a beamlet in figure 13.1(d).

The sparing of organs-at-risk (OARs) should also be included in the optimization as applicable. Radiosensitive organs proximal to the tumor can be included in the objective functions to limit their doses or simply remove spots that pass through them. If OARs are close to the target in the lateral direction, careful spot placement should be considered and in some cases, the use of an aperture can be beneficial. In the distal longitudinal direction, OARs can be spared by taking advantage of the distal falloff of a proton beam. Plans should be carefully evaluated for potential setup errors and range errors. For proton GRID treatment of shallow tumors, it is recommended to limit the skin dose and particularly to avoid hot spots on the skin.

### 13.2.3 Optimal spot spacing

Spot size and spot spacing are analogous to the hole diameter and hole separation of the photon GRID block commonly used in linac SFRT treatments. When protons are used, the PVDR increases as the spot spacing increases or as the spot size decreases. The spot size is an intrinsic property of a PBS delivery system and varies significantly among vendors. Figure 13.2 compares the spot sizes of five commercially available PBS delivery systems. Due to the observed differences in spot size among vendors, the optimal spot spacing of a proton GRID plan depends on the

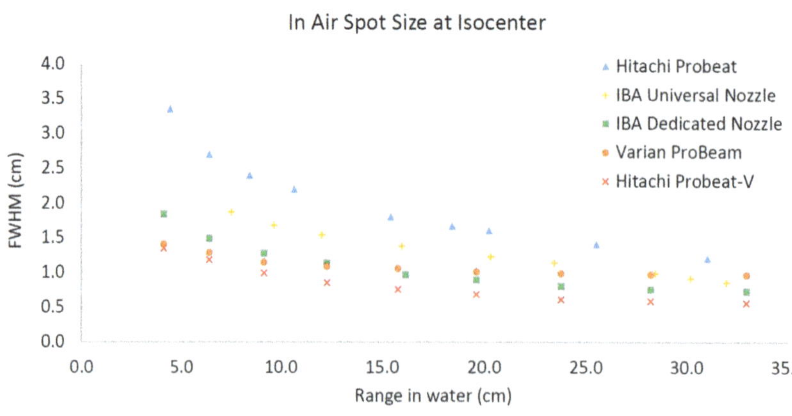


**Figure 13.2.** Typical spot size in terms of the FWHM as a function of the proton range of five popular commercial PBS delivery systems.

hardware system in use. In addition, the spot size further varies with the treatment depth, as seen in figure 13.2. As a result, a different spot spacing may be required when treating a shallow tumor compared to the spot size used to treat a deep tumor in order to achieve a similar PVDR.

The PVDR is a parameter that is essential in order to maintain consistency across different treatment modalities and is thought to correlate with the biological effects of SFRT. To achieve the desired PVDR, the choice of spot spacing can be guided by prior photon experiences. In a photon GRID treatment with a commercial block, the PVDR is in the range of 3–5.9, depending on photon energy and depth [3]. The PVDRs of MLC-based GRID treatments are slightly lower due to the higher transmission though MLCs [6]. To mimic the spatial fractionation of historical photon GRID therapies, Mohiuddin *et al* [19] chose a spot spacing that gave a PVDR from 3.3 to 5 in the region of normal tissue in their practice of proton beam GRID treatments. Normal tissue refers to the skin for tumors touching the surface or the tissue in the beam path between the patient surface and the upper border of the target for deep tumors.

The optimal spot spacing can also be determined by calculating the therapeutic advantage of a GRID treatment over a conventional treatment based on radiobiological models, as proposed in [24, 25]. Given a GRID treatment plan, its equivalent uniform dose (EUD) can be computed. The EUD is defined as the absorbed dose that, if homogeneously delivered to a tumor, would cause the same expected number of clonogens to survive as the actual inhomogeneous dose distribution does [26]. A conventional treatment plan that covers the same tumor with a uniform dose that equals this EUD value is then created. The GRID plan and the uniform dose plan have the same tumor killing rate but may have different normal tissue survival rates which can be quantified by evaluating a parameter called the therapeutic ratio (TR).

The TR of a GRID treatment is defined as:

$$\mathrm{TR} = \frac{\mathrm{SF_{normal}(GRID)}}{\mathrm{SF_{normal}(conventional)}}, \tag{13.1}$$

where $\mathrm{SF_{normal}(GRID)}$ and $\mathrm{SF_{normal}(conventional)}$ are the survival fractions of normal tissue in the GRID plan and in the conventional uniform plan, respectively. A TR of more than one means that the GRID plan is advantageous over the conventional plan, since it results in more normal tissue sparing at the same level of tumor killing.

Because of the 'high dose in a single fraction' nature of GRID therapy, the modified linear–quadratic (MLQ) model should be used in the calculation of the survival rate [27, 28]. In the MLQ model, the overall survival fraction (SF) of a structure receiving an inhomogeneous dose can be calculated as the average survival fraction of all the cells in the volume:

$$\overline{\mathrm{SF}} = \sum V_i \cdot \mathrm{e}^{-\alpha \cdot D_i - \beta \cdot G(t) \cdot D_i^2}, \text{ where } \sum V_i = 1. \tag{13.2}$$

Here, $V_i$ represents a subvolume $i$ that receives a dose $D_i$, $\alpha$ and $\beta$ are the radiosensitivity parameters of the cell type, and $G(t)$ is a dose protraction factor related to cell repair. The MLQ model reduces to the classic LQ model when $G(t) = 1$. For the purposes of the EUD and TR calculations, the LQ model may be used, as the difference between the two models is minimal even though the prescription dose of GRID is as high as 20 Gy [29].

The value of the TR takes into account the effects of spot size and spot spacing. The TR also depends on the tissue type, the prescription dose or desired tumor killing rate, the tumor size, and the tumor depth [29]. For a given tumor and PBS delivery system, the optimal spot spacing results in the maximal TR and the TR must be more than one.

As an example, figure 13.3 shows the calculated TR as a function of spot spacing for two PBS delivery systems: an IBA dedicated nozzle and an IBA universal nozzle (Ion Beam Applications SA, Belgium). A cuboid structure of 8 cm (length) × 8 cm (width) × 6 cm (depth) in a water phantom, centered at a depth of 6 cm, was treated as the tumor. A structure of 10 cm (length) × 10 cm (width) × 3 cm (depth) between the phantom surface and the tumor was contoured as the normal tissue. Figure 13.3(a) shows the dose distribution of a conventional proton plan using

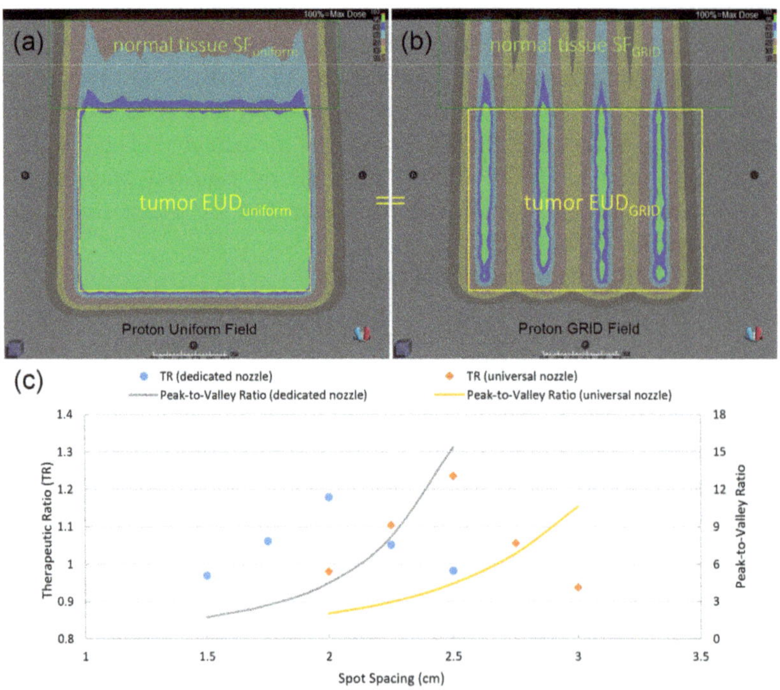


**Figure 13.3.** (a) Dose distribution of the conventional PBS proton plan. (b) Dose distribution of a proton GRID plan. The isodoses of each plan are normalized to their respective maximal doses. The two plans have the same tumor EUD. The yellow contour represents the tumor and the green contour represents normal tissue to be spared. The dotted line shows the depth at which the PVDR is calculated. (c) The TR and the PVDR as a function of spot spacing.

PBS technology, in which the tumor receives a uniform dose of 4.3 Gy. This dose level was derived using the approximation equation given in [28], and corresponds to the EUD of a photon GRID treatment using the standard brass block on a linac with a prescription of 20 Gy. Figure 13.3(b) shows the dose distribution of a proton GRID plan whose prescription was set so that it has the same tumor killing rate as the plan in figure 13.3(a). The following tissue types and LQ parameters from [29] were assumed in the SF calculation: Melanoma RPM17951 cells ($\alpha$ = 0.27, $\beta$ = 0.0468, $\alpha/\beta$ = 5.77) and moderately radiosensitive normal tissue ($\alpha$ = 0.211, $\beta$ = 0.0680, $\alpha/\beta$ = 3.1). Figure 13.3(c) shows the calculated TR for various spot spacing settings. Also shown are the PVDRs in the center of the normal tissue, i.e. at a depth of 1.5 cm, as a function of spot spacing. For the proton GRID treatment of the tumor in this example, the optimal spot spacing was found to be about 2 cm with the IBA dedicated nozzle and around 2.5 cm with the IBA universal nozzle.

### 13.2.4 Dosimetric verification and QA

As in intensity-modulated treatment plans, pretreatment quality assurance (QA) is a recommended practice before any PBS treatment commences. This is typically carried out by computing the plan and delivering the treatment to a water phantom. The QA of a proton beam SFRT plan requires a measurement device with a spatial resolution of a millimeter or less, due to the presence of very high dose gradients.

Film dosimetry has been the method of choice in the past for SFRT dose measurements. When carefully calibrated, film provides absolute dose information at the highest resolution. Commercial devices in the form of 2D ionization chamber arrays are excellent for absolute dose comparisons, but their resolution is on the order of several millimeters. They should be combined with another high-resolution device, such as a scintillation detector that provides relative dose comparisons in addition [18, 30].

## 13.3 Use of parallel opposed beams

Thus far, the discussion has centered on proton beam SFRT using a single-portal PBS field. In the single-portal field case, the optimal entry angle of a proton GRID beam would be one that passes through the fewest critical organs; little attention is paid to tissues beyond the tumor. In some cases, parallel opposed beams are required or may be considered to achieve the required dose distributions. Anatomy and tumor location with respect to critical organs may limit the use of opposed beams.

### 13.3.1 Opposed beams with a matched pattern

When the spot patterns of two opposed beams are matched, their beamlets overlap in 3D space but from opposite directions. An example of such a 'matched' opposed GRID plan is shown in figure 13.4. This case is a good candidate for the use of opposed beams, because the entry angles of both beams are equally optimal. Figure 13.4 (left) shows the dose distribution of a single-beam GRID plan. One beam delivers 20 Gy (the peak dose) inside the tumor. Figure 13.4 (middle) shows the dose distribution of the opposed field GRID plan with a matched pattern. Each

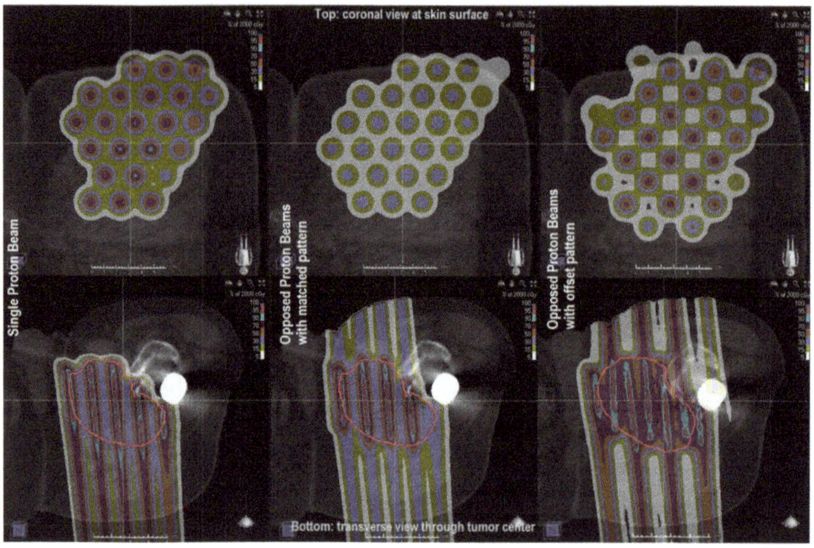


**Figure 13.4.** Dose distribution in a coronal view at the level of the skin (top row) and in a transverse view through the center of the tumor (bottom row) produced by a single-beam proton GRID plan (left), a proton GRID plan of two opposed beams with a matched pattern (middle), and a proton GRID plan of two opposed beams with an offset pattern (right). The prescription is 20 Gy at the maximal dose point for all plans.

**Table 13.1.** Dosimetric comparison of three proton GRID plans: single-beam, opposed beams with a matched pattern, and opposed beams with an offset pattern.

| | Single beam | Matched opposed beams | Offset opposed beams |
|---|---|---|---|
| Tumor mean dose | 9.5 Gy | 10.1 Gy | 14.8 Gy |
| Tumor $V_{10Gy}$ | 36.5% | 39.0% | 98.4% |
| Peak-to-valley ratio at tumor | 3.48 | 3.81 | 1.86 |
| Max skin dose | 18.3 Gy | 10.3 Gy | 17.3 Gy |
| Peak-to-valley ratio at skin | 5.83 | 6.15 | 21.33 |

beam delivers 10 Gy and the composite peak dose is again 20 Gy. A hexagonal grid pattern is used in both plans.

The tumor doses and skin doses of both plans are summarized in table 13.1. The two plans have similar PVDRs. In comparison with the single-beam GRID treatment, when the opposed proton beams with a matched pattern are used, the skin dose is reduced to nearly half while keeping a similar tumor dose.

### 13.3.2 Opposed beams with an offset pattern

We can also use opposed beams but shift the spot pattern of one beam by half a spot spacing. As a result, the beamlets are opposed but non-overlapping in 3D space. One field's beamlet (peak) is thus aligned with the other field's valley. An example of such an 'offset' opposed GRID plan is shown in figure 13.4. A square grid pattern was used in this plan. Figure 13.4 (right) shows the dose distribution of the opposed GRID plan with the offset pattern. Each beam delivers 20 Gy (the peak dose) inside the tumor.

When opposed proton beams with an offset pattern are used, the tumor dose is significantly increased. As shown in table 13.1, the mean tumor dose is about 50% higher than those of the other two plans. The percentage of the tumor volume receiving at least 10 Gy ($V_{10Gy}$) is 98.4% in the 'offset' plan versus 36.5% in the single-beam plan and 39.0% in the 'matched' plan. Although the 'offset' plan has a maximal skin dose similar to that of the single-beam plan, skin sparing is greatly improved with the 'offset' plan, because the PVDR at the skin is now 21.33 compared with 5.83 in the single-beam plan.

This 'cross-firing' technique was proposed by Henry *et al* [17]. They reported the planning of proton beam SFRT with two or four opposing PBS fields. Eclipse version 13 was used as the treatment planning system. Their goal was different from that in the above example, in which the maximal tumor dose was normalized to the prescription dose. Instead, they aimed to cover the planning target volume (PTV) with the prescription dose, allowing a much higher maximal dose. Manual spot editing was utilized to achieve their desired GRID pattern. The following objectives were used for plan optimization: 100% of the PTV should receive 100% of the prescribed dose (priority = 100); only 5% of the PTV was allowed to receive more than 120% of the prescribed dose (priority = 50). They found that it is possible to produce target doses ranging from 100% to 130% of the prescribed dose by cross-firing beam grids that are incident from four directions. Robustness analysis showed that setup errors had only a limited influence on the dose distribution produced in the target if four beam arrays were used for the irradiation. Because this technique has a different dose coverage and a much smaller PVDR than that of traditional SFRT (usually, 50% of the target volume receives about 50% of the prescription dose), its clinical benefits arising from SFRT need to be further studied.

### 13.3.3 Extremely thick tumors

The maximal depth in a patient that most proton machines can currently treat is about 32 cm. The use of a range shifter decreases this depth even more. For tumors whose distal portion is beyond the reach of a single proton beam, another beam from the opposite direction can be used. Half of the tumor is then treated by one GRID beam and the other half treated by the opposing GRID beam. If a matched pattern is used, a small gap should be left between the distal ends of each beam to avoid possible hot spots arising from range uncertainty.

## 13.4 Proton GRID versus proton lattice therapy

Conventional GRID therapy is considered to be two-dimensional SFRT, in which isolated high-dose 'columns' are formed. Lattice radiotherapy (LRT) is a type of three-dimensional SFRT [31] in which a very high dose of radiation is concentrated in small isolated spheres called 'vertices' within the tumor volume. LRT therapy is covered in in detail in chapter 10. In this section, we perform a dosimetric comparison between proton LRT therapy and proton GRID therapy.

### 13.4.1 Proton lattice therapy planning

A case of retroperitoneal liposarcoma (940 cc) was selected for this retrospective comparison study (figure 13.5). The proton GRID plan used one field. Its dose distribution is shown in figure 13.5 (left).

For the LRT planning, a 3D cluster of small spheres (vertices) was first created. The lattice pattern using hexagonal closest packing was adopted and the spheres were set 2.5 cm apart. Only spheres inside the tumor volume were used as optimization targets. The effect of lattice orientation was investigated by applying various degrees of pitch, roll, and yaw of the cluster with respect to the patient. To evaluate the effect of the number of fields, LRT plans with one, two, four, and six fields were created respectively for each lattice orientation.

The orientation of the lattice was found to be critical; the best results were obtained when the number of co-planar vertices was minimized. When protons interact with tissue, the dose gradually increases from about one third of the maximum at the surface to the maximum at the Bragg peak. Therefore, one or two fields could not yield the desired three-dimensional dose falloff due to the pileup of entrance doses from various layers in the lattice. The plan with six equally spaced fields achieved a good LRT dose distribution with 62 vertices inside the tumor. The lattice orientation in this plan was chosen so that the spheres overlap the least in all beam's eye views. Its dose distribution is shown in figure 13.5 (right).

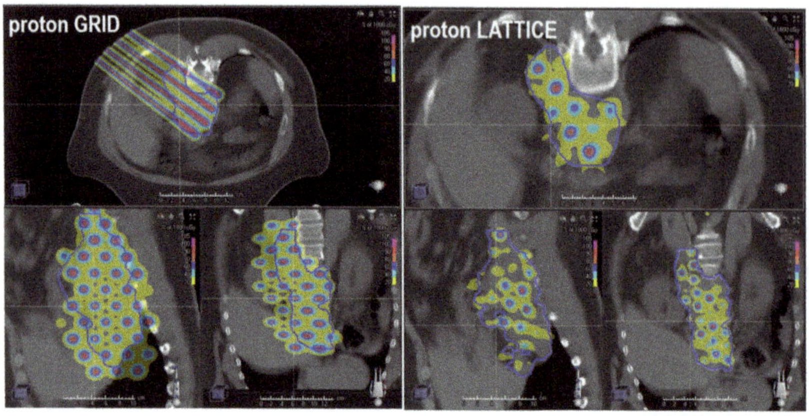


**Figure 13.5.** Dose distribution in transverse, sagittal, and coronal views from the single-field proton GRID plan (left) and the six-field proton LATTICE plan (right). The prescription is 18 Gy to the maximal dose point for both plans.

**Table 13.2.** Comparison of the doses given to critical organs by the proton GRID plan and the proton LATTICE plan.

| | | Dose at 0.5 cc on DVH ($D_{0.5cc}$) | | Volume receiving at least 3 Gy ($V_{3Gy}$) | |
|---|---|---|---|---|---|
| | Location w.r.t. GRID beam | GRID plan | LATTICE plan | GRID plan | LATTICE plan |
| Liver | Proximal | 17.80 Gy | 3.34 Gy | 16.1% | 0.2% |
| Right kidney | | 17.19 Gy | 3.09 Gy | 42.3% | 0.2% |
| Bowels | Distal | 1.05 Gy | 3.39 Gy | 0.0% | 0.3% |
| Left kidney | | 0.14 Gy | 3.24 Gy | 0.0% | 0.8% |
| Spinal cord | Lateral | 0.45 Gy | 1.61 Gy | 0.0% | 0.0% |

### 13.4.2 Dosimetric comparison

The maximal tumor dose is 18 Gy (prescription) for both plans, occurring at peaks or vertices respectively. The mean tumor doses are 8.1 Gy (GRID) and 4.7 Gy (LRT), respectively.

Organs within 1.5 cm of the tumor were investigated and categorized according to their location with respect to the GRID field: proximal, distal, and lateral to the tumor, respectively. The doses given to these organs by both the GRID plan and the LRT plan are summarized in table 13.2. In terms of the maximum dose ($D_{0.5cc}$), GRID gives a higher dose than LRT to the proximal organs (the liver and right kidney), but gives a lower dose to the distal organs (the bowels, and left kidney) and a slightly lower dose to the lateral organ (the spinal cord). In terms of irradiated volume ($V_{3Gy}$), LRT gives <1% of volume to any organ, but GRID gives up to 42% of volume to proximal organs.

This comparison suggests that when a good beam entry angle is available, proton GRID delivers a higher dose to the tumor and a minimal dose to the distal organs. If the tumor is surrounded by critical organs, proton LRT helps to limit the peripheral organs' doses.

### 13.4.3 Plan robustness

Range uncertainty is an unavoidable issue in proton therapy. The robustness of both SFRT plans was evaluated by analyzing the PVDR through shifting the range of protons by ±3%. The PVDR of the LRT plan is 4.76, but this may deteriorate to 3.23 in the worst case of range error. The PVDR of the GRID plan is 4.17, and it remains robust against range uncertainty.

## 13.5 The advantages and challenges of proton GRID therapy

The benefits of SFRT using protons have been discussed in the literature through dosimetric comparisons and early clinical findings [18, 19] (see also chapter 8). As shown in figure 13.1(d), the depth–dose profile of a proton GRID plan is relatively uniform within the target and drops quickly to a zero dose beyond the target. The curve also shows that the beam delivers a lower dose to regions proximal to the target. In contrast, the depth–dose profile of photon GRID treatments decreases continuously within the target, and a photon beam not only deposits the majority of the dose at a shallow depth but also delivers a significant dose to tissues beyond the target [3]. Thus, GRID therapy with a proton beam may be advantageous over a megavoltage photon beam in terms of distal organ sparing and greater tumor doses, and it may be preferred for deep-seated tumors.

The existence of critical structures beyond the tumor but in the beam path always presents a challenge in GRID therapy using megavoltage photons. Part of the tumor has to be blocked in order to avoid severe complications to these distal critical structures due to the high exit dose. Although the use of a megavoltage electron beam has been proposed [32] (as described in chapter 12), taking advantage of its fast dose falloff after a certain depth, it has poorer PVDR and is limited to superficial tumors extending no further than 5 cm deep. In such cases, proton GRID therapy, whose distal dose falls to a negligible level at only 1–2 cm beyond the tumor, is a preferred treatment option.

Proton GRID can achieve a relatively uniform dose along a beamlet inside the tumor, regardless of the depth of the tumor. As a comparison, the depth–dose profile of a 6 MV photon beam decreases by about 3.5% per centimeter in tissue [28]. As a result, the mean tumor dose is higher when a proton beam is used for GRID therapy, assuming the same PVDR. In fact, the larger the tumor, the more advantageous proton GRID may be.

Another advantage of proton GRID is in the treatment of deep-seated tumors. It has been shown that, for deep targets, proton GRID results in better PVDRs and much smaller doses to the proximal normal tissues than conventional photon GRID [18]. This eliminates the need for parallel opposed photon beams using the standard block [33]. New approaches making use of modern linac technologies (3D-CRT, VMAT, and helical tomotherapy) (see chapters 10 and 11) have been investigated for deep tumors, in which the PVDRs are in the range of 1.5–2.8 [10]. Because of the involvement of arc radiation delivery, these approaches give a higher integral dose to the patient than the proton GRID approach.

Two uncertainties have been associated with proton therapy since its inception: range and relative biological effectiveness (RBE). The consequences of these issues must be considered when applying proton beam SFRT clinically. Robustness evaluation, as we demonstrated in section 13.4, suggests that the range error does not change the quality of a proton GRID plan by much. However, caution must be taken if the distal end of the proton beam is near a radiosensitive structure, whose dose may be significantly higher if protons stop deeper than expected. It must also be considered that the RBE at the distal end is actually enhanced due to the higher linear energy transfer (LET) at the Bragg peak's distal edge [34]. A generic constant of 1.1 is widely adopted as the RBE factor for proton therapy. In reality, the RBE varies with tissue type, clinical endpoint, depth, LET, and the fractionation scheme. Available experimental data suggest that, in the case of GRID therapy whose fractional dose is much higher than the common 2 Gy/fraction, the RBE value would be smaller [35]. Henry *et al* [36] investigated the effects of assuming a constant RBE versus assuming a variable RBE on proton GRID plans. They found that clinical goals for the OARs, which were fulfilled by assuming the RBE = 1.1, failed at least one goal when they assumed a variable RBE.

Proton beam SFRT is still in its early stage of implementation. More physical studies, practice, and clinical data are necessary to guide its future development.

## 13.6 Summary

Proton beam SFRT can be achieved with proton PBS by properly guiding the treatment planning system in its spot placement and dose optimization. Based on available proton technology, the planning techniques presented in this chapter can be readily implemented at most proton centers. The use of protons produces a more uniform beamlet dose within the tumor, completely spares normal tissues located beyond the tumor, and gives a smaller dose to proximal organs when treating deep-seated tumors. We focused on the creation of a SFRT dose distribution with similar properties to those of historical photon GRID therapy. Thanks to the flexibility in spot pattern design, unconventional SFRT dose distributions can be also achieved using customized spot patterns or multiple proton beams.

## References


[1] Mohiuddin M, Fujita M and Regine W F *et al* 1999 High-dose spatially-fractionated radiation (GRID): a new paradigm in the management of advanced cancers *Int. J. Radiat. Oncol. Biol. Phys.* **45** 721–7

[2] Billena C and Khan A J 2019 A current review of spatial fractionation: back to the future? *Int. J. Radiat. Oncol. Biol. Phys.* **104** 177–87

[3] Buckey C, Stathakis S and Cashon K *et al* 2010 Evaluation of a commercially-available block for spatially fractionated radiation therapy *J. Appl. Clin. Med. Phys.* **11** 3163

[4] Nobah A, Mohiuddin M and Devic S *et al* 2015 Effective spatially fractionated GRID radiation treatment planning for a passive grid block *Br. J. Radiol.* **88** 20140363

[5] Ha J K, Zhang G and Naqvi S A *et al* 2006 Feasibility of delivering grid therapy using a multileaf collimator *Med. Phys.* **33** 76–82

[6] Stathakis S, Esquivel C and Gutiérrez A N *et al* 2009 Dosimetric evaluation of multi-pattern spatially fractionated radiation therapy using a multi-leaf collimator and collapsed cone convolution superposition dose calculation algorithm *Appl. Radiat. Isot.* **67** 1939–44

[7] Neuner G, Mohiuddin M M and Vander Walde N *et al* 2012 High-dose spatially fractionated GRID radiation therapy (SFGRT): a comparison of treatment outcomes with Cerrobend vs. MLC SFGRT *Int. J. Radiat. Oncol. Biol. Phys.* **82** 1642–9

[8] Jin J Y, Zhao B and Kaminski J M *et al* 2015 A MLC-based inversely optimized 3D spatially fractionated grid radiotherapy technique *Radiother. Oncol.* **117** 483–6

[9] Zhang X, Penagaricano J and Yan Y *et al* 2016 Spatially fractionated radiotherapy (GRID) using helical tomotherapy *J. Appl. Clin. Med. Phys.* **17** 396–407

[10] Sheikh K, Hrinivich W T and Bell L A *et al* 2019 Comparison of treatment planning approaches for spatially fractionated irradiation of deep tumors *J. Appl. Clin. Med. Phys.* **20** 125–33

[11] Newhauser W D and Zhang R 2015 The physics of proton therapy *Phys. Med. Biol.* **60** R155–209
[12] Paganetti H (ed) 2019 *Proton Therapy Physics* 2nd edn (Boca Raton, FL: CRC Press)
[13] Charyyev S and Wang C K 2020 Assessment of ambient neutron dose equivalent in spatially fractionated radiotherapy with protons using physical collimators *Radiat. Prot. Dosim.* **189** 190–7
[14] Paganetti H, Beltran C J and Both S *et al* 2021 Roadmap: proton therapy physics and biology *Phys. Med. Biol.* **66** 05RM01
[15] Gao M, Mohiuddin M M and Hartsell W F *et al* 2015 Spatially fractionated (GRID) radiation therapy using proton pencil beam scanning (PBS): a feasibility study [abstract] *Int. J. Radiat. Oncol. Biol. Phys.* **93** E562
[16] Fair J 2016 Spatially fractionated proton therapy: a Monte Carlo verification *Master Thesis.* (Atlanta, GA, USA: Georgia Institute of Technology)
[17] Henry T, Ureba A and Valdman A *et al* 2017 Proton grid therapy: a proof-of-concept study *Technol. Cancer Res. Treat.* **16** 749–57
[18] Gao M, Mohiuddin M M and Hartsell W F *et al* 2018 Spatially fractionated (GRID) radiation therapy using proton pencil beam scanning (PBS): feasibility study and clinical implementation *Med. Phys.* **45** 1645–53
[19] Mohiuddin M, Lynch C and Gao M *et al* 2020 Early clinical results of proton spatially fractionated GRID radiation therapy (SFGRT) *Br. J. Radiol.* **93** 20190572
[20] Martínez-Rovira I, Fois G and Prezado Y 2015 Dosimetric evaluation of new approaches in GRID therapy using nonconventional radiation sources *Med. Phys.* **42** 685–93
[21] Prezado Y and Fois G R 2013 Proton-minibeam radiation therapy: a proof of concept *Med. Phys.* **40** 031712
[22] Dilmanian F A, Eley J G and Krishnan S 2015 Minibeam therapy with protons and light ions: physical feasibility and potential to reduce radiation side effects and to facilitate hypofractionation *Int. J. Radiat. Oncol. Biol. Phys.* **92** 469–74
[23] Alshaikhi J, Doolan P J and D'Souza D *et al* 2019 Impact of varying planning parameters on proton pencil beam scanning dose distributions in four commercial treatment planning systems *Med. Phys.* **46** 1150–62
[24] Zwicker R D, Meigooni A S and Mohiuddin M 2004 Therapeutic advantage of GRID irradiation for large single fractions *Int. J. Radiat. Oncol. Biol. Phys.* **58** 1309–15
[25] Meigooni A S, Dou K and Meigooni N J *et al* 2006 Dosimetric characteristics of a newly designed grid block for megavoltage photon radiation and its therapeutic advantage using a linear quadratic model *Med. Phys.* **33** 3165–73
[26] Henríquez F C and Castrillón S V 2011 A quality index for equivalent uniform dose *J. Med. Phys.* **36** 126–32
[27] Guerrero M and Li X A 2004 Extending the linear-quadratic model for large fraction doses pertinent to stereotactic radiotherapy *Phys. Med. Biol.* **49** 4825–35
[28] Zhang H, Wu X and Zhang X *et al* 2020 Photon GRID radiation therapy: a physics and dosimetry white paper from the Radiosurgery Society (RSS) GRID/LATTICE, microbeam and FLASH Radiotherapy Working Group *Radiat. Res.* **194** 665–77
[29] Zhang H, Zhong H and Barth R F *et al* 2014 Impact of dose size in single fraction spatially fractionated (grid) radiotherapy for melanoma *Med. Phys.* **41** 021727

[30] Pedroni E, Scheib S and Böhringer T *et al* 2005 Experimental characterization and physical modelling of the dose distribution of scanned proton pencil beams *Phys. Med. Biol.* **50** 541–61

[31] Wu X, Ahmed M M and Wright J *et al* 2010 On modern technical approaches of three-dimensional high-dose lattice radiotherapy (LRT) *Cureus.* **2** e9

[32] Meigooni A S, Parker S A and Zheng J *et al* 2002 Dosimetric characteristics with spatial fractionation using electron grid therapy *Med. Dosim.* **27** 37–42

[33] Meigooni A S, Gnaster M and Dou K *et al* 2007 Dosimetric evaluation of parallel opposed spatially fractionated radiation therapy of deep-seated bulky tumors *Med. Phys.* **34** 599–603

[34] Matsumoto Y, Matsuura T and Wada M *et al* 2014 Enhanced radiobiological effects at the distal end of a clinical proton beam: *in vitro* study *J. Radiat. Res.* **55** 816–22

[35] Gerweck L E and Kozin S V 1999 Relative biological effectiveness of proton beams in clinical therapy *Radiother. Oncol.* **50** 135–42

[36] Henry T and Ödén J 2018 Interlaced proton grid therapy—linear energy transfer and relative biological effectiveness distributions *Phys. Med.* **56** 81–9

# Chapter 14

# Radiobiological modeling and equivalent uniform dose for spatially fractionated radiation therapy

**Stefan H Bartzsch, Robert D Stewart and Juergen Meyer**

Numerous approaches to spatially fractionated radiation therapy (SFRT) are under investigation, including different beam geometries and radiation qualities. Quantitative comparisons of treatment effectiveness are needed to optimize SFRT and to assess its benefits relative to conventional radiation therapy (RT). This chapter highlights the challenges of utilizing the physical dose alone for the comparison and assessment of SFRT treatments using established radiobiological concepts. A framework is presented that combines the equivalent uniform dose (EUD), the equivalent dose in 2 Gy fractions (EQD2) and radiation relative biological effectiveness (RBE) to correct for known dose, dose rate, and linear energy transfer (LET) effects. The shortfalls of using the physical dose for SFRT dosimetry are illustrated and representative preclinical and clinical examples are shown to demonstrate the application of the proposed framework. We acknowledge that the EUD and related concepts derived from the linear–quadratic (LQ) cell survival model may not fully capture all relevant biological effects. However, we show that an incomplete system of radiobiological models that captures well-known biological mechanisms may still be superior to comparison metrics based solely on the physical dose. This is because it serves as a reference to known biological effects independent of SFRT and conventional RT parameters. EUD, with corrections for dose, dose rate, and RBE effects, is a useful metric for the optimization of SFRT, and a convenient way to standardize the reporting of experimental parameters for preclinical and clinical studies.

## 14.1 Introduction

SFRT is an emerging treatment approach characterized by large dose gradients across milli- and submillimeter spatial scales and large doses per fraction (>10–20 Gy).

doi:10.1088/978-0-7503-4046-5ch14

These characteristics pose challenges to established models for outcome prediction, assessment, and treatment comparison. As highlighted and discussed in chapter 16, what are the most appropriate dose metrics with which to compare the biological effects of daily doses of RT delivered with close-to-uniform radiation fields with those of highly modulated SFRT fields delivered in a single fraction? Preclinical SFRT research indicates that the peak and valley doses, the beamlet width, and the center-to-center (CTC) spacing are important factors when modeling biological effects at the tissue level [1]. However, further advances in SFRT research and the associated large variations in beam parameters [2–4] demand quantitative concepts and metrics to enable the comparison and optimization of treatment parameters and patient plans. Quantitative biological models that account for known biology are also essential in the effort to identify and quantify *new* biological mechanisms in preclinical and prospective clinical studies of treatment outcomes. Such parameters would also greatly advance the interpretation of existing studies correlating SFRT with clinical outcome (which are described in chapters 5 through 8). For example, do the differences in biological effects seen in SFRT and treatments delivered with more uniformity in dose reflect novel biological mechanisms? Or, can the physical parameters and established radiobiology models explain the observed biological response? The answers to these questions are important for treatment optimization and the translation of SFRT into clinical practice.

Different ways exist to assess the equivalence of SFRT and other treatment modalities. One approach is to measure the toxicity of SFRT beams and correlate them to uniform doses such that they achieve equivalent toxicity levels [5]. This pragmatic and empirical approach intrinsically includes all biological effects without the need to know the significance and magnitude of less well-understood phenomena, such as bystander signaling, vascular repair mechanisms, or immune response. However, the vast parameter space in SFRT and corresponding tissue responses makes such an approach impractical for comparative studies of patient-specific treatment planning. The main alternative to this empirical approach is to develop quantitative metrics that capture well-documented biological mechanisms and then test the accuracy of these models and metrics against measured laboratory and clinical data. The LQ cell survival model [6, 7] and related concepts are currently the best established and clinically useful framework for the estimation of radiotherapy toxicity and efficacy.

In this chapter, we discuss the equivalent uniform dose (EUD) concept as a potential measure that can be used to compare spatially fractionated and conventional RT. The EUD was introduced in the 1990s to account for moderate dose variations in conventional radiation therapy [1]. We outline how to combine the EUD concept with the equivalent dose in 2 Gy fractions (EQD2) to account for differences in treatment schedules. The EUD and EQD2 concepts are generalized to explicitly account for the RBE of intermediate and high-LET radiations relative to low-LET x-rays. We view the EUD concept as a best-effort approach to compare conventional RT with SFRT, although we expect deviations from experimental observations. Such deviations may highlight the need to account for new biological mechanisms that may possibly be unique to SFRT. Alternatively, these deviations may simply reflect the inevitable uncertainties in laboratory dosimetry (see e.g.

chapter 15) and response assessment. The ability to separate known from unknown biological mechanisms is needed to guide the formulation of refinements to the standard LQ model [8] and related concepts, including EQD2. The limitations of the system of models reviewed in this chapter are discussed, especially with respect to clinical endpoints. In preclinical examples, we highlight the advantages of data analysis based on the EUD and LQ formalism in SFRT. Moreover, we use the LQ approach for treatment planning to illustrate its clinical application in contrast to purely physics-based dose concepts, which are often reported in the SFRT literature.

## 14.2 Dosimetric and biophysical concepts

### 14.2.1 Physical dose

The radiation dose is the key parameter used in radiation oncology to relate the physical properties of a radiation field to energy absorption and biological effects at the molecular, cellular, and tissue levels. Since radiation interactions are an intrinsically stochastic process, energy deposition is also a stochastic process. The specific energy, defined as the energy imparted per unit mass $z \equiv \varepsilon/m$, follows a probability distribution that depends on the size and shape of the biological target as well as the types and energy distributions of ionizing particles passing through the target. The absorbed dose at a certain point in a medium is defined as the mean specific energy in the limit of an infinitely small mass [9], i.e. $D \equiv \lim_{m\to 0}\bar{z} = d\bar{\varepsilon}/dm$. The value of $D$ at a point in a medium can also be expressed as the product of the expected number $v$ of particles passing through a biological target multiplied by the frequency-mean specific energy, $\bar{z}_F \propto$ LET [9]. The frequency and severity of biological damage is determined by the distribution of the number and size of the individual events. Differences in biological damage for one type of radiation relative to another at the same dose, usually quantified by the radiation's RBE, largely arise from differences in the distribution of radiation events and the DNA damage caused by the radiation of interest relative to a low-LET radiation [10].

### 14.2.2 LQ cell survival model

The surviving fraction, $S$, refers to the proportion of cells retaining their reproductive integrity after irradiation. The logarithm of $S$ is usually well approximated as a linear–quadratic function of the absorbed dose $D$, i.e. $-\ln(S) = \alpha D + \beta G D^2$. Here, the parameters $\alpha$ ($Gy^{-1}$) and $\beta$ ($Gy^{-2}$) are specific to the cell, tissue, or tumor as well as the radiation type, kinetic energy, and, therefore, the LET. The Lea–Catcheside dose protraction factor, $G$, corrects for DNA repair during and after treatment [11, 12]. For any arbitrary temporal pattern of radiation delivery, $G$ falls within the range $0 < G \geq 1$. For $n$ sequential doses of size $d$ well separated in time, such that sublethal damage repair is complete between fractions, the dose protraction factor becomes $G = g/n$ [12]. Here, $g$ is the protraction factor for a single dose of radiation delivered over the time interval $\Delta$; for exponential repair kinetics with the rate constant $\mu$, $g$ is given by

$$g = 2(e^{-x} + x - 1)/x^2, \text{ where } x \equiv \Delta \ln(2)/\mu. \tag{14.1}$$

For SFRT treatments delivered in a single fraction of short duration (i.e., $\Delta$ is small compared to $\mu$), $G = g \cong 1$.

Apart from the radiation dose, the ionization density and the distribution of radiation events impact molecular and cellular responses. The most common way to quantify the biological effects arising from different types of radiation is to compute the ratio of the dose of a reference radiation $R$, $D_R$, that produces the same biological effect as a dose $D$ of another type of radiation, i.e. RBE $\equiv D_R/D$. While the LQ model is usually formulated in the literature to relate dose $D$ to $S$, it can be generalized to include RBE effects by replacing $D$ with the RBE-weighted dose (RWD), i.e.

$$S(\text{RWD}) = \exp(-\alpha \cdot \text{RWD} - G \cdot \beta \cdot \text{RWD}^2). \tag{14.2}$$

Here, RWD is the total dose $D$ multiplied by a particle-, LET-, and dose-specific RBE value, and the values of $\alpha$ (Gy$^{-1}$) and $\beta$ (Gy$^{-2}$) are the LQ model parameters for a low-LET reference radiation. As a first approximation, it is assumed in equation (14.2) that the kinetics of DNA repair are the same for low- and high-LET radiations, i.e. the rate constant $\mu$ is considered the same regardless of LET. However, reports in the literature suggest that the rate of DNA damage repair becomes slower with increasing LET [13–15]; in general, $G$ increases toward unity as the rate of DNA repair decreases.

### 14.2.3 Iso-effective dose

Since SFRT is often given in a single fraction, it is useful to have a formalism that relates single-fraction SFRT to more conventional RT schedules. Using the LQ model, two treatment scenarios 1 and 2 will kill the same overall number of cells if they satisfy the iso-effect relationship $-\ln(S_1) = -\ln(S_2)$, which implies that

$$\text{RWD}_1\left(1 + \frac{G_1 \cdot \text{RWD}_1}{\alpha/\beta}\right) = \text{RWD}_2\left(1 + \frac{G_2 \cdot \text{RWD}_2}{\alpha/\beta}\right). \tag{14.3}$$

The temporal and fraction-size effects of treatments 1 and 2 are captured in equation (14.3) by the dose protraction factors $G_1$ and $G_2$, respectively. Because daily doses of 2 Gy are a convenient historical standard for RT, it is useful to define and compute EQD2 as follows:

$$\text{EQD2} \equiv \text{RWD}\frac{\left(1 + \frac{G \cdot \text{RWD}}{\alpha/\beta}\right)}{\left(1 + \frac{2\ \text{Gy}}{\alpha/\beta}\right)}. \tag{14.4}$$

In equation (14.4), the standard 2 Gy per day treatment is delivered with a low-LET reference radiation; therefore, $D$ = RWD because the RBE = 1; also, the Lea–Catcheside dose protraction factor $G$ equals unity for short RT delivery times. It is important to note that EQD2 is a nonlinear function of dose and the RWD only depends on $\alpha/\beta$; it is independent of the value of the LQ parameter $\alpha$.

**Biologically equivalent dose (BED) and EQD2:** BED is defined as $-\ln(S)/\alpha$. Conceptually, the BED corresponds to the total dose administered in a series of infinitely small fractions or as an infinitely protracted exposure. As with EQD2, the BED concept is used in the literature to compare the effectiveness of alternate treatments [16]. That is, any two treatments that have the same BED will kill approximately the same number of cells. Iso-BED calculations are equivalent to iso-EQD2 calculations because EQD2 = BED/[1 + 2 Gy/($\alpha/\beta$)]. Of note, BED is *always* greater than the EQD2. We prefer EQD2 to BED because EQD2 values correspond to clinically used treatment doses.

## 14.3 Nonuniform dose distributions

In laboratory studies and in preclinical and clinical applications of SFRT, dose distributions are purposely modulated on scales ranging from micro- to centimeters in an effort to exploit multicellular and tissue-level recovery processes with the aim of increasing the therapeutic ratio, i.e. decreasing organ at risk (OAR) toxicity while achieving the same or better local tumor control. The EUD concept as formulated by Niemierko [17] is premised on the idea that any two dose distributions are considered equivalent if they cause the same radiobiological effect. Most of the published EUD models are based on cell survival as the clinically relevant endpoint, although some of the larger-scale serial or parallel OAR models use the so-called generalized EUD (gEUD). In this subsection, we focus solely on EUD with some generalizations of the commonly used formula reported in the literature to better account for dose, dose rate, dose fractionation, and RBE effects using the models and formulas summarized in section 14.2.

**Generalized equivalent uniform dose (gEUD):** For normal tissue control probability (NTCP) modeling of OAR responses, the larger-scale (>few millimeters) distribution of dose across the entire tissue has a well-recognized impact on clinical response [18–20]. For conventional RT, the clinical response of some OARs, such as the spine or brain stem, is more closely related to the maximum OAR dose, whereas in other tissues, such as the liver, clinical responses are more closely correlated with the average OAR dose. A simple, empirical way to relate clinical observations to the partial or nonuniform irradiation of an OAR is to define a gEUD [21] as

$$\text{gEUD} = \left( \sum_i v_i \cdot \text{EQD2}_i^{1/a} \right)^a .$$

Here, $v_i$ is the $i$th volume of an OAR receiving $\text{EQD2}_i$ as computed using equation (14.4). In this empirical dose–response model, $a$ is a tissue-specific parameter that reflects the aggregate response of an OAR to an inhomogeneous dose distribution. In the limit as $a \to +\infty$, gEUD equals the maximum EQD2, and in the limit as $a \to -\infty$, gEUD equals the minimum EQD2. For the special case when $a = 1$, gEUD is the arithmetic average EQD2.

The EUD of a dose distribution, $\{D\}$, is the homogeneous (uniform) dose that leads to an equal clonogenic survival in the same tissue region, i.e. $S_{\text{hom}}(D = \text{EUD}) = S_{\text{inhom}}(D = \{D\})$. With the LQ cell survival model, EUD is therefore defined by the iso-survival relationship

$$\begin{aligned}\overline{S} &= \exp(-\alpha \cdot \text{EUD} - \beta \cdot \text{EUD}^2) \\ &= \sum_i \nu_i \exp(-\alpha \cdot \text{RWD}_i - G \cdot \beta \cdot \text{RWD}_i^2)\cdot\end{aligned} \tag{14.5}$$

Here, $v_i$ is the fraction of cells receiving a dose $\text{RWD}_i$. In the left-hand side of equation (14.5), the dose protraction factor is set *a priori* to $G = 1$ (single-fraction delivery in a short time interval) and RBE = 1 to correspond to a low-LET radiation, such as MV x-rays. The right-hand side of equation (14.5) explicitly accounts for the temporal and spatial pattern of radiation delivery and the increased biological effectiveness, per unit dose, of a higher-LET radiation (RBE $\geq$ 1).

Taking the logarithm of both sides of equation (14.5) and solving for EUD yields

$$\text{EUD} = \frac{1}{2}(\alpha/\beta)\left(-1 + \sqrt{1 - \frac{4\ln(\overline{S})}{\alpha(\alpha/\beta)}}\right), \tag{14.6}$$

The EUD computed using equation (14.6) is the dose of a low-LET radiation uniformly delivered as a single dose of radiation in a very short time interval that kills the same number of cells as a nonuniform {RWD} distribution delivered with an arbitrary temporal pattern, e.g. $n$ fractions with intrafraction dose-rate effects modeled by $g$, as computed using equation (14.1). To compare the EUD to a conventional treatment delivered as daily doses of 2 Gy, replace RWD in equation (14.4) with the EUD and then compute the EQD2 as

$$\text{EQD2(EUD)} = \text{EUD}\frac{1 + \frac{\text{EUD}}{\alpha/\beta}}{1 + \frac{2\text{Gy}}{\alpha/\beta}}. \tag{14.7}$$

It is useful to note that the EQD2 computed from the EUD for cell survival is *exactly* the same as computing the EUD from the distribution of EQD2 values, i.e. $\text{EQD2}(\text{EUD}=\{RWD_i\}) = \text{EUD}(\{\text{EQD2}_i\})$. The equivalence of EQD2(EUD) and $\text{EUD}(\{\text{EQD2}_i\})$ arises because EUD and EQD2 are both derived from an iso-survival relationship based on the LQ model.

## 14.4 The uses of EUD and EQD2 in SFRT

To illustrate the differences between, and trends of physical and biological dose metrics, we consider a representative preclinical example: figure 14.1 shows the Monte-Carlo-generated dose profile of the University of Washington 50 MV proton minibeam at a depth of 6 mm [22–24]. The geometry of the physical collimator used to produce this beam has a slit width of 300 μm and a CTC of 1 mm [25]. The left-hand panel of figure 14.1 shows the physical dose profile modeled with TOPAS [26] using a peak dose $D_{\text{Peak}}$=20 Gy. The right-hand panel depicts the corresponding

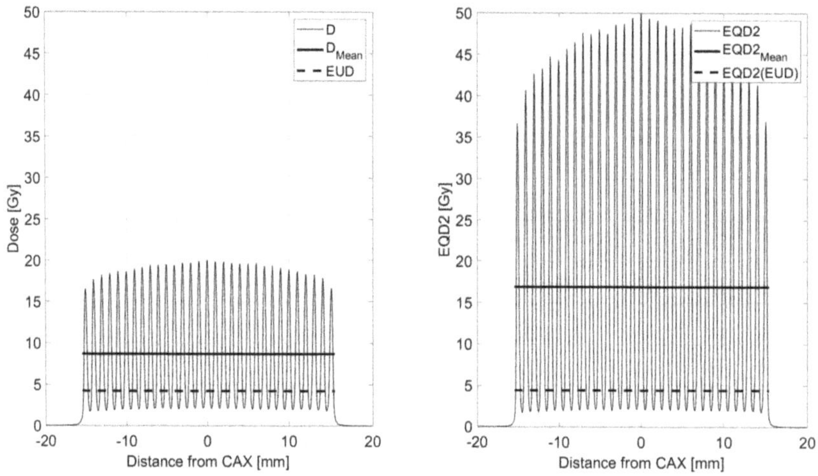


**Figure 14.1.** Illustration of the effects of biological metrics on the SFRT profile. Left: Monte Carlo simulations of a minibeam profile for a 50 MeV proton beam with a peak dose of 20 Gy at the central axis (CAX) and a peak-to-valley dose ratio (PVDR) of ten [23]. The mean dose is 8.7 Gy and the EUD = 4.2 for an $\alpha/\beta = 10$ Gy and $\alpha = 0.3$ Gy$^{-1}$, which corresponds to $S(2$ Gy$) = 0.49$. Right: corresponding EQD2 dose. The peak EQD2 dose is 50 Gy and the PVDR increases to 24. The mean of the EQD2 profile increases accordingly to 16.9 Gy and the EQD2(EUD) to 4.3 Gy.

EQD2 profile with $\alpha/\beta = 10$ Gy. The resulting EQD2 in the peak is 50 Gy. Also shown are the mean dose, $D_{\text{Mean}}$, the EUD, and the corresponding values for the EQD2 dose profiles.

At shallow depths, the mean proton kinetic energy is large, and the RBE for endpoints such as double-strand break (DSB) induction and reproductive cell survival is close to unity, i.e. RBE $\cong$ 1, and therefore $D \cong$ RWD. This irradiation geometry results in $D_{\text{Mean}} = 8.7$ Gy and an EUD and EQD2(EUD) of 4.2 Gy and 4.3 Gy, respectively, as indicated by the dashed lines. Of note, the peak-to-valley dose ratio (PVDR) in the left panel is ten and, when expressed in terms of EQD2, increases to 24 as shown in the right panel. While the mean dose expressed in EQD2 increases proportionally to the peak and valley doses, the EQD2(EUD) remains nearly constant. This is because the mean dose increases linearly with all physical dosimetric parameters, whereas the surviving fraction, see equations (14.5) and (14.6), is a nonlinear function of the dose. The close agreement in the EUD values for the left and right panels and the increase in the PVDR for the dose and EQD2 values reflect the importance of the valley dose and valley EQD2 in determining the iso-effective doses. In the calculation of EUD, it is the survival of cells in the valleys that dominates the overall survival response in the region of interest. Cells within the peak dose region receive such a high dose that there is a very small chance for them to survive in the reproductive sense. It has been reported in the literature that the OAR tolerance dose is more closely correlated with the valley dose than with the mean or maximum doses [1]. This observation is consistent with the hypothesis that the survival of cells in the valley regions of an SFRT treatment largely determines the ability of an OAR to recover.

To elucidate this effect, the profile in the left panel of figure 14.1 was utilized to compute the physical and biological dose metrics over a range of mean doses. This is shown in figure 14.2, with the profile shown in figure 14.1 highlighted for reference. The behavior of the mean dose and EUD, as well as the corresponding values of EQD2, reveal that at doses up to approximately 2 Gy, the EUD and $D_{\text{Mean}}$ are nearly identical. With increasing overall dose, $D_{\text{Mean}}$, $D_{\text{Valley}}$, and $D_{\text{Peak}}$ increase in a proportional fashion, whereas the EUD and EQD2(EUD) asymptotically trend towards the valley dose.

To further illustrate the larger asymptotic trends for a range of $(\alpha/\beta)$ values, we simulated the change in EUD(RWD) and EQD2(EUD) for valley doses from 0.01 Gy to 100 Gy. In figure 14.3, EUD values are shown as multiples of $D_{\text{Valley}}$ (left panel) or $\text{EQD2}_{\text{Valley}}$ (right panel). EUD and EQD2(EUD) approach the valley dose in the limit of very large values of $D_{\text{Valley}}$, reflecting the observation that the overall survival response of cells within a SFRT treatment is largely determined by the surviving cells in the lower-dose ('valley') regions. In the limit of small valley doses, EUD and EQD2(EUD) approach the mean dose and mean EQD2 values, respectively.

A further nonlinear dimension of the analysis of this preclinical proton beam is the change in LET along the beam path, which is most significant along the central axis (CAX). Since the mean proton kinetic energy decreases with depth, proton RBE tends to increase up to and beyond the Bragg peak (BP), resulting in a variable RBE along the CAX. This is illustrated alone and in combination with the other biological effects in figure 14.4. The top left panel shows the depth–dose profiles along the peak (at the CAX with reference to figure 14.1) and valley (at $\frac{1}{2}\times$ CTC = 0.5 mm off-axis). The depth of the profile in figure 14.1 is shown for reference at a depth of 6 mm with a peak dose of 20 Gy. The proton minibeam collimator used for this example was designed to result in a quasi-uniform dose at a BP [25] depth of 17 mm, which can be seen by the near-identical doses for the peak and valley.

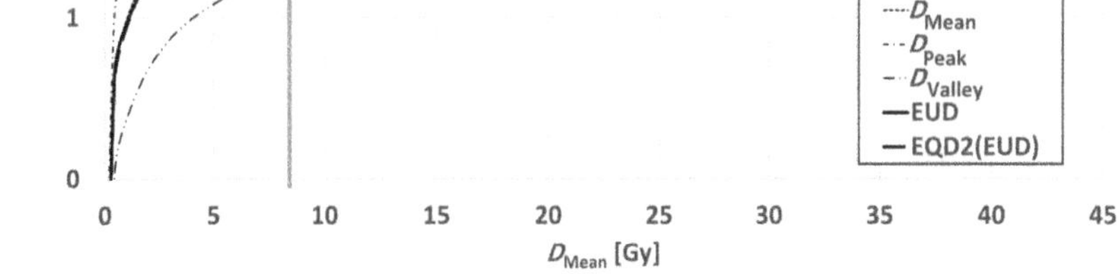


**Figure 14.2.** Changes in EUD and EQD2(EUD) as a function of the profile mean dose. The vertical line indicates the reference to figure 14.1.

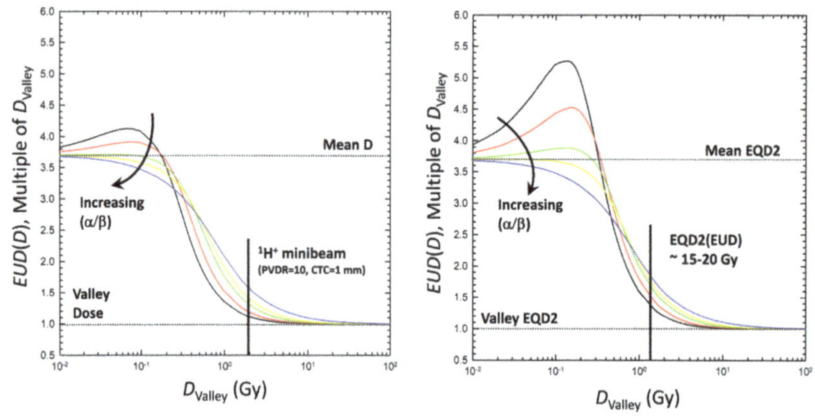


**Figure 14.3.** Asymptotic trends in EUD (RBE=1) and EQD2(EUD) for a representative proton SFRT treatment (CTC =1 mm, slot width = 300 µm, $\alpha = 0.3\ \mathrm{Gy}^{-1}$, and $\alpha/\beta = 1$–$100$ Gy). The vertical lines at 2 Gy in the left and right panels correspond to the proton minibeam data shown in figure 14.1.

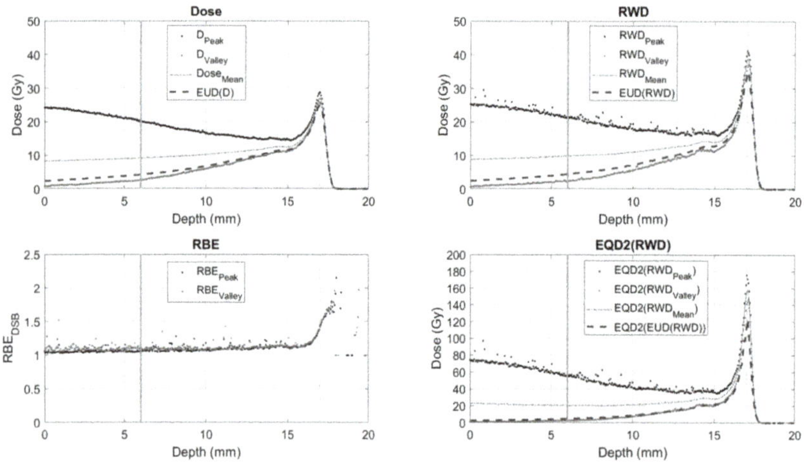


**Figure 14.4.** Depth–dose profiles and the effects of the RBE on dose and EUD for a Monte-Carlo-simulated 50 MeV proton minibeam (using the same parameters as in figure 14.1). The vertical line indicates the depth of the profile shown in figure 14.1. Top left panel: percentage depth–dose curve along the peak at the CAX and the adjacent valley. Bottom left: $RBE_{DSB}$ as a function of depth along the CAX. Top right: corresponding RBE-weighted depth–dose profile. Bottom right: corresponding RBE-weighted depth–dose profile expressed in EQD2.

The corresponding $RBE_{DSB}$ (the RBE required to induce DNA double-strand breakage) is shown in the bottom left panel, both along the peak and along the valley. At the beam entrance, the RBE is close to unity, gradually increasing to 1.1 at a depth of 15 mm before sharply rising to a value of 1.4 at the tip of the BP. While both RBE plots follow a similar trend, the RBE values in the valley are slightly higher at depths of up to about 10 mm. The RWD, which is the product of the spatially correlated dose and corresponding RBE value, is shown in the top right panel.

The effect of the higher RBE values around the BP corresponds to a 40% increase in the RWD. For both the dose and RWD, the mean dose, EUD, and EUD(RWD) follow similar trends with depth, with the latter being close to the valley dose. Applying equation (14.4) results in the EQD2(RWD), which is shown in the bottom right panel. The peak EQD2(RWD) at the reference depth of 6 mm increases from 20 to 55 Gy, whereas at the tip of the BP it increases by a factor of about six from around 30 to nearly 180 Gy. The EQD2[EUD(RWD)] closely follows the valley dose.

## 14.5 Preclinical and clinical studies

Most of the early SFRT research was carried out using synchrotron x-rays [27]. The most commonly reported geometric beam parameters are the width of the micro-planar beams (~25–75 μm), the center-to-center spacing (~100–400 μm), the x-ray energy (~50–600 keV), the peak dose (~50–600 Gy), a PVDR of up to 800 or more [28], and dose rates up to a few tens of kGy $s^{-1}$ [29]. With recent advances in technology and the availability of new facilities and irradiators [30, 31], the variety of SFRT beam parameters has further increased. The beam types now being considered for SFRT encompass a wide range of beam qualities, including kV and MV x-rays, low- and high-energy protons [2], as well as other charged particles, such as lithium, carbon, and oxygen beams [3, 4, 32]. The geometrical differences as well as the LET differences of the different beam types and vastly different dose rates make it extremely challenging to compare and reproduce experimental results among labs and facilities with different SFRT setups [33]. It is important to understand the biological significance of the relevant beam parameters when designing experiments to compare the efficacy of SFRT relative to uniform-dose RT.

### 14.5.1 Examples from the literature

In one laboratory study by Girst *et al* [34], the same mean dose was given using 20 MeV protons uniformly delivered by a minibeam (no corrections for variations in proton RBE). The mean absorbed dose given to the ear of BALB/c mice was 60 Gy, and the minibeam exhibited very large peak doses of 6000 Gy. Significantly reduced adverse effects were found in the SFRT arm. While this demonstrates that normal tissues can sustain enormous doses to very small tissue volumes, the overall result is not surprising when considering the EUD, which predicts that cell killing is largely dominated by the valley doses as illustrated in figures 14.1 through 14.4. The high-dose region in this study only covered ~4% of the entire irradiation area.

The findings reported by Girst *et al* were largely confirmed in a study by Prezado *et al* [35]. They irradiated rat brains with a 100 MeV proton minibeam. A single fraction uniformly delivered at 25 Gy was compared to a proton minibeam with $D_{\mathrm{Mean}} = 25$ Gy in the volume of interest at a depth of 1 cm. The nominal peak and valley doses for the proton minibeam were 57 and 8.8 Gy, respectively. To put this in context, the EUD for this beam at a depth of 1 cm was less than 25 Gy. For illustration purposes, the use of the same generic parameters as those shown above ($\alpha = 0.3$ $\mathrm{Gy}^{-1}$ and $\alpha/\beta = 10$ Gy) results in an EUD of 9.3 Gy, which is close to the reported valley dose of 8.8 Gy.

Both examples illustrate the challenges and inadequacy of using the physical dose (especially the peak dose) alone to understand and model the biological effects of SFRT.

In another study, Smyth *et al* [36] compared the toxicities of a synchrotron microbeam and conventional treatments of mice. They compared the doses needed to cause toxicity in 50% of the probands (TD50) for the head, thorax, and abdomen and total body irradiation. Peak and valley doses were reported for 50 μm wide beams spaced 400 μm apart. Table 14.1 shows a comparison of the SFRT and conventional RT TD50 values for physical dose parameters and the EUD to the head and abdomen.

The average SFRT dose that causes toxicity in 50% of the mice is more than three times higher than the uniform dose, whereas the corresponding EUD values fall between $D_{\text{Valley}}$ and a uniform RT dose. The EUD is closer to $D_{\text{Valley}}$ than to the uniform RT dose and is much lower than either $D_{\text{Peak}}$ or $D_{\text{Mean}}$ for the SFRT treatment. The data shown in table 14.1 suggests that the normal tissue sparing effects of SFRT are largely explained by the known biology embedded in the EUD metric, i.e. by cell killing in the LQ cell survival model. Regardless, the peak and mean doses are clearly not suitable parameters for comparing SFRT to uniform RT dose distributions. While it is difficult to pinpoint the reason for the modest mismatch in the EUD and the uniform RT dose that produces the same toxicity level, a possible explanation may simply involve inaccuracies in microbeam dosimetry. The accurate determination of mini- and microbeam doses is challenging [37], especially for the valley doses that largely govern estimates of the EUD.

Steel *et al* [38] compared *in vitro* cell survival of tumor and normal tissue cells for uniform and microbeam RT. Although the EUD was not reported in their publication, they did compare their data with the LQ model. Figure 14.5 shows their observed cell survival plotted as a function of the EUD using estimates of $\alpha$ and $(\alpha/\beta)$ derived from the uniform-dose experiments. For the non-tumor cell lines MRC5 and HUVEC, the data shown in this figure indicate that cell survival after uniform and microbeam radiotherapy (MRT) irradiation is largely and reasonably well explained by the LQ model with the EUD as the dose metric instead of the mean or peak dose. It is interesting to note that cell survival after MRT is slightly lower for all four cell lines, i.e. normal and tumor cell lines, compared to that of conventional radiation therapy.

**Table 14.1.** Comparison of TD50 dose and EUD parameters for SFRT and conventional RT. Data extracted from Smyth *et al* [36].

| | SFRT | | | | |
|---|---|---|---|---|---|
| TD50 | $D_{\text{Peak}}$ | $D_{\text{Mean}}$ | $D_{\text{Valley}}$ | EUD | Conventional RT Dose |
| Head | 268 Gy | 39.8 Gy | 7.2 Gy | 7.8 Gy | 12.7 Gy |
| Abdomen | 257 Gy | 38.9 Gy | 7.7 Gy | 8.4 Gy | 12.3 Gy |

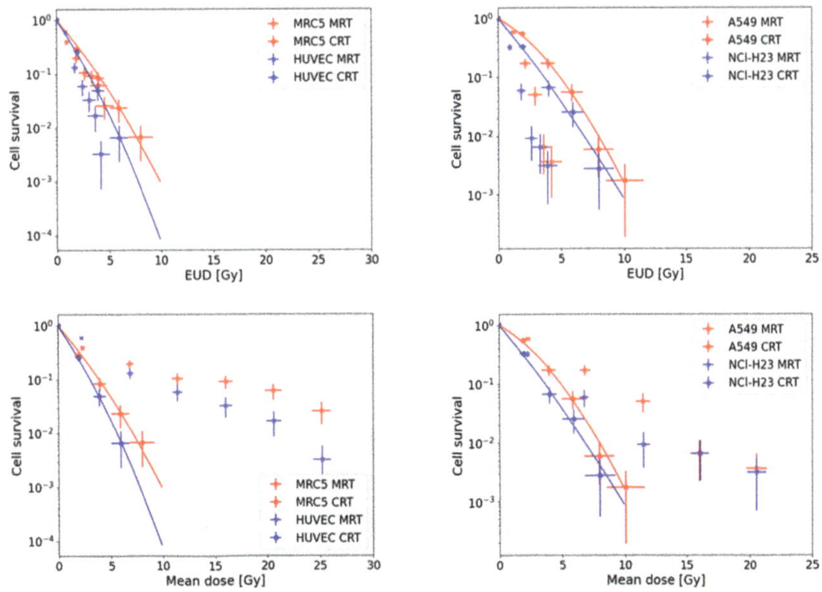


**Figure 14.5.** Left-hand panels: survival of non-tumor MRC5 (human lung fibroblasts, $\alpha = 0.52$ Gy$^{-1}$, $\alpha/\beta = 29$) and HUVEC (human endothelial cells, $\alpha = 0.67$ Gy$^{-1}$ $\alpha/\beta = 24$ Gy) cells after microbeam (MRT) and conventional radiation therapy (CRT). Right-hand panels: survival for two tumor cell lines: A549 (human lung carcinoma, $\alpha = 0.29$ Gy$^{-1}$, $\alpha/\beta = 8$ Gy) and NCl-H23 (human lung adenocarcinoma, $\alpha = 0.59$ Gy$^{-1}$, $\alpha/\beta = 49$ Gy). The top row shows the survival as a function of EUD, the bottom row as a function of mean dose. The solid lines show LQ fits to the measured data for CRT irradiation conditions. Adapted from [38], with permission from MDPI.

### 14.5.2 Treatment planning

An important step toward the first clinical applications of SFRT would be to carry out case studies to determine which patients would most likely benefit from SFRT treatment. As table 14.1 and figure 14.5 illustrate, EUD is potentially a much more useful metric for the comparison of SFRT and conventional RT than the mean or peak doses. Today, no commercial treatment planning system offers dose calculations for SFRT, but several research groups have developed treatment planning tools [39, 40]. Treatment planning in SFRT faces additional challenges compared to conventional RT due to the micrometer resolution required to capture the steep dose gradients. For MRT in particular, dose calculations are computationally expensive and the visualization of doses on the micrometer scale is challenging. Common dose parameters, such as the peak and valley doses, as well as dose–volume histograms (DVH) may be calculated using the larger, millimeter-sized voxel grids used for CT imaging.

Donzelli *et al* [40] computed the DVH within each voxel as illustrated in figure 14.6, which can then be transformed into an EUD if the parameters $\alpha$ and $\beta$ are known. An example of the application of this approach is depicted in figure 14.7. It shows the dose calculation of synchrotron microbeams for a lung tumor case comparing the peak dose, valley dose, and the EUD. The treatment plan

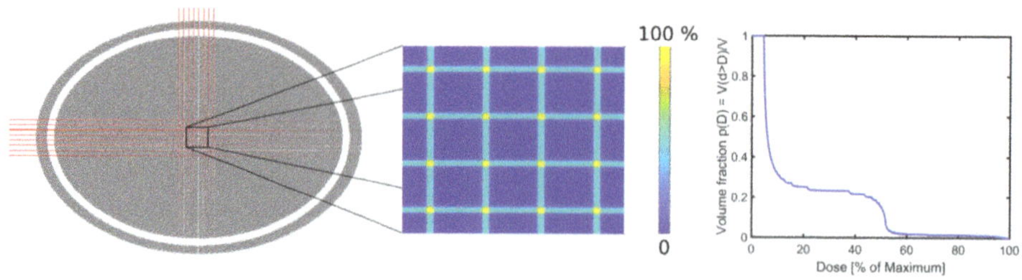


**Figure 14.6.** Dose calculation in SFRT: For each CT voxel, the microscopic dose distribution is calculated (left and center). From the shown dosimetric quantities, peak and valley doses can be determined along with the corresponding DVH (right-most panel). The EUD can then be calculated from the DVH for each voxel using predetermined values of $\alpha$ and $\alpha/\beta$. Reproduced from [40]. © 2018 Institute of Physics and Engineering in Medicine. Reproduced with permission. All rights reserved.

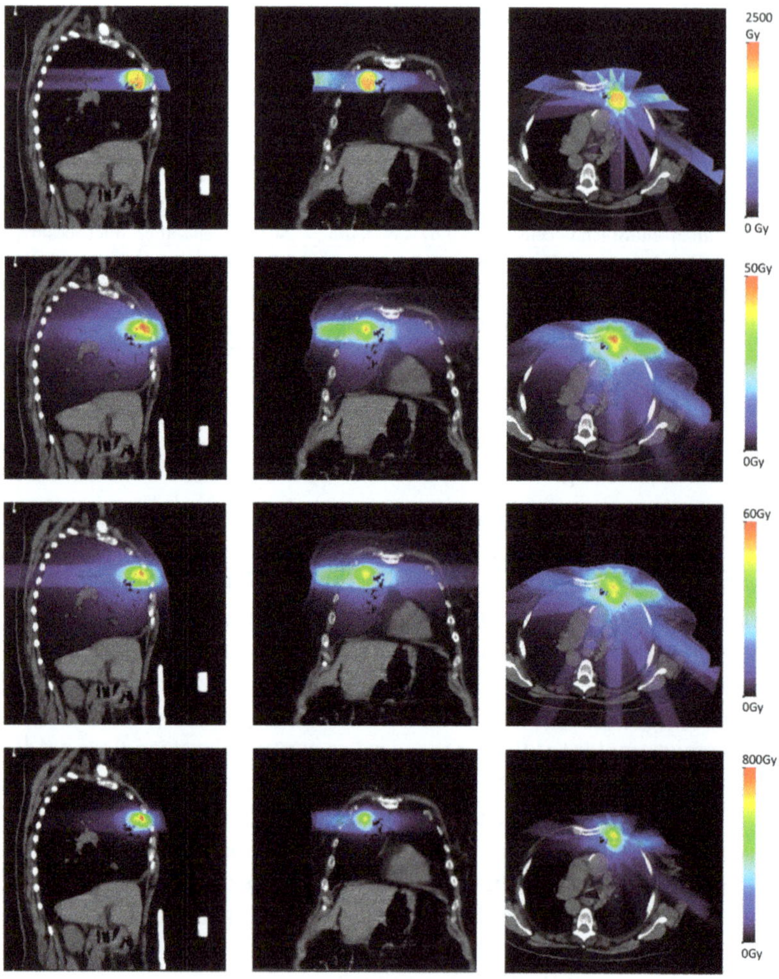


**Figure 14.7.** Treatment plan for a lung tumor SFRT treatment with eight microbeam fields (50 μm wide planar beams and 400 μm spacing). The beams are aligned such that all planes intersect in the target. First row: cumulative peak dose distribution. Second row: cumulative valley dose distribution. Third row: EUD dose distribution. Fourth row: EQD2(EUD) dose distribution. Note the different dose ranges in each row.

incorporates eight beam directions and facilitates the use of tumor-conforming treatment fields with planar beams 50 μm wide and 400 μm apart. The EUD was calculated from the DVH for each CT voxel by assuming $\alpha$ = 0.1 $Gy^{-1}$ and $\beta$ = 0.05 $Gy^{-2}$ ($\alpha/\beta$ =10 Gy). Peak and valley dose maps are superimposed on doses for each contributing field as an aid to visualization. Note the different *y*-axis scales for each scenario. The individual microbeams were aligned such that a cross-firing pattern evolves in the target region. Alternatively, beams could be aligned in an interlaced order, creating a homogeneous field in the target. The corresponding EUDs would be different in each case.

As expected, the EUD distribution in figure 14.7 differs from the peak and valley dose distributions. However, the EUD dose is similar to the valley dose distribution map. The nonlinear, quadratic EQD2 transformation of the EUD leads to an amplification of the high-dose regions relative to the low-dose regions (bottom row in figure 14.7). The EUD and EQD2 calculations in figure 14.7 employ generic $\alpha$ and $\beta$ values rather than tissue- or tumor-specific values. If these parameters used to compute EUD are assigned tissue-specific values, the EUD and EQD2 distributions would become discontinuous at the organ boundaries.

## 14.6 Discussion

To advance our understanding of micro- and minibeam treatment approaches, it is useful and important to compare laboratory results to well-established biophysical mechanisms of action, such as the breakage (i.e., DSB induction) and reunion theory of chromosome aberration formation [41]. Radiation damage to the nuclear DNA of mammalian cells remains the most widely accepted mechanism for the initiation of reproductive cell death, regardless of the mode of cell death (e.g. apoptosis, mitotic catastrophe, or senescence). All forms of radiation damage to a cell's DNA, including DNA DSB and single-strand break (SSB) induction increase linearly with the absorbed dose up to at least several hundred Gy [42, 43]. However, even for doses on the order of 1 or 2 Gy, *cell survival is a nonlinear function of dose, and therefore the mean surviving fraction of cells for an inhomogeneous dose distribution generally does not equal the surviving fraction of the mean of the dose distribution.* Furthermore, this effect is amplified at higher doses because of the nonlinear $\beta D^2$ term in the LQ model. A large and increasing body of laboratory evidence indicates that mean dose is not predictive of tissue responses to SFRT. The maximum dose delivered to submillimeter regions of tissue also seems irrelevant in predicting the clinical outcomes of SFRT, because the aggregate response in larger (>$cm^3$) regions of tissue is determined by the surviving cells rather than reproductively inactivated cells in high-dose, peak SFRT regions on a very small scale (<$mm^3$).

In this chapter, we introduced the EUD as a concept derived from the LQ model, which considers reproductive cell survival to be independent from damage to, or the survival of nearby cells. The LQ model has proven itself valuable in the clinic when comparing alternate treatment schedules through iso-effect calculations. It is also useful for comparing the relative toxicities of low- and high-LET radiations vis-à-vis RBE modeling. However, it is important to note that attempts to directly predict the *absolute* probability of local tumor control are inaccurate and of very limited value because of uncertainties in biological parameters and dosimetry [44]. In terms of SFRT, uncertainties in the biological parameters used for plan comparison and assessment are further compounded by the extreme spatial variations in dose gradients and high dose rates compared to more conventional RT. It is an open question as to whether or not the highly modulated dose patterns used in SFRT trigger different, so far undetected biological mechanisms than those triggered in conventional RT using lower doses per fraction and dose gradients that vary over centimetres of tissue rather than in submillimeter regions of tissue. It is also important to ask how robust the reported valley dosimetry is and what influence any uncertainties in dosimetry and the assessment of biological response have on the dose metrics, such as EUD and EQD2.

In the clinical applications of the LQ model, the transformation of dose distributions into a biologically equivalent dose distribution largely depends on the cell and tissue-specific value(s) of $\alpha/\beta$, which is most appropriately derived from clinical observations. However, it is important to recognize that the value of $\alpha/\beta$ is endpoint specific and different regions of an OAR or tumor target may respond to radiation with an $\alpha/\beta$ that reflects the local environment (e.g. with or without vasculature damage and $O_2$ within a tumor target) and the functional aspects of the OAR. Clinical experience in conventional RT shows that the OAR toxicities of some tissues, such as the skin, lung and liver, are mainly determined by the volume of tissue that receives large doses, whereas the toxicities of other tissues, such as the spinal cord or brain stem, are determined by the maximum dose regardless of the volume of irradiated tissue ('serial organs'). It remains an open question as to whether or not the OAR response to SFRT treatments will obey these classical dose–volume relationships.

The accuracy of the LQ model is well established in the dose range between approximately 1 and 10 Gy and perhaps higher [45]. At doses below 1 Gy, low dose hypersensitivity tends to decrease cell survival more than predicted by the LQ model [46]. At doses much larger than the value of $\alpha/\beta$, observations show a higher survival than predicted by the LQ model, if the dose protraction factor ('$G$') is not used to correct for intrafractional dose-rate effects. The accuracy of the LQ model is improved through the use of the dose protraction factor to account for dose-rate effects [6, 11, 47–49] and other refinements to account for deviations from the Poisson distribution of lethal DNA damage [11, 50, 51]. A number of alternatives to the standard LQ model [6, 48, 52–54] have been proposed, but they all require the introduction of additional parameters into the modeling process beyond the determinations of the two-parameter LQ model, i.e. the values of $\alpha$ and $(\alpha/\beta)$.

SFRT is characterized by peak doses of up to several hundreds or thousands of Gray [34], with even higher EQD2 doses. The peak doses in SFRT are usually well beyond the dose range in which the LQ model is considered accurate. However, as shown in figure 14.2, the high doses in the peak regions do not substantially contribute to the dose that determines equivalent levels of cell survival; therefore, uncertainties in $\alpha$ and $\alpha/\beta$ are unlikely to affect estimates of the overall EUD. On the other hand, valley doses may exceed 10 Gy, decreasing the accuracy of the LQ and related EQD2 and EUD estimates. As shown in figure 14.2, the general trend is for the EUD to approach the valley dose at high doses, and therefore the difference between the EUD and valley doses that are >10 Gy may be negligible. The LQ model is notably robust to predictions of dose–time relationships with regards to uncertainties in biological parameters and mechanisms when compared to models that introduce additional parameters to improve the accuracy of dose–response modeling for doses that are large compared to $(\alpha/\beta)$ [6]. Still, it may be worthwhile to consider EUD calculations based on cell survival models that better capture trends in cell survival for doses that are very large compared to $(\alpha/\beta)$, such as the modified linear–quadratic (MLQ) model [53] and the universal survival curve (USC) model [54].

A wealth of preclinical data demonstrates that SFRT irradiations exhibit an OAR sparing effect relative to conventional RT while being equally effective at local tumor control [55, 56]. Experimental evidence shows that differences in the vasculature, inflammatory and immune reactions, and bystander signaling are responsible for these observations [57–60], although uncertainties in dosimetry may also be a factor, especially in the valley regions. Intercellular mechanisms are not explicitly considered in LQ model of cell survival or related concepts such as the EUD, RBE, and EQD2 concepts summarized in this chapter. Therefore, these concepts are most useful as well-defined and easy-to-compute metrics for the reporting of SFRT results rather than as definitive metrics that predict absolute treatment outcomes.

The EUD is a best-effort approach to compare SFRT treatment fields to conventional RT based on established radiobiology models. Reporting EUD values for SFRT experiments is a starting point for the discovery and quantification of novel biological mechanisms. The inclusion of EUD, EQD2, and RBE into treatment planning systems can help to identify the clinical cases that are most likely to benefit from SFRT. An understanding of tumor control and OAR toxicity after SFRT treatment is essential for future clinical applications, and the EUD is a useful metric for optimized, patient-specific SFRT treatments.

## 14.7 Knowledge gaps and future perspectives

This chapter highlights the need for SFRT to report the biological dose in addition to the physical dose. This does not come without challenges, given the uncertainties in SFRT dosimetry and the biological parameters. Here, we have presented a conceptual basis for a multiscale modeling approach to the assessment and comparison of SFRT and conventional RT using established radiation biology models and concepts. Careful validation of the presented biological dose in SFRT should be done at several levels. The easiest and quickest is to retrospectively analyze experimental results in terms of EUD, with corrections for dose and RBE effects that have already been published, similar to the material presented in this chapter. How would the interpretation of the results of published studies change if presented in the context of EUD with corrections for dose rate, dose, and RBE effects? The next level of testing should be prospective *in vitro* and *in vivo* studies to quantify deviations from uniform irradiation and to relate the results of these studies to fundamental mechanisms of action.

It remains possible that SFRT and treatments that deliver more uniform doses will lead to comparable biological effects when compared using EUD, EQD2, and RBE. We are aware of the fact that a wealth of preclinical observations suggests effects beyond such a simple EUD/geometrical advantage of SFRT. However, only careful experiments that quantify these effects relative to established radiation biology concepts can lead us to a deeper understanding and more complex outcome modeling. Any SFRT-specific effects that modify tumor control and OAR toxicities relative to conventional RT may be incorporated into the presented system of models.

One of the potential advantages of SFRT that has not been sufficiently explored in planning studies is the fact that tissues may cope well with very high doses to small (<$mm^3$) volumes, as demonstrated by e.g. Girst *et al* [34]. Taking advantage of the physical dose deposition characteristics around the BP for proton minibeams, leading to a uniform dose distribution at depth (see, for example, figure 1 in Girst *et al* [34]), could help to identify potential advantages of SFRT over conventional RT. The EUD and related concepts presented in this chapter are potentially useful for studies comparing the multitude of SFRT approaches to more conventional RT.

In addition to institutional validation of treatment planning systems for SFRT, it is important to compare and assess the accuracy of biological parameters in an interinstitutional setting. Are the biological and toxicity parameters used in conventional RT equally appropriate for the modeling of SFRT responses in different facilities and with different SFRT delivery parameters? Or, are the biology and the associated dose–response parameters different for SFRT and conventional RT? The presented biological dose concepts provide a logical extension of concepts that have proven useful in conventional RT and will help us to differentiate effects in a radical, new treatment modality. The use of EUD and related concepts will help to identify the patient cohorts that are most likely to benefit from SFRT and is likely to be more useful for SFRT plan optimization of beam geometries than purely physical dose concepts.

## 14.8 Conclusion and recommendations

For SFRT to gain acceptance by the wider community and to become a clinically valuable tool in the fight against cancer, models that can predict outcomes and toxicities in relation to established approaches are needed. This chapter highlights the limitations of utilizing conventional physical dose metrics for plan comparison and optimization. The EUD concept, while it may not account for all of the most significant biological and systemic dose–response effects, is a metric that can help the community better compare and reproduce laboratory results among facilities and serve as a useful tool for patient-specific optimization of SFRT.

### 14.8.1 Glossary of selected concepts and notation

**RBE** (*dimensionless*)—the relative biological effectiveness of one type of radiation relative to another type of radiation, usually $^{60}$Co γ-rays or MV x-rays. Varies with dose, particle type, kinetic energy (and LET), the biological endpoint of interest and the cell-, tissue-, and tumor-specific responses to radiation.

**RWD** (*units of Gy*)—RBE-weighed dose, i.e. the product of absorbed dose and RBE, which depends on multiple biological factors and the particle type and kinetic energy (i.e. LET).

**EUD** (*units of Gy*)—equivalent uniform dose. The dose (or EQD2 or RWD) distribution to a region of tissue that has the same biological effects as a nonuniform dose distribution.

**gEUD** (*units of Gy*)—generalized EUD. An empirical, tissue-level concept that is sometimes useful for capturing the larger-scale functional aspects of heterogeneous dose distributions. The gEUD and EUD concepts are only equivalent for special cases and biological endpoints.

**EQD2** (*units of Gy*)—equivalent (biological) dose to a region of tissue delivered as daily 2 Gy fractions. From a historical perspective, radiation therapy treatments were often delivered as daily doses of radiation that helped to spare low ($\alpha/\beta$) organs at risk (OARs) without decreasing local control of tumor targets with a large ($\alpha/\beta$). The EQD2 concept is a convenient way to convert (renormalize) alternate treatment schedules, often for a small number of large doses as used in SFRT, to a treatment that kills the same number of cells as a treatment delivered using a conventional, 2 Gy per day, dose (or RWD). Much of the published data on OAR tolerance doses are for conventional radiation therapy treatment schedules (a dose per day less than or equal to 2 Gy). The EQD2 values for MV x-ray treatments are easily generalized to low-energy x-rays and particle therapy (RBE > 1) by replacing the absorbed dose with the RWD.

**EQD2(D)**—Value of the EQD2 computed from the absorbed dose distribution with RBE = 1, regardless of the particle type and kinetic energy (LET).

**EQD2(RWD)**—Value of the EQD2 computed from the RWD distribution with RBE > 1 (or varies with LET). Because EQD2 is a nonlinear function of dose and depends on ($\alpha/\beta$) for the reference radiation, EQD2(RWD) is not equal to RWD (EQD2), i.e. the sequences in which the models are applied are not equivalent. Because ($\alpha/\beta$) is based on the reference radiation (RBE = 1), EQD2 should be computed in terms of RWD rather than dose for scenarios in which RBE > 1 (or varies with LET).

**EUD(EQD2) = EQD2(EUD)**—For the endpoint of cell survival, the sequence in which EQD2 and EUD are computed is exactly the same within the framework of the LQ cell survival model. EUD depends on $\alpha$ and ($\alpha/\beta$) for the reference radiation (RBE = 1), whereas EQD2 only depends on ($\alpha/\beta$) for the reference radiation.

**gEUD(EQD2) ≠ gEUD(EQD2)**—The gEUD concept is an empirical formula that gives preferential weight to small and larger doses of radiation across a region of tissue or tumor target. Because EQD2 is a nonlinear function of the absorbed dose and the RWD, the sequences in which EQD2 and gEUD are computed are different.

## References

[1] Smyth L M L, Senthi S, Crosbie J C and Rogers P A W 2016 The normal tissue effects of microbeam radiotherapy: what do we know, and what do we need to know to plan a human clinical trial? *Int. J. Radiat. Biol.* **92** 302–11

[2] Meyer J, Eley J, Schmid T E, Combs S E, Dendale R and Prezado Y 2019 Spatially fractionated proton minibeams *Br. J. Radiol.* **92** 20180466

[3] González W, Peucelle C and Prezado Y 2017 Theoretical dosimetric evaluation of carbon and oxygen minibeam radiation therapy *Med. Phys.* **44** 1921–9

[4] Martínez-Rovira I, González W, Brons S and Prezado Y 2017 Carbon and oxygen minibeam radiation therapy: an experimental dosimetric evaluation *Med. Phys.* **44** 4223–9

[5] Ibahim M J, Crosbie J C, Yang Y, Zaitseva M, Stevenson A W and Rogers P A W *et al* 2014 An evaluation of dose equivalence between synchrotron microbeam radiation therapy and conventional broadbeam radiation using clonogenic and cell impedance assays *PLoS One* **9** e100547

[6] Brenner D J, Hlatky L R, Hahnfeldt P J, Huang Y and Sachs R K 1998 The linear-quadratic model and most other common radiobiological models result in similar predictions of time-dose relationships *Radiat. Res.* **150** 83–91

[7] McMahon S J 2018 The linear quadratic model: usage, interpretation and challenges *Phys. Med. Biol.* **64** 01TR01

[8] Peng V, Suchowerska N, Rogers L, Claridge Mackonis E, Oakes S and McKenzie D R 2017 Grid therapy using high definition multileaf collimators: realizing benefits of the bystander effect *Acta Oncol. Stockh. Swed.* **56** 1048–59

[9] Booz J, Braby L, Coyne J, Kliauga P, Lindborg L and Menzel H-G *et al* 1983 ICRU report 36 *J. Int. Comm. Radiat. Units Meas.* **os19** https://journals.sagepub.com/toc/crub/os-19/1

[10] Stewart R D, Carlson D J, Butkus M P, Hawkins R, Friedrich T and Scholz M 2018 A comparison of mechanism-inspired models for particle relative biological effectiveness (RBE) *Med. Phys.* **45** e925–52

[11] Sachs R K, Hahnfeld P and Brenner D J 1997 The link between low-LET dose–response relations and the underlying kinetics of damage production/repair/misrepair *Int. J. Radiat. Biol.* **72** 351–74

[12] Stewart R D and Li X A 2007 BGRT: biologically guided radiation therapy-the future is fast approaching! *Med. Phys.* **34** 3739–51

[13] Stewart R D 2001 Two-lesion kinetic model of double-strand break rejoining and cell killing *Radiat. Res.* **156** 365–78

[14] Nikitaki Z, Nikolov V, Mavragani I V, Mladenov E, Mangelis A and Laskaratou D A *et al* 2016 Measurement of complex DNA damage induction and repair in human cellular systems after exposure to ionizing radiations of varying linear energy transfer (LET) *Free Radic. Res.* **50** S64–78

[15] Okayasu R 2012 Repair of DNA damage induced by accelerated heavy ions—a mini review *Int. J. Cancer* **130** 991–1000

[16] Fowler J F 2010 21 Years of biologically effective dose *Br. J. Radiol.* **83** 554–68

[17] Niemierko A 1997 Reporting and analyzing dose distributions: a concept of equivalent uniform dose *Med. Phys.* **24** 103–10

[18] Emami B, Lyman J, Brown A, Coia L, Goitein M and Munzenrider J E *et al* 1991 Tolerance of normal tissue to therapeutic irradiation *Int. J. Radiat. Oncol. Biol. Phys.* **21** 109–22

[19] Bentzen S M, Constine L S, Deasy J O, Eisbruch A, Jackson A and Marks L B *et al* 2010 Quantitative analyses of normal tissue effects in the clinic (QUANTEC): an introduction to the scientific issues *Int. J. Radiat. Oncol. Biol. Phys.* **76** S3–9

[20] Grimm J, Marks L B, Jackson A, Kavanagh B D, Xue J and Yorke E 2021 High dose per fraction, hypofractionated treatment effects in the clinic (HyTEC): an overview *Int. J. Radiat. Oncol. Biol. Phys.* **110** 1–10

[21] Niemierko A 1999 A generalized concept of equivalent uniform dose (EUD) *Med. Phys.* **26** 1100

[22] Ford E, Emery R, Huff D, Narayanan M, Schwartz J and Cao N *et al* 2017 An image-guided precision proton radiation platform for preclinical *in vivo* research *Phys. Med. Biol.* **62** 43–58

[23] Meyer J, Stewart R D, Smith D, Eagle J, Lee E and Cao N *et al* 2017 Biological and dosimetric characterisation of spatially fractionated proton minibeams *Phys. Med. Biol.* **62** 9260–81

[24] Seco J and Verhaegen F (ed) 2021 Monte Carlo modelling of proton beams for small animal irradiation *Monte Carlo Techniques in Radiation Therapy: Applications to Dosimetry, Imaging, Preclinical Radiotherapy.* 2nd edn (Boca Raton, FL: CRC Press), ch 9 pp 143–60

[25] Lee E, Meyer J and Sandison G 2016 Collimator design for spatially-fractionated proton beams for radiobiology research *Phys. Med. Biol.* **61** 5378–89

[26] Perl J, Shin J, Schumann J, Faddegon B and Paganetti H 2012 TOPAS: an innovative proton Monte Carlo platform for research and clinical applications *Med. Phys.* **39** 6818–37

[27] Microbeam Radiation Therapy (MRT) (https://esrf.fr/home/UsersAndScience/Experiments/CBS/ID17/mrt-1.html)

[28] Siegbahn E A, Stepanek J, Bräuer-Krisch E and Bravin A 2006 Determination of dosimetrical quantities used in microbeam radiation therapy (MRT) with Monte Carlo simulations *Med. Phys.* **33** 3248–59

[29] Eling L, Bouchet A, Nemoz C, Djonov V, Balosso J and Laissue J *et al* 2019 Ultra high dose rate Synchrotron Microbeam Radiation Therapy. Preclinical evidence in view of a clinical transfer *Radiother. Oncol.* **139** 56–61

[30] Hadsell M, Zhang J, Laganis P, Sprenger F, Shan J and Zhang L *et al* 2013 A first generation compact microbeam radiation therapy system based on carbon nanotube X-ray technology *Appl. Phys. Lett.* **103** 183505

[31] Bartzsch S, Corde S, Crosbie J C, Day L, Donzelli M and Krisch M *et al* 2020 Technical advances in x-ray microbeam radiation therapy *Phys. Med. Biol.* **65** 02TR01

[32] Dilmanian F A, Eley J G, Rusek A and Krishnan S 2015 Charged particle therapy with mini-segmented beams *Front. Oncol.* **5** 269

[33] Bennett G F 1997 International basic safety standards for protection against ionizing radiation and for the safety of radiation sources: International Atomic Energy Agency, Vienna, Safety Series No. 115, 1996, 353pp *J. Hazard. Mater.* **54** 134–5

[34] Girst S, Greubel C, Reindl J, Siebenwirth C, Zlobinskaya O and Walsh D W M *et al* 2016 Proton minibeam radiation therapy reduces side effects in an *in vivo* mouse ear model *Int. J. Radiat. Oncol. Biol. Phys.* **95** 234–41

[35] Prezado Y, Jouvion G, Hardy D, Patriarca A, Nauraye C and Bergs J *et al* 2017 Proton minibeam radiation therapy spares normal rat brain: long-term clinical, radiological and histopathological analysis *Sci. Rep.* **7** 14403

[36] Smyth L M L, Donoghue J F, Ventura J A, Livingstone J, Bailey T and Day L R J *et al* 2018 Comparative toxicity of synchrotron and conventional radiation therapy based on total and partial body irradiation in a murine model *Sci. Rep.* **8** 12044

[37] Crosbie J C, Svalbe I, Midgley S M, Yagi N, Rogers P A W and Lewis R A 2008 A method of dosimetry for synchrotron microbeam radiation therapy using radiochromic films of different sensitivity *Phys. Med. Biol.* **53** 6861–77

[38] Steel H, Brüningk S C, Box C, Oelfke U and Bartzsch S H 2021 Quantification of differential response of tumour and normal cells to microbeam radiation in the absence of FLASH effects *Cancers* **13** 3238

[39] Day L R J, Donzelli M, Pellicioli P, Smyth L M L, Barnes M and Bartzsch S *et al* 2021 A commercial treatment planning system with a hybrid dose calculation algorithm for synchrotron radiotherapy trials *Phys. Med. Biol.* **66** 055016

[40] Donzelli M, Bräuer-Krisch E, Oelfke U, Wilkens J J and Bartzsch S 2018 Hybrid dose calculation: a dose calculation algorithm for microbeam radiation therapy *Phys. Med. Biol.* **63** 045013

[41] Hlatky L, Sachs R K, Vazquez M and Cornforth M N 2002 Radiation-induced chromosome aberrations: insights gained from biophysical modeling *BioEssays News Rev. Mol. Cell Dev. Biol.* **24** 714–23

[42] Stewart R D 2018 Induction of DNA damage by light ions relative to 60Co γ-rays *Int. J. Part. Ther.* **5** 25–39

[43] Stewart R D, Yu V K, Georgakilas A G, Koumenis C, Park J H and Carlson D J 2011 Effects of radiation quality and oxygen on clustered DNA lesions and cell death *Radiat. Res.* **176** 587–602

[44] Tucker S L, Thames H D and Taylor J M G 1990 How well is the probability of tumor cure after fractionated irradiation described by poisson statistics? *Radiat. Res.* **124** 273–82

[45] Brenner D J 2008 The linear-quadratic model is an appropriate methodology for determining isoeffective doses at large doses per fraction *Semin. Radiat. Oncol.* **18** 234–9

[46] Joiner M C, Marples B, Lambin P, Short S C and Turesson I 2001 Low-dose hypersensitivity: current status and possible mechanisms *Int. J. Radiat. Oncol. Biol. Phys.* **49** 379–89

[47] Wang J Z, Li X A, D'Souza W D and Stewart R D 2003 Impact of prolonged fraction delivery times on tumor control: a note of caution for intensity-modulated radiation therapy (IMRT) *Int. J. Radiat. Oncol. Biol. Phys.* **57** 543–52

[48] Carlson D J, Stewart R D, Li X A, Jennings K, Wang J Z and Guerrero M 2004 Comparison of *in vitro* and *in vivo* alpha/beta ratios for prostate cancer *Phys. Med. Biol.* **49** 4477–91

[49] Huang Z, Mayr N A, Lo S S, Wang J Z, Jia G and Yuh W T C *et al* 2012 A generalized linear-quadratic model incorporating reciprocal time pattern of radiation damage repair *Med. Phys.* **39** 224–30

[50] Sachs R K, Hlatky L, Hahnfeldt P and Chen P L 1990 Incorporating dose-rate effects in Markov radiation cell survival models *Radiat. Res.* **124** 216–26

[51] Carlson D J, Stewart R D, Semenenko V A and Sandison G A 2008 Combined use of Monte Carlo DNA damage simulations and deterministic repair models to examine putative mechanisms of cell killing *Radiat. Res.* **169** 447–59

[52] Guerrero M, Stewart R D, Wang J Z and Li X A 2002 Equivalence of the linear-quadratic and two-lesion kinetic models *Phys. Med. Biol.* **47** 3197–209

[53] Guerrero M and Li X A 2004 Extending the linear-quadratic model for large fraction doses pertinent to stereotactic radiotherapy *Phys. Med. Biol.* **49** 4825–35

[54] Park C, Papiez L, Zhang S, Story M and Timmerman R D 2008 universal survival curve and single fraction equivalent dose: useful tools in understanding potency of ablative radiotherapy *Int. J. Radiat. Oncol. Biol. Phys.* **70** 847–52

[55] Bouchet A, Lemasson B, Le Duc G, Maisin C, Bräuer-Krisch E and Siegbahn E A *et al* 2010 Preferential effect of synchrotron microbeam radiation therapy on intracerebral 9L gliosarcoma vascular networks *Int. J. Radiat. Oncol. Biol. Phys.* **78** 1503–12

[56] Serduc R, Bouchet A, Bräuer-Krisch E, Laissue J A, Spiga J and Sarun S *et al* 2009 Synchrotron microbeam radiation therapy for rat brain tumor palliation-influence of the microbeam width at constant valley dose *Phys. Med. Biol.* **54** 6711–24

[57] Sabatasso S, Laissue J A, Hlushchuk R, Graber W, Bravin A and Bräuer-Krisch E *et al* 2011 Microbeam radiation-induced tissue damage depends on the stage of vascular maturation *Int. J. Radiat. Oncol. Biol. Phys.* **80** 1522–32

[58] Bouchet A, Sakakini N, El Atifi M, Le Clec'h C, Brauer E and Moisan A *et al* 2013 Early gene expression analysis in 9L orthotopic tumor-bearing rats identifies immune modulation in molecular response to synchrotron microbeam radiation therapy *PLoS One* **8** e81874

[59] Ibahim M J, Yang Y, Crosbie J C, Stevenson A, Cann L and Paiva P *et al* 2016 Eosinophil-associated gene pathways but not eosinophil numbers are differentially regulated between synchrotron microbeam radiation treatment and synchrotron broad-beam treatment by 48 hours postirradiation *Radiat. Res.* **185** 60–8

[60] Brönnimann D, Bouchet A, Schneider C, Potez M, Serduc R and Bräuer-Krisch E *et al* 2016 Synchrotron microbeam irradiation induces neutrophil infiltration, thrombocyte attachment and selective vascular damage *in vivo Sci. Rep.* **6** 33601

# Chapter 15

# Spatially fractionated radiation therapy field calibration and commissioning

**Michael Grams and Hualin Zhang**

A rigorous commissioning process is required prior to implementing spatially fractionated radiation therapy (SFRT) techniques in the clinic. This chapter describes suggested calibration, commissioning, and quality assurance procedures for SFRT treatments involving a physical block as well as an advanced lattice delivery method. Treatments using a physical block require water tank measurements to characterize the dosimetric characteristics of the block. Additionally, it is helpful to integrate the block within the user's treatment planning system. Techniques such as lattice SFRT are similar to stereotactic body radiation therapy (SBRT) treatments with specialized planning methods. Since all SFRT treatments typically involve the delivery of high localized doses of radiation, radiation oncology teams should follow dedicated workflows and implement specific safety checks as part of each treatment.

## 15.1 Introduction/overview

The safe and accurate delivery of SFRT depends on a complete and thorough commissioning process. While the characteristically heterogeneous dose distributions are indeed non-typical compared to conventional radiotherapy, the commissioning process for an SFRT treatment program follows concepts that parallel standard commissioning procedures. These include mechanical integrity checks, water tank beam scanning, treatment planning system (TPS) verification, patient-specific quality assurance, and the development of safety checks and treatment workflows. This chapter focuses on commissioning and calibration procedures for GRID treatments involving both physical blocks and lattice SFRT based on a volumetric modulated arc therapy (VMAT) approach. However, the concepts and procedures described here should apply to other SFRT delivery modalities as well if the modality-specific features are fully considered.

doi:10.1088/978-0-7503-4046-5ch15

## 15.2 GRID block calibration and commissioning

Physical blocks made of brass or other suitably attenuating materials were developed for the first GRID treatments using megavoltage (MV) linear accelerators. Over the years, treatments using GRID blocks have been shown to be clinically effective for a variety of disease sites [1, 2]. These treatments are simple to deliver and often involve a single static field. The physical blocks can be commercially obtained [3] at a relatively low cost compared to the cost of other radiotherapy equipment. Because of these attractive qualities, GRID treatments with physical blocks are a commonly used delivery method for SFRT in many treatment centers.

The calibration and commissioning of a GRID block involves basic mechanical integrity checks and the characterization of the dosimetric properties of the block through water tank measurements; it should also include integration of the block within the user's TPS. Integrating the GRID block into the TPS allows the dose distribution in the patient to be visualized and also allows the doses to the target and surrounding organs at risk to be calculated. This can make clinical implementation easier, as the resulting treatment planning process is likely to be similar to existing clinical workflows.

### 15.2.1 Mechanical integrity checks

GRID blocks can have a mass of 22 kg or more and care must be taken to ensure they can be safely and securely mounted on the head of the linear accelerator. They are usually attached to a plastic or metal tray, and the user must confirm the integrity of both the hardware used to attach the block to the tray as well as the tray itself. A visual inspection of the tray to look for cracks or other signs of wear and verification that the mounting bolts are tight are recommended prior to every treatment. It is also recommended to have a spare mounting tray on hand in the event that the tray is broken or damaged.

Once the block is mounted on the tray, an assessment of block movement due to gravity at different gantry positions should be made. This can easily be accomplished using the portal imaging capability of the linear accelerator. At a minimum, portal images should be taken at the four cardinal gantry angles (0°, 90°, 180°, 270°). Measurements of the center of the GRID block relative to the isocenter can then be made as an assessment of block motion with gantry position. It is recommended that the block should not move more than 2 mm at any gantry position, otherwise the block tray and the accessory mount which attaches the assembly to the linear accelerator should be inspected. Figure 15.1 shows examples of this process using portal images taken with the block in place. Small deviations of the central hole due to the weight of the block can be seen at 90° and 270°.

### 15.2.2 Dosimetric characterization of physical GRID blocks

Once the mechanical integrity of the GRID block and mounting tray has been established, the user must characterize its dosimetric properties. This process should include measurements of dose profiles at various depths, percentage depth–dose

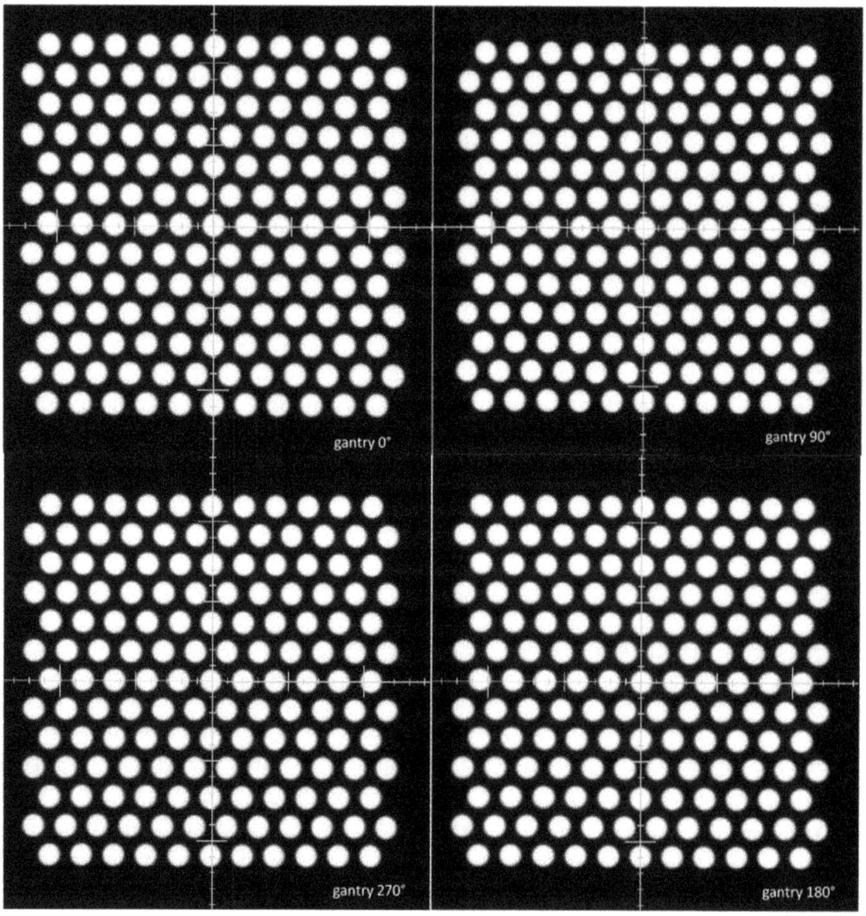


**Figure 15.1.** Portal dosimetry images of a GRID block taken at the four cardinal gantry angles. Deviations of the central hole relative to the isocenter (indicated by the green crosshair) due to the weight of the block can be seen at 90° and 270°.

(PDD) curves, and output factors. It is recommended that these measurements should initially be made in a water tank; once established, subsequent checks can be made in a solid water phantom. A detector with suitable spatial resolution is required for these measurements, as the holes of the GRID block are small (~1 cm) and the resulting dose gradients are quite steep. Examples of acceptable detectors are small-volume ionization chambers, diamond detectors, diodes, and radiochromic film.

Water tank scans of PDDs and both crossline and inline profiles must be obtained for each beam energy that is expected to be used clinically. In addition to providing basic dosimetric data, these measurements can be used to verify TPS calculations. It is common for treatments based on GRID blocks to use a source-to-surface distance (SSD) setup; therefore, the scans taken should correspond to the clinically used SSD (usually 100 cm). The PDDs should be taken for various field sizes up to and

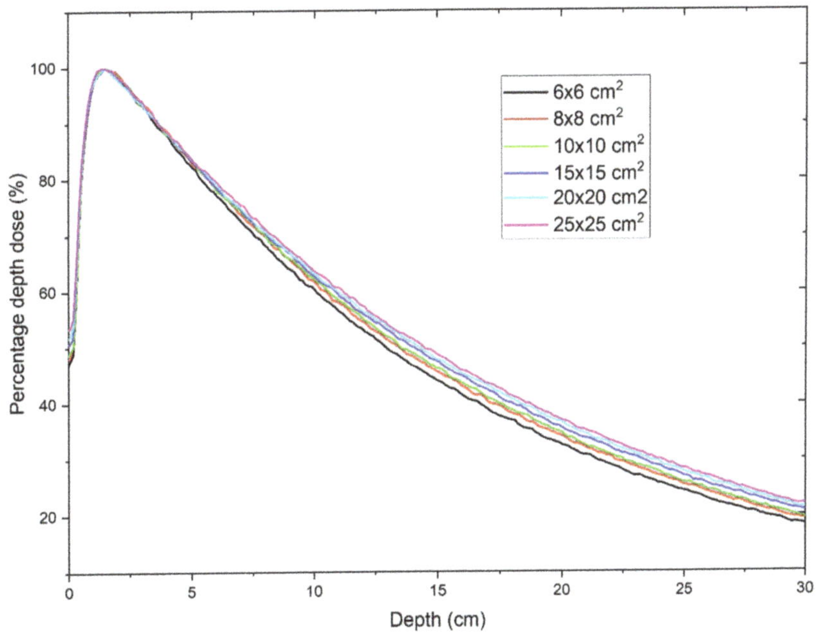


**Figure 15.2.** PDD scans of commercially available brass blocks of various field sizes and a 6 MV beam. PDDs must be measured for all beam energies that are used clinically.

including the largest possible field size with the detector properly aligned along the central axis of the field and within the central GRID block hole. Example PDDs for various field sizes using a 6 MV beam are shown in figure 15.2 for a commercially available (.decimal, Sanford, FL, USA) brass GRID block. It can be seen in figure 15.2 that the smallest field size ($6\times6$ cm$^2$) has the lowest PDD curve and the largest field ($25\times25$ cm$^2$) has the largest PDD curve, but the depth of dose maximum ($d_{max}$) remains the same for all field settings. It is recommended that only flattened beams should be commissioned and the use of flattening filter free (FFF) beams should be avoided. While the higher dose rates typically associated with FFF beams could be advantageous, the biologic consequences of the variable peak-to-valley ratio that would result as a function of off-axis distance are not known.

Inline and crossline profiles are useful to characterize the peak-to-valley ratio of the physical block and should be taken at $d_{max}$ and several depths beyond it. 'Inline' is defined as the direction parallel to the accelerator waveguide and crossline is perpendicular to it. These scans can also be useful for commissioning the block within the TPS, as they provide useful information about the attenuation of the block material. It is sufficient to take all scans at the maximum usable field size for the block being used. Example profiles are shown in figure 15.3. The profiles were taken using a PTW (Freiburg, Germany) microdiamond Type 60019 detector with a a sensitive volume of 0.004 mm$^3$.

In addition to PDDs and profile measurements, output factor measurements must also be made. The output factor measurements should be made at a depth

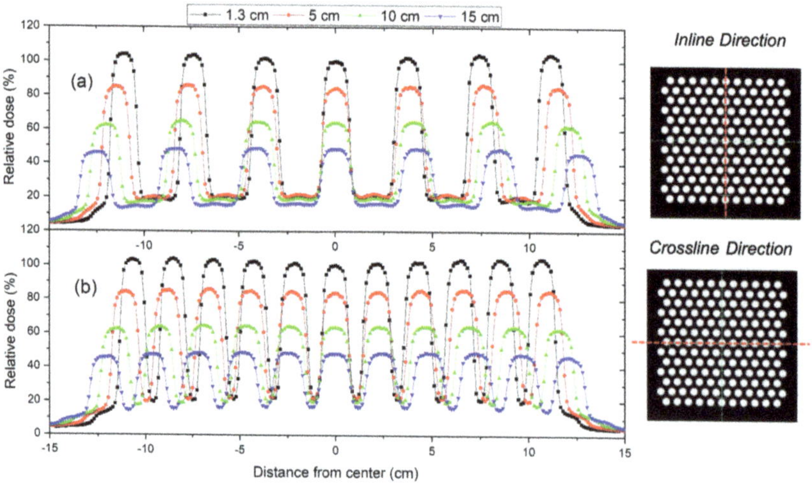


**Figure 15.3.** Inline (a) and crossline (b) profiles of a commercially available brass GRID block taken at various depths (indicated at the top of the figure) in a water tank for a 6 MV beam. The measurements are normalized to the central axis value at $d_{max}$. The images on the right-hand side of the figure indicate the direction of inline and crossline relative to the hole pattern of the GRID block.

corresponding to the point at which the dose is prescribed. For GRID treatments using physical blocks, this is most often $d_{max}$ and therefore the output factor measurements should be made at this depth along the central axis for each beam energy used clinically. These measurements can be used to verify calculations performed within the TPS through secondary monitor unit (MU) calculations.

### 15.2.3 Implementation of the physical block within the treatment planning system

Ideally, the dose distributions resulting from use of the physical block should be visible within the TPS in order to evaluate the dose delivered to the target as well as the surrounding organs at risk (OARs). The TPS requires the fundamental characteristics of the block such as its spatial dimensions and the transmission of the block material at each clinically used energy. The water tank measurements described in section 15.2.2 can be used to help verify and determine these characteristics. Additionally, integration within the user's record and verification of the system and the linear accelerator must be established. While it would be impossible to completely summarize the steps needed for all planning systems, we describe here the general concepts for integrating a physical grid block within a commonly used TPS. These concepts should also apply to other systems with appropriate TPS-specific modifications.

#### *15.2.3.1 Varian Eclipse TPS*

In the Varian Eclipse (Varian Medical Systems, Palo Alto, CA) environment, both the physical block and the tray on which it is mounted need to be defined within the external beam configuration settings of the TPS. Both the block and tray are configured as 'Add-On Materials.' The tray is associated with an 'Internal Code' corresponding to a numerical value used by the treatment unit to identify the add-on. Once the tray and block are defined within the TPS, the user must then define dosimetric properties for the block material, which for Varian Eclipse is simply the transmission.

A critical feature for the successful implementation of the grid block is that the hole size, pattern, and spacing must be accurate within the TPS. While in principle this can be done manually [4], a more convenient alternative for commercially available blocks is to acquire a DICOM file containing the exact block configuration. At least one commercial vendor (.decimal, Sanford, FL, USA) can provide such a DICOM file. The file consists of a treatment plan containing a field with the physical block. This plan must be anonymized each time prior to use, as the same plan cannot be used in more than one patient within Varian Eclipse. Commercially available software such as MIM (MIM Software Inc., Cleveland, OH, USA) or other available software packages can be used for anonymization. The anonymized plan is then imported into Eclipse where the block can be copied and pasted into a treatment field associated with the patient's plan. Figure 15.4 shows images of a commercially available brass grid block (.decimal, Sanford, FL, USA) along with a beam's eye view and a 3D rendering of the block orientation within the Eclipse TPS.

Once the block geometry is established within Eclipse, the block transmission must be determined so that measured and Eclipse-calculated profiles are in agreement. The water tank scans described in section 15.2.2 can be used for this purpose. Eclipse calculations can be obtained by creating a virtual water phantom that has the same dimensions as the water tank in which the profiles were obtained. After setting the SSD in Eclipse to be the same as that used for the acquired water tank measurements, the dose that passes through the GRID block can be calculated for various field sizes. Eclipse-calculated profiles at various depths for different field sizes can then be exported for comparison with the measured water tank profiles. Both the measured data from the water tank and the calculated data within the TPS should be normalized to an identical point for meaningful comparison. An appropriate choice of normalization would be at $d_{max}$ along the central axis for each clinical energy. The block transmission value should be varied within the TPS so that the best possible agreement with the calculations is obtained. Example crossline and inline profile comparisons for a 10 MV beam at $d_{max}$ are shown in figure 15.5.

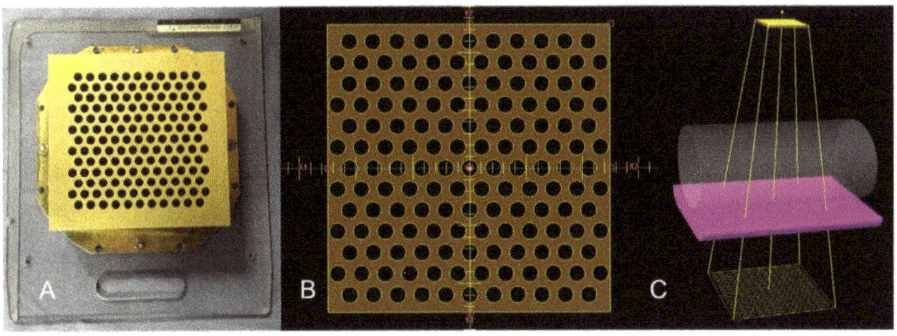


**Figure 15.4.** (A) Photograph of a commercially available brass grid block mounted on a block tray. (B) Beam's eye view of the same block imported within the Eclipse TPS. (C) 3D rendering of a GRID block treatment field on a cylindrical phantom.

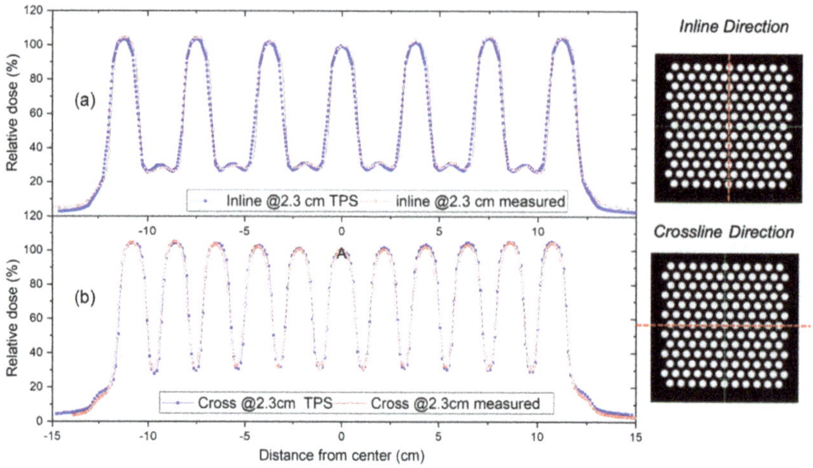


**Figure 15.5.** Inline (a) and crossline (b) profile comparison of measured water tank data (red line) and Eclipse TPS calculations (blue line) for a 10 MV beam passing through a commercially available brass GRID block. All data is normalized to 100% at $d_{max}$. The transmission of the block within the Eclipse TPS was varied to optimize the agreement between the measured and calculated dose profiles. The images on the right-hand side of the figure indicate the direction of inline and crossline relative to the hole pattern of the GRID block.

### *15.2.3.2 Output factors and comparison with TPS*

In addition to profiles measured using a water tank, output factor (OF) measurements should also be made. This data is useful both for secondary MU calculations used for patient treatments as well as for comparison with TPS-calculated output factors. OFs can be measured using the water tank and subsequently verified with additional measurements in a solid water phantom if desired. Comparison with a TPS can be made using a virtual water phantom. It is simplest to measure OFs at the prescription depth for the physical block, which normally is $d_{max}$. It is again imperative to use a detector with a suitably small active volume which is appropriate for the small openings of the block. Care should be taken to align the detector on the central axis of the beam and in the middle of the central hole of the GRID block. For comparison with TPS calculations, a measurement point must be placed at the same location within the virtual phantom. Table 15.1 shows OFs measured using a water tank and acquired using a PTW (Freiburg, Germany) microdiamond Type 60019 detector along with Varian Eclipse TPS-calculated results for both 6 MV and 10 MV energies at $d_{max}$. The OFs were normalized to the OF for a $10 \times 10$ cm$^2$ field size with the GRID block in place. The OF for these measurements is defined as

$$\text{OF} = \frac{\text{Output with GRID block in place for any field size}}{\text{Output with GRID block in place for } 10 \times 10 \text{ cm}^2 \text{ field}}.$$

These measurements were acquired using a commercially available brass GRID block (.decimal, Sanford, FL, USA) and measured for various field sizes at $d_{max}$ values of 1.3 and 2.3 cm for 6 and 10 MV, respectively. The agreement between the

**Table 15.1.** Comparison of measured and Varian Eclipse TPS-calculated 6 MV and 10 MV output factors for various field sizes using a brass GRID block. The OFs were normalized to the OF for a 10 × 10 $cm^2$ field size with the GRID block in place.

| | Field size ($cm^2$) | | | | | |
|---|---|---|---|---|---|---|
| 6 MV output factors | 6 × 6 | 8 × 8 | 10 × 10 | 15 × 15 | 20 × 20 | 25 × 25 |
| PTW microdiamond (measured) | 0.981 | 0.990 | 1.000 | 1.023 | 1.042 | 1.061 |
| TPS (calculated) | 0.977 | 0.990 | 1.000 | 1.013 | 1.024 | 1.034 |
| % Difference | 0.41% | 0.00% | 0.00% | 0.98% | 1.73% | 2.54% |
| | Field size ($cm^2$) | | | | | |
| 10 MV output factors | 6 × 6 | 8 × 8 | 10 × 10 | 15 × 15 | 20 × 20 | 25 × 25 |
| PTW microdiamond (measured) | 0.975 | 0.986 | 1.000 | 1.027 | 1.049 | 1.069 |
| TPS (calculated) | 0.970 | 0.987 | 1.000 | 1.017 | 1.028 | 1.040 |
| % Difference | 0.51% | −0.10% | 0.00% | 0.97% | 2.00% | 2.71% |

measurements and the TPS is within 3% for all output factors; the greatest discrepancies are seen at the largest field sizes.

The measured OF data can be used to formulate a simple secondary MU calculation that can be used to check subsequent TPS calculations for patient treatment plans. This requires the additional step of getting a 'normalization factor' (NF); the NF is defined as the ratio of the detector signal for a 10×10 $cm^2$ field with the GRID block in place to the detector signal for a 10×10 $cm^2$ open field (without the GRID block in place):

$$\text{NF} = \frac{\text{Output with GRID block in place for } 10 \times 10\ \text{cm}^2 \text{ field}}{\text{Output for open } 10 \times 10\ \text{cm}^2 \text{ field}}$$

The measured OFs can be plotted as a function of field size and fitted with a polynomial to provide a function with which the corresponding OFs for intermediate field sizes can be estimated. The secondary MU check can then be calculated as

$$\text{MU} = \frac{\text{Prescription Dose [cGy]}}{\text{NF} \times OF(\text{Field Size}) \times D_o \left[\frac{\text{cGy}}{\text{MU}}\right]}.$$

In the expression above, OF (Field Size) indicates that the appropriate OF should be obtained based on the field size used for treatment and can be determined through a polynomial fit of the measured OF data. $D_o$ is the dose per MU of the user's beam under normalization conditions. For example, for a linac which is calibrated to deliver 1 cGy/MU at 100 SSD using a 10×10 $cm^2$ field size, $D_o$ = 1 cGy/MU. For actual patient treatments, the field size may not be square, so an equivalent field size should be calculated using, for example, the common $4A/P$ formalism [5], where $A$ is the area of the treatment field and $P$ its perimeter. Additionally, part of the field is

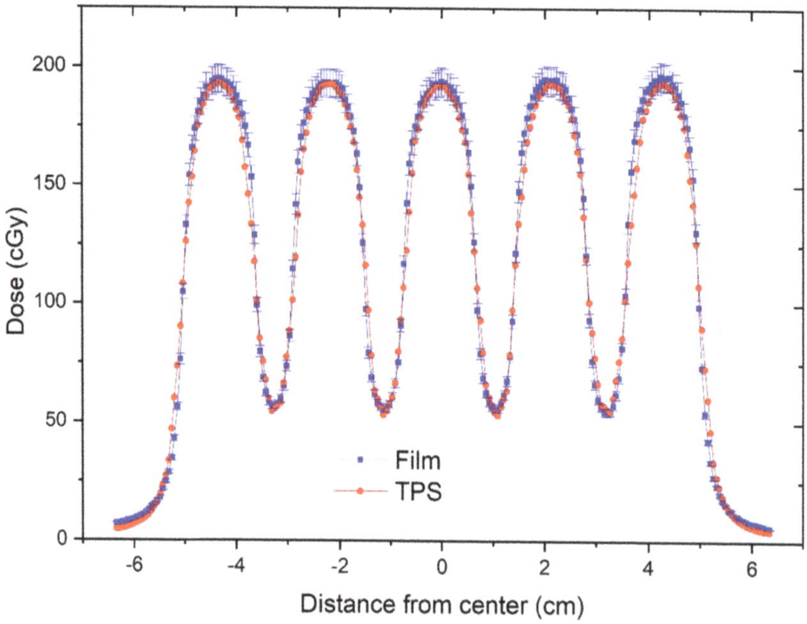


**Figure 15.6.** Dose profile comparison between TPS (red line) and radiochromic film measurement (black line) for a 10 × 10 $cm^2$ field made at a depth of 5 cm in solid water for a 10 MV beam. Radiochromic film measurements can be made for additional checks of TPS calculations and MU verification. The 3% error bars were added into the film measurement.

likely to be blocked with multileaf collimators (MLCs) for treatment in order to conform the field to the target. The percentage area of the field which is blocked can be estimated and used to reduce the overall treatment field size, from which an OF is further refined and used for MU calculations. An acceptable agreement between the simple MU calculation and the TPS should be determined by the user and should be verified by experimental measurement, particularly when the field shape is irregular. In general, the agreement can be expected to be within 5%.

MUs can be verified prior to treatment by measurement using an appropriately sized detector, such as a small ion chamber, a diode, or a diamond detector. Alternatively, radiochromic film or another high-resolution planar detector can be used to verify the overall two-dimensional dose distribution compared to the TPS. Figure 15.6 shows an inline dose profile comparison from a radiochromic (EBT3, Ashland, Bridgewater, NJ, USA) film measurement for a 10×10 $cm^2$ field size made at a depth of 5 cm in solid water with a 10 MV beam.

## 15.3 Commissioning and quality assurance for lattice SFRT

While GRID treatments using physical blocks and a single static field are inherently simple to plan and deliver, more advanced SFRT techniques using intensity-modulated radiation therapy (IMRT) or VMAT are also commonly used. These approaches focus the high-dose regions into vertices or spherical 'lattice' points within the tumor while simultaneously reducing the dose given to the regions around these points to create the heterogeneous dose distributions characteristic of GRID therapy. Several different lattice SFRT planning methods have been published and used clinically [6–9].

As with any treatment planning approach, it is important to ensure the TPS is capable of providing accurate dose calculations. As the lattice points are generally on the order of 1–2 cm in diameter, a TPS which has been adequately commissioned for IMRT or VMAT SBRT treatments should be suitable for lattice SFRT treatments. When commissioning a lattice SFRT program, the user should follow published guidelines for both delivery and treatment planning as they relate to SBRT/stereotactic radiosurgery (SRS) treatments [10, 11] due to the high doses and steep dose gradients delivered.

Because lattice SFRT plans can be quite complex, a verification that the planned dose is safely delivered to the patient is extremely important. Patient-specific QA should be performed prior to each patient's treatment using a method with adequate spatial resolution to resolve the high dose gradients [12, 13]. A variety of suitable detectors are available, such as high-resolution diode arrays, electronic portal imaging devices (EPIDs), and radiochromic film. The chosen method is arbitrary and is likely to be a matter of personal choice as long the technique has sufficient spatial resolution. The following sections discuss general considerations for the QA methods of SFRT treatment plans. As it can be an excellent dosimeter for SFRT QA but has a number of details to consider for successful measurements, the use of radiochromic film (RCF) is discussed in detail.

### 15.3.1 General considerations for patient-specific SFRT QA

At least eight commercial vendors currently offer IMRT QA devices: 3DVH and SNC Patient for MapCHECK and ArcCHECK (Sun Nuclear Corporation, Melbourne, FL, USA), Portal Dosimetry with EPID (Varian Medical Systems, Palo Alto, CA, USA), RIT 113 (Radiological Imaging Technology, Inc., Colorado Springs, CO, USA), IMSure (Standard Imaging Inc., Middleton, WI, USA), Delta4 (ScandiDos, Uppsala, Sweden), VeriSoft with Seven29 2D array (PTW, Freiburg, Germany), COMPASS and OmniPro-IMRT with MatriXX (IBA dosimetry, Schwarzenbruck, Germany). In principle, any of these IMRT QA devices can be used for patient-specific SFRT QA as long as the limitations of each system are understood and appropriately addressed. Examples of limitations include, but are not limited to, the influence of the treatment couch on measurements [14], the angular response variations of array detectors [15], and the dose per pulse and field size correction factors for diodes [16]. As for TPS commissioning, a patient-specific QA process which has been found to be suitable for SBRT treatments should be sufficient for SFRT treatments.

### 15.3.2 Radiochromic film dosimetry for lattice SFRT QA

RCF is an excellent dosimeter for lattice SFRT verification as it has extremely high spatial resolution, is nearly energy independent throughout the range of clinically relevant MV photon beams, and has negligible angular or dose-rate dependence [17]. However, a consistent and accurate RCF dosimetry protocol must be established and adhered to. A useful resource outlining fundamental concepts needed for accurate film dosimetry is given in the references [18].

While RCF can be an excellent choice for patient-specific lattice SFRT QA, there are several associated challenges to be aware of. First, lattice SFRT generally involves the delivery of peak doses of 15–20 Gy or more, so a film capable of accuracy at such high doses is required. Second, tumors treated with lattice SFRT can be quite large, making film dosimetry challenging due to the limited size of the film as well its interaction with the scanner system used for analysis. Finally, lattice SFRT plans may comprise many lattice points that require multiple measurements to sample all lattice points, which can be a time-consuming process. Each of these challenges is discussed and addressed below.

#### *15.3.2.1 High-dose RCF dosimetry*

The slope of the dose–response curve for RCFs generally decreases as the dose increases and can saturate at high values. Therefore, for high-dose applications such as lattice SFRT, a film with appropriate sensitivity should be used [17]. A commercially available solution for high-dose RCF dosimetry is EBT-XD film (Ashland, Bridgewater, NJ, USA) which has been validated in the literature and is recommended for dose measurements above 10 Gy [19–21]. This film is therefore recommended for lattice SFRT QA measurements as well.

#### *15.3.2.2 Large field RCF dosimetry and scanner limitations*

Flatbed document scanners are commonly used for RCF dosimetry and present one of the largest potential sources of error in the so-called lateral response artifact (LRA) [22, 23]. When flatbed scanners are used to analyze RCF, the measured response of the scanner for a uniformly irradiated film will vary with distance from the center of the scanner bed along an axis parallel to the light source. For low doses on the order of 1–2 Gy, the error is quite small (~1%) when RCFs are placed within 5–7 cm of the center of the scanner bed. However, the magnitude of this error can increase substantially with dose and distance from the center of the scanner bed and can be as large as 10%–30% for some RCF types [24]. If an RCF measurement of a lattice SFRT plan involves sampling lattice points across a wide lateral distance, the high-dose regions measured by the film are likely to be affected by the LRA. Fortunately, there are multiple options to mitigate or eliminate dosimetric errors due to the LRA. First, the use of an appropriate high-dose film, such as EBT-XD, substantially reduces the LRA compared to those of other RCF film types [19, 25]. Secondly, a lateral correction can be implemented for the scanner, which eliminates the LRA entirely [24]. The easiest solution, however, is to use EBT-XD film and simply scan the highest-dose regions of the film so that they are within 5–7 cm of the center of the scanner bed. For large field size measurements which are done on a full sheet of film, this requires multiple scans, each one placing a different region of interest near the center of the scanner bed. While somewhat inefficient, simply keeping the exposed portions of the film near the center of the scanner can mitigate the LRA and reduce dosimetric errors to acceptable levels. The user should determine the extent of the LRA for their particular application and scanner as a function of dose and lateral scan position. This can be done by exposing films to different dose levels and scanning them at different lateral positions on the scanner. From these measurements, useful information about the magnitude of the LRA can be determined and the user can then determine appropriate steps for correction.

*15.3.2.3 Measurements of multiple lattice points*

The large tumors typically treated with lattice SFRT may contain many individual high-dose regions. As with any two-dimensional dosimeter, a single RCF measurement may not sample all lattice points. However, with additional methods of QA such as secondary dose calculations and log file analysis, measurements through every lattice point may not be considered necessary once the TPS and delivery systems have been properly commissioned [26]. In this scenario, a subset of lattice points could be sampled with one to three RCF measurements. With appropriate equipment such as a cylindrical film phantom which can rotate, a single measurement can sample multiple lattice points and thus increase the efficiency of the process [27]. An example is illustrated in figure 15.7. Figure 15.7(A) shows a 3D rendering of a patient with a left-sided breast tumor (shown in light green) in which six lattice points (shown in red) have been placed for a lattice SFRT treatment. Figure 15.7(B) is an axial view of a cylindrical film phantom which indicates that the six lattice points can be sampled by rotating the plane of measurement by 36° from the horizontal. Figure 15.7(C) shows the resulting dose plane to be exported from the TPS for comparison to the film measurement. The full details of this process were described in detail by a recent study [27]. Alternatively, multiple measurements made in the coronal or sagittal planes could sample the lattice points if a phantom with rotational symmetry were not available. Figure 15.8 shows a dose profile comparison through three lattice points for the clinical patient plan shown in figure 15.7.

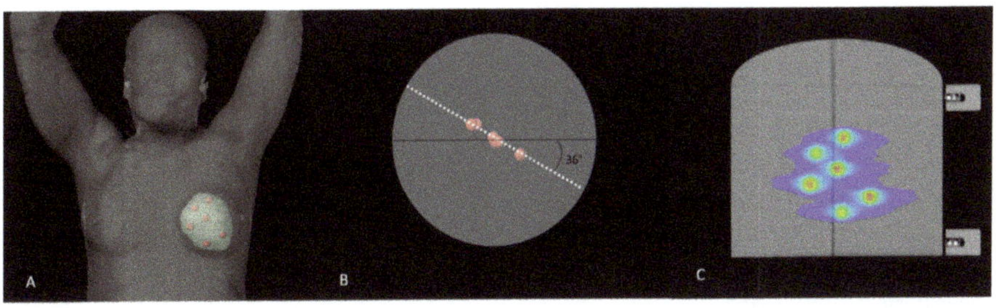


**Figure 15.7.** (A) 3D rendering of a patient with a left-sided breast tumor (light green) in which six lattice points (red) have been placed for a lattice SFRT treatment. (B) Axial representation of a cylindrical phantom showing that the six lattice points can be sampled with a single film measurement if the plane of measurement is rotated 36° from the horizontal. (C) The resulting dose distribution shown in colorwash, which can be exported and compared to the film measurement.

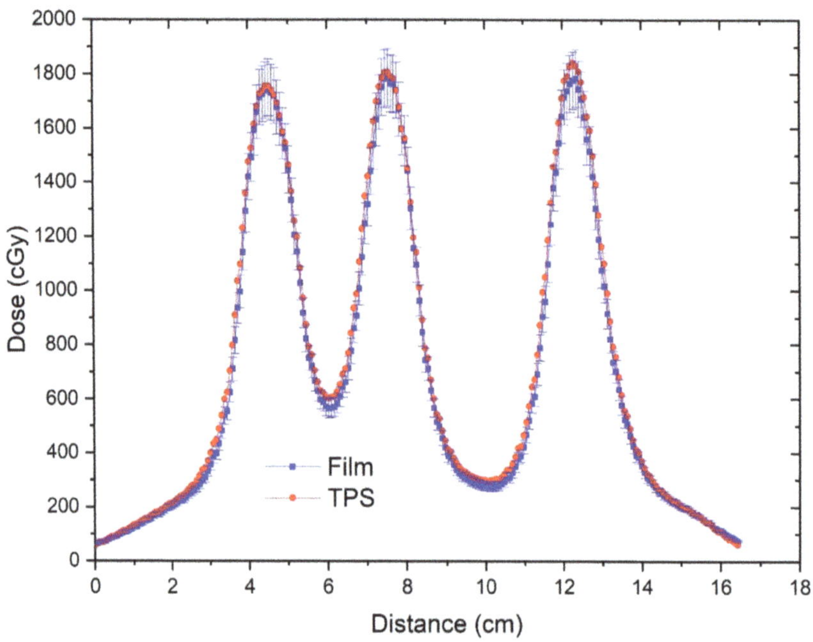


**Figure 15.8.** Dose profile comparison between a film measurement (blue line) and TPS calculation (red line) for the clinical case shown in figure 15.7. The 3% error bars were added into the film measurement.

## 15.4 Suggested treatment workflows and safety checks

Once the appropriate calibration, commissioning, and patient-specific QA procedures for SFRT treatments have been completed, the clinical team should establish standard treatment workflows and safety checks.

### 15.4.1 Suggested treatment workflow and safety checks for GRID treatments using blocks

For a treatment using a physical GRID block, the main considerations are safely mounting the block, ensuring the patient and target are localized correctly (e.g. the patient surface is at the appropriate SSD) and that the radiation field is appropriate for the target size. The following steps may form the basis of a potential workflow and safety checks for treatment.

1. Prior to treatment, inspect the integrity of the GRID block and tray assembly. Make sure there are no cracks or other signs of wear and that all bolts are tight.
2. The patient ID is verified with a standard time-out process.
3. The patient should be set up and immobilized per standard protocols for treating specific tumor sites.
4. Perform image guidance and apply shifts.

   a. With the gantry at the treatment angle and without the block in place, the physicist, therapist, and physician should verify the appropriate SSD and patient positioning.
   b. Without the block in place, the physicist, therapist, and physician should verify the treatment field is appropriate for the target using the light field.
5. Insert the physical block into the head of the linear accelerator.
   a. Prior to insertion, rotate the gantry as needed so that the block is not lifted over the patient.
   b. Make sure the GRID block is securely mounted and will not move when the gantry is rotated to its treatment angle.
6. With the block in place and the gantry at the treatment angle, the physicist, therapist, and physician verify that the light field is appropriate for the target.
   a. Make sure the jaws do not extend beyond the physical block and are appropriate for the field size defined by the target volume.
   b. Make sure the MLCs conform to the target.
7. Exit the treatment room; the physicist, therapist, and physician verify the treatment parameters:
   a. Prescription dose
   b. Beam energy
   c. Gantry angle and field size
   d. Monitor units
8. Treat.

### 15.4.2 Suggested treatment workflow and safety checks for lattice SFRT treatments

Lattice SFRT treatments may use the same procedures as standard SBRT treatments [28]. This involves appropriate immobilization and image-guidance procedures to ensure the high-dose treatment is accurately delivered. An important consideration which may however differ from standard SBRT treatments is to ensure that the various separate high-dose regions are delivered within the tumor and away from OARs. Three-dimensional cone beam computed tomography (CBCT) imaging is required to ensure that no changes in internal anatomy have occurred which would place an OAR near or within a high-dose region defined by the lattice points. A structure which contains all the lattice points should be available for review and overlaid on the CBCT. The physician, therapist, and physicist should confirm all lattice points are safely within the tumor and away from OARs prior to treatment through a comprehensive review of the CBCT image.

The following steps may form the basis of a potential workflow and safety checks for treatment.

1. The patient should be set up and immobilized per standard protocols for treating specific tumor sites.
2. Perform image guidance and apply shifts.
   a. A CBCT is required as part of the image-guidance procedure in order to evaluate potential changes in internal anatomy.

b. The physician, therapist, and physicist should evaluate the CBCT and a structure containing all lattice points to make sure that all high-dose regions are safely within the tumor and away from OARs.

3. Perform the standard final pause procedure and safety checks prior to treatment.
4. Treat.

## 15.5 Knowledge gaps and future perspectives

This chapter has focused on SFRT calibration and commissioning procedures for treatments using a physical block as well as lattice methods. While these are two commonly used treatment methods, other SFRT modalities exist, such as proton GRID [29, 30] and other MLC-based photon methods [31–33]. However, no clinical evidence exists that suggests one SFRT therapy technique is superior to another; in addition, the biologic mechanisms responsible for the effectiveness of SFRT are still not understood. A common theme of all SFRT approaches is the characteristically heterogenous dose distribution. This dose heterogeneity may play a role in inducing the selective killing of cancer cells [34], bystander effects [35], and changes in tumor vasculature [36] and immune-mediate responses [37]. However, dose heterogeneity is likely to change with different planning approaches and plan characteristics such as the size and spacing of high-dose regions. Furthermore, there is also evidence suggesting the importance of the low-dose regions of SFRT plans in terms of biologic effectiveness [38]. The impact of variable SFRT planning parameters such as the size and spacing of both high- and low-dose regions and the resulting dose heterogeneity represents a significant knowledge gap and its investigation is an opportunity for future research.

## 15.6 Conclusions

Accurate calibration and thorough commissioning procedures are essential for the safe and effective delivery of SFRT treatments. Treatments involving a GRID block have special considerations for both commissioning and calibration due to the unique features of the collimating block. Advanced SFRT techniques such as VMAT lattice treatments need similar attention to that given to high-dose SBRT treatments with specialized planning methods. All SFRT treatments require quality assurance procedures, which may include secondary MU checks as well as patient-specific QA measurements. Careful and methodical treatment workflows and safety checks are needed for accurate localization and the safe delivery of SFRT treatments.

## References

[1] Mohiuddin M, Park H, Hallmeyer S and Richards J 2015 High-dose radiation as a dramatic, immunological primer in locally advanced melanoma *Cureus* **7** e417

[2] Kaiser A, Mohiuddin M M and Jackson G L 2012 Dramatic response from neoadjuvant, spatially fractionated GRID radiotherapy (SFGRT) for large, high-grade extremity sarcoma *J. Radiat. Oncol.* **2** 103–6

[3] Buckey C, Stathakis S, Cashon K, Gutierrez A, Esquivel C and Shi C *et al* 2010 Evaluation of a commercially-available block for spatially fractionated radiation therapy *J. Appl. Clin. Med. Phys.* **11** 2–11
[4] Nobah A, Mohiuddin M, Devic S and Moftah B 2015 Effective spatially fractionated GRID radiation treatment planning for a passive grid block *Br. J. Radiol.* **88** 20140363
[5] Khan F M 2003 *The Physics of Radiation Therapy* 3rd edn (Philadelphia, PA: Lippincott Williams & Wilkins)
[6] Duriseti S, Kavanaugh J, Goddu S, Price A, Knutson N and Reynoso F *et al* 2021 Spatially fractionated stereotactic body radiation therapy (Lattice) for large tumors *Adv. Radiat. Oncol.* **6** 100639
[7] Grams M P, Owen D, Park S S, Petersen I A, Haddock M G and Jeans E B *et al* 2021 VMAT grid therapy: a widely applicable planning approach *Pract. Radiat. Oncol.* **11** E339–47
[8] Jin J Y, Zhao B, Kaminski J M, Wen N, Huang Y and Vender J *et al* 2015 A MLC-based inversely optimized 3D spatially fractionated grid radiotherapy technique *Radiother. Oncol.* **117** 483–6
[9] Wu X, Perez N C, Zheng Y, Li X, Jiang L and Amendola B E *et al* 2020 The technical and clinical implementation of LATTICE radiation therapy (LRT) *Radiat. Res.* **194** 737–46
[10] Halvorsen P H, Cirino E, Das I J, Garrett J A, Yang J and Yin F F *et al* 2017 AAPM-RSS medical physics practice guideline 9.a. for SRS-SBRT *J. Appl. Clin. Med. Phys.* **18** 10–21
[11] Smilowitz J B, Das I J, Feygelman V, Fraass B A, Kry S F and Marshall I R *et al* 2015 AAPM medical physics practice guideline 5.a.: commissioning and QA of treatment planning dose calculations—megavoltage photon and electron beams *J. Appl. Clin. Med. Phys.* **16** 14–34
[12] Miften M, Olch A, Mihailidis D, Moran J, Pawlicki T and Molineu A *et al* 2018 Tolerance limits and methodologies for IMRT measurement-based verification QA: recommendations of AAPM Task Group No. 218 *Med. Phys.* **45** e53–83
[13] Ezzell G A, Burmeister J W, Dogan N, LoSasso T J, Mechalakos J G and Mihailidis D *et al* 2009 IMRT commissioning: multiple institution planning and dosimetry comparisons, a report from AAPM Task Group 119 *Med. Phys.* **36** 5359–73
[14] Masi L, Casamassima F, Doro R and Francescon P 2011 Quality assurance of volumetric modulated arc therapy: evaluation and comparison of different dosimetric systems *Med. Phys.* **38** 612–21
[15] Mayo C, Fong de los Santos L, Kruse J, Blackwell C R, McLemore L B and Pafundi D *et al* 2013 Report on use of a methodology for commissioning and quality assurance of a VMAT system *PLoS One* **8** e58877
[16] Banos-Capilla M C, Lago-Martin J D, Gil P and Larrea L M 2021 Sensitivity and specificity analysis of 2D small field measurement array: patient-specific quality assurance of small target treatments and spatially fractionated radiotherapy *J. Appl. Clin. Med. Phys.* **22** 104–19
[17] Niroomand-Rad A, Chiu-Tsao S T, Grams M P, Lewis D F, Soares C G and Van Battum L J *et al* 2020 Full report of AAPM Task Group 235 radiochromic film dosimetry: an update to TG-55 *Med. Phys.* **47** 5986–6025
[18] Howard M E, Herman M G and Grams M P 2020 Methodology for radiochromic film analysis using FilmQA pro and ImageJ *PLoS One* **15** e0233562

[19] Grams M P, Gustafson J M, Long K M and de los Santos L E F 2015 Technical note: initial characterization of the new EBT-XD gafchromic film *Med. Phys.* **42** 5782–6

[20] Miura H, Ozawa S, Hosono F, Sumida N, Okazue T and Yamada K *et al* 2016 Gafchromic EBT-XD film: dosimetry characterization in high-dose, volumetric-modulated arc therapy *J. Appl. Clin. Med. Phys.* **17** 312–22

[21] Palmer A L, Dimitriadis A, Nisbet A and Clark C H 2015 Evaluation of gafchromic EBT-XD film, with comparison to EBT3 film, and application in high dose radiotherapy verification *Phys. Med. Biol.* **60** 8741–52

[22] Schoenfeld A A, Wieker S, Harder D and Poppe B 2016 The origin of the flatbed scanner artifacts in radiochromic film dosimetry-key experiments and theoretical descriptions *Phys. Med. Biol.* **61** 7704–24

[23] van Battum L J, Huizenga H, Verdaasdonk R M and Heukelom S 2016 How flatbed scanners upset accurate film dosimetry *Phys. Med. Biol.* **61** 625–49

[24] Lewis D and Chan M F 2015 Correcting lateral response artifacts from flatbed scanners for radiochromic film dosimetry *Med. Phys.* **42** 416–29

[25] Lewis D F and Chan M F 2016 Technical Note: On GAFChromic EBT-XD film and the lateral response artifact *Med. Phys.* **43** 643–9

[26] Basavatia A K, Fiedler D A, Ritter J, Brodin P, Goddard L C and Jeong K *et al* 2021 Comprehensive patient-specific intensity-modulated radiation therapy quality assurance comparing Mobius3D/FX to conventional methods of evaluation *Cureus* **13** e14910

[27] Grams M P and de Los Santos L E F 2018 Design and clinical use of a rotational phantom for dosimetric verification of IMRT/VMAT treatments *Phys. Med* **50** 59–65

[28] Benedict S H, Yenice K M, Followill D, Galvin J M, Hinson W and Kavanagh B *et al* 2010 Stereotactic body radiation therapy: the report of AAPM Task Group 101 *Med. Phys.* **37** 4078–101

[29] Gao M, Mohiuddin M M, Hartsell W F and Pankuch M 2018 Spatially fractionated (GRID) radiation therapy using proton pencil beam scanning (PBS): feasibility study and clinical implementation *Med. Phys.* **45** 1645–53

[30] Mohiuddin M, Lynch C, Gao M and Hartsell W 2020 Early clinical results of proton spatially fractionated GRID radiation therapy (SFGRT) *Br. J. Radiol.* **93** 20190572

[31] Costlow H N, Zhang H and Das I J 2014 A treatment planning approach to spatially fractionated megavoltage grid therapy for bulky lung cancer *Med. Dosim.* **39** 218–26

[32] Ha J K, Zhang G, Naqvi S A, Regine W F and Yu C X 2006 Feasibility of delivering grid therapy using a multileaf collimator *Med. Phys.* **33** 76–82

[33] Zhang X, Penagaricano J, Yan Y, Sharma S, Griffin R J and Hardee M *et al* 2016 Application of spatially fractionated radiation (GRID) to helical tomotherapy using a novel TOMOGRID template *Technol. Cancer Res. Treat.* **15** 91–100

[34] Zhang H, Zhong H, Barth R F, Cao M and Das I J 2014 Impact of dose size in single fraction spatially fractionated (grid) radiotherapy for melanoma *Med. Phys.* **41** 021727

[35] Asur R, Butterworth K T, Penagaricano J A, Prise K M and Griffin R J 2015 High dose bystander effects in spatially fractionated radiation therapy *Cancer Lett.* **356** 52–7

[36] Sathishkumar S, Boyanovsky B, Karakashian A A, Rozenova K, Giltiay N V and Kudrimoti M *et al* 2005 Elevated sphingomyelinase activity and ceramide concentration in serum of patients undergoing high dose spatially fractionated radiation treatment: implications for endothelial apoptosis *Cancer Biol. Ther.* **4** 979–86

[37] Johnsrud A J, Jenkins S V, Jamshidi-Parsian A, Quick C M, Galhardo E P and Dings R P M *et al* 2020 Evidence for early stage anti-tumor immunity elicited by spatially fractionated radiotherapy-immunotherapy combinations *Radiat. Res.* **194** 688–97
[38] Rivera J N, Kierski T M, Kasoji S K, Abrantes A S, Dayton P A and Chang S X 2020 Conventional dose rate spatially-fractionated radiation therapy (SFRT) treatment response and its association with dosimetric parameters-a preclinical study in a Fischer 344 rat model *PLoS One* **15** e0229053

**IOP** Publishing

Spatially Fractionated, Microbeam and FLASH Radiation Therapy
A physics and multi-disciplinary approach
**Hualin Zhang and Nina A Mayr**

# Chapter 16

# SFRT dose prescription

**Nina A Mayr, Beatriz E Amendola, James S Welsh, Hualin Zhang, Naipy C Perez, Xiaodong Wu and Simon S Lo**

While spatially fractionated radiation therapy (SFRT) is increasingly practiced using various techniques and platforms, the dose prescription in SFRT is a profound departure from the current concepts of conventional dosing strategies in radiation therapy.

The complex dose parameters of SFRT are being defined, and recommendations —extrapolated from early clinical results and preclinical observations—continue to evolve as dose reporting recommendations are being formulated. An important aspect of the evolving field of SFRT is the need to establish close linkage between the parameters of the physically heterogeneous dose and the treatment outcome through rigorous study of experimental *in vivo* models and the accumulation of clinical results. Therefore, the prescription parameters of the heterogeneous dose must be clearly defined, consistently employed throughout clinical trial study populations, and consistently reported in order to achieve meaningful treatment outcome correlations.

This chapter reviews the current status and recommendations for dose prescription strategies from the clinical perspective and their application in terms of physical principles. The chapter provides a practical guide to reporting guidelines for SFRT dose prescription with respect to the target and critical normal tissues.

## 16.1 Introduction

The dose prescription used in SFRT represents a profound departure from the concepts of conventional dosing strategies in radiation therapy. In conventional radiation therapy, the highest possible volume of the target is covered with a dose as uniform as possible across the target at the highest achievable dose required for the specific tumor. In contrast, SFRT applies intentionally *non*-uniform, heterogeneous dose patterns to the target [1–6]. These contain both peak doses, delivered in the ablative dose range of stereotactic radiosurgery (SRS) or stereotactic body radiation

doi:10.1088/978-0-7503-4046-5ch16

therapy (SBRT) in one or very few fractions, and low-dose 'valleys' that alternate with the 'peaks' within the target [4]. The profound tumoricidal effects observed in SFRT are thought to be related to this highly inhomogeneous dose pattern [4, 7, 8], as further described in chapters 2 and 3.

These heterogeneous dose patterns of SFRT are unfamiliar to practitioners and require dosing and prescription parameters beyond current concepts that are not captured by conventional common dose–volume histogram (DVH)-derived dose metrics. Additional heterogeneity dose metrics have to be determined and compared with the biological effects for ultimate translation into clinically actionable prescription regimens. Some of these parameters have been defined and are represented in the published literature. Many others have been proposed and recommended or are in development; their clinical significance is under investigation, or is yet be investigated.

While some of this information is available, based on published studies, much of the correlation of the dose metrics with outcome is yet to be interrogated and defined.

Meanwhile, in this fast-progressing field, clinicians practicing SFRT have to closely follow the evolving progress and must adapt their treatment planning strategies to these transforming dose metrics. Investigators designing clinical trials must be cognizant of the changing and continuously evolving SFRT dose prescription paradigms. The designs of clinical trials and clinical therapy regimens still rely on and take into account dose prescription strategies that have demonstrated clinical effects, leveraging extrapolation from both tumor control and toxicity data to design advanced SFRT dose schedules.

## 16.2 SFRT, brachytherapy, and ablative stereotactic radiotherapy/ radiosurgery

SFRT dosing has many properties in common with both SRS/SFRT and brachytherapy. While these commonalities are only partial, both the brachytherapy-like and SRS/SBRT-like properties of SFRT may be related to its high clinical responses. Brachytherapy and SRS/SBRT can provide important insights into dose prescription principles of SFRT.

### 16.2.1 Brachytherapy

The heterogeneous dose distributions of SFRT most closely resemble those of brachytherapy, particularly high-dose-rate interstitial brachytherapy. As in SFRT, interstitial brachytherapy exhibits a highly heterogeneous dose pattern characterized by alternating high-dose (surrounding the interstitial needles/seeds) and low-dose regions in a fairly regular pattern. The dose of the high-dose regions can exceed that of the interspersed low-dose regions by as much as four- to fivefold. From a clinical point of view, brachytherapy exhibits similarly high response rates, and it has been speculated that the heterogeneous dose pattern of interstitial brachytherapy might contribute to its high local tumor control.

However, in contrast to SFRT, which is *purposefully* prescribed at the peak dose, interstitial brachytherapy prescribes the dose *not* at the dose peaks but at the encompassing peripheral, much lower isodose line, aiming for a prescription dose that is deemed tolerable to normal tissues. Dose heterogeneity within the target has been accepted as an unavoidable property of brachytherapy.

### 16.2.2 SRS and SBRT

The magnitude of the SFRT prescription dose is overall similar to the ablative high-fraction dose range employed in SRS and some SBRT regimens. The 15–20 Gy fraction sizes commonly employed in SFRT [1–4, 9–16] are akin to ablative SRS single fractions. The less common multifraction SFRT [5] has similarities to oligo-fraction SBRT. High-fraction ablative SBRT dose regimens are well known to produce higher response rates than the doses given in conventionally fractionated (1.8–2 Gy) radiation therapy [17, 18]. In contrast to SFRT, but akin to brachytherapy, in SRS/SBRT planning, the dose is prescribed at a lower isodose line encompassing the target. While large expected hotspots and potentially peripheral cold spots (for organ-at-risk (OAR) sparing) are considered acceptable and potentially desirable in SRS/SBRT [19], dose heterogeneity from alternating high-dose and low-dose regions is *not* intentionally designed in SRS/SBRT. In SRS/SBRT, the dose is prescribed at the target periphery ideally encompassing the target, whereas, in contrast, SFRT is prescribed with intent heterogeneously at the dose peaks, while leaving a large proportion of the target in the low-dose domain.

## 16.3 The principles of SFRT dosing

The SFRT dose has been initially prescribed as a *peak dose*, defined at the prescription depth within the tumor at the field center. With the initial GRID collimator technologies, the dose heterogeneity pattern was largely standardized through the fixed configuration of the GRID collimators (as further described in chapter 9). While a seemingly ‘simple’ parameter, the GRID dose, defined as the peak dose, has become a robust dose metric that is solidly linked to the dose–response relationship and tumor control in clinical correlation studies. [2, 3].

As the field of SFRT has advanced to 3D conformal and intensity-modulated radiation therapy (IMRT) techniques, more complex *volumetric dose prescription* approaches have evolved [4–6, 10, 11, 15] while building on the early foundational 2D GRID experience [1–3]. The D10/D90 ratio, defined as the ratio of the doses that cover 90% and 10% of the target volume, has been favored as a more field-size- and depth-independent measure of dose heterogeneity in GRID therapy compared to the peak dose and valley–peak dose ratio (VPDR) [20, 21]. In Lattice radiotherapy (LRT), the dose covering 95% of the volume of the high-dose spheres (vertices) has been proposed as a prescription parameter [22]. SFRT heterogeneity parameters used for planning and dose reporting are discussed in more detail in section 4.1, table 16.1 and chapters 9 and 10.

The fixed geometry of the GRID collimators resulted in consistency of the dose heterogeneity across studies and patient cohorts. Despite the limitations of non-volumetric dose prescription and the initially shallow prescription depth (e.g. $D_{max}$ or a depth of 3 cm), often delivered with a single field, high clinical response rates

**Table 16.1.** Recommended dosimetric parameters.

| Dosimetric Parameters—GRID | Dosimetric Parameters—LRT |
|---|---|
| **Prescription dose:** | |
| Prescription dose ($D_p$, in Gy): Peak dose of the central GRID hole at the prescription depth(1) | Prescription dose ($D_p$, in Gy) (covering 95% of the volume of the vertices): covering 1%–10% of the gross tumor volume (GTV) |
| **Heterogeneity (DVH-derived) parameters:** | |
| Peak dose(2): D10 | Peak dose(2): $D_{max}$ (maximum vertex dose) |
| Valley dose(3): D90 | Valley dose(3): $D_{mean}$ (95–100), defined as the mean dose of the 5% of the lattice volume ($V_L$) that receives the lowest range of doses. |
| VPDR: D90/D10(4) | VPDR(5): $D_{mean}$ (95–100)/$D_p$ |
| D90, D50, D20, D10, D5 (percentage doses covering 90%, 50%, 20%, 10%, and 5% of the GTV) | D90, D50, D20, D10, D5 (percentage doses covering 90%, 50%, 20%, 10%, and 5% of the GTV) |
| V100, V90, V50 (percentage of volumes covered by 100%, 90% and 50% of the prescription dose) | |
| Mean dose given to target ($D_{mean}$) | Mean dose given to target ($D_{mean}$) |
| — | GTV peripheral dose(6) |
| **Geometric parameters:** | |
| Peak width (defined at 50% of the max peak dose) | Vertex diameter (d), including mean and range |
| Peak-to-peak distance | Center-to-center vertex separation (D) |
| — | Total number of vertices |
| **Modeling:** | |
| EUD(7): $EUD = D_{ref} \times \frac{\ln\left\{\frac{\sum_{i=1}^{N} \Delta V_i \times \rho_i \times (SF_2)^{\frac{D_i}{D_{ref}}}}{\sum_{i=1}^{N} \Delta V_i \times \rho_i}\right\}}{\ln(SF_2)}$ | EUD(7): $\mathrm{EUD}_a = \left[\sum_i (v_i D_i{}^a)\right]^{1/a}$ |

Note: Selected common dosimetric parameters are presented based on recent white papers [21, 22], and these continue to evolve. The parameters are different between GRID and LRT, as shown by the differences in their planning processes; the harmonization of GRID and LRT parameters is ongoing and part of the SFRT standardization efforts. The parameters are still variably used, particularly in LRT. A discussion of the full set of planning parameters is beyond the scope of this chapter. The reader is referred to chapters 9 and 10.

(1) In selected cases, the prescription dose may be defined at a depth of $D_{max}$ (as per early GRID practice).

(2) Differences currently exist between the interpretations of peak dose used by GRID and LRT SFRT.

(3) While the optimal valley dose is not sufficiently defined at this time, a dose of no more than 5–6 Gy has been favored as the valley dose limit.

(4) Originally defined as VPDR, i.e. the ratio of the valley dose to the peak dose at the prescription depth. More recently, D90/D10 has been suggested as the definition of SFRT heterogeneity patterns due to its better robustness in terms of depth and field size [20, 21].

(5) In LRT, the VPDR is determined from the *vertex* volume ($V_L$), not the entire GTV, as described in more detail in chapter 10.

(6) The GTV peripheral dose (used to reduce the normal tissue dose) is a characteristic of LRT planning and prescription. The peripheral GTV volume is distinct from the lattice volume ($V_L$), which encompasses all vertices and intervening structures (chapter 10).

[7] The $\alpha/\beta$ ratios for the EUD computations must be consistent with the specific tissue (tumor, specific normal tissues). If the normal tissue type and cancer cell radiosensitivities are unknown, normal tissue $\alpha/\beta$=3.3, cancer cell $\alpha/\beta$ = 10 Gy. For radiosensitive cells, SF (2 Gy)=0.3, for radioresistant cells, SF (2 Gy)=0.7. Response modeling is further discussed in chapter 14.
*Abbreviations:* D10 = the percentage dose covering 10% of the target volume. D90 = the percentage dose covering 90% of the target volume. V100, V90, V50 = the percentages of the volume covered by 100%, 90%, and 50%, respectively, of the prescription dose.
Terms in equations: For GRID therapy, $D_{\text{ref}}$ is a reference dose of 2 Gy. $SF_2$ is a reference survival fraction of the specific clonogen when treated with $D_{\text{ref}}$. $D_i$ is the local dose, $\Delta V_i$ is the local volume, and $\rho_i$ is the local clonogen density [21].
For LRT, $v_i$ is the fraction of the $i$th subvolume receiving the dose $D_i$, and $a$ is a scaling factor that is unique to the tissue's characteristics and radiation sensitivity [22].

with low toxicity have consistently been observed in palliatively treated patients [2–4]. These early outcome studies, in which the GRID prescription doses ranged from 10 to 20 Gy in a single fraction, laid the foundation for an important clinical SFRT dose–response relationship [2, 3], as described in more detail in chapter 5. In the early landmark study by Mohiuddin *et al*, a peak dose of >15 Gy was significantly more effective in generating symptomatic tumor response than lower doses (100% versus 79%) [3]. The outcomes and dose–response relationship of this early GRID experience were independently reproduced in a second cohort (symptomatic tumor response 94% vs 62%) [2]. Overall, the observed tumor response, tumor control, and toxicity results have been corroborated across different GRID block and collimator platforms and across multiple institutions [4, 9, 11].

GRID technology subsequently advanced to multileaf collimator (MLC)-based methods that use IMRT to generate GRID heterogeneity dose distributions that emulate those of collimator-based GRID therapy [4, 23]. The MLC-based SFRT heterogeneity also allows for the individualization of the beamlet profiles to further reduce the OAR dose, as described in chapter 9.

Despite differences in the heterogeneity pattern, the clinical outcomes of MLC-based GRID therapy are consistent with those of collimator-based GRID with respect to tumor control and toxicity in a large palliatively/definitively treated cohort of predominately lung and head and neck (H&N) cancer patients, in which these two delivery techniques were compared [4]. Subsequent studies employing collimator-based techniques [9], MLC-based techniques [10], or both [11], have also demonstrated overall reproducible results. Similar clinical results have been observed with LRT, a 3D form of SFRT [5, 6, 12, 24–26], as reviewed in chapter 7.

These observations show that while the dose heterogeneity profiles generated by various GRID blocks, commercially available collimators, MLCs, and LRT are variable (see chapters 9 and 10), the clinical tumor responses and toxicity results produced by SFRT, as reported in studies to date, are remarkably consistent. This overall reproducibility of clinical response across GRID platforms suggests that the dose heterogeneity patterns of SFRT generated with GRID-based technologies are clinically robust in terms of their tumoricidal and normal tissue sparing effects.

With the recent accumulation of preclinical studies (chapters 2, 3, and 17), it is also becoming increasingly recognized that not only the peak dose but also the low (valley) dose levels contained within the heterogeneous dose distribution in the tumor target may be relevant for tumor response [27]. At this time, it remains unknown precisely where the 'sweet spot' of optimal heterogeneity distribution resides within the spectrum of heterogeneity and dose gradients between the peak and valley doses, i.e. the distribution that produces the highest probability of tumor control. Therefore, as the field moves from the largely standardized dose distributions of the fixed GRID collimator geometries [1–3, 9] to the more variable and complex MLC-based GRID [4, 10, 11, 15] and the 3D SFRT dose designs used in LRT [5, 6], the meticulous modeling of SFRT dose, the standardization of implementation and dose delivery, and the standardization of the reporting of SFRT dose heterogeneity profiles are critically important in order to derive meaningful clinical results for correlation with tumor control. In this context, the equivalent uniform dose (EUD) is an important aspect of dose modeling that can guide SFRT dose prescription, as detailed in chapter 9 and by Zhang *et al* [21] and Wu *et al* [22]. A brief overview of response modeling is given in table 16.1 and a comprehensive discussion of SFRT dose–response modeling is presented in chapter 14.

## 16.4 Current data and recommendations—target dose and fractionation

### 16.4.1 SFRT dose regimens

*GRID therapy.* Dose/fractionation regimens for palliative treatment have been in the range of 15–20 Gy in a single fraction, based on the initial 2D GRID studies of palliation using GRID blocks [1–3]. The dose is generally prescribed as the peak dose (see section 3) at the $D_{\max}$ of a beam which is typically set to 6 MV or to the depth of the tumor center.

The peak dose has generally been defined as the dose at the open-dose spot of the central hole of the GRID, or the central axis of the field [21]. Studies from the 3D GRID era used the geometric pattern of peak and valley doses that was determined by the diameter and spacing of the GRID holes and the resulting proportion (percentage) of open field (vs. blocked field) to define the dose heterogeneity pattern.

SFRT doses can vary, depending on the use of conventional external beam radiation therapy (cERT). If no cERT is given, the SFRT dose tends to be higher, e.g. 20 Gy in one fraction in metastatic patients with very short survival, compared to lower SFRT doses, commonly 15 Gy in one fraction, when SFRT is combined with cERT regimens for longer-term local control.

Based on encouraging results in palliatively treated tumors and with technological advances for better OAR dose reduction therapy, e.g. improved 3D conformal therapy and IMRT techniques, SFRT has been increasingly explored for the treatment of bulky, advanced but potentially curable primary tumors in non-metastatic patients. For these indications, the prescription doses are generally in the range of 15–18 Gy in one fraction [4, 6, 9–11, 15]. Summaries of the reported dose schedules for definitive radiation in non-metastatic primary disease sites are presented in tables 16.2–16.4.

**Table 16.2.** Dose prescriptions used for SFRT and cERT in H&N cancer - outcome studies.

| | Study/year | Huhn *et al* (2006)[1] | Pengaricano *et al* (2010) | Choi *et al* (2019) |
|---|---|---|---|---|
| **Demogr.** | **Years treated** | 1995–2002 | 2005–2007* | 2007–2015 |
| | **Patient numbers** | 13 (RT), 14 (RT + surgery) | 14 (8 pts: + neck dissection) | 21 (9 definitive) |
| **SFRT** | **Technique** | GRID block, 6 MV | MLC (50% open), 6 MV | MLC, GRID Block, 6 MV or 18 MV |
| | **Target dose/ fractionation** | 15 Gy/one (26), 20 Gy/one (1) | 20 Gy/one | 15 Gy/one (16), 20 Gy/one (5) |
| | **Prescribed to** | $D_{max}$ Involved neck LN | GRID GTV, no expansion Involved LN (8) or primary site (6)[2] | $D_{max}$ |
| | **Target periphery dose** | n/r | n/r | n/r |
| | **OAR dose** | Exclusion of cord | Exclusion of cord, brain stem | Maximal avoidance of mandible, cord, brain, brain stem, brachial plexus. Traversing smallest possible skin-to-GTV separation |
| **cERT** | **Technique** | Three-field neck, electron boost to posterior neck | IMRT with simultaneous integrated boost (SIB) | IMRT |
| | **Target dose/ fractionation** | RT, curative (8): median 70 (68–79) Gy; RT, palliative (6): median 59 (54–60) Gy; RT + surgery: median 59.4 (54–72) Gy[3] | Planning target volume (PTV): 66 Gy/30; intermediate-risk PTV: 60 Gy; low-risk PTV: 54 Gy | Definitive:69.96–72.08 Gy at 2.12 Gy/fr; palliative:25 Gy/10 fr to 78 Gy/39 fr |
| | **Prescribed to** | Lateral upper neck, anterior lower neck, posterior neck electron fields | Gross tumor, intermediate risk, and low-risk PTVs | n/r |
| | **OAR's** | Cord ⩽45 Gy | n/r | n/r |

(*Continued*)

**Table 16.2.** *(Continued)*

| | Study/year | Huhn *et al* (2006)[(1)] | Pengaricano *et al* (2010) | Choi *et al* (2019) |
|---|---|---|---|---|
| **Conc. tx** | **Concurrent chemotherapy** | In 7/27 patients during cERT. Type n/r | All patients, including SFRT, most Carboplatin/Docetaxel | During cERT in definitively treated pts. Cisplatin (9), Cispl+Taxol or Etoposide (5), Cetuximab (2) |
| **Outcomes** | **Response** | pCR 85% | pCR 80% | CR 4/9, PR 1/9 (definitive pts) |
| | **Local control** | Neck: 93% (RT); 92% (RT + surgery) | 79% (in-field), no recurrence in GRID volume | n/r |
| | **Survival** | 3-y DSS: 50% (RT); 85% (RT + surg) | DSS 79% | 7/9 (definitive) alive at 7 mo. |
| | **Toxicity (early/acute)** | Gr 2–3 (skin) wound healing delay: 3/13 (RT + surg pts) | Gr 3 (skin): 7/14; gr 3 (mucosal): 4/14 | Gr 3 (skin): 1/21; gr 4 (skin): 4/21; gr 3 bleeding: 3 |
| | **Toxicity (long-term)** | Gr 3: none | Gr 3 (fibrosis): 1/14; trismus (PEG-dependent) 2/14; gr 5: carotid blowout (after surgery, skin flap): 1 | None (short follow-up) |
| | **Follow-up (mo.)** | RT: 10 (3-44) Pre-op RT: 38 (5-116) | 19 (2-38) 10/14 pts >1 yr | 7 (4-16) |

Note: Numbers in parenthesis are numbers of patients.
*Abbreviations:* cERT = conventional external beam radiation therapy; DSS = disease-specific survival; gr = grade; LN = lymph nodes; MLC = multileaf collimator; mo. = months; n/r = not reported, pts = patients; pCR = pathologic complete response; PR = partial response; RT = radiation therapy; surg = surgery; tx = treatment; y = year.
[*] Information obtained from personal communication with author.
[(1)] Similar dosing and outcomes were reported in an update by Edwards *et al* [33].
[(2)] Primary site lesions treated included base of tongue (one patient), retromolar trigone (one), tonsils (one), parotid gland (one), and maxillary sinus (two).
[(3)] Hyperfractionation in six of the 27 patients.
All patients had SFRT first, followed by cERT after one to three days.

**Table 16.3.** Dose prescriptions for SFRT and cERT in sarcoma - outcome studies.

| | Study/Year | Mohiuddin *et al* (2009)[(1)] | Mohiuddin *et al* (2014)[(1)] | Snider *et al* (2020) |
|---|---|---|---|---|
| **Demogr** | **Years treated** | n/r | n/r | 2005–2019 |
| | **Patient numbers** | 33 (bulky unresectable, recurrent, median: 13 cm)[(2)] | 14 (extremity STS >8 cm) preoperative | 26[(3)] (all except 2 pts >10 cm) |
| **SFRT** | **Technique** | GRID block, 6 MV | GRID block, 6 MV | GRID block 6–18 MV and MLC 6–18 MV, protons (2 pts) IGRT |
| | **Target dose/fractionation** | 15 Gy/one | 18 Gy/one | 15 Gy/one |
| | **Prescribed to** | $D_{\max}$ | n/r | GTV |
| | **Target periphery dose** | n/r | n/r | n/r |
| | **OAR dose** | n/r | n/r | n/r |
| **cERT** | **Technique** | n/r | n/r | n/r |
| | **Target dose/fractionation** | 22-70 Gy (median: 50 Gy) (4 pts: GRID alone) | 50 Gy | 45 to 50.4 Gy |
| | **Prescribed to** | n/r | n/r | n/r |
| | **OAR's** | n/r | n/r | n/r |
| **Conc. tx** | **Concurrent chemotherapy** | None | Iphosfamide/Mesna every three weeks | No concurrent chemotherapy (prior chemotherapy followed by progression in 4 pts) |
| **Outcomes** | **Response** | CR: 26%, PR: 50%. cERT>50 Gy: RR 95%, CR 45% cERT<50 Gy: RR 59%, CR 10% | RR:>90% tu necrosis: 65% >80% tu necrosis: 2/14; pCR: 2/14; limb salvage surgery: 93% (13/14) | pCR (>80% tu necrosis): 32%; high gr STS: 35% (6/17) pCR, hi gr extremity sarcoma: 50% (4/8) pCR. R0/R1 resection in all pts; pathologic stage: ypT2a (3 pts), ypT2b (23 pts) |
| | **Local control** | n/r | 100% | 85% (2-yr): |
| | **Survival** | 3/33 pts alive >1 yr | 86% | 65% (2-yr) |
| | **Toxicity (early/acute)** | Early gr 3 (skin): 2/33 | One grade 3 skin reaction (treatment interruption/ discontinuation), two delayed wound healing | 35% major wound complications |
| | **Toxicity (long-term)** | None | None | n/r |
| | **Follow-up (mo.)** | 9 (2–44) | 14 (3-43) | 25 (7–109*) |

Note: Numbers in parenthesis are numbers of patients.
*Abbreviations:* cERT = conventional external beam radiation therapy; CR = complete response; DSS = disease-specific survival; gr = grade; IGRT = image-guided radiation therapy; MLC = multileaf collimator; mo. = months; n/r = not reported, pts = patients; pCR = pathologic complete response; PR = partial response; RR = response rate; RT = radiation therapy; STS = soft tissue sarcoma; tu = tumor; tx = treatment.
* Information obtained from personal communication with author.
(1) Data presented in abstract form.
(2) Multiple sites treated; 20 treatments to the abdomen/pelvis, three to head and neck, seven to the thorax and 15 to extremities.
(3) Soft tissue sarcoma: 21; extra-osseous osteosarcoma: four; chondrosarcoma: one. Prior treatment: resection (followed by progression):three; chemotherapy (followed by progression): four.

**Table 16.4.** Dose prescriptions for SFRT and cERT in lung cancer - outcome studies.

| | Study/year | Somaiah *et al* (2008)[(1)] | Amendola *et al* (2019) | Larrea *et al* (2022)[(1)] |
|---|---|---|---|---|
| **Demogr** | **Years treated** | n/r | 2012–2018 | n/r |
| | **Patient numbers** | Ten (locally advanced, >6 cm NSCLC, palliatve) | Ten (bulky NSCLC, median 8 cm)[(2)] | 11 (unresectable, GTV >45 $cm^3$, unfit for chemotherapy) |
| **SFRT** | **Technique** | GRID (block), 10 MV | LRT, VMAT, 6 MV, daily IGRT | LRT, VMAT daily IGRT |
| | **Target dose/ fractionation** | 15 Gy/one | 18 Gy/one | 15 Gy/one |
| | **Prescribed to** | Tumor center | Vertex tumor volume | Vertex tumor volume |
| | **Target periphery dose** | n/r | 3 Gy/one | n/r |
| | **OAR dose** | n/r | ⩽3 Gy/one | Exclusion of bronchus, large vessels |
| **cERT** | **Technique** | n/r | IMRT, VMAT | IMRT, VMAT |
| | **Target dose/ fractionation** | 36 Gy/12 | 45-58 Gy/25-29; boost: 7 pts (range: 12.5 Gy/5–24 Gy/3) | 55 Gy/20 |
| | **Prescribed to** | n/r | PTV | PTV |
| | **OARs** | n/r | RTOG constraints | n/r |
| **Conc. tx** | **Concurrent chemotherapy** | n/r | No concurrent chemotherapy | Concurrent chemotherapy: 9 |
| **Outcomes** | Response | Symptomatic response (chest pain): CR: 71%, PR: 29%; imaging PR: 9/10 | RR: 9/10; PET/CT: metabolic CR: 3/10, PR: 2/10 | CR (PET/CT): 2; response (>50% by CT): 6; stable disease: 2; progression: 1 |
| | Local control | n/r | 9/10 | n/r (short follow-up) |
| | Survival | n/r | 5/10 alive (3/5 NED) | 7/11 (short follow-up) |
| | Toxicity (early/acute) | No grade >2 | No grade >2 | None, one death from immunotherapy toxicity |
| | Toxicity (long-term) | Grade 2 lung (moderate symptomatic fibrosis: 2) | No late toxicity | None |
| | Follow-up (mo.) | 4 (2–24) | 6 (1-71) | 8 (4–13) |

Note: Numbers in parenthesis are numbers of patients.
*Abbreviations:* cERT = conventional external beam radiation therapy; DSS = disease-specific survival; gr = grade; IGRT = image-guided radiation therapy; LRT = Lattice radiation therapy; MLC = multileaf collimator; mo. = months; NED = no evidence of disease; n/r = not reported, NSCLC = non-small cell lung cancer; pts = patients; pCR = pathologic complete response; PR = partial response; RR = response rate; RT = radiation therapy; RTOG = Radiotherapy Oncology Group; tx = treatment.
(1) Data presented in abstract form.
(2) Five patients with metastatic disease.

Based on recent consensus guidelines for clinical trial design, which critically evaluated the outcome studies of SFRT for definitive radiation therapy, the recommended GRID prescription dose for *primary H&N cancer* is 15 Gy in one fraction [28]. This recommendation is largely aimed at the treatment of stage N3 (>6 cm) bulky neck lymph nodes, while published experience with SFRT administered to the H&N primary tumor sites is minimal to date [10]. The SFRT dose is prescribed to the GTV consisting of the gross nodal mass by imaging and without a margin (table 16.2) Tracking of the peripheral GTV dose is recommended.

In the preoperative treatment of *sarcoma*, a higher dose of 15–18 Gy in one fraction is customary (table 16.3). The higher dose of this range is favored, particularly in extremity sarcomas [28], where the toxicity profile allows a higher dose because of the general absence of an aerodigestive tract and neural structures, except for peripheral nerves. However, caution is required with respect to skin dose in the preoperative setting (see section 7.2).

For *primary lung cancer*, the consensus (unpublished data) determined an SFRT dose of 18 Gy in one fraction, based on the toxicity profiles of early outcome experience with GRID therapy and LRT in both palliatively and definitively treated patients. A dose of 10–20 Gy has been used for GRID therapy in palliative or mixed cohorts with favorable symptomatic response [2, 4]. In definitively treated bulky non-small cell lung cancer (NSCLC) patients, a GRID dose of 15 Gy in one fraction was given successfully [29]. The only fully published case series of definitively treated NSCLC patients used an LRT dose of 18 Gy [6], followed by cERT. A recently presented cohort used an LRT dose of 15 Gy followed by hypofractionated cERT [30] (table 16.4). The SFRT target is the GTV (consisting of the primary lung tumor and bulky nodal mass shown by imaging) without any additional expansion, and including consideration of motion management (as described in section 5.2).

*Lattice radiotherapy (LRT).* Dosing in LRT is overall consistent with GRID therapy. Dose prescription and planning are generally more complex in LRT than in GRID techniques. Because of the highly variable positioning of the high-dose vertices in LRT, guidelines for multiple dosimetric parameters have been developed, including the vertex size and spacing, the total vertex volume, and the ratio of the vertex volume to the GTV; these are reviewed in more detail in chapter 10. Active reduction of the peripheral GTV dose using dose constraints in the peripheral subvolume of the GTV, while prescribing the SFRT dose to the lattice volume (table 16.1) which encompasses the region of the vertices, is a characteristic of LRT, as further reviewed in chapter 10. For example, in primary lung cancer, this peripheral GTV is constrained to 3 Gy, while the peak dose is prescribed at 18 Gy to cover at least 95% of the lattice volume.

In *gynecologic cancer*, the clinical trial consensus (unpublished data) recommends a dose of either 24 Gy in three fractions based on current outcome experience with LRT [5, 24] in cervical cancer or alternatively a single-fraction dose of 16.5 Gy, the dose equivalent of the three-fraction regimen. In a recent cervical cancer study, 24 Gy was prescribed to cover 95% of the vertex volume (VTV). The vertices were evenly spread throughout the VTV and adjusted to reduce the dose at the periphery of the target (determined by a 3 mm inner margin) to the limit of ⩽9 Gy in three fractions.

### 16.4.2 SFRT fractionation

The vast majority of SFRT dose schedules are single-fraction regimens, but multifraction schedules have occasionally been used. As an example, the only published case series in cervical cancer (see section 4.1) used an SFRT dose of 24 Gy in three fractions [5].

The potential inconsistency of geometric positioning in between fractions is a possible disadvantage of multifraction schedules. Even small-scale shifts in geometry in between the positioning of the peak and valley dose regions from fraction to fraction may be detrimental, although their consequences have not been explored. The current literature does not describe any outcome correlation comparing single-versus multifraction schedules. However, SFRT with more than one fraction has also demonstrated high local control [5], and major volumetric and geometry-altering changes within the tumor generally tend to occur later during treatment. Tumoral changes triggering adaptive therapy have been reported after a range of 11–23 (median: 16) fractions (SFRT plus cERT) in cervical cancer [5] and within ten fractions in lung cancer [30]. Although this scant data is early and limited, in conjunction with the reported favorable local control outcomes, these results suggest that image-guided radiation therapy (IGRT) delivery may at least partly overcome geometric positional variation between fractions. Further investigations are needed to elucidate potential interfraction changes of tumor volume, configuration, and dose pattern in SFRT.

High single-fraction regimens of 15–20 Gy are safe and feasible, based on the SRS/SBRT experience [31, 32], with the use of state-of-the-art advanced delivery technologies, including stereotactic immobilization, motion management, and meticulous IGRT technique. Conversely, multifraction SFRT regimens may have the advantage of reducing toxicity in anatomic sites where OARs are closely approximated to the tumor and thereby pose high risks for large ablative single fractions. These tradeoffs have to be carefully considered when designing regimens, particularly those intended for the treatment of potentially curable primary tumors.

## 16.5 SFRT target and delivery

### 16.5.1 Target volume definition

While prescription to a specified depth can still be used for shallow targets, the SFRT dose is generally prescribed to a volumetric target (chapters 9 and 10). In most disease sites, this target is the GTV without an added PTV margin (tables 16.2–16.4). This is a major departure from the current practice of target definition, which employs the clinical target volume (CTV) to include microscopic involvement and PTV expansion to account for setup motion. However, in SFRT, particularly in LRT, the dose in the GTV periphery tends to be generally low, and the addition of cERT can provide coverage of microscopic disease. The high local control rates observed in the outcome studies [1–6, 16, 33, 34] support this concept.

In tumor sites with close approximation to critical normal tissues, active dose reduction in the periphery of the target can be employed and has been recommended by some for the purpose of meeting OAR constraints [5, 6]. This is particularly feasible in MLC-based GRID therapy and LRT, albeit with different approaches (see section 7).

For gynecologic cancer, frequently characterized by both a mobile target and mobile sensitive OARs in the immediate vicinity, such OAR dose reduction has been incorporated into the dosimetry process by reducing the dose in the periphery of the target (GTV) to 9 Gy for an SFRT dose of 24 Gy. This is achieved by creating an inner margin within the GTV that is subject to the corresponding dose constraint. In LRT, peripheral target dose reduction is commonly facilitated by individualized placement of the high-dose spheres (vertices) at a distance from the GTV periphery, which is achieved by creating a vertex volume, ($V_L$, table 16.1) [5, 6, 22]. Similar principles have been applied in SFRT for lung cancer.

However, strategies for dose reduction in the SFRT target periphery have generally been used inconsistently. Therefore, in future prospective outcome studies, meticulous guidance and careful reporting of the dose to the target periphery are important parameters for study design [28].

### 16.5.2 Delivery and motion control

Image-guided therapy delivery with stereotactic alignment, immobilization, immediate pre-fraction imaging and IGRT are critical for SFRT delivery. In mobile targets in close vicinity to sensitive OARs, such as targets in the pelvis, abdomen, and lung, target motion control is of utmost importance in view of the high dose delivered in SFRT. Motion control strategies (such as respiratory control) that achieve the best possible immobilization of the target are ideally preferred over target expansion using an internal target volume (ITV). If an ITV is used, additional peripheral target dose reduction that takes into consideration the motion of OARs is highly recommended.

## 16.6 SFRT dose and conventionally fractionated external beam radiation dose

Very soon after the development of megavoltage GRID technology, clinical outcome data demonstrated that the addition of cERT, i.e. conventionally fractionated 'homogenous' intent radiation, to the entire tumor volume is indispensable in order to achieve durable symptom control and tumor response [2, 3].

In the palliative treatment of metastatic tumors, the decision to add cERT is generally individualized based on the patient's goal of care and expected survival time. SFRT alone without cERT may thus be acceptable in some palliative cases. However, the overall paradigm of palliation has changed in the era of greatly improved and expanded systemic chemo- and targeted therapies that have lengthened patients' survival and enhanced quality of life in patients with metastatic tumors. Along with this paradigm change, palliative radiation has evolved from a largely short-term palliative care modality to the treatment of patients for more durable (and often permanent) symptom control and improved quality of life, which can also be associated with longer survival [35]. For the definitive treatment of potentially curable patients with advanced and bulky primary tumors, the addition of cERT to SFRT is the standard.

In these definitive treatment regimens for primary tumors, full-dose cERT, *without* any dose adjustments or reductions because of the SFRT dose, has generally been employed. There is subtle evidence that tumor response in H&N cancer may be impaired if the cERT dose is reduced to less than 75% of the definitive dose level [11].

Therefore, the design of dose schedules for clinical trials in new disease entities should carefully consider the current best standard-of-care cERT dose appropriate for the specific disease, stage, and tumor extent. It is imperative to carefully plan and document the doses used for both the SFRT and cERT components of the treatment, including the target and normal tissue doses for each component.

## 16.7 The doses to critical normal structures (organs at risk)

### 16.7.1 Strategies for OAR dose reduction

In the early GRID era, strategies for OAR dose reduction relied on the complete exclusion of critical normal tissues from the beam (for example, exclusion of the neural structures and mandible in H&N cancer) [9–11]. However, with extensive tumor involvement, these methods may be insufficient, as not all OARs can simply be excluded from the SFRT target volume while still delivering an adequate target dose.

In MLC-based GRID therapy and particularly in LRT, the flexibility to adapt the SFRT heterogeneity pattern to reduce the dose given to OAR structures has much improved. With MLC-based GRID, MLC-generated 'GRID holes' that would otherwise deliver an entry or exit dose to OARs, such as the spinal cord, peripheral nerves, brain, and others, can be selectively blocked [4, 23], resulting in a reduced OAR dose while somewhat altering the SFRT pattern. In IMRT or VMAT-based LRT the heterogeneity pattern can be further manipulated by strategically positioning the high-dose spheres (vertices) to reduce the peripheral target dose and thereby meet the defined dose constraints for OARs.

### 16.7.2 SFRT dose prescription parameters for OARs

SFRT constraints for OARs continue to evolve. Outcome data with respect to toxicity in palliative SFRT case series are reassuring but should still be viewed with some caution because of the frequently short survival times of these patients and the resulting lack of long-term toxicity data. Therefore, more recent case series of definitively treated patients are better suited to provide guidance for the tolerance dose to OARs in SFRT. A summary of the dose reduction used for OARs in studies of specific tumor types together with toxicity outcomes is given in tables 16.2–16.4.

In definitively treated H&N cancer, OARs, including the spinal cord, the brain stem, and optic chiasm structures must be excluded from the SFRT volume based on the recent consensus [28] and published outcome experience [4, 9–11]. The spinal cord, brain stem, brachial plexus, carotid artery, and mandible should be considered as OARs (table 16.2). Caution has been strongly advised in the consensus that patients with carotid artery involvement *and* skin involvement or carotid involvement *and* prior irradiation should not receive SFRT because of observed fatal carotid bleeding under these conditions [10, 28].

In *sarcoma*, the exclusion of sensitive neural structures (e.g. the brachial plexus) from the SFRT volume and beam path should be strongly considered whenever possible. An exclusion with a 1 cm OAR margin will achieve a negligible SFRT dose. Particular attention should be given to the skin surface dose in this frequently preoperative setting and the tendency for skin stretching (from the tumor bulk) with ensuing vascular compromise. The SFRT dose given to the skin surface should be <150% of the prescribed GRID dose or a maximum of 30 Gy (150% of 20 Gy) [28].

In *lung cancer*, the management of OARs relies heavily on the exclusion of critical normal structures, including the spinal cord, heart, esophagus, and trachea/carina from the SFRT target volume, and it is important to consider normal organ motion. In addition, particularly with LRT-based SFRT, the dose given to the periphery of the GTV is reduced to 3 Gy in one fraction by adapting the vertex positioning. Similarly, in *cervical cancer*, it is recommended to reduce the dose to 9 Gy in three fractions at the target periphery (for an SFRT dose of 24 Gy in three fractions) and to take account of organ motion.

However, despite these guidelines [28] based on the published series [5, 6, 9–11, 15], *volumetric* parameters for specific normal tissue doses in SFRT are still largely elusive in the SFRT literature (tables 16.2–16.4), and there is a dearth of reported toxicity outcomes correlating 3D OAR volumes with SFRT doses. Therefore, in the absence of a large body of toxicity–SFRT dose correlation data, we have to resort to SRS/SBRT to extrapolate from this similarly large/ablative fractionation experience. While peripheral SFRT doses are generally low and thereby often much closer to the conventional fractionation range, in situations of gross tumor involvement around critical normal structures (such as the brachial plexus, brain stem, bowel, and others), these tissues may receive high-dose fractions from SFRT that can approach ablative hypo-fraction size. In this scenario, it is reasonable to base the limits of normal tissue tolerances on those used in SRS and SBRT [19, 36–41], which represent the major available data set for this question. These SRS/SBRT-derived tolerance doses, however, have to be considered in conjunction with the OAR dose contributions from the cERT portion of the treatment, which generally includes no reduction in target dose.

Ample experience exists for the combination of the dose parameters for normal tissue limits from conventionally fractionated regimens with those of ablative-fraction schemes, initially in external beam and high-dose-rate brachytherapy combinations, and more recently in the combination of conventional dose schedules with dose intensification through ablative-fraction stereotactic boosts [42, 43]. However, for the estimation of OAR dose limits for combinations of ablative SFRT fractionation and conventional fractionation schemes, the re-irradiation experience [37, 44, 45] should be viewed with caution, because the intervening time interval between the initial treatment course and the re-irradiation course can mitigate the normal tissue toxicity, thus potentially overestimating the normal tissue tolerance.

The variability of the fraction sizes received from the SFRT and cERT portions of treatment by specific organs calls for meticulous dose–response modeling using various models, including LQ, modified LQ, gLQ, and others, in order to define normal tissue dose limits for the combination of SFRT with conventional external radiation. Dose modeling in SFRT is reviewed in more detail in chapter 14.

### 16.7.3 SFRT dose and systemic chemotherapy and targeted therapy

Concurrent chemo- and targeted therapies are in wide use for definitive treatment, and these are generally given without significant reductions in the radiation dose. Currently the majority of SFRT regimes in definitive non-metastatic patients limit the use of concurrent chemotherapy to the cERT portion of treatment [5, 6, 9–11, 30]. While one study in H&N cancer patients has included concurrent chemotherapy during single-fraction SFRT [10], current recommendations advise that chemotherapy in H&N and lung cancer should be limited to the cERT phase [28]. In fractionated SFRT, concurrent Cisplatin has been given concurrently with an SFRT regimen of 8 Gy each for a total of three fractions in cervical cancer. Toxicity in this series was minimal [5].

## 16.8 Recommendations for dose reporting

Consistent and comprehensive dose reporting is of paramount importance. It is essential to clearly standardize and implement dose prescription parameters that define the relevant DVH properties for both clinical trials and clinical practice. Such standardization is currently being defined for both GRID therapy and LRT, and the reader is referred to the respective white papers [21, 22] and to the rapidly evolving recommendations for more detail. Among the dose heterogeneity parameters, the concept of VPDR, which commonly relied on peak and valley point doses, is developing into a volumetric paradigm (table 16.1). At present, parameters still differ somewhat between GRID therapy and LRT techniques, as shown in table 16.1. While some of this variation is related to differences in heterogeneity configurations and planning strategies between GRID and LRT, some will likely be resolved through further harmonization.

In addition, response modeling of variable heterogeneity dose distributions with EUD modeling for the target lesion and critical normal structures are recommended, particularly in view of the differing heterogeneity patterns produced by different SFRT platforms and techniques [28], and these also require further development. Detailed considerations for SFRT dose–response modeling are discussed in chapter 14.

## 16.9 Conclusions and future directions

While the published experience provides important guidance for the dosing of target and dose limits to normal tissues, dose schedules and parameters for SFRT in specific disease sites continue to evolve. Rigorous studies with larger patient cohorts and with precise definitions and implementation of dose reporting linked to tumor control and toxicity outcomes will be needed to refine prescription metrics for SFRT, particularly in definitively treated diseases.

SFRT poses an increased level of complexity for dose prescription and planning strategies. While dose–volume histograms have long defined summary statistics for the dose within the target volume, their focus has been on high-dose coverage of the target and the minimization of OAR exposure. Differential histograms instead of the cumulative DVHs that are familiar to clinicians may better reflect and describe peak and valley dose populations within the tumor target. Additional advanced dose statistics describing the dose heterogeneity are needed to define specific heterogeneity properties and perhaps their geographic distribution, so that outcome correlations can be established and further refined.

Only a thoughtful design of heterogeneity dose properties that can be consistently applied across patients and institutions and is well modeled in terms of biological effects, while grounded in the published experience, can further elucidate and optimize the heterogeneity dose–response correlation.

## References

[1] Mohiuddin M, Curtis D L and Grizos W T *et al* 1990 Palliative treatment of advanced cancer using multiple nonconfluent pencil beam radiation: A pilot study *Cancer* **66** 114–8

[2] Mohiuddin M, Fujita M and Regine W F *et al* 1999 High-dose spatially-fractionated radiation (GRID): a new paradigm in the management of advanced cancers *Int. J. Radiat. Oncol. Biol. Phys.* **45** 721–7

[3] Mohiuddin M, Stevens J H and Reiff J E *et al* 1996 Spatially fractionated (GRID) radiation for palliative treatment of advanced cancer *Radiat. Oncol. Investig.* **4** 41–7

[4] Neuner G, Mohiuddin M M and Vander Walde N *et al* 2012 High-dose spatially fractionated GRID radiation therapy (SFGRT): a comparison of treatment outcomes with Cerrobend vs. MLC SFGRT *Int. J. Radiat. Oncol. Biol. Phys.* **82** 1642–9

[5] Amendola B E, Perez N C and Mayr N A *et al* 2020 Spatially fractionated radiation therapy using lattice radiation in far-advanced bulky cervical cancer: a clinical and molecular imaging and outcome study *Radiat. Res.* **194** 724–36

[6] Amendola B E, Perez N C and Wu X *et al* 2019 Safety and efficacy of lattice radiotherapy in voluminous non-small cell lung cancer *Cureus* **11** e4263

[7] Griffin R J, Ahmed M M and Amendola B *et al* 2020 Understanding high-dose, ultra-high dose rate, and spatially fractionated radiation therapy *Int. J. Radiat. Oncol. Biol. Phys.* **107** 766–78

[8] Johnsrud A J, Jenkins S V and Jamshidi-Parsian A *et al* 2020 Evidence for early stage anti-tumor immunity elicited by spatially fractionated radiotherapy–immunotherapy combinations *Radiat. Res.* **194** 688–97

[9] Huhn J L, Regine W F and Valentino J P *et al* 2006 Spatially fractionated GRID radiation treatment of advanced neck disease associated with head and neck cancer *Technol. Cancer Res. Treat.* **5** 607–12

[10] Penagaricano J A, Moros E G and Ratanatharathorn V *et al* 2010 Evaluation of spatially fractionated radiotherapy (GRID) and definitive chemoradiotherapy with curative intent for locally advanced squamous cell carcinoma of the head and neck: initial response rates and toxicity *Int. J. Radiat. Oncol. Biol. Phys.* **76** 1369–75

[11] Choi J I, Daniels J and Cohen D *et al* 2019 Clinical outcomes of spatially fractionated GRID radiotherapy in the treatment of bulky tumors of the head and neck *Cureus* **11** e4637

[12] Amendola B E, Perez N C and Wu X *et al* 2018 Improved outcome of treating locally advanced lung cancer with the use of Lattice Radiotherapy (LRT): a case report *Clin. Transl. Radiat. Oncol.* **9** 68–71

[13] Mohiuddin M, Memon M and Nobah A *et al* 2014 Locally advanced high-grade extremity soft tissue sarcoma: response with novel approach to neoadjuvant chemoradiation using induction spatially fractionated GRID radiotherapy (SFGRT) (abstr) *J. Clin. Oncol.* **32** 10575

[14] Mohiuddin M, Miller T and Ronjon P *et al* 2009 Spatially fractionated grid radiation (SFGRT): a novel approach in the management of recurrent and unresectable soft tissue sarcoma (abstr) *Int. J. Radiat. Oncol. Biol. Phys.* **75** S526

[15] Snider J W, Molitoris J and Shyu S *et al* 2020 Spatially fractionated radiotherapy (GRID) prior to standard neoadjuvant conventionally fractionated radiotherapy for bulky, high-risk soft tissue and osteosarcomas: feasibility, safety, and promising pathologic response rates *Radiat. Res.* **194** 707–14

[16] Kudrimoti M, Regine W F and Huhn J L *et al* 2002 Spatially fractionated radiation therapy (SFR) in the palliation of large bulky (>8 cm) melanomas (abstr) *Int. J. Radiat. Oncol. Biol. Phys.* **54** 342–3

[17] Ball D, Mai G T and Vinod S *et al* 2019 Stereotactic ablative radiotherapy versus standard radiotherapy in stage 1 non-small-cell lung cancer (TROG 09.02 CHISEL): a phase 3, open-label, randomised controlled trial *Lancet Oncol.* **20** 494–503

[18] Mossa-Basha M, Gerszten P C and Myrehaug S *et al* 2019 Spinal metastasis: diagnosis, management and follow-up *Br. J. Radiol.* **92** 20190211

[19] Benedict S H, Yenice K M and Followill D *et al* 2010 Stereotactic body radiation therapy: the report of AAPM Task Group 101 *Med. Phys.* **37** 4078–101

[20] Zhang H, Grams M and Foy J *et al* 2022 A dosimetric parameter reference look-up table for GRID collimator-based spatially fractionated radiation therapy *Cancers* **14** 1037

[21] Zhang H, Wu X and Zhang X *et al* 2020 Photon GRID radiation therapy: a physics and dosimetry white paper from the Radiosurgery Society (RSS) GRID-Lattice-Microbeam-FLASH Radiotherapy Working Group *Radiat. Res.* **194** 665–77

[22] Wu X, Perez N and Zheng Y *et al* 2020 The Technical and Clinical Implementation of LATTICE Radiation Therapy (LRT *Radiat. Res.* **194** 737–46

[23] Ha J K, Zhang G and Naqvi S A *et al* 2006 Feasibility of delivering grid therapy using a multileaf collimator *Med. Phys.* **33** 76–82

[24] Amendola B E, Perez N and Amendola M *et al* 2010 Lattice radiotherapy with RapidArc for treatment of gynecological tumors: dosimetric and early clinical evaluations *Cureus* **2** e15

[25] Amendola B E, Perez N and Amendola M A *et al* 2020 The use of Lattice radiation therapy in patients with voluminous tumors (abstract) *Int. J. Radiat. Oncolo. Biol. Phys.* **108** e520

[26] Blanco Suarez J M, Amendola B E and Perez N *et al* 2015 The use of lattice radiation therapy (LRT) in the treatment of bulky tumors: a case report of a large metastatic mixed Mullerian ovarian tumor *Cureus* **7** e389

[27] Rivera J N, Kierski T M and Kasoji S K *et al* 2020 Conventional dose rate spatially-fractionated radiation therapy (SFRT) treatment response and its association with dosimetric parameters—a preclinical study in a Fischer 344 rat model *PLoS One* **15** e0229053

[28] Mayr N, Snider J W and Regine W F *et al* 2022 An international consensus on the design of prospective clinical-translational trials in spatially fractionated radiation therapy *Adv. Radiat. Oncol.* **7** 100866

[29] Somaiah N, Warrington J and Taylor H *et al* 2008 High dose spatially fractionated radiotherapy (SFR) using a megavoltage GRID in advanced lung tumors: preliminary experience in UK (abst) *Int. J. Radiat. Oncol. Biol. Phys.* **72** S490

[30] Larrea L, Gonzalez V and Antonini P *et al* 2021 Lattice radiotherapy (LRT)-spatially fractionated radiotherapy (SFRT): advanced non-small cell lung cancer (NSCLC): early experience (abstr) *Int. J. Radiat. Oncol. Biol. Phys.* **111** e443

[31] Bartl A J, Mahoney M and Hennon M W *et al* 2022 Systematic review of single-fraction stereotactic body radiation therapy for early stage non-small-cell lung cancer and lung oligometastases: how to stop worrying and love one and done *Cancers (Basel)* **14** 790

[32] Siva S, Bressel M and Mai T *et al* 2021 Single-fraction vs multifraction stereotactic ablative body radiotherapy for pulmonary oligometastases (SAFRON II): the Trans Tasman Radiation Oncology Group 13.01 phase 2 randomized clinical trial *JAMA Oncol* **7** 1476–85

[33] Edwards J M, Shah P H and Huhn J L *et al* 2015 Definitive GRID and fractionated radiation in bulky head and neck cancer associated with low rates of distant metastasis (abst) *Int. J. Radiat. Oncol. Biol. Phys.* **93** E334

[34] Kudrimoti M, Regine W F and Meigooni A S *et al* 2001 High dose spatially fractionated radiation (GRID): a new paradigm in the management of advanced cancers (abstr) *Int. J. Radiat. Oncol. Biol. Phys.* **51** 50–1

[35] Palma D A, Olson R and Harrow S *et al* 2020 Stereotactic ablative radiotherapy for the comprehensive treatment of oligometastatic cancers: long-term results of the SABR-COMET phase II randomized trial *J. Clin. Oncol.* **38** 2830–8

[36] Gerhard S G, Palma D A and Arifin A J *et al* 2021 Organ at risk dose constraints in SABR: a systematic review of active clinical trials *Pract. Radiat. Oncol.* **11** e355–65

[37] Grimm J, Vargo J A and Mavroidis P *et al* 2021 Initial data pooling for radiation dose–volume tolerance for carotid artery blowout and other bleeding events in hypofractionated head and neck retreatments *Int. J. Radiat. Oncol. Biol. Phys.* **110** 147–59

[38] Kapitanova I, Biswas S and Divekar S *et al* 2021 Estimating the tolerance of brachial plexus to hypofractionated stereotactic body radiotherapy: a modelling-based approach from clinical experience *Radiat. Oncol.* **16** 98

[39] Lo S S, Sahgal A and Chang E L *et al* 2013 Serious complications associated with stereotactic ablative radiotherapy and strategies to mitigate the risk *Clin. Oncol. (R. Coll. Radiol.)* **25** 378–87

[40] Sahgal A, Chang J H and Ma L *et al* 2021 Spinal cord dose tolerance to stereotactic body radiation therapy *Int. J. Radiat. Oncol. Biol. Phys.* **110** 124–36

[41] Timmerman R 2022 A story of hypofractionation and the table on the wall *Int. J. Radiat. Oncol. Biol. Phys.* **112** 4–21

[42] Higgins K A, Pillai R N and Chen Z *et al* 2017 Concomitant chemotherapy and radiotherapy with SBRT boost for unresectable stage III non-small cell lung cancer: a phase I study *J. Thorac. Oncol.* **12** 1687–95

[43] Wang S C, Ting W C and Chang Y C *et al* 2020 Whole pelvic radiotherapy with stereotactic body radiotherapy boost vs. conventionally fractionated radiotherapy for patients with high or very high-risk prostate cancer *Front. Oncol.* **10** 814

[44] Doi H, Tamari K and Oh R J *et al* 2021 New clinical data on human spinal cord re-irradiation tolerance *Strahlenther. Onkol.* **197** 463–73

[45] Nieder C, Grosu A L and Andratschke N H *et al* 2006 Update of human spinal cord reirradiation tolerance based on additional data from 38 patients *Int. J. Radiat. Oncol. Biol. Phys.* **66** 1446–9

**IOP** Publishing

Spatially Fractionated, Microbeam and FLASH Radiation Therapy
A physics and multi-disciplinary approach
**Hualin Zhang and Nina A Mayr**

# Chapter 17

# SFRT dosimetric parameters and their associations with treatment response

**Sha X Chang and Robert J Griffin**

The essence of spatially fractionated radiation therapy (SFRT) is the coexistence of intentional dose hot spots and cold spots distributed throughout the tumor volume. Clinical treatments and preclinical research in recent decades have clearly demonstrated that SFRT is very different than conventional radiation therapy and that SFRT is capable of a potentially high therapeutic ratio. A significant amount of work is needed to realize the potential power of SFRT for broad clinical application including work toward a solid understanding of the association between SFRT dosimetric parameters and treatment responses, which is a premise for SFRT treatment optimization. This chapter summarizes our current and limited understanding of SFRT dosimetry and treatment response associations, and reveals the urgency of reducing this significant knowledge gap. The chapter also offers specific suggestions for future research.

## 17.1 Introduction/overview

In recent years, SFRT has received well-deserved renewed attention in the radiation oncology community as a treatment with a potentially high therapeutic ratio, especially for cancer patients with bulky and late-stage tumors that are challenging to manage safely and effectively with conventional radiation therapy. Despite its decades-long history of clinical application and preclinical research and the impressive treatment outcomes demonstrated, SFRT remains unorthodox in radiation therapy [1–3]. This is partly due to the fact that the essence of SFRT, namely the coexistence of many small hot spots and cold spots throughout the tumor volume, seems to contravene the long-held concept of our understanding of tumor control in conventional radiation therapy—that the entire tumor volume must be covered by a therapeutic dose level in order to achieve tumor local control [4–6].

doi:10.1088/978-0-7503-4046-5ch17

Today, the impressive SFRT treatment responses reported so far (see chapters 5–8) have led to a surge in preclinical SFRT research and have caused an unprecedented number of additional radiotherapy clinics to implement SFRT clinically. However, in order for SFRT to gain broader acceptance in clinical application, we need to significantly improve our understanding of SFRT's underpinning mechanisms and the association between SFRT dosimetric parameters and treatment responses. An understanding of the latter association is vital for SFRT treatment parameter optimization and for clinical study design that compares SFRT with conventional radiation therapy in terms of tumor control and toxicity outcomes.

In conventional radiation therapy, we have gained a solid understanding of the dosimetry and treatment outcome associations based on decades-long clinical studies, as summarized in 'Quantitative Analyses of Normal Tissue Effects in the Clinic (QUANTEC): an introduction to the scientific issues' by Bentzen *et al* [7] for normal tissue dose tolerance and the clinical practice in which the prescription dose covers the entire treatment volume [8]. Today, this understanding of the association of dose–volume histogram (DVH) parameters and treatment response is routinely used to review patient treatment plan quality and optimize the therapeutic ratio of treatments. For instance, lung V20 (the percentage of normal lung volume receiving at least a 20 Gy dose) is identified as the dosimetric parameter that is closely associated with the risk of pulmonary radiation toxicity [7], and a low minimum tumor dose is associated with lack of local control [9]. For SFRT, we do not yet have the understanding needed to evaluate and optimize patient treatment; as stated in a review paper by Billena and Khan [10]: 'more clinical and biological data are needed to specify ideal dosimetry parameters and to formulate robust clinical indications and guidelines for optimal standardized care.' Without a solid understanding of the clinical impact of SFRT dosimetric parameters, we are unable to fully unleash the potential power of radiation with spatial fractionation in cancer treatment. The challenges we are facing include: (1) the very limited clinical application of SFRT to date; (2) the lack of good-quality documentation on SFRT dosimetric parameters; (3) the complexity of SFRT dosimetry; and (4) the fact that most SFRT clinical treatments have consisted of a single fraction followed by a full course of conventional chemoradiation therapy, making the study of the treatment response association with SFRT dosimetry alone challenging. In this chapter, we intend to focus on this poorly understood but crucial issue and shed some light on how we may gain a better understanding of this association in clinical applications using findings from preclinical studies. We will also discuss potential approaches and challenges in conducting this important research.

## 17.2 SFRT-specific dosimetric parameters

SFRT has a complex dosimetry compared to that of conventional radiation therapy. Table 17.1 lists dosimetric parameters that can be used to characterize all forms of SFRT including GRID, lattice, microbeam, and minibeam. Seven of the parameters in table 17.1 are specific to SFRT: peak dose, valley dose, peak–valley dose ratio (PVDR), peak width, valley width, peak-to-peak distance, and the percentage

**Table 17.1.** Commonly used dosimetric paramters in SFRT and non-SFRT plans.

| | Peak dose | Valley dose | PVDR | Peak width | Valley width | Peak-to-peak distance | % volume directly irradiated | Min. target dose | DVHs (organs at risk and targets) | Equivalent uniform doses (organs at risk and targets) |
|---|---|---|---|---|---|---|---|---|---|---|
| SFRT parameters<br>– Dosimetric<br>– Geometric | x | x | x | x | x | x | x | | | |
| Non-SFRT parameters | | | | | | | | x | x | x |

volume that is directly irradiated. There can be variations of the parameters used to characterize SFRT, such as a valley–peak dose ratio instead of a PVDR. These SFRT-specific dosimetric parameters depict the essence of SFRT treatment: the coexistence of both high-dose and low-dose subregions throughout the treatment volume. Thus, as a major identifying feature of this therapeutic approach, the dosimetric parameters used should be accurately reported in SFRT studies. However, in many SFRT publications, the reporting of the dosimetric parameters is often incomplete. Some of the reported dosimetric parameters may not be accurate, as they were not verified in a similar way to that used for practically all dosimetric parameters in conventional radiation therapy. For instance, one of the authors (Chang) found that the treatment planning system dose calculation for the valley dose may be significantly lower (by ~20%) in GRID therapy delivered by MLC segments (a convenient approach to delivering GRID therapy using modern accelerators). The GRID therapy irradiation configuration is drastically different from the irradiation configurations used to commission treatment planning software dose models; therefore, the computed dose of a GRID beam may have a much larger error compared to dose calculations for conventional radiation therapy beams. It is important to validate the accuracy of SFRT dose calculations using actual dose measurements before clinical implementation and dosimetric documentation take place. It is also important that the documentation should state the depth at which the reported SFRT parameters are measured, as the parameter values may vary with the depth–peak/valley dose and thus PVDRs are all depth dependent. For traditional 2D SFRT (GRID therapy, microbeam, and minibeam), the depth of the SFRT-specific dosimetry parameters is either the surface or the depth of the maximum dose [11]. For lattice therapy, the 3D form of SFRT, the SFRT-specific parameters are commonly referred to as the depth(s) of the high-dose vertices and of the valleys between the adjacent vertices within the target volume [12]. The depth difference and thus the value difference in the SFRT-specific dosimetric parameters should be noted when comparing different SFRT treatments.

In addition to the SFRT-specific parameters, table 17.1 also includes non-SFRT-specific dosimetric parameters used in conventional external beam radiation therapy (cERT)—the minimum target volume dose, dose–volume histograms (DVHs), the equivalent uniform doses (EUDs) given to organs at risk (OARs), and the treatment targets. The minimum target volume dose together with the vertex dose has been used to prescribe lattice therapy [12]. An unanswered question remains, which is whether radiobiological models, including the EUD model developed for cERT, are still suitable for SFRT, a topic which will be discussed in more detail later in this chapter. A variety of studies have considered whether a calculation of the EUD based on a cERT 2 Gy fraction may not accurately estimate the EUD for inhomogeneous dose applications [9, 13].

## 17.3 SFRT dosimetric parameters and their association with treatment responses

Today we lack a good understanding of how different aspects of the complex SFRT dosimetry are associated with treatment response in both clinical and preclinical SFRT applications. Without this understanding, we are unable to meaningfully optimize SFRT treatment for each individual patient. The good news is that the increasing popularity of SFRT in clinical applications and preclinical research promises a significant advancement in knowledge. It is reasonable to assume that the dosimetric parameters that capture the essence of SFRT (a coexistence of many high-dose and low-dose subregions within the treatment target) may have a stronger association with the treatment response compared to unrelated parameters. In a recently published preclinical study by Rivera *et al* [10], the authors illustrated that not all SFRT-specific dosimetric parameters have the same association with treatment response. We will discuss below each of the dosimetric parameters listed in table 17.1 in terms of their association with the treatment response.

### 17.3.1 SFRT-specific dosimetric parameters

There are seven SFRT-specific parameters in table 17.1. Three of them are dose parameters (peak dose, valley dose, and PVDR) and four are geometric parameters (peak width, valley width, peak-to-peak distance, and % volume directly irradiated). Note that in a given study, not all dosimetric parameters are independent variables. This was well illustrated by Rivera *et al* in a rat fibrosarcoma tumor model study that used a large variety of radiation spatial fractionation schemes—uniform tumor radiation, half-tumor radiation, 2 mm-wide SFRT, and minibeam SFRT [10]. The authors reported that in their study, seven pairs of dosimetric parameters were strongly correlated. The peak width is strongly correlated with the valley width (a Pearson correlation coefficient of 1.0), and the volume directly irradiated is closely correlated with the valley width and peak width (Pearson correlation coefficients above 0.9). Therefore, before concluding that an association exists between a dosimetric parameter and the treatment response, an analysis of self-correlation among SFRT dosimetric parameters should be performed. Note that dosimetric parameter variation in most clinical applications is intentionally limited for reasons of treatment standardization. As a result, the self-correlation among all SFRT dosimetric parameters can be very strong. For instance, if the same GRID radiation pattern is used in a study, there will be a very strong self-correlation among all the SFRT-specific geometric parameters (table 17.1). For this reason, most clinical studies are not designed to study the associations of individual dosimetric parameters with treatment response.

*Peak dose*: the peak dose has perhaps been regarded as the most important and thus best-reported SFRT dosimetric parameter. Its importance is reflected by the fact that it is used to prescribe all SFRT treatments. For instance, clinical GRID therapy using a MV photon beam prescribes a 15–20 Gy peak dose at the depth of the maximum dose [11], and preclinical microbeam therapy using a kV photon beam prescribes a ~100 Gy peak dose at the surface [3]. In lattice therapy, the treatment dose prescribed is the dose at the vertex, i.e. the 3D peak dose [12]. An early GRID study by Mohiuddin *et al* [14] indicated that peak doses of more than 15 Gy are associated with better therapeutic responses than peak doses of less than 15 Gy. However, the peak dose represents only part of the essence of SFRT (the coexistence of many small hot spots and cold spots within treatment volume) and we simply do not yet understand whether the peak dose is the dosimetric parameter that has the closest association with SFRT-induced tumor control and toxicity. A solid understanding of the clinical impact of each SFRT dosimetric parameter is crucial for clinical SFRT treatment design and reporting. In an attempt to unravel this and other unknowns in the association of SFRT dosimetry with treatment response, we designed and conducted a preclinical study using a large range of SFRT dosimetric parameter values, as shown in figure 17.1 [10]. In this study, the dosimetric approach is that the peak/maximum dose varies from 34 Gy to 225 Gy and the peak width varies from 0.3mm to 10mm in addition to uniform tumor treatment, half-tumor treatment, and the control (no radiation) using a rat fibrosarcoma tumor model. Animal survival, tumor volume change, and body weight change (an indication of toxicity) were recorded and associated with the dosimetric parameters. As shown in figure 17.2, the peak dose has no association with survival, which is also an indicator of tumor control, since no animal died of toxicity in the study. Because the peak dose has routinely been used to prescribe SFRT treatment, the potential implication of this finding is significant if proven true in clinical settings. For the reason previously stated (treatment standardization), there are no clinical studies on this subject. To validate the finding in other preclinical studies, the coauthor Chang partnered with Prezado *et al* of the Curie Cancer Institute of France and Fernandez *et al* at the University of Bern of Switzerland to review previously published preclinical SFRT work in the literature and our unpublished work in terms of SFRT dosimetric parameters and treatment response. Only seven of the reviewed studies have sufficient information to associate the dosimetric parameters with the treatment outcome, defined as an extended life span relative to the no-treatment group (personal communication).

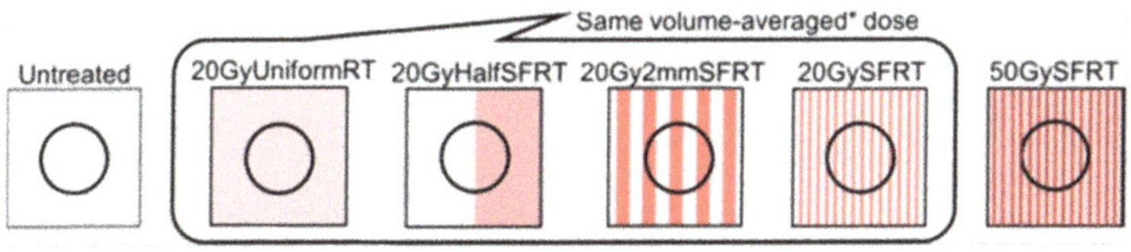


**Fig 1. Illustration of the SFRT spatial fractionation study design.** A very large range of radiation spatial fractionation scale was used to derive the impact of radiation spatial fractionation. Four arms share the same 20 Gy volume-average dose. The high dose 50GySFRT arm is added because 20GySFRT is not known to have tumor control. The dosimetric parameters studied and number of animals per study arm are listed in Table 1.

**Table 1. Summary of nine SFRT dosimetric parameter specifications in the six-arm study.**

| Treatment Arm | # of Animals | Vol-Avg Dose[a] (Gy) | Peak Surface Dose (Gy) | Valley Surface Dose (Gy) | EUD (T[e]/N[e]) | PVDR[f] | Valley Width (mm) | Peak Width (mm) | % Volume Irradiated |
|---|---|---|---|---|---|---|---|---|---|
| Untreated | 8 | 0 | 0 | 0 | 0 | N/A | 0 | 0 | 0 |
| 20GyUniformRT | 8 | 20 | 20.8 | 20.8 | 19.9/20.1 | 1 | 20 | 20 | 100 |
| 20GyHalf-SFRT | 5 | 20 | 39 | 3.1 | 2.9/30.5 | 12.6 | 10 | 10 | 47.8(±2.2)[d] |
| 20Gy2mmSFRT[c] | 6 | 17.6[b] | 34.5 | 6.2 | 5.2/25.1 | 5.6 | 2 | 2.2 | 51.5(±11.6) |
| 20GySFRT | 9 | 20 | 91 | 6.8 | 5.3/47.4 | 13.3 | 0.9 | 0.31 | 20.3 |
| 50GySFRT | 6 | 50 | 225 | 16.8 | 13.1/117.3 | | | | |

**Table 2. Pearson Correlation coefficient matrix for the eight SFRT dosimetric parameters relevant for tumor treatment response.**

| | Valley Dose | Peak Dose | AVG Dose | Tissue EUD | Tumor EUD | Peak Width | Valley Width | PVDR | % Vol. Irradiated |
|---|---|---|---|---|---|---|---|---|---|
| Valley Dose | 1.00 | | | | | | | | |
| Peak Dose | 0.38 | 1.00 | | | | | | | |
| AVG Dose | 0.63 | 0.91 | 1.00 | | | | | | |
| Tissue EUD | 0.44 | 0.99 | 0.95 | 1.00 | | | | | |
| Tumor EUD | 0.99 | 0.26 | 0.53 | 0.32 | 1.00 | | | | |
| Peak Width | 0.63 | -0.36 | 0.00 | -0.28 | 0.72 | 1.00 | | | |
| Valley Width | 0.65 | -0.34 | 0.02 | -0.25 | 0.74 | 1.00 | 1.00 | | |
| PVDR | -0.57 | 0.64 | 0.40 | 0.61 | -0.67 | -0.78 | -0.77 | 1.00 | |
| % Vol. Irradiated | 0.70 | -0.26 | 0.13 | -0.17 | 0.78 | 0.93 | 0.93 | -0.91 | 1.00 |

https://doi.org/10.1371/journal.pone.0229053.t002

**Figure 17.1.** SFRT study design (top), dosimetric parameters (middle), and the Pearson correlation coefficients among the parameters (bottom) of a rat fibrosarcoma tumor model study. Reprinted from [10], with permission of PLOS One.

The preliminary results of the preclinical study review confirm that the peak dose has little or no association with an extended life span. The final results of this meta-analysis are under preparation for publication at the time of writing.

Although the preclinical studies can shed some light on the association between SFRT peak dose and tumor control in the clinical application, we cannot directly apply their conclusions to clinical patient care without validation in the clinical setting. In addition to the substantial difference between human cancer patients and lab animals in general, another important difference is that in preclinical studies, the treatment response is observed after single-fraction SFRT, while in the clinical application the treatment response is observed after single-fraction SFRT followed by a full course of conventional radiation therapy. In the latter case, the treatment outcome cannot be attributed to SFRT dosimetry alone, and therefore it may not have a similar association with dosimetric parameters to that observed in preclinical studies.

*Valley dose*: there have been several preclinical studies of valley dose in terms of its association with treatment responses. In a review paper on synchrotron-based microbeam radiation research by the late Brauer-Krisch and colleagues, the valley dose was considered to have the same association with normal tissue toxicity as the minimum dose in cERT [5]. In a synchrotron-based microbeam study by Nakayama

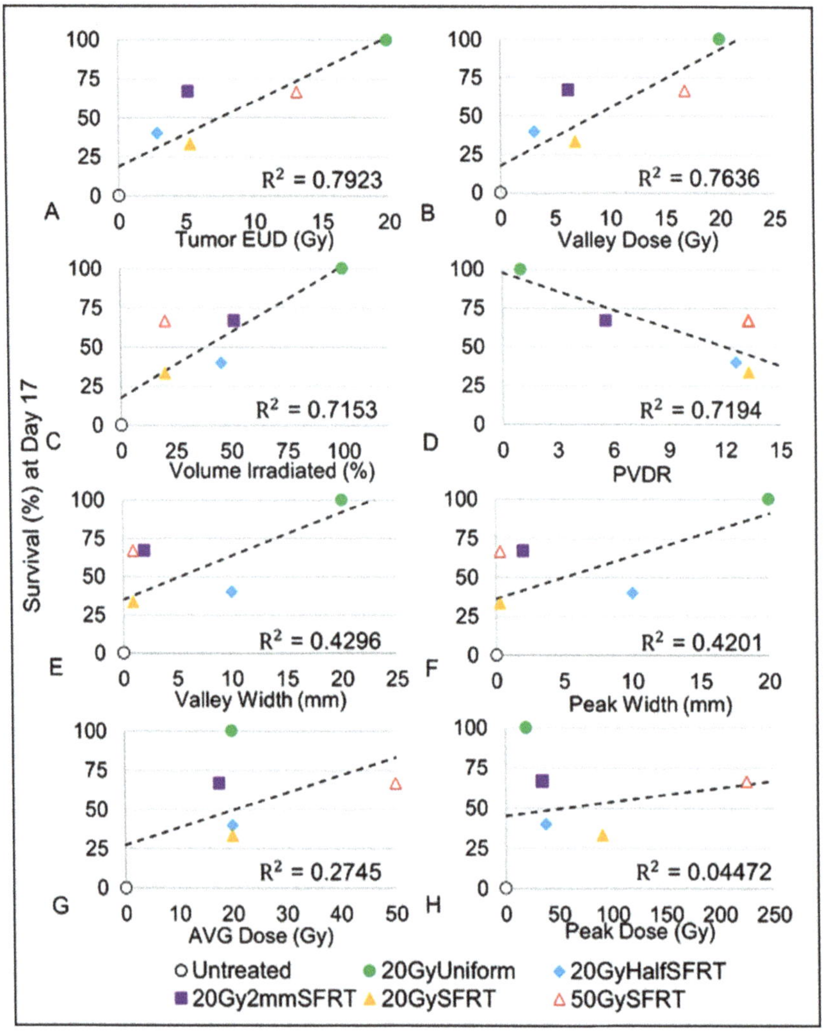


**Figure 17.2.** Association between survival (day 17) and eight SFRT dosimetric parameters in a rat fibrosarcoma tumor model study. Reprinted from [10] with permission of PLOS One.

*et al* [6], the authors reported that the valley dose has the closest correlation with normal brain toxicity; their study used a fixed 25 micron peak width separated by 100, 200, and 300 microns. They found that the corresponding 50% lethal peak doses were 244, 533, and 792 Gy, which confirms the finding that peak dose lacks an association with the treatment outcome. Since the valley doses were similar (13, 14, 13 Gy) for 50% survival, this study shows that the valley dose is closely associated with survival. This finding was also well demonstrated by Rivera *et al* [10]; as seen in figure 17.2, the valley dose exhibited the closest association with survival (tumor control) among the eight dosimetric parameters studied. In the same study, the valley dose also exhibited the strongest (but still weak—$R^2$ = 0.3814) association with body weight change among the dosimetric parameters studied; this is an indication of treatment toxicity in animal studies. In a cellular study of dose equivalence between microbeam radiation therapy (MRT) and broad beam (BB) radiotherapy [7], the authors experimentally determined the MRT's BB dose through cell clonogenic studies. The BB equivalence dose was found to be equal or less than the valley dose calculated by Monte Carlo simulation, and the dose equivalence was cell line dependent and peak dose dependent. These results from cellular and preclinical studies must be reexamined to determine their clinical relevance under SFRT clinical application conditions, in which SFRT is followed by conventional radiation therapy. It appears that the valley dose is highly important to avoid toxicity in a given SFRT regimen. At the same time, new data using conventional radiation suggest that low-dose exposures may turn on beneficial biology such as immune activation [15, 16], as further discussed in chapters 2 and 3. Although further research is needed to identify the relevance of the dosimetric parameters in SFRT, the valley dose likely plays an important role in the biological control of the tumor, the toxicity to organs at risk, and in complementing the massive cell killing expected to occur in the peak dose regions to enhance the systemic anticancer immune response.

*PVDR:* the PVDR captures an important aspect of the essence of SFRT, i.e. the dose difference between the dose hot spots and cold spots that coexist in the treatment volume. It is rational to assume that a high PVDR value, which indicates greater dose heterogeneity, is desirable in order to achieve a high therapeutic ratio in SFRT. However, PVDR's association with the treatment response is still largely unknown, especially in clinical applications. For preclinical SFRT, Rivera *et al* reported a negative-slope association between the PVDR value and animal survival (figure 17.2), which was supported by the preliminary finding of the preclinical SFRT literature review by Fernandez-Palomo, Chang and Prezado [17]. The negative-slope association between the PVDR and survival can be explained by the close and positive association between the valley dose and survival and the inverse relation between the valley dose and the PVDR value (the higher the valley dose, the smaller the PVDR). The benefit of a high PVDR value for interlacing microbeam beam pair irradiation is straightforward: tissue outside the tumor volume is exposed to only a single microbeam, and a high PVDR reduces valley dose and thus toxicity for a given peak dose. Inside the tumor volume, the two microbeam beams interlace and the peak dose superimposes with the valley dose to form a uniform high-dose distribution [18]. For single SFRT beam radiation, the benefit of a high PVDR value is less understood. In theory, a high PVDR value can be very important to SFRT's ability to stimulate radiation-induced *in situ* antigen production, and a high PVDR suggests that optimal low-dose volumes exist, which might further assist the immunologic reactions against residual tumor volume [16]. The high dose in the peak subregions induces a high level of tumor antigen presentation and the low dose in the valley subregions allows the survival of immune cells such as antigen-presenting cells that carry the tumor antigens to nearby lymph nodes to initiate a systemic anticancer immune response [8]. Growing numbers of reports on the combination of radiotherapy and immunotherapy suggest that there could be an optimal association between PVDR and treatment response if SFRT treatment goals are correctly tailored.

#### *17.3.1.1 SFRT geometric parameters*

The peak width, valley width, peak-to-peak distance, and the percentage of volume directly irradiated characterize the geometrical and spatial aspects of SFRT. The latter two parameters can be derived from the former two and there are often close correlations among the SFRT geometric parameters (figure 17.2). The association between the geometric parameters and the treatment response has been studied preclinically. In terms of local control, preclinical studies indicate that the higher the percentage of the tumor that is directly irradiated and receives a high peak dose, the lower the cellular survival [7] and the better the tumor control [9]. The higher the percentage of the tumor volume that is irradiated by the peak dose, the more the treatment is like conventional radiation therapy, which is known to result in better local control for the SFRT treatment using the same volume-averaged dose [9]. It is reasonable to assume that the geometric parameters may be important for the radiation-induced *in situ* immunomodulatory effects discussed in the paragraph on PVDR. The geometric parameters may affect the quantity of tumor antigen produced and the quantity of tumor-infiltrating immune cell sparing, both of which are essential for the radiation-induced antitumor immune response. In clinical application, the SFRT geometric parameters used tend to be very similar to those in preclinical studies due to the desire for standardization. In GRID therapy, the peak width is approximately 1cm and the valley width is 1.7 cm [11], and similar values are used in 3D lattice therapy [12]. There are self-correlations between the dosimetric parameters and geometric parameters in SFRT, especially in MV photon therapy, in which the valley dose is strongly influenced by the peak width due to large amounts of tissue scatter radiation. The clinical impact of the SFRT geometric parameters is complex and challenging to unravel, and it can be different for different SFRT clinical applications (tumor local control or radiation-induced *in situ* immunomodulatory effects).

### 17.3.2 Conventional RT dosimetric parameters

In addition to the SFRT-specific parameters, cERT dosimetric parameters are also used to characterize clinical SFRT treatment plan dosimetry. The main conventional dosimetric parameters we discuss here are the volume-averaged dose (integral dose), DVHs of the target and OARs, and their EUDs. Although EUDs are used in SFRT, the suitability of existing radiobiological models for use in clinical SFRT has been challenged.

*Volume-averaged dose:* the volume-averaged dose is the dosimetric parameter that does not capture the essence of SFRT dosimetry, where dose varies significantly and frequently in space; it has the least association with treatment response. This is clearly demonstrated in the preclinical study by Rivera *et al*, in which a large variety of spatial fractionation geometry was used at a constant volume-averaged dose [9].

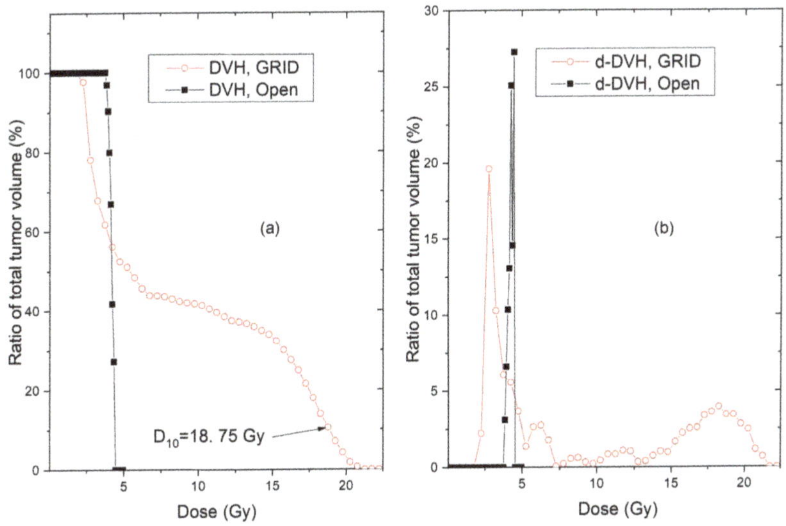


**Figure 17.3.** An example of a cumulative DVH (left) and an example of a differential DVH (d-DVH) (right) for GRID therapy. Compared to DVH, the d-DVH curve is a more intuitive representation of the radiation spatial fractionation of GRID dosimetry. The two peaks in d-DVH represent the dose valley and dose peak with a PVDR of approximately six. Figure: courtesy, Dr Hualin Zhang, University of Southern California, USA.

As shown in figure 17.2, no association was observed in this study between the volume-averaged dose and survival and body weight changes post radiation (not shown), an indication of treatment toxicity in animal research.

*DVHs:* there are two forms of the DVH. The most-used form in radiation therapy is the integral DVH, in which the $y$-axis represents the structural volume and the $x$-axis represents the minimum dose received by the structural volume. The other form can be referred to as differential DVH, in which the percentage of the organ volume that receives the specific dose is plotted. Figure 17.3 illustrates the two tumor DVH forms for a GRID therapy by Zhang *et al* [19], in which 5% of the target volume received 18 Gy and 17% of the volume received 3 Gy in a GRID therapy study. Compared to the integral DVH, the differential DVH more directly depicts the spatial (volume) fractionation essence of SFRT and is thus the more informative DVH form for SFRT plan evaluation.

*EUDs*: tumor and normal organ EUDs are commonly used in conventional radiation therapy clinical treatment plan evaluation. At present, the suitability of EUD and other radiobiological models for use in SFRT remains an unanswered question. This is because EUD and other radiobiological models are based on a cell survival exponential equation that calculates the probability of cell death from the radiation dose it directly receives. In SFRT, the majority of the cells in the treatment volume are outside areas exposed to direct radiation and thus receive only the valley dose, which is typically one to two orders of magnitude smaller than the dose received by the cells in the peak regions. Relative to the peak dose, the valley dose is much higher in clinical megavoltage photon SFRT (in which the PVDR is often less than five) [14, 20] than that in preclinical kV photon microbeam SFRT (in which the PVDR is often more than 20) [21]. The radiobiological models developed for conventional radiation therapy are unable to model the bystander effect (cell death not caused by directly received radiation but by radiation received by cells nearby) [1, 2], the abscopal effect (cell death away from the treatment region) [3, 4], and drastic microvasculature modulation in the entire tumor due to SFRT radiation [22]. These secondary effects that occur in low- or no-dose regions in SFRT are most likely initiated in the high-dose subregions, but the mechanisms involved remain poorly understood and are not modeled by the existing radiobiological models. More research is needed to understand the unique cellular, tissue, and systemic responses to SFRT radiation, which are the foundation for the development of reliable radiological models for SFRT. A recent study by Cahoon *et al* [23] used mathematical modeling to take account of both the cytotoxic effect of direct radiation on cells and the radiation-induced bystander effect, which is expected to play a more important role in SFRT than in conventional radiation. The authors investigated the impact of the bystander effect on cell survival *in vitro* and concluded that the SFRT exhibited higher apparent tumor EUDs but a similar normal tissue complication probability (NTCP) to that of conventional radiation. Using a rat fibrosarcoma tumor model, Rivera *et al* evaluated the association of tumor EUD ($a = -10$) and normal tissue EUD ($a = 5$) with tumor control and body weight change post radiation (an indication of treatment toxicity). They found that the tumor EUD and the valley dose had the closest association with survival (figure 17.2). Note that there is a high self-correlation between the valley dose and the tumor EUD, as the valley dose is heavily weighted in the tumor EUD calculation (Pearson correlation coefficient of 0.99, figure 17.1). Existing models of EUD calculations for non-homogeneous doses need to be studied in the context of SFRT to confirm or deny their relevance (see references to EUD above).

## 17.4 Current knowledge gaps in our understanding of the clinical impact of SFRT dosimetric parameters and research opportunities

The gap between our current understanding and the knowledge required to optimize clinical SFRT for a given treatment outcome is significant. For conventional radiation therapy, we have such knowledge and use it routinely to optimize patient treatment and increase the treatment therapeutic ratio. For SFRT, we do not yet know which dosimetric parameters have a close association with a given treatment outcome on which we should focus and which can be ignored. Without this knowledge, we cannot fully unleash the potential power of radiation spatial fractionation for patient treatment. Fortunately, we have begun to understand the impact of SFRT dosimetric parameters on treatment response in preclinical studies and found that among the seven dosimetric parameters studied, the peak dose is not a dosimetric parameter that is closely associated with treatment response when the peak dose is maintained at a high enough level to achieve stereotactic body radiation therapy (SBRT)-level cell killing. Moreover, the interpretation of preclinical study results for clinical SFRT treatment, in which SFRT is followed by a conventional course of radiation therapy, is unknown. There are significant challenges in studying the association in clinical application because (1) most clinical SFRT treatment is followed by a course of conventional radiation therapy and in many cases by chemotherapy—thus, both treatments contribute to the treatment response; and (2) the SFRT-specific dosimetric parameters used in clinical application are strongly self-correlated largely due to the desire for treatment standardization and the aim of containing high-dose regions within the tumor volume.

One way to move forward is to design preclinical studies that mimic clinical reality—a single SFRT treatment followed by a course of cERT or alternatively, other clinical SFRT+cERT or SFRT+cERT/chemotherapy schemes. The availability of commercial image-guided small animal irradiation technologies makes it easier to conduct animal studies to investigate the role of SFRT in priming immunotherapy and chemotherapy, as we and others have demonstrated [24–26]. Early treatment responses can be evaluated through biomarkers, such as the immune profile of infiltration cells, at different time points (before and after SFRT, during and after the following conventional radiation therapy). In addition, tumor blood flow/oxygenation has been found to greatly react to SFRT approaches, and this change in the tumor microenvironment may have a marked effect on follow-on conventional chemo- or radiation therapy. These aspects have been documented in our prior studies [22, 27]. The early responses should be used to monitor the treatment response observed later and should be correlated with it. It is likely that some of the early responses, especially those monitored before the impact of the following conventional therapy, can be associated with SFRT dosimetric parameters for potential SFRT dosimetric parameter optimization.

## 17.5 Conclusions

At this early stage of SFRT clinical application and research development, the association between treatment response and SFRT dosimetry is not well understood in both clinical and preclinical studies. SFRT dosimetry is far more complex than that of conventional radiation therapy, and preclinical data have clearly demonstrated that SFRT dosimetry has a unique association with treatment response that is very different than that seen in conventional radiation therapy. Furthermore, the heterogeneous coexistence of extreme hot spots and cold spots throughout the tumor volume, which is the core of SFRT dosimetry, may initiate robust nonlocal effects (the cellular bystander effect, tumor microenvironment modulation, and the abscopal effect) that may be very different or absent in conventional radiation therapy. Therefore, the knowledge we have gained in decades of conventional radiation therapy research and clinical application may not be directly applicable to SFRT. Understanding the association between the treatment response and SFRT dosimetry for a given treatment intent is vital for treatment design and optimization and also to elucidate the working mechanisms of SFRT. There is now a sense of urgency related to improving our understanding of the clinical impact of SFRT dosimetric parameters, because practically all SFRT treatments have been prescribed using the peak dose, while preclinical studies have clearly shown a consistent lack of association between the peak dose and the treatment outcome. If this is true in clinical SFRT applications, it may be a contributing factor to the fact that the same SFRT treatment prescription dose leads to different treatment responses. To move forward, we suggest three approaches: (1) high-quality, standardized recording of SFRT dosimetric parameters, especially the SFRT-specific parameters, in SFRT studies in clinical patients; (2) more preclinical research into the association between SFRT dosimetry and treatment response under clinical SFRT application conditions (SFRT + cERT/chemotherapy/immunotherapy); and (3) the use of appropriate biomarkers as surrogates for treatment outcomes in the study of response association with SFRT dosimetry.

## References


[1] Griffin R J, Ahmed M M, Amendola B, Belyakov O, Bentzen S M and Butterworth K T *et al* 2020 Understanding high-dose, ultra-high dose rate, and spatially fractionated radiation therapy *Int. J. Radiat. Oncol. Biol. Phys.* **107** 766–78

[2] Billena C and Khan A J 2019 A current review of spatial fractionation: back to the future? *Int. J. Radiat. Oncol. Biol. Phys.* **104** 177–87

[3] Brauer-Krisch E, Serduc R, Siegbahn E A, Le Duc G, Prezado Y and Bravin A *et al* 2010 Effects of pulsed, spatially fractionated, microscopic synchrotron X-ray beams on normal and tumoral brain tissue *Mutat Res.* **704** 160–6

[4] Tome W A and Fowler J F 2002 On cold spots in tumor subvolumes *Med. Phys.* **29** 1590–8

[5] Mavroidis P, Lind B and Brahme A 2001 Biologically effective uniform dose for specification, report and comprison of dose response relations and treatment plans *Phys. Med. Biol.* **46** 2607–30

[6] Niemierko A 1997 Reporting and analyzing dose distributions: a concept of equivalent uniform dose *Med. Phys.* **24** 103–10

[7] Bentzen S M, Constine L S, Deasy J O, Eisbruch A, Jackson A and Marks L B *et al* 2010 Quantitative Analyses of Normal Tissue Effects in the Clinic (QUANTEC): an introduction to the scientific issues *Int. J. Radiat. Oncol. Biol. Phys.* **76** S3–9

[8] Niemierko A 1998 Radiobiological models of tissue response to radiation in treatment planning systems *Tumori* **84** 140–3

[9] Gonzalez S J and Carando D G 2008 A general tumour control probability model for non-uniform dose distributions *Math. Med. Biol.* **25** 171–84

[10] Rivera J N, Kierski T M, Kasoji S K, Abrantes A S, Dayton P A and Chang S X 2020 Conventional dose rate spatially-fractionated radiation therapy (SFRT) treatment response and its association with dosimetric parameters—a preclinical study in a Fischer 344 rat model *PLoS One* **15** e0229053

[11] Zhang H, Wu X, Zhang X, Chang S X, Megooni A and Donnelly E D *et al* 2020 Photon GRID radiation therapy: a physics and dosimetry white paper from the Radiosurgery Society (RSS) GRID/LATTICE, microbeam and FLASH Radiotherapy Working Group *Radiat. Res.* **194** 665–77

[12] Wu X, Perez N C, Zheng Y, Li X, Jiang L and Amendola B E *et al* 2020 The technical and clinical implementation of LATTICE Radiation Therapy (LRT) *Radiat. Res.* **194** 737–46

[13] Terahara A, Niemierko A, Goitein M, Finkelstein D, Hug E and Liebsch N *et al* 1999 Analysis of the relationship between tumor dose inhomogeneity and local control in patients with skull base chordoma *Int. J. Radiat. Oncol. Biol. Phys.* **45** 351–8
[14] Mohiuddin M, Fujita M, Regine W F, Megooni A S, Ibbott G S and Ahmed M M 1999 High-dose spatially-fractionated radiation (GRID): a new paradigm in the management of advanced cancers *Int. J. Radiat. Oncol. Biol. Phys.* **45** 721–7
[15] Herrera F G, Irving M, Kandalaft L E and Coukos G 2019 Rational combinations of immunotherapy with radiotherapy in ovarian cancer *Lancet Oncol.* **20** e417–33
[16] Herrera F G, Ronet C, Ochoa de Olza M, Barras D, Crespo I and Andreatta M *et al* 2022 Low-dose radiotherapy reverses tumor immune desertification and resistance to immunotherapy *Cancer Discov.* **12** 108–33
[17] Fernandez-Palomo *et al* 2022 Should peak dose be used to prescribe spatially fractionated radiation therapy? - A review of preclinical studies *Cancers (Basel)* **14** 3625
[18] Serduc R, Brauer-Krisch E, Siegbahn E A, Bouchet A, Pouyatos B and Carron R *et al* 2010 High-precision radiosurgical dose delivery by interlaced microbeam arrays of high-flux low-energy synchrotron X-rays *PLoS One* **5** e9028
[19] Zhang H, Zhong H, Barth R F, Cao M and Das I J 2014 Impact of dose size in single fraction spatially fractionated (grid) radiotherapy for melanoma *Med. Phys.* **41** 021727
[20] Zhang H, Grams M P, Foy J J and Mayr N A 2022 A dosimetric parameter reference look-up table for GRID collimator-based spatially fractionated radiation therapy *Cancers (Basel)* **14** 1037
[21] Brauer-Krisch E, Serduc R, Siegbahn E A, Le Duc G, Prezado Y and Bravin A *et al* 2010 Effects of pulsed, spatially fractionated, microscopic synchrotron X-ray beams on normal and tumoral brain tissue *Mutat. Res.* **704** 160–6
[22] Fontanella A N, Boss M K, Hadsell M, Zhang J, Schroeder T and Berman K G *et al* 2015 Effects of high-dose microbeam irradiation on tumor microvascular function and angiogenesis *Radiat. Res.* **183** 147–58
[23] Cahoon P, Giacometti V, Casey F, Russell E, McGarry C K and Prise K M *et al* 2021 Investigating spatial fractionation and radiation induced bystander effects: a mathematical modelling approach *Phys. Med. Biol.* **66** 225007
[24] Johnsrud A J, Jenkins S V, Jamshidi-Parsian A, Quick C M, Galhardo E P and Dings R P M *et al* 2020 Evidence for early stage anti-tumor immunity elicited by spatially fractionated radiotherapy–immunotherapy combinations *Radiat. Res.* **194** 688–97
[25] Kanagavelu S, Gupta S, Wu X, Philip S, Wattenberg M M and Hodge J W *et al* 2014 In vivo effects of lattice radiation therapy on local and distant lung cancer: potential role of immunomodulation *Radiat. Res.* **182** 149–62
[26] Price L S L, Rivera J N, Madden A J, Herity L B, Piscitelli J A and Mageau S *et al* 2021 Minibeam radiation therapy enhanced tumor delivery of PEGylated liposomal doxorubicin in a triple-negative breast cancer mouse model *Ther. Adv. Med. Oncol.* **13** 17588359211053700
[27] Griffin R J, Koonce N A, Dings R P, Siegel E, Moros E G and Brauer-Krisch E *et al* 2012 Microbeam radiation therapy alters vascular architecture and tumor oxygenation and is enhanced by a galectin-1 targeted anti-angiogenic peptide *Radiat. Res.* **177** 804–12

**IOP** Publishing

Spatially Fractionated, Microbeam and FLASH Radiation Therapy
A physics and multi-disciplinary approach
**Hualin Zhang and Nina A Mayr**

# Chapter 18

## Monte Carlo simulation of photon beam spatially fractionated radiotherapy

**Immaculada Martínez-Rovira and José M Fernández-Varea**

Monte Carlo (MC) calculations are widely used for accurate dose computation in radiotherapy. They have played a key role in the dose assessment for photon spatially fractionated radiotherapy (SFRT) due to the distinct irradiation characteristics of these novel modalities with respect to conventional radiotherapy. MC simulations have been employed to prove the performance of the existing dose calculation algorithms implemented in commercial treatment planning systems for megavoltage GRID therapy, as well as to optimize irradiation configurations and the design of beam modifiers, including collimators. In addition, the specific irradiation characteristics of synchrotron-based microbeam radiation therapy (MRT) and minibeam radiation therapy (MBRT) in terms of energy spectrum, machine geometry, and beam polarization demanded the development of dedicated MC-based calculation engines able to compute dose distributions at the micrometric scale. In this chapter, an overview of the MC studies performed in photon SFRT is presented, with a special focus on the MC dose computation challenges of photon SFRT with respect to dose computation in standard radiotherapy.

### 18.1 Introduction/overview

Accurate dose computation is a requisite for a successful outcome in radiotherapy. Within this context, MC simulations have become an essential tool to accurately determine absorbed dose distributions. In photon SFRT, dose computation implies further challenges compared to dose computation in standard radiotherapy, especially when submillimeter beam sizes and multiple beamlets are used. The commercial treatment planning systems (TPSs) employed in conventional radiotherapy must be adapted and benchmarked prior to their use in GRID therapy. Moreover, the energy spectrum of synchrotron-based microbeam radiation therapy (MRT) and minibeam radiation therapy (MBRT) is far below the typical

doi:10.1088/978-0-7503-4046-5ch18

megavoltage photon energies used in conventional radiotherapy; thus, the fast dose computation algorithms implemented in TPSs are not applicable to these techniques. This feature and the need to assess peak and valley doses at the micrometer scale has rendered MC simulations the gold standard for determining absorbed dose distributions in SFRT.

This chapter first includes a brief overview of the relevant photon and electron interactions in photon SFRT (sections 18.2 and 18.3) as well as a short summary of the MC simulation of radiation transport (section 18.4). Sections 18.5, 18.6, and 18.7 report MC dose computation for megavoltage GRID therapy, synchrotron-based MRT, and MBRT, respectively. Finally, some reflections on future perspectives and the main conclusions are presented in sections 18.8 and 18.9.

## 18.2 Photon interactions

Beams of x-rays are used for the applications covered in the present chapter. The energies of interest span the range from around 1 keV to 10 MeV. In this energy range, the possible photon–atom interaction processes are the photoelectric effect, Rayleigh scattering, Compton scattering, pair production, and triplet production. Photonuclear reactions can be disregarded. The article by Hubbell [1] is an excellent source of information on this topic. Another reference that might be consulted is the review paper by Salvat and Fernández-Varea [2].

### 18.2.1 Photoelectric effect

In the photoelectric effect, an incident photon is absorbed by one of the bound atomic electrons, which is ejected. This can happen only if the photon's energy is larger than the binding energy of the atomic (sub)shell from which the photoelectron is expelled. The quantum-mechanical details of this interaction mechanism can be described at several levels, ranging from the simple nonrelativistic Born approximation for an electron subject to a Coulomb potential [3] to the rigorous relativistic partial-wave treatment of an electron in a screened atomic potential [4].

### 18.2.2 Rayleigh scattering

In this type of collision, the incident photon is absorbed, and a photon is emitted with the same energy but in a different direction. The interaction is called elastic because the atom remains in its initial quantum state. In the form-factor approximation, the atomic differential cross section (DCS) for Rayleigh scattering is expressed as the product of the Thomson DCS and the form factor. The Thomson DCS describes the angular distribution of a photon colliding elastically with a free electron at rest. In turn, the form factor is the Fourier transform of the atomic electron density, thus taking account of the fact that the electron distribution is bound to the target atom. Hubbell *et al* [5] tabulated the form factors of all atoms along with the corresponding integrated Rayleigh cross sections. More refined descriptions of Rayleigh scattering have been proposed, but the associated calculations are difficult. Nevertheless, the ensuing DCSs can be parameterized by adding a complex anomalous form factor to the usual form factor; see, for instance, the work of Salvat and Fernández-Varea [2].

### 18.2.3 Compton scattering

This is an inelastic process whereby the photon is absorbed by the target atom and another photon is emitted in a different direction with a lower energy. The energy transfer is taken by an atomic electron, which is ejected. The simplest description of a Compton collision considers that the struck electron is initially unbound and stationary. The angular distribution of the scattered photon is then given by the Klein–Nishina DCS. Binding effects can be incorporated in the so-called Waller–Hartree approximation, which multiplies the Klein–Nishina DCS by the incoherent scattering function [6]. Tables of the incoherent scattering functions of all atoms can be found in [5] together with the corresponding integrated Compton cross sections. More advanced formalisms exist to describe Compton collisions. For instance, the relativistic impulse approximation accounts for both the binding and the motion of the target electron; see, for example, [7] and the references therein.

### 18.2.4 Pair and triplet production

High-energy photons may decay into an electron and a positron in the presence of a massive, charged particle. The presence of the latter is required to fulfill conservation of energy and linear momentum. If the massive particle is an atomic nucleus, the process is called pair production, and the threshold is $2m_ec^2$ because the nucleus absorbs linear momentum but a negligible amount of recoil energy. If the decay occurs in the vicinity of one of the atomic electrons, the corresponding threshold is shifted to $4m_ec^2$, since the spectator electron receives both linear momentum and energy, being ejected from the atom. The process is then accordingly termed triplet production. The description of both processes is involved even in the simplest approach, the Born approximation, in which the created electron and positron are described as plane waves, disregarding their electrostatic interaction with the atom. The tabulation of Hubbell *et al* [8] is the most used source of information on this topic. More recently, Hubbell and Seltzer [9] and Hubbell [1] discussed the status of cross-section data for electron–positron pair production.

### 18.2.5 Photon–atom interaction databases

The most comprehensive information on photon–atom interaction cross sections (or, equivalently, mass attenuation coefficients) is the Evaluated Photon Data Library EPDL97 [10] from the Lawrence Livermore National Laboratory. Alternatively, the National Institute of Standards and Technology (NIST) maintains the XCOM database [11]. These databases pertain to *isolated* atoms; cross sections for molecules or compounds can be generated by resorting to the additivity rule. In the case of a low-atomic-number material such as water, the photoelectric effect is the dominant interaction process for photon energies of up to around 30 keV, and Compton scattering prevails at larger energies. Rayleigh interactions and pair or triplet production play lesser roles.

## 18.3 Electron interactions

As already mentioned, the applications addressed in this chapter concern photons with energies ranging from around 1 keV to 10 MeV. However, electrons are set in motion in photoelectric and Compton interactions, and electron–positron pairs can be created at energies greater than $2m_ec^2$. These electrons and positrons become ionizing particles whose interactions with the medium should be considered in order to provide a complete picture of the radiation transport and associated energy deposition. Compact surveys of electron– and positron–atom interactions have been written by Berger and Wang [12] and Seltzer [13]. The review article of Salvat and Fernández-Varea [2] contains further references.

### 18.3.1 Elastic scattering

In electron–atom or positron–atom elastic collisions, the projectile changes its direction of flight and does not lose kinetic energy. Classical physics and non-relativistic quantum mechanics both lead to the famous Rutherford DCS, which describes the elastic collision of an electron or positron with a bare nucleus. Screening effects can be straightforwardly incorporated within the Born approximation, yielding the screened Rutherford DCS when the projectile–atom interaction is modeled as an exponentially screened Coulomb potential [12]. More advanced approaches sideline the assumption of plane waves and model the screening effects more faithfully within a fully relativistic formalism. ICRU Report 77 [14] provides an overview of the various theoretical frameworks employed to describe the elastic scattering of electrons and positrons.

### 18.3.2 Inelastic scattering

In these interactions, the incident electron or positron loses part of its kinetic energy, which is invested to excite or ionize the target atom. If the collision is modeled as occurring with a free electron at rest, the inelastic DCS admits analytical formulas, namely the Møller and Bhabha DCSs pertaining to electron or positron inelastic scattering, respectively. These DCSs diverge for small energy losses [13]. The plane-wave Born approximation avoids this shortcoming by adopting a realistic wave function for the target electron, and the distorted-wave Born approximation additionally improves the wave function of the projectile electron or positron. However, these *ab initio* formalisms are numerically cumbersome. The review by Llovet *et al* [15] summarizes various semi-empirical models and the aforementioned formalisms employed to calculate inner-shell ionization by electron impact, and it includes a comprehensive comparison of distorted-wave Born cross sections for the ionization of the K, L, and M (sub)shells, including experimental data.

### 18.3.3 Bremsstrahlung emission

Electrons and positrons can lose kinetic energy by emitting an x-ray when they are accelerated close to a nucleus or an atomic electron, processes that are called electron–nucleus bremsstrahlung and electron–electron bremsstrahlung, respectively. A simple analytical DCS for electron–nucleus bremsstrahlung can be deduced in the nonrelativistic Born approximation; however, in the relativistic Born approximation the analytical formula (Bethe–Heitler DCS) is quite lengthy, and beyond these simplified approaches the DCS must be calculated numerically but convergence is only achieved for kinetic energies of a few MeV at most. Seltzer and Berger [16] devised a calculation scheme that combines numerical DCSs at low energies with Bethe–Heitler DCSs at high energies and interpolates between them. Electron–nucleus bremsstrahlung has been revisited by Mangiarotti and Martins [17], and electron–electron bremsstrahlung has been addressed by Tessier and Kawrakow [18].

### 18.3.4 Positron annihilation

In addition to the elastic, inelastic, and bremsstrahlung interaction mechanisms summarized above, a positron may experience annihilation with an atomic electron, resulting in the emission of one or more photons. The most likely process is the production of two photons. Positron annihilation with an electron at rest is described by the analytical Heitler DCS. Annihilation may happen while the positron is moving, but the largest probability of annihilation occurs once the positron has slowed down to rest. Then, owing to the conservation of linear momentum and energy, the two photons are emitted 'back-to-back' with energies equal to $m_e c^2$.

## 18.4 Monte Carlo simulation of radiation transport

MC methods are numerical techniques that employ stochastic (i.e., non-deterministic) algorithms to simulate the behavior of a variety of systems by modeling individual object–object relationships. This offers conceptual simplicity and great flexibility in solving complex problems. The MC solution to the considered problem demands the random sampling of many such object–object interactions to obtain the average values and associated (type A) uncertainties of the quantities of interest. For this repetitive task, computers rely on pseudorandom number generators which are invoked by sampling methods adapted to probability distribution functions that are specific to the problem at hand.

MC techniques are extensively used in radiation physics to model the transport (that is, propagation and interaction) of ionizing radiation through matter. In the mid-1930s, Fermi pioneered the MC study of neutron diffusion and, during the late 1940s, Ulam and von Neumann systematized the use of MC methods. MC simulation is superior to the numerical solution of the (deterministic) Boltzmann transport equation in two respects: (i) MC software can incorporate more accurate radiation–matter interaction cross sections as they become available, and (ii) it can track radiation through complex geometries. On the contrary, the transport equation is limited to tracking radiation through simple geometries using simplistic cross sections. In turn, the cross-section databases implemented in a specific MC program are used to derive the probability distribution functions from which the random variables that define the trajectories of the tracked radiation are sampled, namely, the distance to the next interaction point, the type of interaction, the energy loss and/or angular deflection, and the initial state of the emitted secondary radiations (if any) [19].

Photons only interact with matter a few times: either their energy is high and pair production is dominant, or after a few Compton collisions, they have lost so much energy that photoelectric absorption becomes the most likely fate. As a consequence, MC programs simulate all photon interactions in a detailed, i.e. event-by-event way. On the other hand, electrons with kinetic energies approaching or exceeding 1 MeV undergo a very large number of elastic or inelastic collisions before being slowed down to rest. In such cases, the associated simulation time becomes prohibitive and alternative strategies are adopted in which the global effect of many interactions is condensed into a smaller number of electron step lengths to improve the simulation speed [12].

The development of the first electronic computers and the continued increase in computational resources have facilitated the wide application of MC simulation to solve a large variety of problems in radiation physics. The success of MC methods is further explained by the availability of general-purpose MC programs, i.e. those that can simulate the coupled transport of photons and electrons with energies in a broad range (from around 1 keV to 1 GeV) and in arbitrary materials (elements, compounds, etc). The choice of MC code (GEometry ANd Tracking 4 (Geant4), Electron Gamma Shower (EGSnrc), PENetration and Energy LOss of Positrons and Electrons (PENELOPE), Monte Carlo N-Particle (MCNP), etc.) should primarily be motivated by the accuracy of the implemented physics models for the intended application. In the case of SFRT, Compton scattering and the photoelectric effect are the dominant interaction mechanisms, and the transport of the ejected Compton recoil electron and photoelectron plays an important role. It is also necessary to assess the sensitivity of the required results to specific interaction processes and the cross sections employed to track them. Examples of such analyses for MRT can be found in the articles by Siegbahn *et al* [20] and Spiga *et al* [21].

## 18.5 Monte Carlo simulation of megavoltage GRID therapy

Commercial TPSs have been previously used to compute dose distributions in GRID therapy. However, the performance of the available algorithms for the calculation of dose distributions in GRID therapy must be evaluated when small beams are employed. Such an evaluation should include comparisons with both independent MC simulations and experimental data. A physics and dosimetry white paper was recently published by the Radiosurgery Society's GRID/LATTICE, Microbeam and FLASH Radiotherapy Working Group; it provides some recommendations for the planning of SFRT dose distributions [22].

The first MC dosimetry evaluation in GRID radiotherapy was published by Zhang *et al* [23] in 2006. Their paper reported a full characterization of a GRID collimator. They showed good agreement between calculated and measured dose distributions. Some differences were reported for the apertures located away from the central axis due to the use of simplified photon source and collimator models. In addition, the source model did not consider electron contamination, leading to lower valley doses than the measured ones. The calculated dose distributions were combined with radiobiological models to assess cell survival and therapeutic ratios [23]. Posterior MC studies by Zhang *et al* [24, 25] investigated the impacts of tumor size and hypofractionation schemes on the therapeutic ratios of several types of tumors.

The influence of the beam size and peak-to-peak distance on different collimators was also evaluated by Gholami *et al* [26, 27], who conducted an extensive analysis of 25 collimators and assessed the therapeutic ratio using radiobiological models. They found that the optimum hole diameter should be between 1 and 1.25 cm, while the peak-to-peak distance should be in the range of 1.7–1.8 cm. Ha *et al* demonstrated the feasibility of generating grid distributions with a multileaf collimator [28]. The photoneutron dose contamination in GRID therapy was also assessed by Chegeni *et al* [29].

The use of smaller beam sizes in GRID therapy could allow the exploration of the dose–volume effects, as in MRT and MBRT. However, the advantages of micrometric field sizes are not preserved using clinical medical linear accelerators (LINACs) owing to the significant lateral scattering of MV x-rays, which reduces the peak–valley dose ratio (PVDR) in healthy tissues [30]. In addition, the beam size must be large so as not to dramatically decrease the dose rate. Martínez-Rovira *et al* [31] proved using MC simulations that the use of flattening-filter-free medical LINACs might offer the possibility of improving the therapeutic index of GRID therapy. This approach provided two main advantages: (i) a shift of the energy spectrum towards lower energies, resulting in an increase in the PVDR in healthy tissues; (ii) an increase in the photon fluence that compensates the loss in the dose rate if smaller field sizes of several millimeters are employed. MC simulations were also used to propose new strategies to improve GRID therapy with other types of beams and energies [32].

## 18.6 Monte Carlo simulation of synchrotron-based microbeam radiation therapy

The x-ray source used in MRT differs significantly from a LINAC. The bright synchrotron radiation used in MRT is produced when the trajectories of electrons that have been accelerated to very high energies (GeV) are deflected in devices consisting of a series of magnets, such as a wiggler. The beam is typically tuned by tens of meters of beam modifiers including filters, slits, diaphragms, and collimators. The final beam is highly linearly polarized in the electrons' orbital plane, the energy spectrum is in the kilovoltage range, and it has very low beam divergence. At the biomedical beamline of the European Synchrotron Radiation Facility (ESRF), the degree of linear polarization at the patient position is 0.994, the horizontal and vertical divergences are 0.5 mrad and 0.02 mrad, respectively, and the energy spectrum is in the kilovoltage range [33]. Figure 18.1 displays the energy spectrum of the MRT beam with respect to the photon beam generated in a conventional 6 MV LINAC, as well as the relevant photon interaction cross sections in water. These distinct beam features (which differ from those of conventional radiotherapy), along with the need for dose calculations at the micrometer scale, have limited the use of

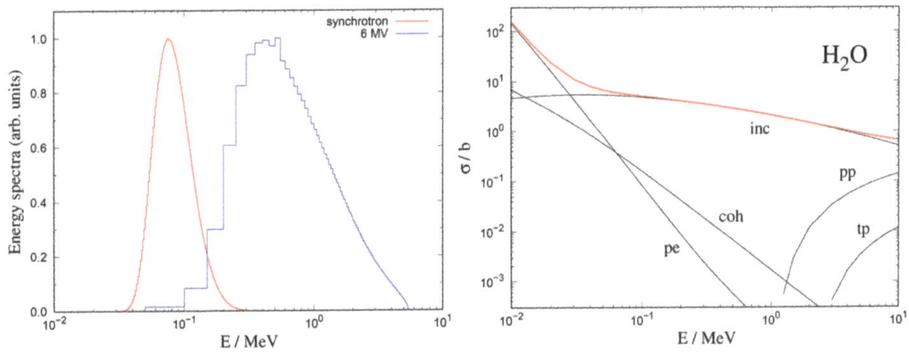


**Figure 18.1.** Left. Simulated energy spectra of the ESRF biomedical line (left histogram) [33] and of the 6 MV beam of a Varian Clinac C accelerator (right histogram) [34]; both spectra have been normalized to the maximum height. Right. Photon interaction cross sections for $H_2O$ as a function of energy; the thin black curves are the contributions of the photoelectric effect (pe), Rayleigh scattering (coh), Compton scattering (inc), pair production (pp), and triplet production (tp), while the thick red curve is the sum.

commercially available TPSs. Given this context, MC simulations play a key role in dose computation for MRT.

The first dosimetry studies ever published in MRT were mostly performed at the computational level [35–37]. In 1992, Slatkin *et al* [35] calculated the first dose distributions for cylindrical microbeams, which produced larger PVDR yields than planar microbeams due to the more rapid lateral dose falloff. However, only the latter have been used in MRT biological studies due to the limitations of manufacturing collimators that can produce micrometer-sized cylindrical beams.

Since then, numerous MC investigations using different MC codes have assessed the effects of the beam energy, beam width, peak-to-peak distance, irradiation geometry, and array size on the main dosimetric parameters in order to optimize MRT irradiation conditions [20, 21, 38–41]. The role of the array (tumor) size is particularly relevant. A clear reduction in PVDR values is observed when the field size (number of beams) increases due to the contribution of the tails of the outer beams to the central valley. As expected, a decrease in PVDR is also observed for tighter peak-to-peak distances due to the increase in the valley dose. Comprehensive MC data comparing several irradiation configurations can be found in [20, 21, 38–41]. The most used MRT configuration and the one retained for future clinical trials at the ESRF consisted of 50 μm wide microbeams spaced at 400 μm.

MC studies also confirmed the most favorable beam energy in terms of PVDR optimization. PVDR values should be low for cancer cells to achieve tumor control with a greater equivalent uniform dose (EUD). For the healthy tissues, PVDR values should be high (with a valley dose as low as possible) to ensure normal tissue sparing and thus, reduce the toxicity level by using a smaller EUD [42]. Shinohara *et al* [40] found that the optimum x-ray energy was in the range of 100–300 keV for the treatment of deep-seated tumors, and Prezado *et al* [43] found that the optimal energy was 175 keV. However, the use of higher energies in MRT still needs to be carefully assessed, since microbeam penumbras increase with the beam energy.

The simplification of the photon source has been a common practice in all these MRT MC studies, since a single parallel rectangular microbeam was typically simulated from the target surface and then a superposition algorithm was employed to retrieve the dose distributions of the full array. This methodology neglected the shape and divergence of the synchrotron source as well as the effect of the collimator. Nettelbeck *et al* [44] reported that simplifications in the source modeling led to important inaccuracies in the assessment of the valley doses, beam penumbra, and PVDR values. The inclusion of beam divergence resulted in penumbra doses up to 26% larger and valley doses up to 10% larger. The modeling of a synchrotron-distributed source showed sharp dose perturbations of up to 30% at the beam edges. The superposition of a single dose profile also led to differences in the valley dose and in the PVDR yields within 4% with respect to the full array modeling. Moreover, the inclusion of the multislit collimator resulted in differences of up to 8% in the beam width [44].

The effect of the beam polarization on the dose distributions was also analyzed through MC simulations by De Felici *et al* [38], Hugtenburg *et al* [45], and Bartzsch *et al* [46]. They results showed a significant influence in the absorbed dose outside the radiation field (dose differences of up to 40%). Within the radiation field, 3% dose differences were observed between simulations that included or excluded beam polarization.

Within this context, detailed source models that considered the beam production in the wiggler device as well as the beam transport through the whole beamline were developed. The work of Martínez-Rovira *et al* [33, 47] reported the first detailed photon source characterization of the ESRF Biomedical Beamline, which included the energy, spatial distribution, divergence, and polarization state of the beam. This information was used to generate a photon source model that was experimentally validated against a comprehensive dataset of radiochromic film measurements in homogenous and heterogeneous phantoms. This model was included in an MC calculation engine based on the PENELOPE code [19] interfaced with SHADOW [48], a synchrotron radiation and x-ray optics simulation tool. The code allowed dose computation in micrometer-sized bins in voxelized structures with adequate timings for radiotherapy treatments in synchrotron facilities. Similar MC calculation engines based on the Geant4 toolkit [49] were developed by Cornelius *et al* [50], Dipuglia *et al* [51], and Day *et al* [52], the latter of which included the beamline modeling at the biomedical beamline of the Australian Synchrotron. The work of Cornelius *et al* [50] included the vertical scanning of the patient that is needed to achieve tumor coverage due to the fact that the vertical dimension of the synchrotron beam is very small.

Among the different techniques used to reduce the computation time of MC simulations, optimization of the particle transport parameters or dose scoring methods is particularly relevant. Previous works showed that the photon and electron absorption energies at which the transport is discontinued should be carefully selected to minimize the computation time while retaining accurate MRT dose distributions [38, 47]. In addition, the dose computation in micrometer-sized voxels requires long calculation times to keep the statistical uncertainties of the computed doses low. Lin *et al* [53] established the maximum mesh dimensions for different microbeam sizes based on the variations of peak and valley doses and PVDR values caused by averaging effects. Hybrid dose calculation algorithms for MRT have recently been implemented in commercial TPSs to further minimize the computation time [54–56]. In these works, MC simulations compute photon transport, whereas convolution-based dose calculations are employed for secondary electron transport estimation.

In order to proceed toward forthcoming clinical trials in MRT, MC calculations have been combined with radiobiological models to establish safe irradiation protocols [57] as well as to identify optimal clinical scenarios for MRT [58]. MC simulations have also been used to explore the possibility of increasing the therapeutic index produced by high-atomic-number dose enhancers in the tumor prior to the administration of MRT [43, 53, 59].

## 18.7 Monte Carlo simulation of photon minibeam radiation therapy

In 2006, Dilmanian *et al* proposed the use of thicker microplanar beams as a novel radiosurgery approach with clinical potential [60]. The limitation of the thin beams (25–75 μm) employed in MRT is that they are constrained to the extremely high dose rates of synchrotrons in order to avoid the blurring of the dose distribution caused by cardio-synchronous pulsations. Instead, the wider beams (500–700 μm) used in MBRT can more easily achieve widespread clinical implementation, since minibeams are not as vulnerable to beam smearing caused by cardiac pulsations. Manchado *et al* [61] used MC simulations to assess the impacts of cardio-synchronous pulsations on MRT and MBRT dose distributions.

The MBRT configuration typically used in radiobiological studies consists of 600 μm wide microbeams spaced at 1200 μm. A few MC studies tried to optimize the irradiation configuration of MBRT [60, 62–64]. Using MC simulations, Dilmanian *et al* [60] technically proved the feasibility of interlacing two orthogonal arrays of minibeams to produce a homogeneous dose in a tumor. The mechanical precision required makes this type of irradiation extremely difficult when using microbeams. In addition, calculations revealed a very sharp dose falloff (30 μm) at the edge of the field compared to that of radiosurgery (2–5 mm), which is of great interest for tumors located near sensitive structures [60]. Moreover, Prezado *et al* [62] opened the door to the use of higher-energy photons for MBRT, which would allow the use of higher penetration powers. MC simulations showed that the optimum energy that maximizes the tumor dose while sparing healthy tissues would be 375 keV.

As was the case for MRT, the peculiar irradiation characteristics of synchrotron-based MBRT (energy, machine geometry, polarization, etc.) compared to those of conventional radiotherapy demanded the development of dedicated MC-based calculation engines able to compute dose distributions in voxelized structures at the micrometer scale. The first MBRT dose calculations in complex structures were published by Gokeri *et al* [65], who assumed that minibeams were parallel beams emerging from a phantom surface. Martínez-Rovira *et al* [66] developed the first

MC calculation engine for MBRT that included an accurate source model and experimentally verified it using heterogeneous phantoms.

As stated, photon MBRT has the potential to be implemented outside synchrotrons using commercially available x-ray equipment [67–69]. For this purpose, MC calculations have helped to implement photon MBRT in small-animal irradiators by optimizing beam modifiers, such as collimators, as well as computing accurate dose distributions using dedicated engines [67–69].

Finally, MC calculations carried out with the Geant4 code [49] and the Geant4-DNA extension [70] have also been employed to study the biological effects of MBRT through their micro- and nanodosimetric characteristics [71].

## 18.8 Knowledge gaps and future perspectives

Emerging radiotherapy techniques such as photon SFRT involve complex biological mechanisms that are not fully known at present. Although MC calculations are the most accurate dose computation tool when used properly, they will not be sufficient to answer some of the open questions in SFRT, such as the definition of the optimum configuration for forthcoming clinical trials in terms of beam energy, beam width, the spacing between beams, PVDRs, EUDs, etc. Further combined multidisciplinary studies will be required to understand how the physical parameters of the radiation impact the biological response and how this impact could be used to benefit the cancer treatments.

Regarding dose calculations, future clinical implementations of SFRT will demand faster calculation algorithms, especially for MRT and MBRT. However, the simulation of a very large number of particle histories is required to achieve the desired statistical accuracy at the micrometer scale and calculation times are too long for SFRT treatment planning and the optimization of beam parameters. These computing power requirements of MC simulations could restrict their routine clinical applicability. The use of hybrid dose calculation algorithms, variance-reduction techniques, parallelization methods, or graphical processing units might pave the way for MC dose calculations to be used in more routine SFRT clinical applications.

## 18.9 Conclusions

MC calculations are the gold standard for photon and electron transport. They play a key role in dose assessment for photon SFRT, in which the absorbed dose distribution must be determined at the micrometric scale. In the case of GRID therapy, the performance of the available dose calculation algorithms implemented in commercial TPSs needs to be evaluated/verified before they can be clinically applied. This process can be completed through validation based on MC calculations and comparisons with experimental data. In the specific cases of MRT and MBRT, the photon energies of the synchrotron beam and as its properties (polarization, divergence, and spatial distribution) render conventional kernel-based dose calculation algorithms inapplicable. Within this framework, MC calculations are essential, not only for the development of dedicated calculation engines able to evaluate (peak and valley) SFRT dose distributions in phantoms and patients, but also for the optimization of irradiation configurations, and the design of beam modifiers and collimators.

## References


[1] Hubbell J H 2006 Review and history of photon cross section calculations *Phys. Med. Biol.* **51** R245–62

[2] Salvat F and Fernández-Varea J M 2009 Overview of physical interaction models for photon and electron transport used in Monte Carlo codes *Metrologia* **46** 112–38

[3] Bransden B H and Joachain C J 2003 *Physics of Atoms and Molecules* (New York: Pearson Education)

[4] Sabbatucci L and Salvat F 2016 Theory and calculation of the atomic photoeffect *Radiat. Phys. Chem.* **121** 122–40

[5] Hubbell J H, Veigle W J, Briggs E A, Brown R T, Cromer D T and Howerton R J 1975 Atomic form factors, incoherent scattering functions and photon scattering cross sections *J. Phys. Chem. Ref. Data* **4** 471–538

[6] Hubbell J H 1997 Summary of existing information on the incoherent scattering of photons, particularly on the validity of the use of the incoherent scattering function *Radiat. Phys. Chem.* **50** 113–24

[7] Stutz G E 2014 Compton scattering cross section for inner-shell electrons in the relativistic impulse approximation *Nucl. Instrum. Methods Phys. Res., Sect.* B **319** 8–16

[8] Hubbell J H, Gimm H A and Overbo I 1980 Pair, triplet, and total atomic cross sections (and mass attenuation coefficients) for 1 MeV–100 GeV photons in elements $Z = 1$ to 100 *J. Phys. Chem. Ref. Data* **9** 1023–148

[9] Hubbell J H and Seltzer S M 2004 Cross section data for electron–positron pair production by photons: a status report *Nucl. Instrum. Methods Phys. Res., Sect.* B **213** 1–9

[10] Cullen D E, Hubbell J H and Kissel L 1997 EPDL97: the evaluated photon data library'97 version https://www.osti.gov/biblio/295438

[11] Berger M J, Hubbell J H, Seltzer S M, Chang J, Coursey J S and Sukumar R *et al* 2010 XCOM: Photon Cross Sections Database National Institute of Standards and Technology

[12] Berger M J and Wang R 1988 Multiple-scattering angular deflections and energy-loss straggling *Monte Carlo Transport of Electrons and Photons* ed T M Jenkins, W R Nelson and A Rindi (New York: Plenum)

[13] Seltzer S M 1988 Cross sections for bremsstrahlung production and electron-impact ionization, in Monte Carlo transport of electrons and photons *Monte Carlo Transport of Electrons and Photons* ed T M Jenkins, W R Nelson and A Rindi (New York: Plenum)

[14] International Commission on Radiation Units & Measurements 2007 *Elastic scattering of electrons and positrons* 77 ICRU https://www.icru.org/report/elastic-scattering-of-electrons-and-positrons-icru-report-77/

[15] Llovet X, Powell C J, Salvat F and Jablonski A 2014 Cross sections for inner-shell ionization by electron impact *J. Phys. Chem. Ref. Data* **43** 013102

[16] Seltzer S M and Berger M J 1986 Bremsstrahlung energy spectra from electrons with kinetic energy 1 keV–10 GeV incident on screened nuclei and orbital electrons of neutral atoms with Z = 1–100 *At. Data Nucl. Data Tables* **35** 345–418

[17] Mangiarotti A and Martins M N 2017 A review of electron–nucleus bremsstrahlung cross sections between 1 and 10 MeV *Radiat. Phys. Chem.* **141** 312–38

[18] Tessier F and Kawrakow I 2008 Calculation of the electron–electron bremsstrahlung cross-section in the field of atomic electrons *Nucl. Instrum. Methods Phys. Res., Sect.* B **266** 625–34
[19] Salvat F 2019 *PENELOPE 2018: A code system for Monte Carlo simulation of electron and photon transport* Nuclear Energy Agency
[20] Siegbahn E A, Stepanek J, Bräuer-Krisch E and Bravin A 2006 Determination of dosimetrical quantities used in microbeam radiation therapy (MRT) with Monte Carlo simulations *Med. Phys.* **33** 3248–59
[21] Spiga J, Siegbahn E A, Bräuer-Krisch E, Randaccio P and Bravin A 2007 The GEANT4 toolkit for microdosimetry calculations: application to microbeam radiation therapy (MRT) *Med. Phys.* **34** 4322–30
[22] Zhang H, Wu X, Zhang X, Chang S X, Megooni A and Donnelly E D *et al* 2020 Photon GRID radiation therapy: a physics and dosimetry white paper from the Radiosurgery Society (RSS) GRID/LATTICE, Microbeam and FLASH Radiotherapy Working Group *Radiat. Res.* **194** 665–77
[23] Zhang H, Johnson E L and Zwicker R D 2006 Dosimetric validation of the MCNPX Monte Carlo simulation for radiobiologic studies of megavoltage grid radiotherapy *Int. J. Radiat. Oncol. Biol. Phys.* **66** 1576–83
[24] Zhang H, Wang J Z, Mayr N, Kong X, Yuan J and Gupta N *et al* 2008 Fractionated grid therapy in treating cervical cancers: conventional fractionation or hypofractionation? *Int. J. Radiat. Oncol. Biol. Phys.* **70** 280–8
[25] Zhang H, Zhong H, Barth R F, Cao M and Das I J 2014 Impact of dose size in single fraction spatially fractionated (grid) radiotherapy for melanoma *Med. Phys.* **41** 021727
[26] Gholami S, Nedaie H A, Longo F, Ay M R, Wright S and Meigooni A S 2016 Is grid therapy useful for all tumors and every grid block design? *J. Appl. Clin. Med. Phys.* **17** 206–19
[27] Gholami S, Nedaie H A, Longo F, Ay M R, Dini S A and Meigooni A S 2017 Grid block design based on Monte Carlo simulated dosimetry, the linear quadratic and Hug–Kellerer radiobiological models *J. Med. Phys.* **42** 213–21
[28] Ha J K, Zhang G, Naqvi S A, Regine W F and Yu C X 2006 Feasibility of delivering grid therapy using a multileaf collimator *Med. Phys.* **33** 76–82
[29] Chegeni N, Karimi A H, Jabbari I and Arvandi S 2018 Photoneutron dose estimation in GRID therapy using an anthropomorphic phantom: a Monte Carlo study *J. Med. Signals Sens.* **8** 175–83
[30] Gokeri G, Kocar C, Tombakoglu M and Cecen Y 2013 Monte Carlo simulation of stereotactic microbeam radiation therapy: evaluation of the usage of a linear accelerator as the x-ray source *Phys. Med. Biol.* **58** 4621–42
[31] Martínez-Rovira I, Puxeu-Vaque J and Prezado Y 2017 Dose evaluation of grid therapy using a 6 MV flattening filter-free (FFF) photon beam: a Monte Carlo study *Med. Phys.* **44** 5378–83
[32] Martínez-Rovira I, Fois G and Prezado Y 2015 Dosimetric evaluation of new approaches in GRID therapy using nonconventional radiation sources *Med. Phys.* **42** 685–93
[33] Martínez-Rovira I, Sempau J and Prezado Y 2012 Development and commissioning of a Monte Carlo photon beam model for the forthcoming clinical trials in microbeam radiation therapy *Med. Phys.* **39** 119–31
[34] Brualla L, Rodriguez M, Sempau J and Andreo P 2019 PENELOPE/PRIMO-calculated photon and electron spectra from clinical accelerators *Radiat. Oncol.* **14** 6

[35] Slatkin D N, Spanne P, Dilmanian F A and Sandborg M 1992 Microbeam radiation therapy *Med. Phys.* **19** 1395–400

[36] Stepanek J, Blattmann H, Laissue J A, Lyubimova N, Di Michiel M and Slatkin D N 2000 Physics study of microbeam radiation therapy with PSI-version of Monte Carlo code GEANT as a new computational tool *Med. Phys.* **27** 1664–75

[37] Orion I, Rosenfeld A B, Dilmanian F A, Telang F, Ren B and Namito Y 2000 Monte Carlo simulation of dose distributions from a synchrotron-produced microplanar beam array using the EGS4 code system *Phys. Med. Biol.* **45** 2497–508

[38] De Felici M, Felici R, Sanchez del Rio M, Ferrero C, Bacarian T and Dilmanian F A 2005 Dose distribution from x-ray microbeam arrays applied to radiation therapy: an EGS4 Monte Carlo study *Med. Phys.* **32** 2455–63

[39] Anderson D, Siegbahn E A, Fallone B G, Serduc R and Warkentin B 2012 Evaluation of dose–volume metrics for microbeam radiation therapy dose distributions in head phantoms of various sizes using Monte Carlo simulations *Phys. Med. Biol.* **57** 3223–48

[40] Shinohara K, Kondoh T, Nariyama N, Fujita H, Washio M and Aoki Y 2014 Optimization of X-ray microplanar beam radiation therapy for deep-seated tumors by a simulation study *J. Xray Sci. Technol.* **22** 395–406

[41] Chicilo F, Hanson A L, Geisler F H, Belev G, Edgar A and Ramaswami K O *et al* 2020 Dose profiles and x-ray energy optimization for microbeam radiation therapy by high-dose, high resolution dosimetry using Sm-doped fluoroaluminate glass plates and Monte Carlo transport simulation *Phys. Med. Biol.* **65** 075010

[42] Dilmanian F A, Button T M, Le Duc G, Zhong N, Peña L A and Smith J A *et al* 2002 Response of rat intracranial 9L gliosarcoma to microbeam radiation therapy *Neuro Oncol.* **4** 26–38

[43] Prezado Y, Fois G, Le Duc G and Bravin A 2009 Gadolinium dose enhancement studies in microbeam radiation therapy *Med. Phys.* **36** 3568–74

[44] Nettelbeck H, Takacs G J, Lerch M L and Rosenfeld A B 2009 Microbeam radiation therapy: a Monte Carlo study of the influence of the source, multislit collimator, and beam divergence on microbeams *Med. Phys.* **36** 447–56

[45] Hugtenburg R P, Adegunloye A S and Bradley D A 2010 X-ray microbeam radiation therapy calculations, including polarisation effects, with the Monte Carlo code EGS5 *Nucl. Instrum. Methods Phys. Res.* A **619** 221–4

[46] Bartzsch S, Lerch M, Petasecca M, Bräuer-Krisch E and Oelfke U 2014 Influence of polarization and a source model for dose calculation in MRT *Med. Phys.* **41** 041703

[47] Martínez-Rovira I, Sempau J and Prezado Y 2012 Monte Carlo-based treatment planning system calculation engine for microbeam radiation therapy *Med. Phys.* **39** 2829–38

[48] Sanchez del Rio M, Canestrari N, Jiang F and Cerrina F 2011 SHADOW3: a new version of the synchrotron X-ray optics modelling package *J. Synchrotron Radiat.* **18** 708–16

[49] Agostinelli S, Allison J, Amako K, Apostolakis J, Araujo H and Arce P *et al* 2003 Geant4—a simulation toolkit *Nucl. Instrum. Methods Phys. Res.* A **506** 250–303

[50] Cornelius I, Guatelli S, Fournier P, Crosbie J C, Sanchez Del Rio M and Bräuer-Krisch E *et al* 2014 Benchmarking and validation of a Geant4-SHADOW Monte Carlo simulation for dose calculations in microbeam radiation therapy *J. Synchrotron Radiat.* **21** 518–28

[51] Dipuglia A, Cameron M, Davis J A, Cornelius I M, Stevenson A W and Rosenfeld A B *et al* 2019 Validation of a Monte Carlo simulation for microbeam radiation therapy on the imaging and medical beamline at the Australian Synchrotron *Sci. Rep.* **9** 17696

[52] Day L R J, Pellicioli P, Gagliardi F, Barnes M, Smyth L M L and Butler D *et al* 2020 A Monte Carlo model of synchrotron radiotherapy shows good agreement with experimental dosimetry measurements: data from the imaging and medical beamline at the Australian Synchrotron *Phys. Medica* **77** 64–74
[53] Lin H, Jing J, Xu L and Mao X 2017 Monte Carlo study of the influence of energy spectra, mesh size, high Z element on dose and PVDR based on 1-D and 3-D heterogeneous mouse head phantom for microbeam radiation therapy *Phys. Med.* **44** 96–107
[54] Debus C, Oelfke U and Bartzsch S 2017 A point kernel algorithm for microbeam radiation therapy *Phys. Med. Biol.* **62** 8341–59
[55] Donzelli M, Bräuer-Krisch E, Oelfke U, Wilkens J J and Bartzsch S 2018 Hybrid dose calculation: a dose calculation algorithm for microbeam radiation therapy *Phys. Med. Biol.* **63** 045013
[56] Day L R J, Donzelli M, Pellicioli P, Smyth L M L, Barnes M and Bartzsch S *et al* 2021 A commercial treatment planning system with a hybrid dose calculation algorithm for synchrotron radiotherapy trials *Phys. Med. Biol.* **66** 055016
[57] Martínez-Rovira I, Sempau J, Fernández-Varea J M, Bravin A and Prezado Y 2010 Monte Carlo dosimetry for forthcoming clinical trials in x-ray microbeam radiation therapy *Phys. Med. Biol.* **55** 4375–88
[58] Smyth L M L, Day L R, Woodford K, Rogers P A W, Crosbie J C and Senthi S 2019 Identifying optimal clinical scenarios for synchrotron microbeam radiation therapy: a treatment planning study *Phys. Med.* **60** 111–9
[59] Martínez-Rovira I and Prezado Y 2011 Monte Carlo dose enhancement studies in microbeam radiation therapy *Med. Phys.* **38** 4430–9
[60] Dilmanian F A, Zhong Z, Bacarian T, Benveniste H, Romanelli P and Wang R *et al* 2006 Interlaced x-ray microplanar beams: a radiosurgery approach with clinical potential *Proc. Natl Acad. Sci.* **103** 9709
[61] Manchado de Sola F, Vilches M, Prezado Y and Lallena A M 2018 Impact of cardiosynchronous brain pulsations on Monte Carlo calculated doses for synchrotron micro- and minibeam radiation therapy *Med. Phys.* **45** 3379–90
[62] Prezado Y, Thengumpallil S, Renier M and Bravin A 2009 X-ray energy optimization in minibeam radiation therapy *Med. Phys.* **36** 4897–902
[63] Deman P, Vautrin M, Stupar V, Barbier E L, Elleaume H and Esteve F *et al* 2011 Monochromatic minibeam radiotherapy: theoretical and experimental dosimetry for preclinical treatment plans *Phys. Med. Biol.* **56** 4465–80
[64] Martínez-Rovira I and Prezado Y 2014 Minibeam radiation therapy for the management of osteosarcomas: a Monte Carlo study *Med. Phys.* **41** 061706
[65] Gokeri G, Kocar C and Tombakoglu M 2010 Monte Carlo simulation of microbeam radiation therapy with an interlaced irradiation geometry and an Au contrast agent in a realistic head phantom *Phys. Med. Biol.* **55** 7469–87
[66] Martínez-Rovira I, Sempau J and Prezado Y 2014 Monte Carlo-based dose calculation engine for minibeam radiation therapy *Phys. Med.* **30** 57–62
[67] Esplen N M, Chergui L, Johnstone C D and Bazalova-Carter M 2018 Monte Carlo optimization of a microbeam collimator design for use on the small animal radiation research platform (SARRP) *Phys. Med. Biol.* **63** 175004

[68] González W, Dos Santos M, Guardiola C, Delorme R, Lamirault C and Juchaux M *et al* 2020 Minibeam radiation therapy at a conventional irradiator: dose-calculation engine and first tumor-bearing animals irradiation *Phys. Med.* **69** 256–61

[69] Treibel F, Nguyen M, Ahmed M, Dombrowsky A, Wilkens J J and Combs S E *et al* 2021 Establishment of microbeam radiation therapy at a small-animal irradiator *Int. J. Radiat. Oncol. Biol. Phys.* **109** 626–36

[70] Incerti S, Baldacchino G, Bernal M, Capra R, Champion C and Francis Z *et al* 2010 The Geant4-DNA project *Int. J. Modeling Simul. Sci. Comput.* **1** 157–78

[71] Dos Santos M, Delorme R, Salmon R and Prezado Y 2020 Minibeam radiation therapy: a micro- and nano-dosimetry Monte Carlo study *Med. Phys.* **47** 1379–90

**IOP** Publishing

Spatially Fractionated, Microbeam and FLASH Radiation Therapy
A physics and multi-disciplinary approach
**Hualin Zhang and Nina A Mayr**

# Chapter 19

## Monte Carlo simulation of proton SFRT

**Tim Schneider, Ludovic De Marzi and Ramón Ortiz**

Monte Carlo (MC) simulations represent an essential tool with which to study the different techniques of proton spatially fractionated radiation therapy (pSFRT). They are used to design collimators, investigate dose distributions, calculate treatment plans, perform radioprotection studies, and also to simulate radiochemical and radiobiological mechanisms. The most commonly used MC simulation platforms are GEometry ANd Tracking 4 (Geant4) and in particular the derived codes Geant4 Application for Emission Tomography (GATE) and TOol for PArticle Simulation (TOPAS); however, pSFRT studies have also been carried out using Monte Carlo N-Particle (MCNP), FLUktuierende KAskade (FLUKA), and RayStation. Despite many similarities to the simulation of conventional uniform fluence proton therapy, MC studies of proton SFRT may require different physics and scoring settings in order to fully resolve the highly heterogeneous dose distributions.

### 19.1 Introduction

Monte Carlo (MC) techniques comprise a broad class of numerical methods that are characterized by their use of random sampling at one or multiple steps during the computational process. Since their introduction to medical physics in the 1960s and 70s [1, 2], MC simulations have become an essential tool for photon and proton therapy studies, with applications ranging from physics research to radiation protection and the development of treatment planning systems.

In the field of pSFRT, MC simulations are mainly used in the context of proton minibeam radiation therapy (pMBRT) which uses lateral beamlet sizes in the range of about 0.1–1 mm; these are often too small to be properly handled by software developed for conventional proton therapy (PT). In addition, MC software has also been used in a few studies of proton GRID (beamlet widths of 1–2 cm) and microbeams (beamlet widths <0.1 mm).

doi:10.1088/978-0-7503-4046-5ch19  

The aim of this chapter is to briefly introduce the principal software, techniques, and simulation settings that have been used for MC studies of pSFRT and to present the most important application fields. Readers who are interested in the basic principles of the MC method are referred to the many comprehensive documents that can be found in the literature (see, for example, Seco and Verhaegen [3], Rogers and Bielajew [4], Rogers [5], and Verhaegen and Seuntjens [6] for general discussions of MC simulation in radiation therapy as well as a dedicated chapter in Paganetti [7] for a summary of MC simulation in proton therapy).

## 19.2 Building and running MC simulations

This section will briefly present the software that is typically used to perform MC simulations for pSFRT studies and sketch out the basic steps used to build and run such simulations. While general principles should apply to most of the different MC software in use today, concrete examples will focus on the two simulation platforms TOPAS and GATE.

### 19.2.1 Commonly used software

In the context of pSFRT studies, the most commonly used MC codes today are TOPAS [8, 9] and GATE [10, 11] which are both based on the open-source simulation toolkit Geant4 [12–14]. Geant4 was designed as a general software package to simulate the passage of particles through matter and is widely used in various domains such as high-energy and nuclear physics as well as astro- and radiation physics. It was first developed in the 1990s and is maintained by the Geant4 collaboration [12, 15].

Geant4 is a library written in the programming language C++, containing building blocks that are common to general particle simulations. In order to build a Geant4 simulation, a user has to write and compile a custom C++ program using building blocks from the library. This makes Geant4 very versatile MC software which can be customized and, due to its open-source code, extended by a user. At the same time, Geant4 may be less accessible to users lacking experience in C++ programming.

To address this usability barrier, GATE and TOPAS were designed as platforms built on top of Geant4. Both toolkits provide a high-level macro language, allowing a more straightforward creation of MC simulations through the definition of simple macro files. In these files, the user defines the geometry, particle source types, and physics to be simulated as well as the desired quantities to be tallied and the output data to be saved (see sections 19.2.2 and 19.2.3).

GATE was first publicly released in 2004 as software dedicated to the simulation of nuclear imaging techniques (specifically single-photon emission computed tomography (SPECT) and positron emission tomography (PET)) but has since been extended to other medical imaging applications and radiation therapy [10, 16]. It is developed and maintained by the OpenGATE collaboration [11]. TOPAS was launched in 2009 as a simulation tool for proton therapy and has since been

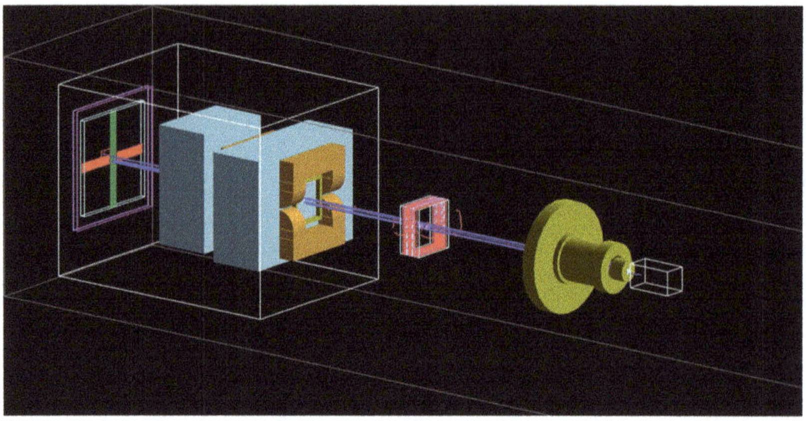

**Figure 19.1.** Examples of a pencil beam scanning nozzle and a minibeam collimator (gold-colored cylindrical structure in the right half of the image) modeled in TOPAS.

expanded to more general radiation therapy applications as well as radiobiological simulations [17]. It is currently maintained and distributed by TOPAS MC Inc. [9].

GATE and TOPAS include very similar feature sets, so the toolkit chosen for a given simulation is generally a question of the user's personal preference. A fundamental difference between the two platforms lies in the distribution methods: GATE, just like Geant4, is an open-source project, whereas TOPAS is a proprietary package requiring executable-only user licenses [18] (free research licenses are available). In the context of proton SFRT, TOPAS, and GATE have been used for pMBRT simulations [19–22] and in particular for the development and optimization of minibeam collimators [23–26] (see section 19.4.1).

Other MC studies of proton minibeams have been carried out using the FLUKA [27–29] software as well as Geant4-generated dose distributions of individual minibeams [30–32], which were further processed using the computational environment Laser Accelerated Particle extension for the Computational Environment for Radiotherapy Research (LAP-CERR) [33, 34]. Furthermore, proton GRID treatment plans [35, 36] have been computed using MCNP [37, 38] and the RayStation MC dose calculation algorithm [39]. Finally, MC software packages dedicated to radiochemical and radiobiological simulations, such as Geant4-DNA [40, 41] TRAX and TRAX-CHEM [42], have also found their first applications in proton SFRT (figure 19.1) (see section 19.4.5).

### 19.2.2 Setting up the simulation

In order to set up an MC simulation for proton therapy, the user has to go through different steps, which may vary from one software package to another. In general, however, four categories must be specified: (i) the geometry to be simulated; (ii) the beam or source of the irradiation; (iii) the data to be recorded or the output to be generated and (iv) the physics processes to be included in the simulation (see section 19.2.3).

In TOPAS and GATE, the simulation geometry can be created using predefined primitive solids (cubes, cylinders, spheres, etc.) which can be nested and stacked to build more complex geometries. Alternatively, geometry components generated with CAD (computer-aided design) software can be imported as well as medical imaging files such as DICOM. Each geometry component is then assigned a material, which can either be chosen from a database of predefined materials and elements or constructed by specifying its chemical composition (element or isotope content) as well as its physical properties (density, aggregate state, etc). Finally, the electromagnetic fields may be attached to geometry components. This can be useful to model the focussing and scanning magnets of pencil beam scanning and proton minibeam nozzles [43, 44].

A typical example of a geometry component used in pSFRT simulations is a collimator. It can be modeled as a solid block, typically made of brass or tungsten, containing multiple air-filled daughter volumes that represent the slits or holes of the collimator. Many MC software products also offer a generic way to model a single hole of an arbitrary shape which can then be replicated and placed at other locations in a parametrized way to easily create entire patterns (see e.g. the *genericRepeater* option in GATE or the *specialized components* in TOPAS).

A central aspect of every radiotherapy MC simulation is the definition of the beam or radiation source. For applications in proton therapy, there are two common approaches: either to create a parametrized beam source or to use a phase space source. A parametrized source requires the definition of the particle type, the particle energy distribution (usually assumed to be Gaussian and specified by the mean energy and the energy spread, i.e. the standard deviation of the Gaussian), and the spatial and angular distributions of the beam particles. The latter two are usually assumed to be Gaussian (especially when working with pencil beams), although flat distributions are also possible. Finally, it may be necessary to also define the beam emittance or alternatively the correlation coefficient between the spatial and angular distributions. These parameters become particularly important in the context of magnetically focussed minibeams, as a small divergence or a strong correlation between the beam's spatial and angular distributions is required to achieve small beam sizes at the focal point [43, 44].

In contrast, phase space sources use long tables (stored in so-called *phase space files*) of particles and their properties (particle type, energy, position, direction of momentum) to define how new particles are created at the source position. Phase space files can sometimes be obtained directly from a manufacturer or a reference database but often have to be constructed through dedicated, preceding MC simulations using e.g. parametrized beam sources. Their advantage is that they can replace the full simulation of complex geometry components by starting the simulated particles at a position closer to the target region, which may result in a drastic reduction in the computation time. On the flip side, phase space files have to contain sufficiently large amounts of data (usually at least several millions of particles) to ensure statistically sound simulation results.

Finally, the user has to specify the quantities to be assessed during the simulation and the output to be generated. Apart from the aforementioned phase space files, typical quantities of interest in proton therapy simulations are the dose, the linear energy transfer (LET), the fluence, and information about the generated secondary particles. TOPAS and GATE provide predefined modules (called *scorers* and *actors*, respectively) for the most commonly considered quantities. Typical output formats are plain text (ASCII characters), comma-separated-value (CSV) tables, binary files, and files following the ROOT framework standard [45].

### 19.2.3 Physics and scoring settings

The definition of the appropriate physics is imperative to ensure that a MC simulation yields correct results. While, in principle, only one *true* physics model exists, in practice it may be advantageous to approximate or exclude certain physical processes in order to speed up the simulation. In many MC software packages, it is therefore left to the user to define the physics to be simulated. The Geant4-based toolkits provide the concepts of *physics list builders* for this task, which allow the user to put together predefined electromagnetic and hadronic *physics lists* containing the physical processes relevant for different application cases.

The physical processes involved in pSFRT are the same as those relevant to conventional PT. Consequently, the same physics lists as those recommended for conventional PT can be used in pSFRT studies [25, 46–49]. As an example, a typical physics list used in TOPAS simulations is built using the *Geant4_Modular* option with *g4em-standard_opt3, g4h-phy_QGSP_BIC, g4decay, g4ion-binarycascade, g4h-elastic_HP, g4stopping,* and *g4radioactivedecay* modules. However, when dealing with the small beamlet sizes of mini- and microbeams, extra care should be taken with respect to resolution parameters such as the *range cut* (the production threshold for secondary particles after EM interactions) and the *step size* (the distance to the next interaction), which may have a significant effect, for example, on the dose deposition calculation.

Figure 19.2 illustrates the influence of the range cut on the lateral dose profiles. Simulations were run for four different range cut values (0.1, 0.05, 0.01, and 0.001 mm) and three different techniques, namely conventional broad beam PT, proton GRID (with a beamlet width of 1 cm) and pMBRT (with a beamlet width of 0.8 mm). The beam source, voxel size, and other physics settings were identical in all

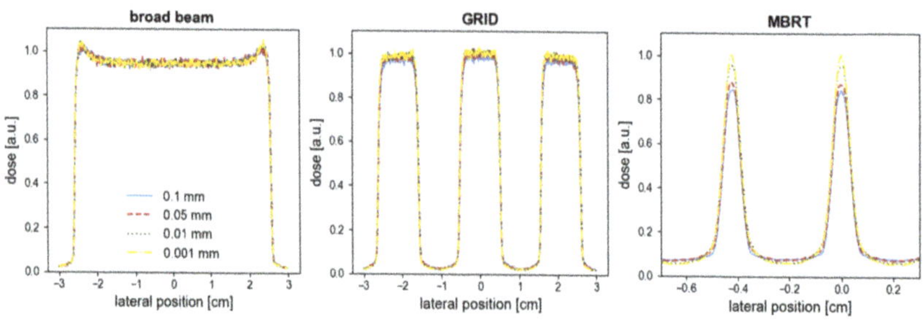


**Figure 19.2.** Lateral dose profiles at different range cuts for broad beam irradiation (left), proton GRID (center), and pMBRT (right).

**Table 19.1.** The influence of the range cut on the peak–valley dose ratio (PVDR).

| Range cut (mm) | PVDR | |
|---|---|---|
| | *GRID* | *MBRT* |
| 0.1 | 41.7 ± 1.7 | 12.1 ± 0.3 |
| 0.05 | 41.6 ± 1.7 | 13.0 ± 0.3 |
| 0.01 | 47.7 ± 2.1 | 17.6 ± 0.5 |
| 0.001 | 50.1 ± 2.2 | 18.4 ± 0.5 |

cases and the GRID and minibeam patterns were produced by collimators. While they had no discernible effect on the broad beam dose, it was found that higher cut values led to a reduction of the peak dose for the SFRT techniques, and for minibeams, they also led to an overestimation of the valley dose. Consequently, large deviations of the peak–valley dose ratio (PVDR) of up to 20%–35% were observed, as shown in table 19.1.

The range cut therefore needs to be tuned to ensure a realistic dose deposition calculation. This value needs to be selected in each particular case, depending on the beamlet size. For proton minibeams, a range cut of 100–500 μm is commonly used [21, 25, 47, 49]. In proton GRID calculations, Henry *et al* [46] considered values of 200 and 400 μm for beamlets of 0.5 and more than 1 cm full width at half maximum (FWHM), respectively. The range cut also influences the proton range calculations, as reported by Grevillot *et al* [50]. When the range cut is sufficiently low, the effect of the step size limitation becomes negligible [50]. Regarding the database binning for electromagnetic interactions, Grevillot *et al* reported that this binning needs to be set to a value larger than 15 bins per decade to ensure that interactions are independent of the range cut and step size values. MC studies of proton SFRT commonly consider values from 20 to 100 bins per decade [48].

Regardless of the definition of the physics processes, the computed dose and LET distributions may be also affected by the resolution of the scoring. Proton GRID and pMBRT fields may require higher spatial resolutions than those of conventional proton fields to accurately score the high- and low-dose regions that characterize SFRT. Figure 19.3 illustrates the effect of the scoring voxel size on the lateral dose profiles. Three voxel sizes (0.1, 0.5, and 1.0 mm) were considered and simulated for the same three techniques mentioned above. Again, while the broad beam distributions seem to be unaffected by the change in voxel size, a significant effect is observed in the GRID and MBRT dose profiles and resulting PVDR values shown in table 19.2. The peak doses are reduced for increasing voxel dimensions. In addition, the homogeneity of the pMBRT profile may be affected by this parameter, since the scoring results of the peak doses are influenced by the position of the peak with respect to the voxel position, leading to a possible volume averaging effect.

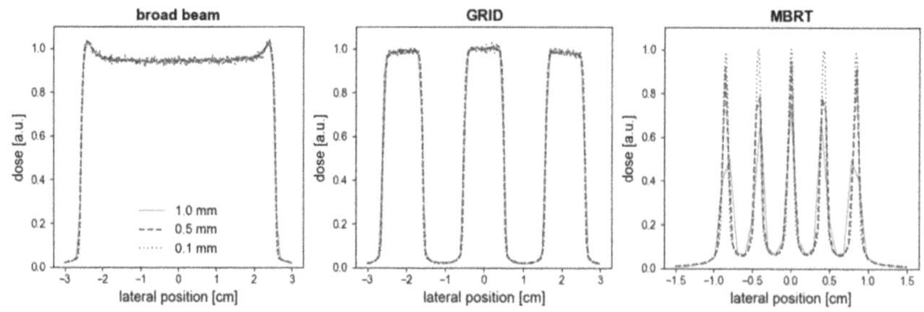


**Figure 19.3.** Lateral dose profiles at different voxel sizes for broad beam irradiation (left), proton GRID (center), and pMBRT (right).

**Table 19.2.** The influence of the voxel size on the peak-to-valley dose ratio (PVDR).

| Voxel size (mm) | PVDR | |
|---|---|---|
| | *GRID* | *MBRT* |
| 1.0 | 44.7 ± 0.7 | 11.8 ± 0.2 |
| 0.5 | 47.5 ± 1.0 | 14.9 ± 0.3 |
| 0.1 | 49.7 ± 2.0 | 18.1 ± 0.5 |

Consequently, the maximum voxel size used to score realistic radiation–matter interactions should be adjusted depending on the beamlet size, spacing, and, by extension, the frequency of the spatial dose modulation. Studies of pMBRT at beamlet widths >0.7 mm FWHM at the scoring volume used typical voxel sizes of typically 0.1 mm and at most 0.2 mm in the direction of spatial fractionation [25, 47, 49, 51], while proton GRID simulations worked with beamlet widths from 0.5 to 3 mm and voxel dimensions greater than 0.1 mm [46].

### 19.2.4 Statistical uncertainties of MC simulations

MC simulations simulate individual particle *histories*, i.e. the trajectories of single particles and their associated secondary particles which can undergo multiple different interactions according to predefined probability density functions. A consequence of this is that each simulated history produces a slightly different result and leads to different values of the investigated quantities. Simulating a large number of particles and combining the results of many histories (e.g. by summing or averaging) eventually allows the scored quantity of interest to converge to a stable value. The accuracy of this value is given by the statistical uncertainty.

The main quantities of interest considered in pSFRT (i.e. the dose, LET, and derived quantities) are typically calculated on a voxel basis. In TOPAS and GATE, the corresponding scoring actors are able to report the statistical measures (such as the variance, standard deviation, and other moments) of the scored quantities in each voxel.

For cumulative quantities, such as the dose, the uncertainty can be calculated using the method described by Chetty *et al* [52]:

$$\bar{s}_{d_k} = \sqrt{\frac{1}{N-1}\left(\frac{\sum_{i=1}^{N} d_{k,i}^2}{N} - \left(\frac{\sum_{i=1}^{N} d_{k,i}}{N}\right)^2\right)},$$

where $\bar{s}_{d_k}$ is the standard error of the mean in the voxel $k$, $d$ is the quantity of interest in the $k$th voxel produced by independent history $i$, and $N$ is the total number of primary histories. With respect to LET uncertainties, the standard deviation of the LET values is calculated by taking the standard deviation of the LET values of each repetition divided by the square root of the number of independent repetitions [43].

The uncertainty of MC simulations is usually not reported at the voxel level, but rather expressed as a global uncertainty over a considered target volume. Different methods are used to compute such a global uncertainty. A common approach is to state the root mean square of the uncertainties of the bins with a dose greater than a certain percentage of the maximum dose (e.g. 50% or 90%). Typical values for a global dose uncertainty computed in this way range from 0.4% to 3% [25, 47, 49, 51]. Alternatively, a limit can be set for the maximum voxel uncertainty in the considered scoring volume [48].

Regarding derived quantities such as the PVDR or peak–valley LET ratio (PVLT), the corresponding uncertainty must be calculated by propagating the uncertainties of each independent variable of the derived quantity according to the following equation:

$$\Delta X(a, b, \ldots, z) = \sqrt{\left(\frac{dX}{da}\right)^2 \Delta a^2 + \left(\frac{dX}{db}\right)^2 \Delta b^2 + \ldots + \left(\frac{dX}{dz}\right)^2 \Delta z^2},$$

where $\Delta X$ is the uncertainty of the derived quantity $X$ and $\Delta a$, $\Delta b$, and $\Delta z$ are the uncertainties of the variables $a$, $b$, and $z$.

## 19.3 Validation of MC simulations

The validation of MC simulations can generally be divided into two types. The first type refers to tests of the simulation code itself and the accuracy of the implemented physics processes. This can be done by simulating geometrically simple setups (e.g. only a beam in air or a water volume) and by individually considering the different physical processes (scattering, secondary production, etc.) and quantities (stopping power, cross sections, etc). The second type arises for the simulation of specific beam delivery or irradiation setups and typically consists of the validation of a specific beam, beamline, or nozzle model.

While many studies have validated general PT simulations in TOPAS [53–56] and GATE [50, 57, 58] (see also the work of the Geant4 Medical Simulation

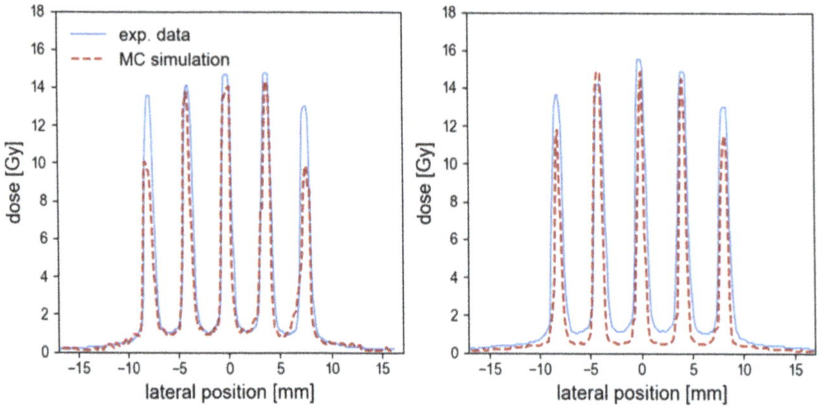


**Figure 19.4.** Simulation of collimated proton minibeams at a PBS nozzle, showing the full nozzle model (left) and a model starting at the nozzle exit with a virtual beam source (right), which leads to an underestimation of the valley doses.

Benchmarking Group [59, 60]), recent studies have also focused on pSFRT cases. In this context, Guardiola *et al* verified a collimator-based proton minibeam implementation installed at a passive scattering beamline modeled with GATE [22]. To validate the model, lateral and longitudinal dose profiles as well as the PVDR were simulated and experimentally measured in a water tank and a solid water phantom. The dose measurements were carried out with radiochromic films and the PTW microDiamond detector [61].

In another study, De Marzi *et al* validated a TOPAS model of a collimator-based pMBRT implementation at a PBS nozzle [21]. Lateral and longitudinal dose profiles as well as the PVDR in a water tank were assessed and compared to measurements performed with the IBA RAZOR diode [62] and a plane parallel chamber. The team evaluated two cases, first modeling the complete PBS nozzle and then starting from a virtual beam source placed at the nozzle exit. A significant underestimation of the valley doses was found in the latter case (the virtual beam source), whereas an excellent agreement of both peak and valley doses could be obtained with the full model (see figure 19.4). This highlights the importance of accurately reproducing the sources for beam scattering and the low-intensity halos of proton pencil beams, in particular when simulating collimator-based SFRT techniques.

## 19.4 Applications of MC simulations for proton SFRT

### 19.4.1 Optimization of collimators

Physical collimators are commonly used in SFRT to attenuate or block the beam in order to create the characteristic spatial fractionation patterns. In particular, the generation of clinically relevant proton minibeams still relies on this technique, since current proton therapy facilities cannot deliver small enough beams. MC simulations play an important role in the design of such collimators, as they provide a means to quickly, cost-effectively, and accurately test different collimator geometries before starting the actual manufacturing process.

In this context, Guardiola *et al* [25] used MC simulations to optimize a collimator design for planar minibeams and to determine the collimator material, thickness, slit shape, intraslit spacing, and collimator-to-phantom distance. Similar studies, also evaluating different slit or hole widths, were performed by Lee *et al* [24] and for pencil-shaped minibeams by Charyyev *et al* [23] and Tobola-Galus *et al* [29].

Considering factors such as the PVDR, dose rate, neutron yield, relative valley, and peak dose as well as ease of manufacture, a reasonable trade-off was achieved with collimators 5–6 cm thick made out of brass and collimator-to-phantom distances of 2–5 cm. Depending on the beam energy and application case, good results were obtained with slit widths ranging from 0.3 to 0.7 mm spaced at interslit distances (measured from center to center) from 1 to 3.5 mm [24, 25].

It should be noted that the aforementioned studies considered static collimators, which are typically optimized for a specific irradiation case. In order to provide a more flexible approach, Sotiropoulos *et al* [26] developed the new concept of dynamic minibeam collimators composed of either one or two collimation layers forming a single, adjustable minibeam slit. Mounting the collimator on a hexapod attached to the exit of a PBS nozzle allows the single-slit collimator to be moved to allow the delivery of dose patterns with multiple planar minibeams. The team used MC simulations performed with TOPAS to evaluate and compare several collimator designs and has already conducted a proof-of-concept experiment.

### 19.4.2 Supporting dosimetry for experiments

In addition to optimizing hardware components such as collimators, MC methods are also important tools that are widely used to support the dosimetry preceding an experiment. A common practice consists of experimental dosimetry campaigns in which lateral dose profiles are measured at different significative depths using high-spatial-resolution detectors, such as radiochromic films or a microdiamond detector. MC simulations, previously benchmarked against experimental data [21], are then performed with the purpose of calculating dose distributions for the target volume in the animal or human patient to be treated. The simulation results, combined with the experimental data acquired for verification of the irradiation conditions, are then used to determine the dose prescription in terms of *monitor units* [63].

MC simulations may be also useful after irradiation, since it is a common practice to measure dose profiles at the time of irradiation using radiochromic films placed around the irradiated samples [64, 65]. MC simulations can then be used to trace back the dose delivered to a given position in the irradiated volume, which may help, for instance, in the interpretation of unexpected observations occurring during a long-term follow-up of irradiated subjects.

### 19.4.3 Treatment planning

To be able to compute the dose distribution for clinical patients, suitable software called a treatment planning system (TPS) is needed. This requires conventional TPS

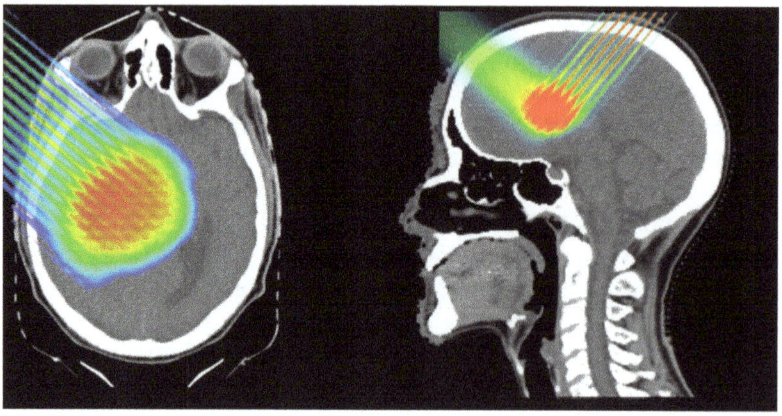

**Figure 19.5.** Examples of a pMBRT plan dose distribution for two different intracranial cases computed with TOPAS.

algorithms to be adapted to: (i) model minibeams (in particular for SFRT with beamlet widths <0.5 mm) and external collimators with submillimetric resolution; (ii) compute the dose distribution generated by these beam geometries with a submillimeter resolution in heterogeneous volumes or patient images; and (iii) optimize the treatment plan, in particular taking into account specific SFRT constraints such as the transverse and longitudinal optimisation of the peak and valley dose profile in healthy tissues and the dose given to the target (figure 19.5).

MC simulations, due to their versatility of use, are very well adapted to this type of calculation and are widely used for the simulation of clinical treatment plans with conventional irradiation techniques. Their use in SFRT irradiation is therefore a logical choice [19], and initial studies have shown that they can be used to simulate SFRT clinical plans in a realistic way.

For now, very few studies have compared possible pSFRT treatment plans with the plans made by current techniques, such as pencil beam scanning (PBS) or intensity-modulated radiation therapy (volumetric modulated arc therapy (VMAT) or stereotactic radiotherapy (RT)) for various clinical cases. In the works of Guardiola *et al* [22] and Kłodowska *et al* [28], hybrid analytical algorithms and Monte Carlo dose calculations (GATE and FLUKA, respectively) were used to optimize the spot positions and relative weights of individual Bragg peaks composing the field and thus produce spread-out Bragg peaks (SOBP) and homogeneous depth–dose distributions. These first studies have shown the possibility of achieving quasi-clinical dose distributions (in 3D in large volumes, with SOBP, and at high proton energies) with very small minibeams (widths <0.5 mm). Proton GRID therapy using a PBS technique was also successfully developed and clinically implemented [35] using a TPS and an analytical pencil beam algorithm which were benchmarked against MCNP Monte Carlo simulations.

Simulations and treatment plans for intracranial cases have shown that pMBRT may provide satisfactory treatment plans with only one or two proton minibeam arrays delivered in a clinical center with little modification of the existing beamlines [47, 66].

Finally, several teams have focused on quantities that are typically accessible through Monte Carlo simulations [20, 47, 67]: indeed, as the LET distributions may be useful for the interpretation of biological effects in proton therapy as well as for the computation of relative biological effectiveness (RBE)-weighted dose distributions, the dose-averaged LET is often computed in Monte Carlo or TPS programs. These types of simulation have revealed variations in the LET distribution from 1 to 3 keV $\mu m^{-1}$ between the peak and valley regions in healthy tissues due to secondary particle scattering effects in the valley dose areas, which could have an impact in terms of RBE [47].

### 19.4.4 Radiation protection

The secondary radiation fields of concern produced by pMBRT irradiators consist mainly of stray neutrons, which are mainly produced inside the patient or by the scattering elements of the nozzle, such as range modulator wheels, scatterers, or beam-shaping devices (brass collimators and compensators). In order to study the potential impact of these neutrons on healthy tissues in patients, experimental measurements, Monte Carlo simulations, or analytical computations can be used to assess the exposure of organs as well as the ambient dose within the treatment room. However, as demonstrated by many studies [68, 69], the secondary neutron dose received by a patient in conventional proton therapy is highly dependent on patient-specific variables such as age, size, tumor morphology, and location as well as irradiation-specific parameters such as the beamline configuration, the SOBP width and depth, and the number of beams. Beyond that, the variation of stray neutrons inside and outside the irradiated area is a complex issue, as external neutrons (from the treatment head or the aperture) are usually a significant component of the secondary dose at a distance from the target, while the dose deposited by internal neutrons may be more significant inside the treatment field.

Since the measurement of the effective neutron dose is challenging, MC simulations are usually parameterized to evaluate the neutron fluence as a function of the energy spectrum, which is then multiplied by a fluence-to-dose equivalent conversion factor to obtain the ambient dose equivalent. Several methods have been proposed to accurately estimate the dose and ambient dose equivalent delivered to the normal tissues of proton therapy patients, and a comprehensive comparison of normal tissue dose and risk across different proton beam delivery methods (in particular passive scattering, PBS, and pMBRT) has been published [66, 69].

One study in particular [66] demonstrated that an increased secondary neutron dose relative to passive or active proton therapy techniques should be expected in planar minibeam proton therapy, which would be more pronounced in organs situated closer to the irradiated target and less pronounced in organs located further away from the target. However, although the neutron yield generated by a multislit collimator might be increased, the biological neutron dose in the phantom or patient is still expected to be less than 1% of the total absorbed dose [25]. In another study, a second type of collimator with holes arranged in a hexagonal pattern was also studied, and the ambient neutron dose equivalent was tallied at different angles and distances from a water phantom [23]. As for a planar arrangement, simulations have shown that the neutron dose could increase by a factor of ten due to the presence of the physical collimator, but it remains less than those produced by conventional passively scattered proton beams.

The different materials used in the mechanical generation of small beamlets (e.g. tungsten, brass, nickel, and iron) as well as their dimensions, shapes, and distances have also been evaluated in the context of SFRT. For example, it has been shown that tungsten offers improved dose distributions (the highest PVDR and lowest penumbra) compared with other lighter materials [25]. However, protons interacting in the collimator generate nuclear reactions, which cause a significant emission of neutrons and can significantly contribute to the secondary dose received by normal tissues. Regarding neutron emission, tungsten leads to neutron yields roughly three to four times greater than those of the other materials [25, 70].

### 19.4.5 The radiobiology of proton SFRT

One of the most recent application fields for MC simulations concerns research into the radiobiological mechanisms underlying the specific effects observed in proton SFRT. Comprehensive radiobiological simulations are still very challenging due to the complexity and, in some cases, still unknown details of biological systems, radiation response, and damage repair pathways. Nevertheless, toolkits such as Geant4-DNA [40, 41], the derived TOPAS-n-Bio platform [71], and the software TRAX-CHEM [42] offer features to simulate not only the primary radiation–matter interaction, down to energies of a few electronvolts, but also the ensuing radiochemical processes, such as the creation and diffusion of solvated electrons and reactive oxygen species. Moreover, endpoints such as single- and double-strand DNA breaks can be quantified and some DNA repair mechanisms may be modeled [72, 73].

In the context of proton SFRT, Dos Santos *et al* [74] used Geant4-DNA to conduct a micro- and nano-dosimetric study comparing pMBRT to x-ray and electron MBRT. They were able to show that protons yield an increased number of complex DNA damage clusters at the end of the range, which, compared to the other considered techniques, could provide a benefit in the treatment of radio-resistant tumors. In another study, Dal Bello *et al* [75] used TRAX-CHEM to propose and investigate a chemical mechanism to explain the efficacy of proton minibeam and x-ray microbeam irradiations. They suggested that the creation of hydrogen peroxide in the peak dose regions and its diffusion to the valley regions could be a possible actor for the improved treatment outcome and successfully tested their model by comparing it with the dosimetric data of previous mini- and microbeam experiments.

## 19.5 Knowledge gaps and future perspectives

Despite the progress of pSFRT in the last decade, in part thanks to the support of MC simulations, there are still several knowledge gaps that should be addressed in the forthcoming years to fully exploit the benefits of pSFRT techniques.

The demand for commercial TPS software to support the clinical implementation of different pSFRT approaches is still unfulfilled. While proton GRID treatments with beamlet widths of 1–2 cm can be planned and optimized using any existing clinical TPS, techniques using submillimeter beamlets, such as pMBRT, require spatial resolutions beyond those offered by currently available solutions. In addition, current clinical TPSs typically do not support the simulation of mechanical collimators, which have been used, for instance, in several minibeam studies. Therefore, dedicated pSFRT TPS software is needed for the clinical implementation of those techniques.

Concerning the validation of the MC software products used for pSFRT, a further benchmark using complex phantoms will be necessary. To date, pSFRT MC simulations have only been validated using simple experimental data measured in water, solid water, or plastic phantoms consisting of rectangular slabs [21, 76]. Studies comparing simulated and experimentally measured data using more complex phantom geometries (e.g. animal and anthropomorphic phantoms) are to be undertaken to further validate MC models of pSFRT techniques and to promote the transition towards clinical implementation.

Finally, it will be imperative to further improve our understanding of the radiobiological mechanisms underlying the distinct effects that pSFRT treatments have on cancerous and healthy tissues through biological and clinical studies. In this context, the few existing studies demonstrate that MC simulations, although still at an early stage for radiobiological applications, could potentially provide a powerful tool with which to advance radiobiology research in this field.

## 19.6 Conclusions

Monte Carlo simulations are an essential tool for research, development, and treatment planning in proton therapy. In the context of pSFRT, they are widely used to design and optimize collimators, compute macro- and microscopic dose distributions, perform radioprotection studies, and even to investigate basic radiochemical and radiobiological processes. Users can choose one of these available software packages and toolkits for research-oriented MC simulations (popular examples include TOPAS, GATE, FLUKA, and MCNP) as well as treatment planning software with MC features (e.g., RayStation). While MC simulations of pSFRT are generally very similar to those of conventional PT techniques, extra care should be taken with respect to resolution parameters such as the range cut and scoring voxel size, as these parameters may have a significant effect on the simulation results. Due to the increasing need for high-precision dose calculation engines and considering the ongoing improvements in computational hardware, it appears that MC simulations will continue to play a central role in pSFRT research and may even find their way into routine clinical practice.

## References

[1] Berger M J, Seltzer S M, Domen S R and Lamperti P J 1975 *Stopping-Power Ratios for Electron Dosimetry with Ionization Chambers International symposium on advances in*

*biomedical dosimetry* (Vienna: IAEA) pp 589–609 https://inis.iaea.org/search/search.aspx?orig_q=RN:7225299

[2] Berger M J 1963 Monte Carlo calculation of the penetration and diffusion of fast charged particles *Methods Comput. Phys.* **1**

[3] Seco J and Verhaegen F (ed) 2016 *Monte Carlo Techniques in Radiation Therapy* (Boca Raton, FL: CRC Press)

[4] Rogers D W O and Bielajew A F 1990 *The Dosimetry of Ionizing Radiation, Volume III* ed K R Kase, B E Bjarngard and F H Attix (San Diego, CA: Academic)

[5] Rogers D W O 2006 Fifty years of Monte Carlo simulations for medical physics *Phys. Med. Biol.* **51** R287–301

[6] Verhaegen F and Seuntjens J 2003 Monte Carlo modelling of external radiotherapy photon beams *Phys. Med. Biol.* **48** R107–64

[7] Paganetti H 2012 *Proton Therapy Physics* ed H Paganetti (Boca Raton, FL: CRC Press)

[8] Perl J, Shin J, Schumann J, Faddegon B and Paganetti H 2012 TOPAS: an innovative proton Monte Carlo platform for research and clinical applications *Med. Phys.* **39** 6818–37

[9] TOPAS MC Inc. www.topasmc.org (accessed 10 January 2022)

[10] Jan S *et al* 2011 GATE V6: a major enhancement of the GATE simulation platform enabling modelling of CT and radiotherapy *Phys. Med. Biol.* **56** 881–901

[11] OpenGATE collaboration http://www.opengatecollaboration.org/ (accessed 10 January 2022)

[12] Agostinelli S *et al* 2003 Geant4 – a simulation toolkit *Nucl. Instrum. Methods Phys. Res.* A **506** 250–303

[13] Allison J *et al* 2016 Recent developments in Geant4 *Nucl. Instrum. Methods Phys. Res.* A **835** 186–225

[14] Geant4 https://geant4.web.cern.ch (accessed 10 January 2022)

[15] Geant4 Collaboration members https://geant4.web.cern.ch/collaboration/members (accessed 10 January 2022)

[16] Sarrut D *et al* 2021 Advanced Monte Carlo simulations of emission tomography imaging systems with GATE *Phys. Med. Biol.* **66** 10TR03

[17] Faddegon B, Ramos-Méndez J, Schuemann J, McNamara A, Shin J, Perl J and Paganetti H 2020 The TOPAS tool for particle simulation, a Monte Carlo simulation tool for physics, biology and clinical research *Phys. Med.* **72** 114–21

[18] TOPAS MC license https://www.topasmc.org/license (accessed 10 January 2022)

[19] Prezado Y and Fois G R 2013 Proton-minibeam radiation therapy: a proof of concept *Med. Phys.* **40** 031712

[20] Meyer J *et al* 2017 Biological and dosimetric characterisation of spatially fractionated proton minibeams *Phys. Med. Biol.* **62** 9260–81

[21] De Marzi L, Patriarca A, Nauraye C, Hierso E, Dendale R, Guardiola C and Prezado Y 2018 Implementation of planar proton minibeam radiation therapy using a pencil beam scanning system: a proof of concept study *Med. Phys.* **45** 5305–16

[22] Guardiola C, De Marzi L and Prezado Y 2020 Verification of a Monte Carlo dose calculation engine in proton minibeam radiotherapy in a passive scattering beamline for preclinical trials *Br. J. Radiol.* **93** 20190578

[23] Charyyev S, Artz M, Szalkowski G, Chang C-W, Stanforth A, Lin L, Zhang R and Wang C-K C 2020 Optimization of hexagonal-pattern minibeams for spatially fractionated radiotherapy using proton beam scanning *Med. Phys.* **47** 3485–95

[24] Lee E, Meyer J and Sandison G 2016 Collimator design for spatially-fractionated proton beams for radiobiology research *Phys. Med. Biol.* **61** 5378–89

[25] Guardiola C, Peucelle C and Prezado Y 2017 Optimization of the mechanical collimation for minibeam generation in proton minibeam radiation therapy *Med. Phys.* **44** 1470–78

[26] Sotiropoulos M and Prezado Y 2021 A scanning dynamic collimator for spot-scanning proton minibeam production *Sci. Rep.* **11** 18321

[27] Böhlen T, Cerutti F, Chin M, Fassò A, Ferrari A, Ortega P, Mairani A, Sala P, Smirnov G and Vlachoudis V 2014 The FLUKA code: developments and challenges for high energy and medical applications *Nucl. Data Sheets* **120** 211–14

[28] Kłodowska M, Olko P and Waligórski M P R 2015 Proton microbeam radiotherapy with scanned pencil-beams – Monte Carlo simulations *Phys. Medica* **31** 621–6

[29] Tobola-Galus A, Swakon J and Olko P 2018 Dosimetric characterization of collimators for spatially fractionated proton therapy of the eye *Radiat. Prot. Dosim.* **180** 351–54

[30] Girst S *et al* 2016 Proton minibeam radiation therapy reduces side effects in an *in vivo* mouse ear model *Int. J. Radiat. Oncol. Biol. Phys.* **95** 234–41

[31] Sammer M, Greubel C, Girst S and Dollinger G 2017 Optimization of beam arrangements in proton minibeam radiotherapy by cell survival simulations *Med. Phys.* **44** 6096–104

[32] Sammer M, Girst S and Dollinger G 2021 Optimizing proton minibeam radiotherapy by interlacing and heterogeneous tumor dose on the basis of calculated clonogenic cell survival *Sci. Rep.* **11** 3533

[33] Deasy J O, Blanco A I and Clark V H 2003 CERR: a computational environment for radiotherapy research *Med. Phys.* **30** 979–85

[34] Schell S and Wilkens J J 2010 Advanced treatment planning methods for efficient radiation therapy with laser accelerated proton and ion beams *Med. Phys.* **37** 5330–40

[35] Gao M, Mohiuddin M M, Hartsell W F and Pankuch M 2018 Spatially fractionated (GRID) radiation therapy using proton pencil beam scanning (PBS): feasibility study and clinical implementation *Med. Phys.* **45** 1645–53

[36] Mohiuddin M, Lynch C, Gao M and Hartsell W 2020 Early clinical results of proton spatially fractionated GRID radiation therapy (SFGRT) *Br. J. Radiol.* **93** 20190572

[37] Werner C J *et al* 2018 MCNP Version 6.2 Release Notes, 2

[38] Fair J L 2016 Spatially fractionated proton therapy: a Monte Carlo verification *Master's Thesis* Georgia Tech http://hdl.handle.net/1853/55045

[39] Schreuder A N, Bridges D S, Rigsby L, Blakey M, Janson M, Hedrick S G and Wilkinson J B 2019 Validation of the RayStation Monte Carlo dose calculation algorithm using realistic animal tissue phantoms *J. Appl. Clin. Med. Phys.* **20** 160–71

[40] Bernal M A *et al* 2015 Track structure modeling in liquid water: a review of the Geant4-DNA very low energy extension of the Geant4 Monte Carlo simulation toolkit *Phys. Med.* **31** 861–74

[41] Incerti S *et al* 2018 Geant4-DNA example applications for track structure simulations in liquid water: a report from the Geant4-DNA Project *Med. Phys.* **45** e722–39

[42] Boscolo D, Krämer M, Durante M, Fuss M and Scifoni E 2018 TRAX-CHEM: a pre-chemical and chemical stage extension of the particle track structure code TRAX in water targets *Chem. Phys. Lett.* **698** 11–8

[43] Schneider T 2020 Advancing the generation of proton minibeams for radiation therapy *PhD Thesis* Université Paris-Saclay https://theses.hal.science/tel-03105944

[44] Schneider T, Patriarca A, Degiovanni A, Gallas M and Prezado Y 2021 Conceptual design of a novel nozzle combined with a clinical proton linac for magnetically focussed minibeams *Cancers (Basel)* **13** 4657
[45] ROOT Data Analysis Framework https://root.cern (accessed 10 January 2022)
[46] Henry T, Bassler N, Ureba A, Tsubouchi T, Valdman A and Siegbahn A 2017 Development of an interlaced-crossfiring geometry for proton grid therapy *Acta Oncol.* **56** 1437–43
[47] Lansonneur P, Mammar H, Nauraye C, Patriarca A, Hierso E, Dendale R, Prezado Y and De Marzi L 2020 First proton minibeam radiation therapy treatment plan evaluation *Sci. Rep.* **10** 7025
[48] Martínez-Rovira I, Fois G and Prezado Y 2015 Dosimetric evaluation of new approaches in GRID therapy using nonconventional radiation sources *Med. Phys.* **42** 685–93
[49] Schneider T, De Marzi L, Patriarca A and Prezado Y 2021 Monte Carlo comparison of proton and helium-ion minibeam generation techniques *Front. Phys.* **9** 35
[50] Grevillot L, Frisson T, Zahra N, Bertrand D, Stichelbaut F, Freud N and Sarrut D 2010 Optimization of GEANT4 settings for proton pencil beam scanning simulations using GATE *Nucl. Instrum. Methods Phys. Res.* B **268** 3295–305
[51] Peucelle C 2016 Spatial fractionation of the dose in charged particle therapy *PhD Thesis* Université Paris Saclay https://theses.hal.science/tel-01432875
[52] Chetty I J, Rosu M, Kessler M L, Fraass B A, Ten Haken R K, Kong F-M S and McShan D L 2006 Reporting and analyzing statistical uncertainties in Monte Carlo-based treatment planning *Int. J. Radiat. Oncol. Biol. Phys.* **65** 1249–59
[53] Testa M, Schümann J, Lu H-M, Shin J, Faddegon B, Perl J and Paganetti H 2013 Experimental validation of the TOPAS Monte Carlo system for passive scattering proton therapy *Med. Phys.* **40** 121719
[54] Liu H, Li Z, Slopsema R, Hong L, Pei X and Xu X G 2019 TOPAS Monte Carlo simulation for double scattering proton therapy and dosimetric evaluation *Phys. Medica* **62** 53–62
[55] Lin L, Ainsley C G, Solberg T D and McDonough J E 2014 Experimental characterization of two-dimensional spot profiles for two proton pencil beam scanning nozzles *Phys. Med. Biol.* **59** 493–504
[56] De Marzi L, Da Fonseca A, Moignier C, Patriarca A, Goudjil F, Mazal A, Buvat I and Hérault J 2019 Experimental characterisation of a proton kernel model for pencil beam scanning techniques *Phys. Medica* **64** 195–203
[57] Resch A F, Elia A, Fuchs H, Carlino A, Palmans H, Stock M, Georg D and Grevillot L 2019 Evaluation of electromagnetic and nuclear scattering models in GATE/Geant4 for proton therapy *Med. Phys.* **46** 2444–56
[58] Winterhalter C *et al* 2020 Evaluation of GATE-RTion (GATE/Geant4) Monte Carlo simulation settings for proton pencil beam scanning quality assurance *Med. Phys.* **47** 5817–28
[59] G4MSBG initiative: G4-Med https://twiki.cern.ch/twiki/bin/view/Geant4/G4MSBG (accessed 10 January 2022)
[60] Arce P *et al* 2021 Report on G4-Med, a Geant4 benchmarking system for medical physics applications developed by the Geant4 Medical Simulation Benchmarking Group *Med. Phys.* **48** 19–56
[61] Marinelli M, Prestopino G, Verona C and Verona-Rinati G 2016 Experimental determination of the PTW 60019 microDiamond dosimeter active area and volume *Med. Phys.* **43** 5205

[62] Liu P Z Y, Reggiori G, Lobefalo F, Mancosu P, Tomatis S, McKenzie D R and Suchowerska N 2016 Small field correction factors for the IBA Razor *Phys. Medica* **32** 1025–9

[63] Bertho A *et al* 2021 First evaluation of temporal and spatial fractionation in proton minibeam radiation therapy of glioma-bearing rats *Cancers (Basel)* **13** 4865

[64] Prezado Y *et al* 2018 Proton minibeam radiation therapy widens the therapeutic index for high-grade gliomas *Sci. Rep.* **8** 16479

[65] Prezado Y *et al* 2019 Tumor control in RG2 glioma-bearing rats: a comparison between proton minibeam therapy and standard proton therapy *Int. J. Radiat. Oncol. Biol. Phys.* **104** 266–71

[66] Maia Leite A, Ronga M G, Giorgi M, Ristic Y, Perrot Y, Trompier F, Prezado Y, Créhange G and De Marzi L 2021 Secondary neutron dose contribution from pencil beam scanning, scattered and spatially fractionated proton therapy *Phys. Med. Biol.* **66** 225010

[67] Henry T and Ödén J 2018 Interlaced proton grid therapy – linear energy transfer and relative biological effectiveness distributions *Phys. Medica* **56** 81–9

[68] Bonfrate A, Farah J, De Marzi L, Delacroix S, Hérault J, Sayah R, Lee C, Bolch W E and Clairand I 2016 Influence of beam incidence and irradiation parameters on stray neutron doses to healthy organs of pediatric patients treated for an intracranial tumor with passive scattering proton therapy *Phys. Medica* **32** 590–9

[69] Sayah R *et al* 2014 Secondary neutron doses received by paediatric patients during intracranial proton therapy treatments *J. Radiol. Prot.* **34** 279–96

[70] Charyyev S and Wang C-K C 2020 Assessment of ambient neutron dose equivalent in spatially fractionated radiotherapy with protons using physical collimators *Radiat. Prot. Dosim.* **189** 190–7

[71] Schuemann J, McNamara A L, Ramos-Méndez J, Perl J, Held K D, Paganetti H, Incerti S and Faddegon B 2019 TOPAS-nBio: an extension to the TOPAS simulation toolkit for cellular and sub-cellular radiobiology *Radiat. Res.* **191** 125–38

[72] McMahon S J, Schuemann J, Paganetti H and Prise K M 2016 Mechanistic modelling of DNA repair and cellular survival following radiation-induced DNA damage *Sci. Rep.* **6** 33290

[73] Henthorn N T, Warmenhoven J W, Sotiropoulos M, Mackay R I, Kirkby N F, Kirkby K J and Merchant M J 2018 In silico non-homologous end joining following ion induced DNA double strand breaks predicts that repair fidelity depends on break density *Sci. Rep.* **8** 2654

[74] Dos Santos M, Delorme R, Salmon R and Prezado Y 2020 Minibeam radiation therapy: a micro- and nano-dosimetry Monte Carlo study *Med. Phys.* **47** 1379–90

[75] Dal Bello R, Becher T, Fuss M C, Krämer M and Seco J 2020 Proposal of a chemical mechanism for mini-beam and micro-beam efficacy *Front. Phys.* **8** 452

[76] Peucelle C, Nauraye C, Patriarca A, Hierso E, Fournier-Bidoz N, Martínez-Rovira I and Prezado Y 2015 Proton minibeam radiation therapy: experimental dosimetry evaluation *Med. Phys.* **42** 7108–13

# Part III

## Physics of microbeam, minibeam SFRT and ultra-high dose rate FLASH therapy

# Chapter 20

## Microbeam SFRT with photons

**Valentin Djonov, Cristian Fernandez-Palomo and Paolo Pellicioli**

This chapter introduces the reader to microbeam radiotherapy (MRT), the spatially fractionated approach with the smallest possible heterogeneous dose distribution. The chapter takes the reader from the development of MRT to the basic concepts in the field. Against this background, the chapter covers the properties of photon microbeams from the basic to the most complex: size, shape, energy, collimators, radiation sources, MRT modalities, and dosimetry. It then discusses the effects of MRT on normal tissues and all the possibilities of MRT for tumor control, such as multidirectional microbeams, high ablative doses, preferential vascular effects, immune responses, temporal fractionation of microbeams, combinations with drugs, and MRT as a drug delivery system.

### 20.1 Introduction

Conventional radiotherapy uses large radiation fields to treat tumors with a homogeneous dose. The limiting factor of such a homogeneous dose is the occurrence of radiotoxicity in normal tissue. To reduce the toxicity of this treatment to normal tissue, the most commonly used strategy is to fractionate the dose over time. However, the dose can also be distributed in space in the form of a heterogeneous radiation field. This inhomogeneous radiation field is the basis of spatially fractionated radiation therapy (SFRT), which treats tumors with a series of multiple beams (figure 20.1). SFRT was introduced by Alban Koehler in 1909 in the form of GRID therapy, in which a grid of centimeter-wide openings was placed in an x-ray beam to produce a series of centimeter-wide beams [1]. Later, in the 1980s, GRID therapy evolved into minibeam radiation therapy, in which the beam width was reduced to a few millimeters, and in the early 1990s, the beam width was reduced to the micrometer range with the introduction of MRT [2].

doi:10.1088/978-0-7503-4046-5ch20

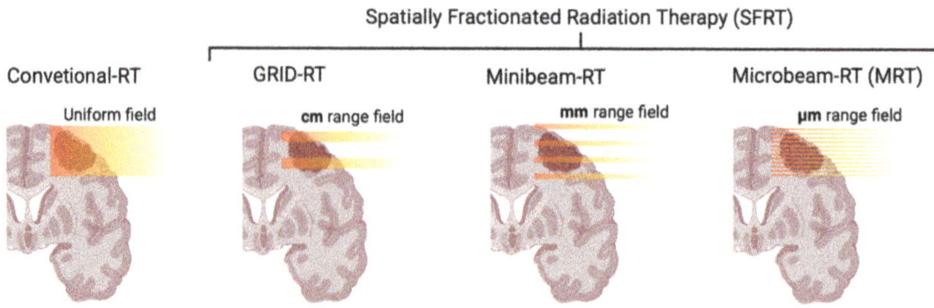


**Figure 20.1.** The evolution of SFRT from a uniform field to an array of micron-wide microbeams. Created with BioRender.com.

### 20.1.1 Basic definitions

The spatial fractionation of radiation in GRID, minibeam, and microbeam radiotherapy has the distinct advantage of reducing the volume of tissue exposed to the dose (figure 20.1), which increases the tolerance of normal tissue. This inversely proportional effect has been defined as the '**dose/volume effect**' and is more pronounced with smaller beams, as used in MRT.

MRT is the SFRT modality that can take full advantage of the dose/volume effect. This advantage results from the extremely thin, 23–100 µm wide microbeams that make up the MRT array [3]. The width of each microbeam is important because, since a mouse cell has an average diameter of 10–20 µm, each microbeam dose, commonly referred to as a '**peak dose**,' can only laterally hit one to ten cells in its path, depending on cell diameter and concentration. This means that the cells outside the microbeam are spared from the peak dose (figure 20.2). However, they still receive a lower dose contribution due to radiation scattered into the target, which is called the '**valley dose**.' Thus, the higher the peak dose, the higher the valley dose.

It is important to remember that the transition from the peak dose to the valley dose is not geometrically perfect due to scattered and secondary radiation. Therefore, there is an area of dose transition in MRT called the **penumbra** (figure 20.2). The penumbra can greatly impact the biological effects of MRT, because thin microbeams 25 µm wide can sometimes show effects equivalent to 50 µm beams due to the penumbra alone [4].

To obtain a large dose/volume effect with MRT, one should try to keep the peak dose high and the valley dose low. The concept known as the **peak–valley dose ratio (PVDR)** is an indicator of this difference. In other words, the PVDR is the ratio between the peak dose and the valley dose and it is understood that the higher the PVDR, the sharper the difference between the peak and the valley.

Since microbeams are so thin, lateral cell damage in their path is not severe as long as the valley dose remains low. The best strategy for keeping the valley dose low is to increase the distance between the microbeams that make up the MRT array. In general, the **spacing** between microbeams is defined as the **center-to-center (c-t-c)** distance between them, and this distance is normally fixed, depending on the collimator (see section 20.2.3).

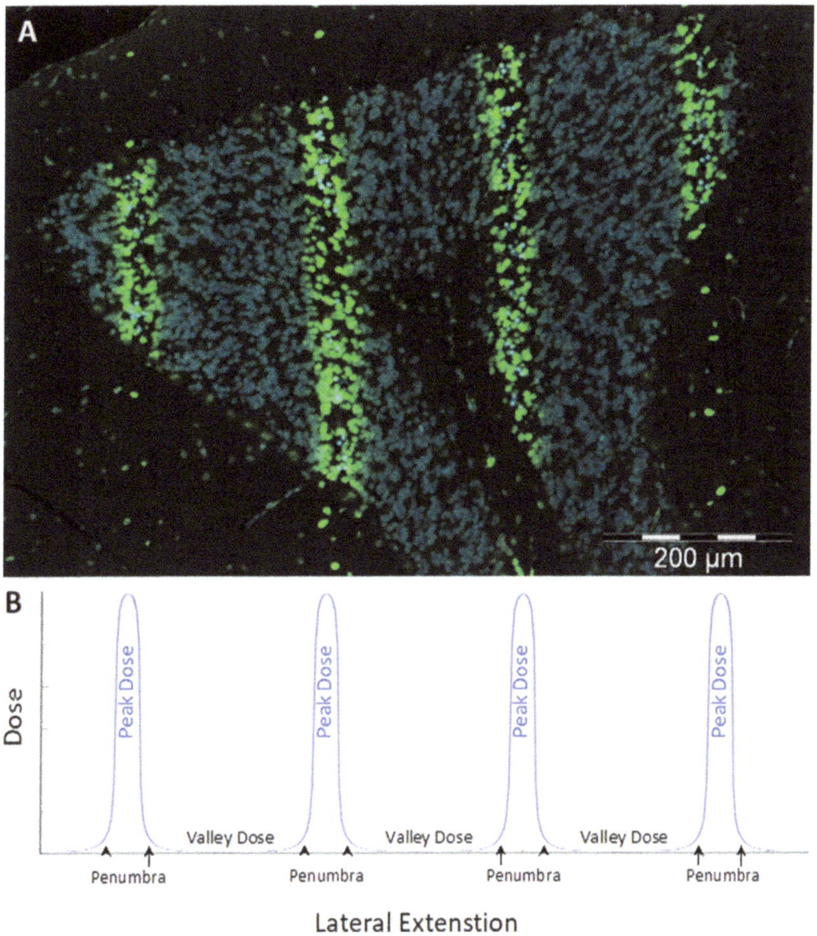


**Figure 20.2.** Dose profile of MRT adjacent to a histologic section showing DNA damage. (A) The cerebellum of a rat 8 h after irradiation with a peak dose of 350 Gy using microbeams of 25 μm spaced at 200 μm at the European Synchrotron Facility (ESRF). The cerebellum shows a variable concentration of green-stained cells in the microbeam path, indicating positivity for $\gamma$-H2AX. The blue color indicates 4',6-diamidino-2-phenyl-indole (DAPI) counterstaining. (B) A graphical representation of the MRT dose profile showing the respective peak and valley doses and penumbra.

## 20.2 Characteristics of photon microbeams

### 20.2.1 Microbeam size and shape

Defining the most effective microbeam geometry was key at the beginning of MRT development, as tissues such as the cerebellum of piglets could withstand peak doses of up to 600 Gy [5]. Research has shown that rats with intracranial 9L gliosarcoma treated with an array of 27 μm wide beams in stepwise mode had increased survival rates when irradiated with beams spaced at 75–100 μm c-t-c [6]. In studies of mouse mammary carcinomas, better tumor control was observed when an array of 50 μm

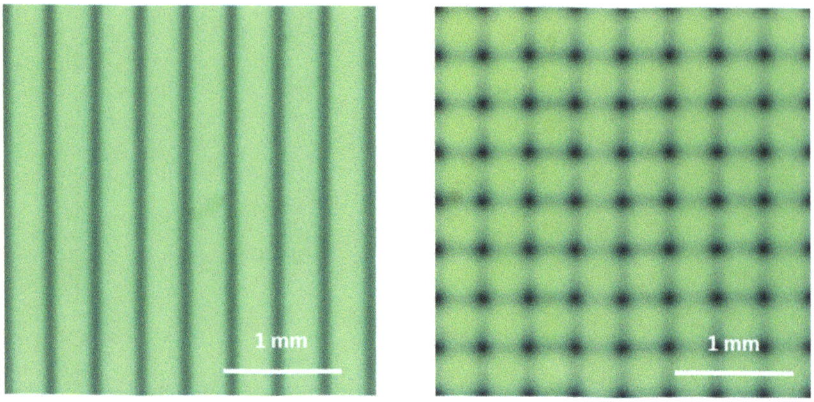


**Figure 20.3.** Two-dimensional dose distribution geometry of an array of microbeams (left) and pencil beams (right) of 50 μm wide beamlets, spaced at 400 μm c-t-c. The radiation fields were recorded using radiochromic films.

wide beams spaced at 200 μm c-t-c was used compared to that obtained using an array of 500 μm wide beams spaced at 2000 μm c-t-c [7]. Following this series of systematic studies, MRT configurations using arrays of 50 μm wide microbeams spaced at 200–400 μm c-t-c have been widely used because they not only provide excellent survival curves and tumor control, but can also be generated and controlled with technical reliability.

An array of microbeams is defined by spatial fractionation of the radiation field in one of the directions perpendicular to the direction of beam propagation. The microbeams are therefore a few tens of micrometers wide and up to a few centimeters long to cover the target extent. More extreme configurations use spatial fractionation in both directions, creating a matrix of beam spots called pencil beams [8]. This geometry further increases the PVDR and allows for better preservation of normal tissue, even with larger irradiated volumes [9]. A visual example of the dose distribution of micro- and pencil beams acquired using radiochromic films can be found in figure 20.3.

One of the main features of MRT is the steep dose gradient at the edge of the microbeams. The penumbra, also known as the extent of the beam shoulder, is usually no more than a few tens of micrometers wide and is usually defined as an 80%–20% [10] or 90%–10% [11] falloff of the peak dose.

A fundamental requirement of microbeam irradiation is to maintain the width of the beams at the micrometer scale as they traverse the target volume. Therefore, **minimal beam divergence** is required to define quasi-parallel microbeams. Beam divergence also affects the extent of the beam penumbra due to scattering and possible total reflection effects that photons may encounter as they traverse beam stoppers and multislit collimators [12, 13] (see section 20.2.3).

### 20.2.2 Photon energy

In MRT, the choice of x-ray radiation energy is a critical issue because the maintenance of high dose gradients and steep penumbras can only be achieved if the secondary electrons generated during irradiation, which are responsible for most of the delivered dose, have a short travel range before slowing down to rest.

Observations of the interaction between x-rays and water [14] for 50 keV photons show that a non-negligible fraction of the high-energy electrons is released by the photoelectric effect. At 100 keV, photons interact mainly by Compton scattering, and about 13 keV is transferred to secondary electrons. At 200 keV, photons transfer about 44 keV to electrons after Compton scattering. Considering these photon energies, electrons at 10 keV, 30 keV, and 50 keV have a travel range of 3 μm, 18 μm, and 43 μm in water, respectively [15]. Photons with an energy of about 100 keV are therefore the most favorable radiation source with which to obtain a steep dose gradient in MRT [16]. Irradiation with MeV photons would produce a cloud of high-energy electrons, resulting in degradation of the spatially fractionated geometry, expansion of the microbeam penumbra, and reduction of the PVDR value.

The disadvantage of using keV photons is the lower penetration depth. With a 100 keV radiation beam, transmittance is only 50% after about 4 cm of water [17]. This can potentially limit the treatment of tumors that are deep in the patient and may not receive enough radiation to be damaged. Fortunately, the high tolerance of mature healthy tissue to micrometric radiation allows the delivery of entrance doses of up to hundreds of Gy, which can produce a therapeutic effect. For clinical applications, the use of photon energies at around 150 keV may be the most effective compromise to preserve the sharp penumbras of the microbeams and the lower photon absorption.

### 20.2.3 Multislit collimators used to shape microbeams

The spatial fractionation of x-ray radiation fields is usually achieved by placing a multislit collimator (MSC) in front of the target. An MSC is a mechanical component that exhibits a periodic variation of radiation attenuation in one of the directions perpendicular to the direction of beam propagation. The homogeneous photon beam arriving from the radiation source is blocked in some areas by absorption in the metal blades of the MSC, so that only part of the radiation is transmitted. While the first MSC models were made with alternating foils of two different materials [18], e.g. aluminum and gold [19], modern machining techniques allow the manufacture of MSCs made of metal blocks designed to create a regular pattern of apertures through which the radiation can pass undisturbed [20].

MSCs can be designed with an adjustable aperture width for versatility or with a geometry defined by a fixed aperture, allowing easier alignment and control during an experiment. At both the European and Australian synchrotrons, the beamlines used to develop MRT are equipped with an MSC with 50 μm wide apertures and a 400 μm spacing c-t-c. Figure 20.4 shows an example of a single-stack MSC. The combination of two MSCs whose periodicity is defined in two perpendicular directions allows the creation of the pencil beam configuration.

When designing a MSC, two critical factors must be considered: radiation absorption capacity and photon–metal interaction at the inner surface of the

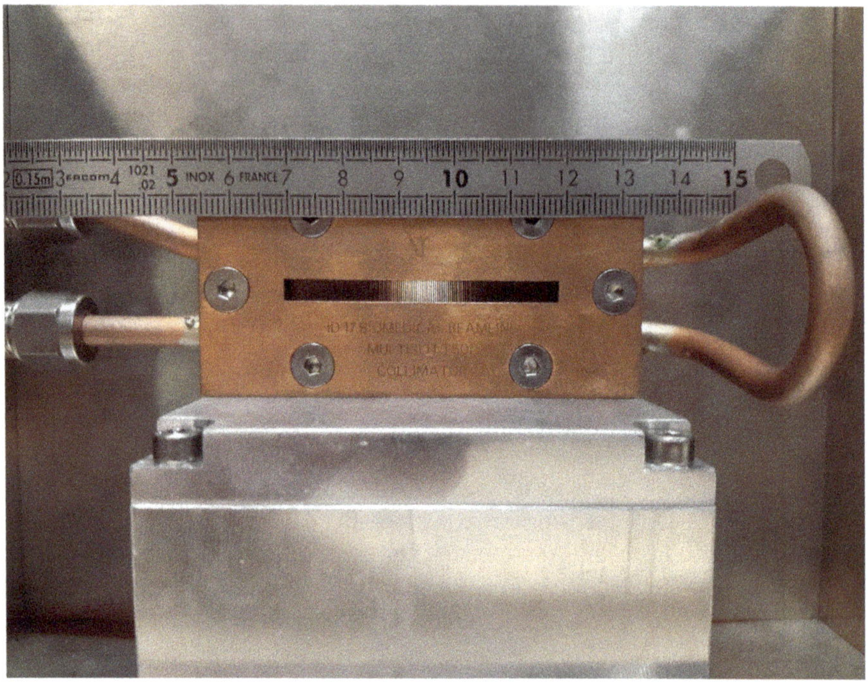


**Figure 20.4.** Picture of the single-stack MSC at the ESRF—ID17 Biomedical Beamline. The aperture pattern defines 50 μm wide beams spaced at 400 μm c-t-c.

MSC [12, 13]. Tungsten-based alloys provide strong absorption for photons at less than 300 keV but can leak radiation at energies above this if the tungsten content in the alloy is not high enough. Significantly increasing the MSC thickness as a mitigation measure can promote the reflection of radiation from the inner walls of the MSC, even for quasi-parallel microbeams, causing deflected photons to reach valley regions. Therefore, the final compromise adopted when fabricating an MSC must consider beam energy, beam divergence, the availability of absorbent materials, and the technical feasibility of producing precise apertures.

## 20.3 Radiation sources of microbeams

### 20.3.1 Synchrotron radiation source

Today, third-generation synchrotron radiation sources are the most suitable x-ray sources for MRT. In a synchrotron, electrons are kept circulating at relativistic speeds in a storage ring. X-rays are produced when the electrons pass through the alternating magnetic field generated by a so-called wiggler installed in one of the straight sections of the storage ring. The x-rays are emitted in a direction tangential to the closed orbit of the electrons, as a cone of radiation with a divergence of a few mrad in the horizontal plane and of the order of μrad in the vertical plane, allowing the generation of quasi-parallel beams. The resulting beam is rectangular and

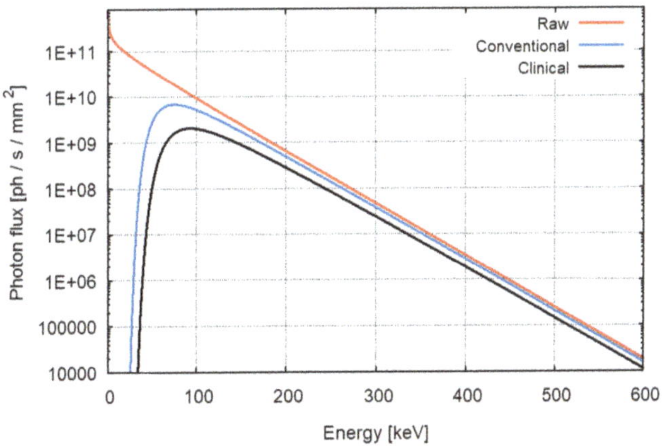


**Figure 20.5.** Spectrum profiles at the European Synchrotron ID17 Biomedical Beamline for the maximum ESRF storage ring current of 200 mA. The red line shows the intensity of the raw spectrum produced by the wiggler source. Two examples of filtered spectra used for MRT irradiations are also displayed. The ESRF storage ring current can also operate at 90 mA or 40 mA.

narrow; it measures a few centimeters in width and only a few millimeters in height at the position of the sample. Therefore, to produce the effect of a larger field, a vertical scan of the target through the beam is required (see section 20.3.1.1).

An average dose rate up to 16 000 Gy $s^{-1}$ can be achieved, i.e. in the ultrahigh-dose-rate range, allowing the delivery of hundreds of Gy of radiation in a fraction of a second. This makes synchrotron sources suitable for both MRT and FLASH radiation therapy. With a short irradiation time, the problem of natural cardio-synchronous movement of tissues that could distort the shape of microbeams in the target volume is drastically reduced [21–23]. Moreover, when the irradiation of biological tissue is completed in less than around 200 ms, the full FLASH effect can also be exploited [24].

Such high radiation intensity is provided by a polychromatic spectrum with main photon energies in the range of 0–300 keV. The low-energy part of the spectrum, which is below 50 keV, is cut off by a series of attenuators. Spectra with an average energy between 100 keV and 200 keV and a dose rate extending over a range of four orders of magnitude can be obtained by further filtering of the x-ray beam. Figure 20.5 shows, as an example, the raw spectra produced by the wiggler device at the ESRF—ID17 Biomedical Beamline and two different configurations of filtered spectra used for MRT experiments. The significant high-energy falloff is due to the emission characteristics of the wiggler source.

*20.3.1.1 The general structure of the synchrotron beamlines used for MRT*

In a synchrotron x-ray research center, the radiation source is located from a few tens to hundreds of meters in advance of the target position. The transport of the x-ray beam from the source to the target takes place in laboratories called beamlines.

The structure of a beamline consists of a front-end section where the wiggler source is located, an optical hutch for beam filtering, and an experimental hutch where sample irradiation takes place. These three sections are enclosed in lead cabins to provide radiation protection. A control room next to the experimental hutch allows remote control of the irradiation by the researchers.

The two most active beamlines in MRT research today are the ESRF—ID17 Biomedical Beamline (Grenoble, France) and the Australian Synchrotron (ANSTO) —Imaging and Medical Beamline (IMBL) (Clayton, Australia). These two beamlines plan to conduct clinical trials in the next few years. Other beamlines also involved in MRT research are at the Canadian Light Source (Saskatoon, Canada), Spring-8 (Hyogo, Japan), and Elettra (Trieste, Italy). A potential new beamline study is currently under development at DESY (Hamburg, Germany).

Along the beamline, a series of mechanical slits define the shape of the synchrotron beam reaching the target. In addition to the MSC and attenuators described in the previous sections, beamlines intended for MRT are equipped with a fast shutter that can define the exposure time with an error of less than one millisecond [25]. This component is of crucial importance because the use of ultrahigh dose rates requires tight controls to avoid overexposure during dose delivery.

Various detectors are used during beamline alignment or to monitor beam intensity during irradiation. The types of detectors used are ionization chambers, Compton chambers [26] and large-area plane-parallel ionization chambers. Radiation stability monitoring components are often implemented as pairs of identical detectors to meet redundancy requirements for projects developing radiation sources from a clinical perspective.

Because the position of the synchrotron beam is fixed and cannot rotate like the radiation sources in conventional hospital equipment, the target moves vertically into the beam, allowing the final size of the irradiation field to be defined. For work in preclinical settings, Kappa-type goniometers are often combined with translational motors to ensure precise alignment of the target in the beam and to allow its vertical movement [27, 28]. Fundamental variables that must be controlled with high precision during irradiation are the vertical velocity, which defines the final delivered dose, and parasitic vibrations of the stage during the scan, which can cause the delivery of microbeams with an oscillatory shape and consequently a degradation of the dose distribution. In preparation for upcoming human clinical studies, a dedicated positioning system capable of accommodating human patients is being developed and commissioned at both Australian and European synchrotron facilities.

Image guidance is key to better positioning of the target volume within the beam and improving RT outcomes. To date, customized setups have been developed for preclinical studies at beamlines. Attenuated synchrotron beams can be used in combination with an indirect detector system based on a scintillator (to convert x-rays into visible light), an optical system, and a CCD camera to perform radiography of the target while delivering doses only on the order of cGy [29–31]. As an alternative to synchrotron radiation, an external x-ray tube can be installed for full-field imaging [32, 33]. External markers placed on the surface of the specimen or anatomical structures can be used to define the position of the irradiation point in space and align it in the beam using graphical user interfaces, in accordance with treatment plans defined starting from a clinical computed tomography (CT) image.

### 20.3.2 Alternative radiation sources

One of the limitations slowing the translation of MRT into clinical applications is the limited number of synchrotron facilities that can provide a radiation source that meets the criteria required for MRT. In addition, synchrotrons are large and expensive research centers, only a small fraction of which are intended for clinical applications. The development of alternative, more compact, and affordable radiation sources is a key factor in the spread of MRT.

Inverse Compton scattering (ICS) sources are based on similar synchrotron principles, but here photons are produced by the interaction of moving electrons with the electric field of a powerful laser. The Munich Compact Light Source (MuCLS) [34] is a working example of such a radiation source; it uses a compact storage ring 4.6 m in circumference and is capable of successfully producing microbeams. Lyncean Technology Inc. is currently developing the next generation of ICS sources capable of delivering x-rays up to 140–180 keV with an interesting dose rate on the order of a few Gy $s^{-1}$ [35].

Radiation sources based on compact x-ray tubes are widely available and have been tested as a possible alternative to synchrotron sources. Bremsstrahlung and characteristic x-ray photons are produced by electrons with a kinetic energy of up to tens of MeV hitting a target of heavy metal, such as tungsten. The very low efficiency of the process, resulting in a dose rate of a few Gy per minute, coupled with the isotropic emission of the radiation, make x-ray tubes useful only for *in vitro* MRT research or for more relaxed geometries, such as minibeams [36–39].

Carbon nanotube (CNT) field emission technology has been investigated because of its ability to extract electrons and produce microbeams with an x-ray tube [40]. CNT uses high electric fields near a nanometer-sized cathode to achieve small emittance and high electron current densities [41]. A prototype based on this technology has demonstrated the ability to produce a dose rate of 2 Gy $s^{-1}$ and 300 μm wide beams, corresponding to a geometry closer to that of a minibeam than that of microbeam irradiation [42, 43].

The latest concept for a compact microbeam radiation source is the line-focus x-ray tube. The idea behind this device is to use a strongly eccentric focal spot on a rapidly rotating target. To achieve dominant energy transport by electron scattering in the target, high acceleration voltages and high rotational speeds of the target surface are required [44]. Models simulating its use in clinical systems suggest the use of a 600 kV accelerating voltage at a power of 1.5 MW. A dose rate of 180 Gy $s^{-1}$ is expected at 0.5 m from the focal spot, with a higher average photon energy of 150 keV [45]. The development of this radiation source is underway.

## 20.4 MRT modalities

When we talk about MRT modalities, we are describing the different ways in which MRT can be delivered to tissue. Most MRT modalities have great similarities to conventional radiotherapy, such as single irradiation, temporal fractionation of the dose, combination with drugs, etc. However, the inherent geometric distribution of the dose in MRT makes the study of its biological effects very challenging.

Studying the dose deposition of a single microbeam array is quite straightforward, as we can observe DNA damage with the $\gamma$H2AX marker. However, things become more complex when more than one irradiation field is used, as the peak dose of the microbeams overlaps with the valley dose.

### 20.4.1 Description of the incident MRT arrays

MRT can be delivered using a single array or as multiple arrays. As shown in figure 20.6, multiple arrays of microbeams fired at the target are referred to as **cross fired** (although they do not necessarily form a cross). However, given the different geometries of the microbeams, it is important to define exactly how cross-fired microbeam arrays are directed and how they converge on the target.

*20.4.1.1 Trajectory of entry*

The MRT arrays can be described in terms of their trajectory or entry point. When two or more arrays with the same trajectory are directed at the target, they are called **unidirectional**. When two or more MRT arrays are directed at the target from different trajectories or entry points, we call them **bidirectional** or **multidirectional**. When the trajectories of the MRT arrays form an angle of 90° at the target, they are called **orthogonal** MRT arrays.

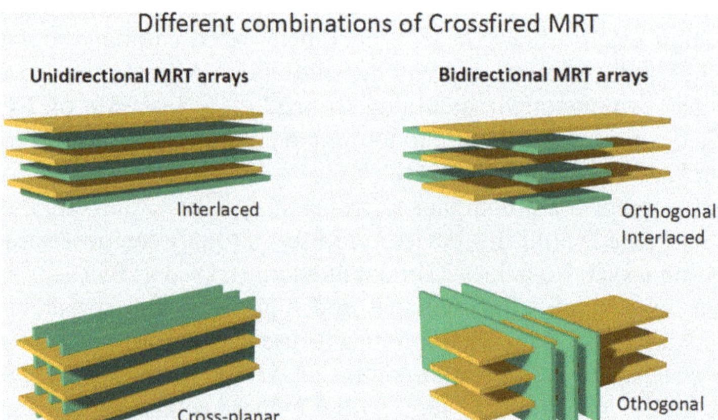


**Figure 20.6.** Different combinations of cross-fired MRT arrays.

*20.4.1.2 Convergence in the target*

The convergence of MRT arrays in the target refers to whether or not the peak doses overlap when two or more microbeam arrays are used. If the peak doses do not overlap at any point, the arrays are said to be **interlaced**. On the other hand, if the peak doses meet at the convergence point, they are referred to as **cross-planar** arrays.

## 20.5 MRT dosimetry

Dosimetry is a current topic in MRT because calculating or measuring the absolute dose delivered by an x-ray source with photons in the keV range and with ultrahigh dose rates on the order of thousands of Gy is a physical challenge. Spatial fractionation of the irradiation field is still non-trivial when coupled with the need to resolve dose features on the scale of a few micrometers.

While protocols for evaluating absolute dosimetry at synchrotron sources for homogeneous fields at ultrahigh dose rates using small-volume ionization chambers [46] and alanine-based detectors [47] have been defined and verified, a large number of detectors based on different physical principles have been tested and are being developed to provide reliable dosimetry at the micrometric scale. Among the most suitable MRT dosimeters, the following deserve a mention: radiochromic films [8, 48–50] and plastics [51–54], silicon-based detectors [55–58], and diamond detectors [59–62]. A more comprehensive list of detectors used in MRT can be found in the literature [63].

Reliable dose calculation is also critical in dosimetry. For MRT, Monte Carlo (MC) techniques implemented with various software packages such as GEometry ANd Tracking 4 (GEANT4), Electron Gamma Shower (EGS), and Penetration and ENErgy LOss of Positrons and Electrons (PENELOPE) have been used extensively to estimate the delivered dose. The choice of scattering cross section libraries for photons in the keV range, electron tracking cutoff values, and synchrotron source polarization effects must be carefully considered in MRT dose calculations. In addition, the need to divide the irradiated volume into small micrometric voxels to resolve the MRT grid features requires large computational power to obtain small statistical uncertainty in each voxel.

Synchrotron radiation sources can be modeled using analytical approaches [64, 65] or by full MC simulations [50, 66]. Both approaches provide the x-ray spectrum that is used as input to the MC dose calculation. Kernel-based dose calculations have been tested to speed up the simulation of the dose calculation inside the target, but they proved to be not as accurate as conventional MC simulations. A new and innovative approach is to combine an analytical (kernel-based) approach for short-range electron transport with the MC technique for photon scattering in what is called a 'hybrid' approach [16]. This approach leads to short simulation times and minimal dose differences compared to pure MC simulations.

The dose calculation model should be properly integrated with treatment planning software capable of selecting the region to be treated and visualizing the treatment plan. The most recent development in MRT treatment planning systems (TPSs) is the integration of the 'hybrid' algorithm into the commercial Varian

Eclipse software [67, 68]. In addition, when working with x-rays in the keV range, the correct conversion of material composition to CT Hounsfield units is essential.

Continuous improvements in the field of micrometer-scale dosimetry for MRT, both on the experimental and simulative side, have made it possible to significantly reduce the differences between measured and calculated doses. These differences and measurement uncertainties are often less than 5%–10% [49, 50], close to the usual 3% required for conventional RT. Although a unique detector and simulation machine for MRT have not been defined as the gold standard, the prerequisites for moving to clinical trials may soon be achieved.

## 20.6 Biological effects of MRT

### 20.6.1 Effects on normal tissue

From a clinical perspective, one of the most important outcomes of MRT is its ability to spare normal tissue. In fact, MRT is currently the only high-dose radiotherapy technique that can spare normal tissue via two mechanisms: (i) volumetric sparing through the spatial fractionation of microbeams (the dose/volume effect) [69–71] and (ii) sparing of normal tissue through the ultrahigh dose rates known as the FLASH effect [3, 72]. The biology responsible for the FLASH effect is rapid local oxygen consumption that avoids or reduces ROS-mediated cellular damage [3, 72], allowing safe delivery of multiple MRT arrays, among other benefits.

### 20.6.2 The effects of single and multiple MRT arrays

Early research into MRT focused on studying the effects of a single array to assess radiation toxicity in normal tissue. Today, the application of multiple MRT arrays to tumors is an area of research that is gaining momentum. Published research indicates that the preclinical models most commonly treated with multiple MRT arrays are rodent brain tumors [73–78] and, to a lesser extent, mammary carcinomas [79, 80] and melanomas [81]. The goal of using multiple arrays is to hit the tumor with a complex geometric pattern of peak doses while always keeping the cumulative valley dose low enough to avoid radiation toxicity. It is imperative that these side effects be kept in check, as they can significantly affect the treatment outcome. It is important to keep valley doses low for multiple arrays, as they are administered on the same day in one session. Therefore, the goal of administering multiple MRT arrays is to achieve an ablative effect in the tumor microenvironment.

#### *20.6.2.1 Extremely high ablative doses to tumors*

MRT targets tumors with an innovative combination of high peak doses ranging from 133 to 1900 Gy [80–82] and valley doses ranging from 2.46 to 30 Gy [80–82]. This breakthrough combination of peak and valley doses has demonstrated remarkable tumor control in several cancer models: brain tumors in rats [75, 83–85], mammary carcinomas in mice [86, 87], and more recently, melanomas in mice [88].

Extrapolating from the results of MRT experiments in chicken embryos, zebrafish, and mouse melanomas, it is clear that the tumor microenvironment is an excellent target, as MRT is particularly efficient in (i) affecting the abnormal tumor vasculature and (ii) transforming the immunosuppressive tumor microenvironment into a 'hot zone' characterized by an influx of immune cells.

*20.6.2.2 Preferential vascular effects of MRT*

MRT has been shown to produce a preferential deleterious effect on tumor vessels rather than healthy vascular tissue. This preferential effect is caused by the rapidly growing immature vasculature [89, 90]. Peak doses act selectively on the rapidly growing 'tortuous' tumor vessels [91], inducing transient tumor ischemia [92, 93] and neutrophil infiltration [89]. Data from studies in birds [94], zebrafish [95], and mice [96] show that peak MRT doses of hundreds of Gy selectively destroy immature tumor neovasculature, disrupting perfusion and leading to tumor hypoxia and necrosis.

*20.6.2.3 Immune responses unique to MRT*

MRT can strongly modulate the immunogenicity of the tumor microenvironment compared with conventional radiotherapy. MRT can significantly activate pathways associated with natural killers and CD8+ T cells in rat brains [97]; it can stimulate persistent macrophage-derived cytokines in mouse plasma [98]; it can induce higher levels of proinflammatory genes in tumors [86] and trigger the release of the monocyte-attracting chemokines MCP-1 and RANTES [99], which are critically involved in leukocyte recruitment in inflamed and malignant tissues [100]. Recently, Djonov's group at the University of Bern discovered how macrophages migrate and collect along the microbeam path and also that MRT elicits significantly greater tumor infiltration by CD8+ T cells than a uniform field of radiation.

### 20.6.3 The effects of temporal fractionation

Temporal fractionation of the MRT array means that multiple arrays are not delivered in one day, but one array per day on consecutive days. Temporal fractionation has been adopted from conventional radiotherapy, so MRT can now benefit from reoxygenation of the tumor and further sparing of normal tissue from radiation damage. However, an additional benefit of the temporal fractionation of MRT is that peak and valley doses no longer need to be as high, which could allow for a better transition from synchrotron facilities to the clinic.

Preclinical research into the temporal fractionation of MRT is still in its infancy, but it is already showing excellent results. Data from the temporal fractionation of three MRT arrays at a peak dose of 133 Gy used to treat radiation-resistant B16-F10 melanoma in mice showed complete remission in 50% of the tumors [88]. The surviving animals lived for 18 months and did not develop metastases. No melanomas were present at the tumor site. In fact, a nevus remained, which was formed only by melanin-laden macrophages, suggesting their involvement in the elimination of melanoma and linking the effect of MRT to the immune system.

### 20.6.4 The effects of MRT in combination with drugs

Combining MRT with drugs was a natural step toward improving treatment outcomes by attempting to create an additive effect between the ablative power of MRT and the chemical effect of the drugs. Research data on this topic are still in their infancy, but show encouraging results. One of the first papers showed that survival of mice with 9L gliosarcomas increased when MRT was combined with intracerebral administration of gadolinium, which acts as a radiation enhancer [101]. Another strategy improved the treatment of 4T1 mammary carcinomas in mice using MRT combined with Anginex, an antiangiogenic peptide [7]. The combination of MRT with chemotherapies has also been studied. In one study, rats with 9L gliosarcomas showed increased survival when MRT was combined with the drug JAI-51, which inhibits microtubule polymerization and thus exerts an antiproliferative effect [74]. In another study, human glioblastomas implanted in mice showed a dramatic reduction in growth when MRT was combined with cisplatin, which cross-links DNA and inhibits cell division [102].

In the above cases, the drugs were administered before MRT because of the desire to achieve an additive effect. However, if MRT is administered before the drugs, it may serve as a means to induce transient vascular permeability to allow greater extravasation of the drugs into the tumors. In essence, MRT could be used as a drug delivery system.

#### *20.6.4.1 The use of MRT as a drug delivery system*

The use of MRT as a drug delivery system is a new approach developed by the Djonov laboratory at the University of Bern in Switzerland. Simply put, when MRT is administered at low peak doses (75–150 Gy), there is a selective effect in which the normal vasculature has a higher tolerance to the dose, while the immature tumor vasculature is temporally perturbed, increasing vascular permeability [94, 95, 103]. The permeability/therapeutic window lasts between 45 min and 4 h after MRT in both avian and mouse models. This type of application of MRT could really promote its use in the clinic, as it would be used as an adjunct to improve currently established treatments, rather than becoming the main treatment.

## 20.7 Summary and key points

- MRT is the SFRT modality that can take full advantage of the dose/volume effect. This advantage results from the extremely thin microbeams that make up the MRT array.
- The microbeams are only a few tens of micrometers wide (23–100 μm), but up to a few centimeters long to cover the target.
- One of the main features of MRT is the steep dose gradient at the edge of the microbeams. However, the transition from the peak dose to the valley dose is not geometrically perfect, due to scattered and secondary radiation; it is called the penumbra.
- Photons with an energy of about 100 keV are the most favorable radiation source with which to obtain a steep dose gradient in MRT. However, the

disadvantage of using keV photons is their lower penetration depth, which may limit the application of MRT in the clinic.

- While the radiation sources of photon MRT are synchrotrons, the narrow shape of the microbeam array is generated by a multislit collimator.
- Synchrotrons are capable of delivering ultrahigh dose rates; these have two functions: they prevent the smearing of microbeams due to cardio-synchronous motion, and they spare normal tissue as a result of the FLASH effect.
- The MRT array has a simple geometry that can easily become complex when multiple microbeam arrays are directed at the tissue. In this cross-fired scenario, the peak and valley doses can overlap, resulting in significant side effects if the doses are too high.
- The use of multiple microbeam arrays goes hand in hand with very precise MRT dosimetry. The most reliable dosimeters are: radiochromic films and plastics, silicon-based detectors, and diamond detectors.
- Reliable dose calculation is also critical in dosimetry. Monte Carlo techniques implemented with software such as GEANT4, EGS, and PENELOPE are widely used.
- The biological effects of MRT arise from the ablative peak doses, which produce a unique set of MRT-related effects on the tumor microenvironment: (i) a preferential deleterious effects on tumor vessels over healthy vascular tissue, and (ii) strong modulation of the immunogenicity of the tumor microenvironment.
- MRT can be fractionated in time, which exploits tumor reoxygenation and further improves tumor control.
- MRT can be combined with drugs to achieve additive effects and with radiation boosters to achieve a synergistic effect.
- MRT can be used as a drug delivery system in which low peak doses temporally disrupt tumor vasculature and create a vascular permeability window for drug or nanoparticle delivery.

## References

[1] Köhler A 1909 A method of deep roentgen irradiation without injury to the skin *Arch. Roentgen Ray* **14** 141–2

[2] Slatkin D N, Spanne P, Dilmanian F A and Sandborg M 1992 Microbeam radiation therapy *Med. Phys.* **19** 1395–400

[3] Fernandez-Palomo C, Fazzari J, Trappetti V, Smyth L, Janka H and Laissue J *et al* 2020 Animal models in microbeam radiation therapy: a scoping review *Cancers* **12** 527

[4] Fernandez-Palomo C, Mothersill C, Bräuer-Krisch E, Laissue J, Seymour C and Schültke E 2015 γ-H2AX as a marker for dose deposition in the brain of wistar rats after synchrotron microbeam radiation *PLoS One* **10** e0119924

[5] Laissue J A, Blattmann H, Michiel M D, Slatkin D N, Lyubimova N and Guzman R *et al* 2001 Weanling piglet cerebellum: a surrogate for tolerance to MRT (microbeam radiation therapy) in pediatric neuro-oncology *Proc. SPIE* **4508** 65–73

[6] Dilmanian F A A, Button T M, le Duc G, Zhong N, Peña L A and Smith J A L L *et al* 2002 Response of rat intracranial 9L gliosarcoma to microbeam radiation therapy *Neuro-Oncol.* **4** 26–38

[7] Griffin R J, Koonce N A, Dings R P M, Siegel E, Moros E G and Bruer-Krisch E *et al* 2012 Microbeam radiation therapy alters vascular architecture and tumor oxygenation and is enhanced by a galectin-1 targeted anti-angiogenic peptide *Radiat. Res.* **177** 804–12

[8] Pellicioli P, Bartzsch S, Donzelli M, Krisch M and Bräuer-Krisch E 2019 High resolution radiochromic film dosimetry: comparison of a microdensitometer and an optical microscope *Phys. Medica* **65** 106–13

[9] Schültke E, Trippel M, Bräuer-Krisch E, Renier M, Bartzsch S and Requardt H *et al* 2013 Pencilbeam irradiation technique for whole brain radiotherapy: technical and biological challenges in a small animal model *PLoS One* **8** 1–9

[10] Dilmanian F A, Qu Y, Feinendegen L E, Peña L A, Bacarian T and Henn F A *et al* 2007 Tissue-sparing effect of x-ray microplanar beams particularly in the CNS: is a bystander effect involved? *Exp. Hematol.* **35** 69–77

[11] Serduc R, Bräuer-Krisch E, Siegbahn E A, Bouchet A, Pouyatos B and Carron R *et al* 2010 High-precision radiosurgical dose delivery by interlaced microbeam arrays of high-flux low-energy synchrotron x-rays *PLoS One* **5** e9028

[12] Pellicioli P, Donzelli M, Davis J A, Estève F, Hugtenburg R and Guatelli S *et al* 2021 Study of the X-ray radiation interaction with a multislit collimator for the creation of microbeams in radiation therapy *J. Synchrotron Radiat.* **28** 392–403

[13] Nettelbeck H, Takacs G J, Lerch M L F F and Rosenfeld A B 2009 Microbeam radiation therapy: a Monte Carlo study of the influence of the source, multislit collimator, and beam divergence on microbeams *Med. Phys.* **36** 447–56

[14] Berger M J, Hubbell J H, Seltzer S M, Chang J, Coursey J S and Sukumar R *et al* 2010 *XCOM: Photon Cross Sections Database (Version 1.5).* (Gaithersburg, MD: National Institute of Standards and Technology)

[15] Berger M J, Coursey J S, Zucker M A and Chang J 2017 *Stopping-Power & Range Tables for Electrons, Protons, and Helium Ions* (Gaithersburg, MD: National Institute of Standards and Technology)

[16] Donzelli M, Brauer-Krisch E, Oelfke U, Wilkens J J and Bartzsch S 2018 Hybrid dose calculation: A dose calculation algorithm for microbeam radiation therapy *Phys. Med. Biol.* **63** 045013

[17] Hubbel J H and Seltzer S M 2004 *X-Ray Mass Attenuation Coefficients* (Gaithersburg, MD: National Institute of Standards and Technology)

[18] Slatkin D N, Dilmanian F A, Nawrocky M M, Spanne P, Gebbers J O and Archer D W *et al* 1995 Design of a multislit, variable width collimator for microplanar beam radiotherapy *Rev. Sci. Instrum.* **66** 1459–60

[19] Bräuer-Krisch E, Bravin A, Zhang L, Siegbahn E, Stepanek J and Blattmann H *et al* 2005 Characterization of a tungsten/gas multislit collimator for microbeam radiation therapy at the European Synchrotron Radiation Facility *Rev. Sci. Instrum.* **76** 064303

[20] Bräuer-Krisch E, Requardt H, Brochard T, Berruyer G, Renier M and Laissue J A *et al* 2009 New technology enables high precision multislit collimators for microbeam radiation therapy *Rev. Sci. Instrum.* **80** 074301

[21] Donzelli M, Bräuer-Krisch E and Oelfke U 2016 Brain motion induced artefacts in Microbeam Radiation Therapy: a Monte Carlo study *Radiother. Oncol.* **118** S34–5

[22] Manchado de Sola F, Vilches M, Prezado Y and Lallena A M 2018 Impact of cardiosynchronous brain pulsations on Monte Carlo calculated doses for synchrotron micro- and minibeam radiation therapy *Med. Phys.* **45** 3379–90

[23] Duncan M, Donzelli M, Pellicioli P, Brauer-Krisch E, Davis J A, Lerch M L F, Anatoly B and Rosenfeld M P 2019 First experimental measurement of the effect of cardio-synchronous brain motion on the dose distribution during microbeam radiation therapy *Med. Phys.* **47** 213–22

[24] Montay-Gruel P, Acharya M M, Petersson K, Alikhani L, Yakkala C and Allen B D *et al* 2019 Long-term neurocognitive benefits of FLASH radiotherapy driven by reduced reactive oxygen species *Proc. Natl Acad. Sci. USA* **166** 10943–51

[25] Renier M, Brochard T, Nemoz C and Thomlinson W 2002 A white-beam fast-shutter for microbeam radiation therapy at the ESRF *Nucl. Instrum. Methods Phys. Res. Sect. Accel. Spectrometers Detect. Assoc. Equip.* **479** 656–60

[26] Berkvens P, Brauer-Krisch E, Brochard T, Nemoz C, Renier M and Fournier P *et al* 2013 Highly robust, high intensity white synchrotron beam monitor *IEEE Nuclear Science Symposium Conference Record.* (Piscataway, NJ: Institute of Electrical and Electronics Engineers Inc.)

[27] Bräuer-Krisch E, Nemoz C, Brochard T, Berruyer G, Renier M and Pouyatos B *et al* 2013 The preclinical set-up at the ID17 biomedical beamline to achieve high local dose deposition using interlaced microbeams *J. Phys. Conf. Ser.* **425** 022001

[28] Wysokinski T W, Chapman D, Adams G, Renier M, Suortti P and Thomlinson W 2015 Beamlines of the biomedical imaging and therapy facility at the Canadian light source – part 3 *Nucl. Instrum. Methods Phys. Res. Sect. Accel Spectrometers Detect. Assoc. Equip.* **775** 1–4

[29] Nemoz C, Kibleur A, Hyacinthe J N, Berruyer G, Brochard T and Brauer-Krisch E *et al* 2016 *In vivo* pink-beam imaging and fast alignment procedure for rat brain tumor radiation therapy *J. Synchrotron Radiat.* **23** 339–43

[30] Donzelli M, Bräuer-Krisch E, Nemoz C, Brochard T and Oelfke U 2016 Conformal image-guided microbeam radiation therapy at the ESRF biomedical beamline ID17 *Med. Phys.* **43** 3157–67

[31] Pelliccia D, Poole C M, Livingstone J, Stevenson A W, Smyth L M L and Rogers P A W *et al* 2016 Image guidance protocol for synchrotron microbeam radiation therapy *J. Synchrotron Radiat.* **23** 566–73

[32] Livingstone J, Adam J F, Crosbie J C, Hall C J, Lye J E and McKinlay J *et al* 2017 Preclinical radiotherapy at the Australian synchrotron's imaging and medical beamline: instrumentation, dosimetry and a small-animal feasibility study *J. Synchrotron Radiat.* **24** 854–65

[33] Barnes M 2018 *A patient-positioning system for synchrotron micro-beam radiotherapy (MRT)* RMIT University Masters by research https://researchrepository.rmit.edu.au/esploro/outputs/9921863984801341

[34] Eggl E, Dierolf M, Achterhold K, Jud C, Günther B and Braig E *et al* 2016 The Munich compact light source: initial performance measures *J. Synchrotron Radiat.* **23** 1137–42

[35] Hornberger B, Kasahara J, Gifford M, Ruth R and Loewen R 2019 A compact light source providing high-flux, quasi-monochromatic, tunable X-rays in the laboratory *Proc. SPIE* **11110** 1111003

[36] Babcock K, Sidhu N, Kundapur V and Ali K 2011 Collimator design for experimental minibeam radiation therapy *Med. Phys.* **38** 2192–7
[37] Bazyar S, Inscoe C R, O'Brian E T, Zhou O and Lee Y Z 2017 Minibeam radiotherapy with small animal irradiators; in vitro and *in vivo* feasibility studies *Phys. Med. Biol.* **62** 8924–42
[38] Bartzsch S, Cummings C, Eismann S and Oelfke U 2016 A preclinical microbeam facility with a conventional x-ray tube *Med. Phys.* **43** 6301–8
[39] Prezado Y, Dos Santos M, Gonzalez W, Jouvion G, Guardiola C and Heinrich S *et al* 2017 Transfer of minibeam radiation therapy into a cost-effective equipment for radiobiological studies: a proof of concept *Sci. Rep.* **7** 1–10
[40] Schreiber E C and Chang S X 2012 Monte Carlo simulation of a compact microbeam radiotherapy system based on carbon nanotube field emission technology *Med. Phys.* **39** 4669–78
[41] Shiffler D, Zhou O, Bower C, LaCour M and Golby K 2004 A high-current, large-area, carbon nanotube cathode *IEEE Trans. Plasma Sci.* **32** 2152–4
[42] Hadsell M, Zhang J, Laganis P, Sprenger F, Shan J and Zhang L *et al* 2013 A first generation compact microbeam radiation therapy system based on carbon nanotube X-ray technology *Appl. Phys. Lett.* **103** 183505
[43] Hadsell M, Cao G, Zhang J, Burk L, Schreiber T and Schreiber E *et al* 2014 Pilot study for compact microbeam radiation therapy using a carbon nanotube field emission micro-CT scanner *Med. Phys.* **41** 061710
[44] Bartzsch S and Oelfke U 2017 Line focus x-ray tubes – a new concept to produce high brilliance x-rays *Phys. Med. Biol.* **62** 8600
[45] Winter J, Galek M, Matejcek C, Wilkens J J, Aulenbacher K and Combs S E *et al* 2020 Clinical microbeam radiation therapy with a compact source: specifications of the line-focus X-ray tube *Phys Imaging Radiat Oncol.* **14** 74–81
[46] Fournier P, Crosbie J C, Cornelius I, Berkvens P, Donzelli M and Clavel A H *et al* 2016 Absorbed dose-to-water protocol applied to synchrotron-generated x-rays at very high dose rates *Phys. Med. Biol.* **61** N349–61
[47] Soliman Y S, Pellicioli P, Beshir W B B, Abdel-Fattah A A, Fahim R A and Krisch M *et al* 2020 A comparative dosimetry study of an alanine dosimeter with a PTW PinPoint chamber at ultra-high dose rates of synchrotron radiation *Phys. Medica* **71** 161–7
[48] Bartzsch S, Lott J, Welsch K, Bräuer-Krisch E and Oelfke U 2015 Micrometer-resolved film dosimetry using a microscope in microbeam radiation therapy *Med. Phys.* **42** 4069–79
[49] Day L R J, Pellicioli P, Gagliardi F, Barnes M, Smyth L M L and Butler D *et al* 2020 A Monte Carlo model of synchrotron radiotherapy shows good agreement with experimental dosimetry measurements: data from the imaging and medical beamline at the Australian Synchrotron *Phys. Medica* **77** 64–74
[50] Dipuglia A, Cameron M, Davis J A, Cornelius I M, Stevenson A W and Rosenfeld A B *et al* 2019 Validation of a Monte Carlo simulation for microbeam radiation therapy on the imaging and medical beamline at the Australian Synchrotron *Sci. Rep.* **9** 1–14
[51] Doran S J, Rahman A T A A, Bräuer-Krisch E, Brochard T, Adamovics J and Nisbet A *et al* 2013 Establishing the suitability of quantitative optical CT microscopy of PRESAGE®radiochromic dosimeters for the verification of synchrotron microbeam therapy *Phys. Med. Biol.* **58** 6279–97

[52] Doran S, Pellicioli P, Adamovics J and Brauer-Krisch E 2017 Enhanced method for determining the low-LET saturation dose of PRESAGE® *J. Phys. Conf. Ser.* **847** 012028
[53] Mcerlean C, Bräuer-Krisch E, Adamovics J, Leach M O O and Doran S J J 2015 High resolution 3D dosimetry for microbeam radiation therapy using optical CT *J. Phys. Conf. Ser.* **573** 5–8
[54] McErlean C M, Bräuer-Krisch E, Adamovics J and Doran S J 2015 Assessment of optical CT as a future QA tool for synchrotron x-ray microbeam therapy *Phys. Med. Biol.* **61** 320–37
[55] Lerch M L F, Petasecca M, Cullen A, Hamad A, Requardt H and Bräuer-Krisch E *et al* 2011 Dosimetry of intensive synchrotron microbeams *Radiat. Meas.* **46** 1560–5
[56] Fournier P, Cornelius I, Donzelli M, Requardt H, Nemoz C and Petasecca M *et al* 2016 X-Tream quality assurance in synchrotron X-ray microbeam radiation therapy *J. Synchrotron Radiat.* **23** 1180–90
[57] Fournier P, Cornelius I, Dipuglia A, Cameron M, Davis J A and Cullen A *et al* 2017 X-Tream dosimetry of highly brilliant X-ray microbeams in the MRT hutch of the Australian Synchrotron *Radiat. Meas.* **106** 405–11
[58] Davis J A, Paino J R, Dipuglia A, Cameron M, Siegele R and Pastuovic Z *et al* 2018 Characterisation and evaluation of a PNP strip detector for synchrotron microbeam radiation therapy *Biomed. Phys. Eng. Express* **4** 044002
[59] Almaviva S, Marinelli M, Milani E, Prestopino G, Tucciarone A and Verona C *et al* 2010 Chemical vapor deposition diamond based multilayered radiation detector: Physical analysis of detection properties *J. Appl. Phys.* **107** 014511
[60] Marinelli M, Prestopino G, Verona C and Verona-Rinati G 2016 Experimental determination of the PTW 60019 microDiamond dosimeter active area and volume *Med. Phys.* **43** 5205–12
[61] Livingstone J, Stevenson A W, Butler D J, Häusermann D and Adam J-F F 2016 Characterization of a synthetic single crystal diamond detector for dosimetry in spatially fractionated synchrotron x-ray fields *Med. Phys.* **43** 4283–93
[62] Butler D J, Beveridge T, Lehmann J, Oliver C P, Stevenson A W and Livingstone J 2018 Spatial response of synthetic microDiamond and diode detectors measured with kilovoltage synchrotron radiation *Med. Phys.* **45** 943–52
[63] Bartzsch S, Corde S, Crosbie J C, Day L, Donzelli M and Krisch M *et al* 2020 Technical advances in x-ray microbeam radiation therapy *Phys. Med. Biol.* **65** 02TR01
[64] Del Río M S and Dejus R J 2004 XOP 2.1 – a new version of the X-ray optics software toolkit *AIP Conf. Proc.* **705** 784–7
[65] Tanaka T and Kitamura H 2001 SPECTRA: A synchrotron radiation calculation code *J. Synchrotron Radiat.* **8** 1221–8
[66] Martínez-Rovira I, Sempau J and Prezado Y 2012 Development and commissioning of a Monte Carlo photon beam model for the forthcoming clinical trials in microbeam radiation therapy *Med. Phys.* **39** 119–31
[67] Poole C M, Day L R J, Rogers P A W and Crosbie J C 2017 Synchrotron microbeam radiotherapy in a commercially available treatment planning system *Biomed. Phys. Eng. Express* **3** 025001
[68] Day L R J, Donzelli M, Pellicioli P, Smyth L M L, Barnes M and Bartzsch S *et al* 2021 A commercial treatment planning system with a hybrid dose calculation algorithm for synchrotron radiotherapy trials *Phys. Med. Biol.* **66** 055016

[69] Smyth L M L, Donoghue J F, Ventura J A, Livingstone J, Bailey T and Day L R J *et al* 2018 Comparative toxicity of synchrotron and conventional radiation therapy based on total and partial body irradiation in a murine model *Sci. Rep.* **8** 12044

[70] Priyadarshika R C U, Crosbie J C, Kumar B and Rogers P A W 2011 Biodosimetric quantification of short-term synchrotron microbeam versus broad-beam radiation damage to mouse skin using a dermatopathological scoring system *Br. J. Radiol.* **84** 833–42

[71] Potez M, Trappetti V, Bouchet A, Fernandez-Palomo C, Güç E and Kilarski W W *et al* 2018 Characterization of a B16-F10 melanoma model locally implanted into the ear pinnae of C57BL/6 mice *PLoS One* **13** e0206693

[72] Montay-Gruel P, Bouchet A, Jaccard M, Patin D, Serduc R and Aim W *et al* 2018 X-rays can trigger the FLASH effect: ultra-high dose-rate synchrotron light source prevents normal brain injury after whole brain irradiation in mice *Radiother. Oncol.* **129** 582–8

[73] Bouchet A, Lemasson B, Le Duc G, Maisin C, Bräuer-Krisch E and Siegbahn E A *et al* 2010 Preferential effect of synchrotron microbeam radiation therapy on intracerebral 9L gliosarcoma vascular networks *Int. J. Radiat. Oncol. Biol. Phys.* **78** 1503–12

[74] Bouchet A, Boumendjel A, Khalil E, Serduc R, Brauer E and Siegbahn E A *et al* 2012 Chalcone JAI-51 improves efficacy of synchrotron microbeam radiation therapy of brain tumors *J. Synchrotron Radiat.* **19** 478–82

[75] Laissue J A, Geiser G, Spanne P O, Dilmanian F A, Gebbers J O and Geiser M *et al* 1998 Neuropathology of ablation of rat gliosarcomas and contiguous brain tissues using a microplanar beam of synchrotron-wiggler-generated X rays *Int. J. Cancer* **78** 654–60

[76] Schültke E, Bräuer-Krisch E, Blattmann H, Requardt H, Laissue J A and Hildebrandt G 2018 Survival of rats bearing advanced intracerebral F 98 tumors after glutathione depletion and microbeam radiation therapy: conclusions from a pilot project *Radiat. Oncol.* **13** 89

[77] Serduc R, Christen T, Laissue J A, Farion R R, Bouchet A and van der Sanden B *et al* 2008 Brain tumor vessel response to synchrotron microbeam radiation therapy: a short-term *in vivo* study *Phys. Med. Biol.* **53** 3609–22

[78] Serduc R, Bouchet A, Bräuer-Krisch E, Laissue J A, Spiga J and Sarun S *et al* 2009 Synchrotron microbeam radiation therapy for rat brain tumor palliation – influence of the microbeam width at constant valley dose *Phys. Med. Biol.* **54** 6711–24

[79] Crosbie J C, Anderson R L, Rothkamm K, Restall C M, Cann L and Ruwanpura S *et al* 2010 Tumor cell response to synchrotron microbeam radiation therapy differs markedly from cells in normal tissues *Int. J. Radiat. Oncol. Biol. Phys.* **77** 886–94

[80] Dilmanian F A, Morris G M, Zhong N, Bacarian T, Hainfeld J F and Kalef-Ezra J *et al* 2003 Murine EMT-6 carcinoma: high therapeutic efficacy of microbeam radiation therapy *Radiat. Res.* **159** 632–41

[81] Fernandez-Palomo C, Trappetti V, Potez M, Pellicioli P, Krisch M and Laissue J *et al* 2020 Complete remission of mouse melanoma after temporally fractionated microbeam radiotherapy *Cancers* **12** 2656

[82] Dilmanian F A, Button T M, Le Duc G, Zhong N, Peña L A and Smith J A L *et al* 2002 Response of rat intracranial 9L gliosarcoma to microbeam radiation therapy *Neuro-Oncol.* **4** 26–38

[83] Bouchet A, Bräuer-Krisch E, Prezado Y, El Atifi M, Rogalev L and Le Clec'h C *et al* 2016 Better efficacy of synchrotron spatially microfractionated radiation therapy than uniform radiation therapy on glioma *Int. J. Radiat. Oncol. Biol. Phys.* **95** 1485–94

[84] Serduc R, Brauer-Krisch E, Siegbahn E A, Bouchet A, Pouyatos B and Carron R *et al* 2010 High-precision radiosurgical dose delivery by interlaced microbeam arrays of high-flux low-energy synchrotron X-rays *PLoS One* **5** e9028
[85] Slatkin D N, Spanne P, Dilmanian F A, Gebbers J O and Laissue J A 1995 Subacute neuropathological effects of microplanar beams of x-rays from a synchrotron wiggler *Proc. Natl Acad. Sci. USA* **92** 8783–7
[86] Yang Y, Swierczak A, Ibahim M, Paiva P, Cann L and Stevenson A W *et al* 2019 Synchrotron microbeam radiotherapy evokes a different early tumor immunomodulatory response to conventional radiotherapy in EMT6.5 mammary tumors *Radiother. Oncol.* **133** 93–9
[87] Dilmanian F A, Kalef-Ezra J, Petersen M J, Bozios G, Vosswinkel J and Giron F *et al* 2003 Could X-ray microbeams inhibit angioplasty-induced restenosis in the rat carotid artery? *Cardiovasc. Radiat. Med.* **4** 139–45
[88] Potez M, Fernandez-Palomo C, Bouchet A, Trappetti V, Donzelli M and Krisch M *et al* 2019 Synchrotron microbeam radiation therapy as a new approach for the treatment of radioresistant melanoma: potential underlying mechanisms *Int. J. Radiat. Oncol. Biol. Phys.* **105** 1126–36
[89] Brönnimann D, Bouchet A, Schneider C, Potez M, Serduc R and Bräuer-Krisch E *et al* 2016 Synchrotron microbeam irradiation induces neutrophil infiltration, thrombocyte attachment and selective vascular damage *in vivo Sci. Rep.* **6** 33601
[90] Sabatasso S, Laissue J A, Hlushchuk R, Graber W, Bravin A and Bräuer-Krisch E *et al* 2011 Microbeam radiation-induced tissue damage depends on the stage of vascular maturation *Int. J. Radiat. Oncol. Biol. Phys.* **80** 1522–32
[91] Bouchet A, Potez M, Coquery N, Rome C, Lemasson B and Bräuer-Krisch E *et al* 2017 Permeability of brain tumor vessels induced by uniform or spatially microfractionated synchrotron radiation therapies *Int. J. Radiat. Oncol. Biol. Phys.* **98** 1174–82
[92] Bouchet A, Lemasson B, Christen T, Potez M, Rome C and Coquery N *et al* 2013 Synchrotron microbeam radiation therapy induces hypoxia in intracerebral gliosarcoma but not in the normal brain *Radiother. Oncol.* **108** 143–8
[93] Potez M, Fernandez-Palomo C, Bouchet A, Trappetti V, Donzelli M and Krisch M *et al* 2019 Synchrotron microbeam radiation therapy as a new approach for the treatment of radioresistant melanoma: potential underlying mechanisms *Int. J. Radiat. Oncol. Biol. Phys.* **105** 1126–36
[94] Sabatasso S, Laissue J A, Hlushchuk R, Graber W, Bravin A and Bräuer-Krisch E *et al* 2011 Microbeam radiation-induced tissue damage depends on the stage of vascular maturation *Int. J. Radiat. Oncol. Biol. Phys.* **80** 1522–32
[95] Brönnimann D, Bouchet A, Schneider C, Potez M, Serduc R and Bräuer-Krisch E *et al* 2016 Synchrotron microbeam irradiation induces neutrophil infiltration, thrombocyte attachment and selective vascular damage *in vivo Sci. Rep.* **6** 1–10
[96] Potez M, Fernandez-Palomo C, Bouchet A, Trappetti V, Donzelli M and Krisch M *et al* 2019 Synchrotron microbeam radiation therapy as a new approach for the treatment of radioresistant melanoma: potential underlying mechanisms *Int. J. Radiat. Oncol. Biol. Phys.* **105** 1126–36
[97] Bouchet A, Sakakini N, El Atifi M, Le Clec'h C, Brauer E and Moisan A *et al* 2013 Early gene expression analysis in 9L orthotopic tumor-bearing rats identifies immune modulation in molecular response to synchrotron microbeam radiation therapy *PLoS One* **8** e81874

[98] Ventura J, Lobachevsky P N, Palazzolo J S, Forrester H, Haynes N M and Ivashkevich A *et al* 2017 Localized synchrotron irradiation of mouse skin induces persistent systemic genotoxic and immune responses *Cancer Res.* **77** 6389–99

[99] Potez M, Fernandez-Palomo C, Bouchet A, Trappetti V, Donzelli M and Krisch M *et al* 2019 Synchrotron microbeam radiation therapy as a new approach for the treatment of radioresistant melanoma: potential underlying mechanisms *Int. J. Radiat. Oncol.* **105** 1126–36

[100] Connolly K A, Belt B A, Figueroa N M, Murthy A, Patel A and Kim M *et al* 2016 Increasing the efficacy of radiotherapy by modulating the CCR2/CCR5 chemokine axes *Oncotarget* **7** 86522–35

[101] Régnard P, Bräuer-Krisch E, Troprès I, Keyriläinen J, Bravin A, Le and Duc G 2008 Enhancement of survival of 9L gliosarcoma bearing rats following intracerebral delivery of drugs in combination with microbeam radiation therapy *Eur. J. Radiol.* **68** S151–5

[102] Sabatasso S, Fernandez-Palomo C, Hlushchuk R, Fazzari J, Tschanz S and Pellicioli P *et al* 2021 Transient and efficient vascular permeability window for adjuvant drug delivery triggered by microbeam radiation *Cancers* **13** 2103

[103] Bouchet A, Lemasson B, Christen T, Potez M, Rome C and Coquery N *et al* 2013 Synchrotron microbeam radiation therapy induces hypoxia in intracerebral gliosarcoma but not in the normal brain *Radiother. Oncol.* **108** 143–8

# Chapter 21

# Spatially fractionated radiation therapy: from photons to charged particles

**Yolanda Prezado**

Although it has existed for more than a century, spatially fractionated radiation therapy (SFRT) is still not widely employed compared to conventional radiotherapy. However, decades of clinical and preclinical data have shown that SFRT has promise as a high-therapeutic-index treatment. The use of photons in SFRT allows its widespread implementation but presents several drawbacks and limitations. Alternatively, the use of charged particles in combination with SFRT promises to overcome these limitations by combining the physical and biological advantages of protons and heavy ions for both normal tissue sparing and tumor control with the benefits of SFRT. Although the exploration of charged-particle SFRT is very recent, the data obtained indicate that this novel approach has the potential to offer radical treatments in some severe cases, such as high-grade gliomas. Moreover, the reduced neurotoxicity of charged-particle SFRT may be of interest in pediatric oncology. Charged-particle SFRT offers several possibilities for both scientific research and potential future clinical practice.

## 21.1 Introduction

Radiotherapy (RT) is one of the most important methods used in cancer treatment. An estimated 2.9 million people will be diagnosed with cancer in the EU-28 in 2030, of whom 50% will receive external beam radiotherapy [1]. Technological advances in RT in recent decades have led to improved tumor dose conformation, thus diminishing the dose given to organs at risk [2]. Despite this, adverse effects of RT are still common, and this is the main limitation of its use: the normal tissue tolerances compromise the effective treatment of radioresistant tumors.

The utilization of highly spatially modulated beams activates different biological mechanisms from those involved when direct damage by ionizing radiation takes

doi:10.1088/978-0-7503-4046-5ch21  

place. This approach, called SFRT, uses a strong spatial modulation of the radiation dose to create alternating regions of high and low doses in contrast to standard RT, which utilizes homogeneous dose distributions. SFRT has been demonstrated to spare normal tissues while still maintaining good local tumor control [3]. There are four main types of SFRT: GRID therapy [4], lattice therapy [5], microbeam radiation therapy (MRT) [6], and minibeam radiation therapy (MBRT) [7]. While a number of patients have been treated with GRID and lattice therapy, MRT and MBRT have only been used at preclinical stages. All four types of SFRT have been mainly explored with x-rays thus far.

Although the first such treatments date back to the early 20th century [8], SFRT is rarely applied clinically compared to standard RT. Nowadays, techniques such as GRID [4] and lattice therapy [5] are mainly used for the palliative treatment of bulky malignant tumors, which cannot otherwise be handled. They provide remarkable relief from severe symptoms and significant tumor regression while being minimally toxic in palliative settings [3]. In both techniques, a high radiation dose is delivered in one fraction (10–20 Gy) using megavoltage x-ray beams produced by clinical medical linear accelerators (linacs).

The advancement of both technology and radiobiology [3] is generating renewed interest in SFRT at many centers worldwide, and newly formed working groups are actively formulating guidelines and protocols [9]. A growing number of clinical trials for palliative SFRT are ongoing or being planned. However, the implementation of SFRT using linacs is a double-edged sword. On the one hand, the widespread availability of these machines facilitates patient access to these techniques. On the other hand, it does not allow patients to fully benefit from the advantages of spatial fractionation, i.e. the reduction of normal tissue complications. The lateral scattering of megavoltage beams reduces the degree of spatial modulation of the dose, which consequently reduces the normal tissue tolerances. In addition, the characteristics and output of conventional linacs require the use of thick beamlets ($>1$ cm$^2$), which limits dose escalation in order to spare normal tissues and restricts the use of this technique to bulky and very advanced tumors.

Since normal tissue radiosensitivity depends on the volume of tissue irradiated [10], a possible way to shift to curative treatment is to combine spatial fractionation of the dose with the use of very narrow beams, which is what MRT and MBRT accomplish. Both originated at large synchrotron sources, which are facilities that provide intense kilovoltage x-ray beams with negligible beam divergence. The irradiation is performed with arrays of parallel, thin beams: 25- to 100 μm wide beams in MRT and 0.5–1.0 mm wide in MBRT. Numerous experiments have shown that MRT and MBRT can spare normal tissues, even at doses of more than 50 Gy in one fraction [7, 11]. Remarkable tumor control has also been observed [12, 13].

The extremely narrow beams used in MRT require (a) the use of very high dose rates ($\geqslant$100 Gy s$^{-1}$) to maintain the peak and valley patterns, (b) low-kilovoltage energies (inadequate for deep-seated tumor treatments) to reduce lateral scattering, and (c) a challenging positioning system and some unique dosimetry protocols. All these requirements hinder MRT's clinical applicability. MBRT helps overcome these limitations, as the thicker beams (0.5–1.0 mm) allow it to be provided by low-cost equipment, such as small animal irradiators [14, 15]. Therefore, MBRT is a technique that offers the best compromise between the thick beams used in GRID and lattice RT, which impose limits due to normal tissue dose tolerances, and the extreme conditions of MRT. Most of the studies of MBRT used kV photon beams. The use of megavoltage (MV) photons would lead to a much-reduced spatial modulation, reducing its benefits.

To develop the concept further, the type of particle can be changed, i.e. charged particles can be used instead of photons. The use of charged particles in combination with SFRT may allow patients to fully benefit from the advantages of spatial fractionation of the dose, while at the same time paving a direct avenue for optimal future patient treatments. In the next sections, we review the rationale, state of the art, and perspectives of charged-particle SFRT.

## 21.2 Charged-particle SFRT: its rationale and the state of the art

The high therapeutic index of SFRT can be further increased by combining it with the superior relative biological effectiveness of charged particles, as they not only allow for more selective depth–dose deposition compared with that of photons but also have negligible dose deposition after the Bragg peak.

Moreover, there are some indications that heavy ions can potentiate the immune response in a more effective manner than photons or even proton beams [16]. This might result in a highly effective synergistic effect with the potential immune activation induced by SFRT [17].

In recent years, different approaches have been explored, which are described in the following subsections.

### 21.2.1 Proton MBRT

Proton MBRT (pMBRT), proposed in 2013 by Prezado *et al* [18] and Zlobinskaya *et al* [19], represents the most evolved experimental form of SFRT with charged particles. It combines the more localized dose distribution of the Bragg peak of protons with the possibility of simultaneously achieving a homogeneous dose distribution in the tumor and a pronounced spatial fractionation of the dose in the normal tissues [18, 20], even with a single field of minibeams (0.5–1.0 mm in width); see figure 21.1. This represents an important advantage over x-ray MBRT wherein multiple interlacing fields are usually required to achieve target dose homogenization, which is both error prone and technically challenging. The Institut Curie–Orsay Proton Therapy Center (ICPO) witnessed the first worldwide technical implementation of pMBRT at a clinical center in 2014 [21]. pMBRT was performed at one of the passive beamlines, and proton minibeams were produced by means of a brass multislit collimator (MScol). A similar implementation was employed by Dilmanian *et al* [21] in 2015 to confirm the physical feasibility of the technique.

Since the first experiments, efforts have concentrated on optimizing the proton minibeam generation at clinical centers. Some studies have reported on the best MScol material, thickness, shape, and distance to the target for pMBRT [23, 24].

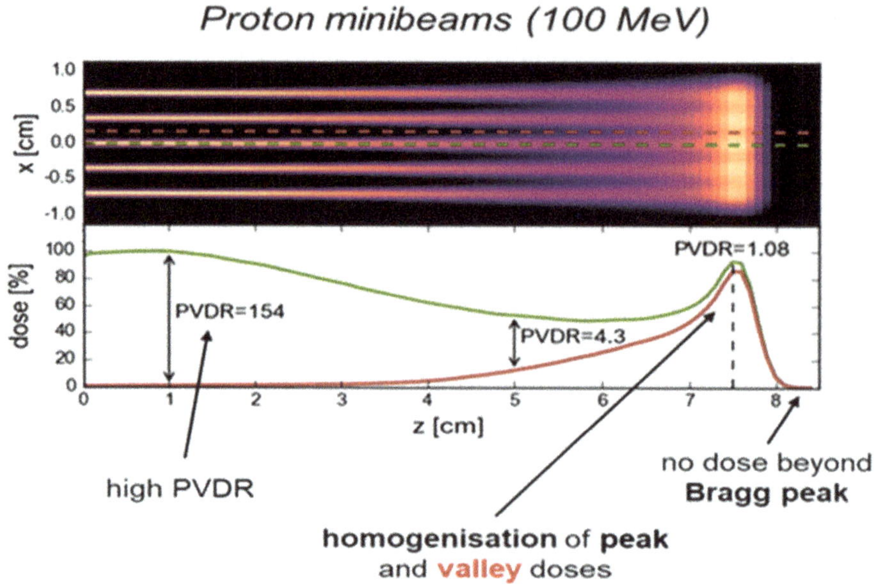


**Figure 21.1.** Dose distributions in pMBRT. Taken with permission from [20].

Other important technological milestones include the implementation of pMBRT using a pencil beam scanning system with an optimized MScol [25], a scanning dynamic collimator for spot-scanning proton minibeam production [26], and a new nozzle design for magnetically focused minibeams [27]. The last approach removes the need for any mechanical collimation, which improves irradiation efficiency and flexibility as well as the degree of spatial fractionation in healthy tissue. Moreover, a recent conceptual design study indicated that the new minibeam nozzle, in combination with proton linacs such as LIGHT (Advanced Oncotherapy PLC), may provide an optimal implementation of pMBRT. In addition, the high irradiation efficiency of magnetically focused minibeams could pave the way toward a combination of pMBRT and FLASH therapy [28]. The next steps will be to perform a technical design study and ultimately the construction and testing of a nozzle prototype.

Dosimetry is one of the main challenges of pMBRT. If pMBRT were to be applied to patients, high-precision dose measurements (2%) would be required, which would be challenging and error prone due to the very small beam sizes involved. For small fields (in terms of physical size), no methodology or correction factors, such as scatter factors, exist. The volume averaging effect, or the lack of secondary electron equilibrium, play non-negligible roles, and the approximations of classical radiation physics tend to be valid to a lesser extent compared to those for larger fields. Ionization chambers, which are the gold standard detectors in RT, do not offer the spatial resolution required to resolve the peak and valley regions. Preclinical dosimetry is currently performed using a two-step protocol [29, 30]: absolute dosimetry is carried out under broad beam (BB) conditions using an

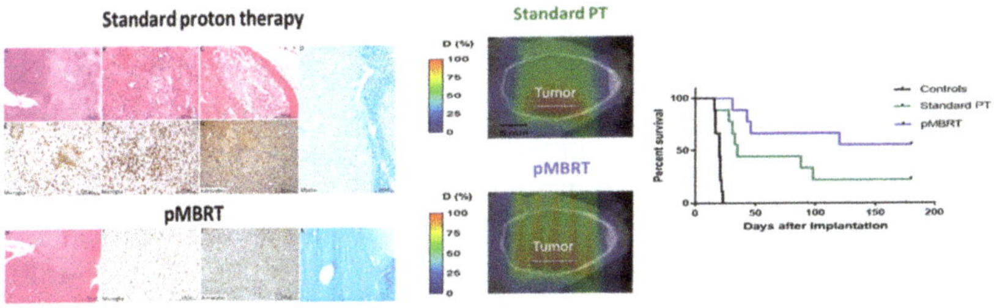


**Figure 21.2.** Illustration of the net gain in the therapeutic index of pMBRT. Left: minimum toxicity in pMBRT. Histopathological and immunohistochemical analyses revealed substantial damage in the conventional group (A–G). *Conventional irradiation*: (A) Multifocal to coalescing lesion characterized by (B) edema, necrosis, and gliosis. (C) More severe lesions with cavitation and mineralization. (D) Destruction of the myelin was also observed. (E, F) Microglial activation and microglial nodules (microgliosis). (G) Astrocyte activation with a marked increase in glial fibrillary acidic protein (GFAP) immunolabeling (astrogliosis). *Minibeam irradiation*: (H) No lesion was observed in most rats (seven out of eight), with (I and J) normal microglial and astrocytic networks, and (K) normal myelin organization. Only one microscopic inflammatory focus was observed in one of the eight rats. Taken with permission from [33]. Center: dose distributions received by the tumor-bearing rats. Right: tumor control. Survival curves of tumor-bearing rats: controls (black line), standard PT (green), and pMBRT with a quasi-homogeneous dose in the target (blue). An enhanced lifespan can be observed. Taken from [34].

ionization chamber, and relative dosimetry is realized with high-resolution detectors, such as Gafchromic films [21, 30], microdiamond detectors [30], or small diodes [25].

A series of radiobiological studies have already demonstrated the remarkable reduction in the normal tissue toxicity caused by pMBRT as compared to that of standard proton therapy [19, 31–33]. The first experiments were devoted to a comparative evaluation of the response of the skin to pMBRT versus its response to homogenous proton BB irradiation. In a three-dimensional human skin model, the latter resulted in significantly higher inflammatory response and cell death than that of pMBRT irradiation [19]. In addition, proton BB irradiation of mouse ears led to a significantly higher degree of edema, erythema, or desquamation than that in a group of animals that received proton MBRT at the same average dose (60 Gy) [31].

Another pioneering experiment reported the remarkable reduction of neurotoxicity caused by pMBRT [33]. The whole brain (excepting the olfactory bulb) of two groups ($n$ = 8/group) of normal rats (seven weeks old) was irradiated: (i) a first group received a seamless (standard) proton irradiation with high doses (25 Gy in one session) and (ii) a second group received pMBRT irradiation with peak doses of 58 Gy/fraction (corresponding to the same average dose of 25 Gy). The animals were then followed up for six months. A longitudinal magnetic resonance imaging (MRI) study was carried out using a 7 T small animal MRI scanner along with histological and immunochemical analyses. The rats treated with conventional proton irradiation presented grade 3 skin damage (moist desquamation) and extensive brain damage, including necrosis, demyelination, astrogliosis, and microglial activation, whereas those who received pMBRT treatments did not have significant tissue damage [33]; see figure 21.2. It has also been demonstrated that pMBRT treatment has no significant impact on the cognitive, motor, or emotional processes [32].

This reduction of neurotoxicity with respect to standard RT may improve the therapeutic index in cases wherein tumor control is accompanied by substantial side effects, such as pediatric astrocytoma. It also opens the door to a more efficient treatment of extremely radioresistant tumors, such as high-grade gliomas (glioblastoma multiforme (GBM)), which are among the most challenging conditions in clinical oncology. In this context, glioma-bearing rats were irradiated in a series of experiments. pMBRT resulted in tumor control that was equal or superior to that of standard RT but without the latter's side effects observed in different rat glioma models, opening the possibility of more aggressive irradiation schemes [34–36]. In addition, in some of the configurations evaluated, 70% of the rats who survived tumor-free for more than six months belonged to the pMBRT group [34]. The mean survival time was significantly higher in the pMBRT group than in the standard PT group, despite the heterogeneous target dose coverage. Tumor sterilization was achieved even in cases in which large areas of the tumor received low (non-tumoricidal) doses [36]. This contradicts the classical paradigm that RT requires the deposition of a lethal dose in every tumor cell for tumor ablation. Recent evaluations point at a determinant role of the immune system in the antitumor response of pMBRT [37]. Moreover, the fact that large areas (or even the whole brain) could be irradiated without significant side effects would allow clinicians to overcome one of the major difficulties in glioma treatment, which is its infiltrative nature.

A recent study has also shown that pMBRT would benefit from hypofractionation schemes [38]. pMBRT was previously delivered in one single fraction to avoid any blurring of the characteristic peak and valley pattern due to repositioning inaccuracies. In this study, crossfire irradiation using two orthogonal arrays delivered on two different days spaced 48 h apart was employed to short-circuit the technical challenges of achieving accurate area irradiation with submillimetric precision. As a result, 83% of the rats that survived tumor-free received crossfire irradiation in two fractions. Compared to the results of some other spatially fractionated techniques, such as MRT, this is one of the best results obtained thus far in glioma-bearing rats treated with pMBRT [39]. These results can facilitate the translation of pMBRT to patient treatment by enabling the dose to be split into several fractions based on entry ports using cross-fired arrays with lower peak doses than those used in single-fraction/single-port studies.

Ultimately, the goal is to translate and reproduce the findings of pMBRT from small animal experiments into clinical treatments. The experimental data gathered thus far indicate that pMBRT can further increase the therapeutic index, allowing clinical practice to move from mostly palliative treatments (e.g. GRID therapy) to curative treatments. pMBRT might offer an efficient treatment method for radiation-resistant tumors, such as GBM, osteosarcomas, chordomas, or chondrosarcomas, as it allows higher and potentially curative doses to be deposited in the tumor. It might also be of interest in pediatric oncology due to its remarkable reduction in neurotoxicity. The first therapeutic trials could include primitive brain tumors with a very poor prognosis, such as recurrent gliomas. Results of the evaluation of two different brain tumors, glioma and meningioma, revealed that pMBRT meets the recommended criteria for clinically acceptable dose–volume histograms in organs at risk. Satisfactory homogeneity was achieved in the target, while a level of spatial dose modulation in normal tissues similar to those in preclinical studies was obtained [40].

In conclusion, pMBRT is a novel cancer therapy approach that promises a high therapeutic index in difficult-to-treat cases such as GBM. Even though it is a novel method, the biological data gathered thus far has challenged the classical paradigm in RT and encouraged the preparation of phase I clinical trials.

### 21.2.2 Proton GRID therapy

Benefiting from the advantages of the newest proton delivery method, namely, pencil beam scanning, the possibility of merging proton therapy with GRID therapy was also recently proposed after pMBRT [41, 42]. The use of protons instead of photons for GRID therapy offers several benefits. As in the case of pMBRT, the use of protons results in a more uniform dose within the tumor (a lower peak–valley dose ratio (PVDR)) while sparing normal tissues located beyond the tumor. In common with photon GRID therapy, proton GRID therapy uses beamlets ~1 cm in diameter and is limited to bulky tumors (mainly palliative treatments).

Proton GRID therapy could benefit patients who can neither be treated with photons nor with standard BB irradiation nor with photon GRID due to the tolerance of normal tissues. In a previous report, ten patients with large tumors were palliatively treated with proton GRID therapy (1 cm wide beams) [43]. The median time to the last follow-up was around six months. At the last follow-up, seven patients were alive, while three had died (figure 21.3). Among the treated patients,

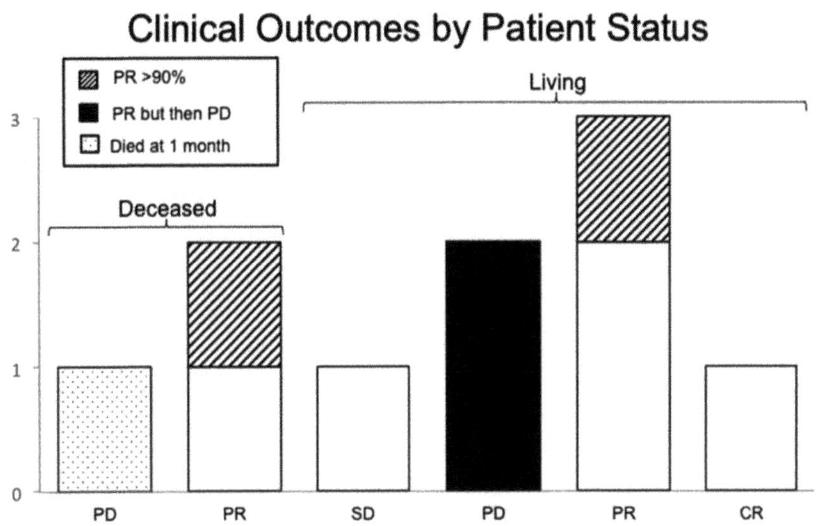


**Figure 21.3.** Clinical outcomes by patient status. CR, complete response; PD, progressive disease; PR, partial response; SD, stable disease. Taken from [43]. © 2020 the authors. Published by the British Institute of Radiology.

60% suffered from pain and 30% experienced a decreased range of motion. Bleeding and hydronephrosis were observed in 20% and 10% of these patients, respectively. More details of proton GRID therapy can be found in chapter 13.

### 21.2.3 Light ion SFRT

The reduced multiple Coulomb scattering (MSC) and nuclear fragmentation of light ions (helium to lithium) compared to those of protons and heavier ions, respectively, make such ions a good candidate for SFRT. Thus far, only theoretical (Monte Carlo) simulations of light ion MBRT have been carried out [22, 44].

Using the Monte Carlo N-Particle extended (MNCPX) software, Dilmanian *et al* [22] assessed the evolution of minibeam width as a function of depth and ion species. As a result of the reduced MSC, a reduction by a factor of three of the full width at half maximum can be expected at a depth of 3 cm when changing from protons to lithium. This implies that at the same center-to-center distance, dose homogenization can be achieved at shallower depths using protons. In addition, the possibility of keeping the beam width narrow at this depth helps to preserve normal tissue.

A deeper comparative evaluation of helium and proton beams was carried out by Schneider *et al* [44]. Using Monte Carlo simulations, they confirmed the advantage of helium ions for MBRT in terms of the PVDR, the Bragg peak-to-entrance dose ratio (BEDR), and linear energy transfer (LET). In particular, helium ion minibeams exhibit significantly improved depth–dose profiles with nearly three times higher BEDRs than that of proton MBRT for 1 mm wide beams. A higher PVDR is achieved in nearly MBRT at identical center-to-center distances, which benefits normal tissue sparing. In contrast, dose homogenization in the target, which today represents the standard practice in clinics, is more complicated when helium ions are used, as opposed to protons. Finally, the LET values in the Bragg peak are about four times higher for helium ion minibeams than for proton minibeams (figure 21.4).

The consequent increased relative biological effectiveness could provide more tumor control. Helium ions also exhibit LET values that are twice as high at shallow depths in normal tissues. This is, however, compensated by the higher BEDR of helium MBRT.

Biological experiments are warranted to confirm the benefits of light ion MBRT.

### 21.2.4 Carbon and oxygen SFRT

Among the different types of ion species, carbon ions are considered to have the most optimal properties in terms of superior physical and biological characteristics [45]. Oxygen ions benefit from a higher LET, which could be of benefit in the treatment of hypoxic tumors.

Several dosimetric studies have assessed the potential benefits and drawbacks of the combination of carbon or oxygen ions and MBRT [46–48]. Gonzalez *et al* [46] showed that carbon and oxygen follow a similar behavior and that similar values of peak and (very low) valley doses are obtained. Extremely high PVDR values of 5000 could be obtained for center-to-center distances of 3500 μm at the entrance, which favors tissue sparing. However, a possible concern is nuclear fragmentation and the

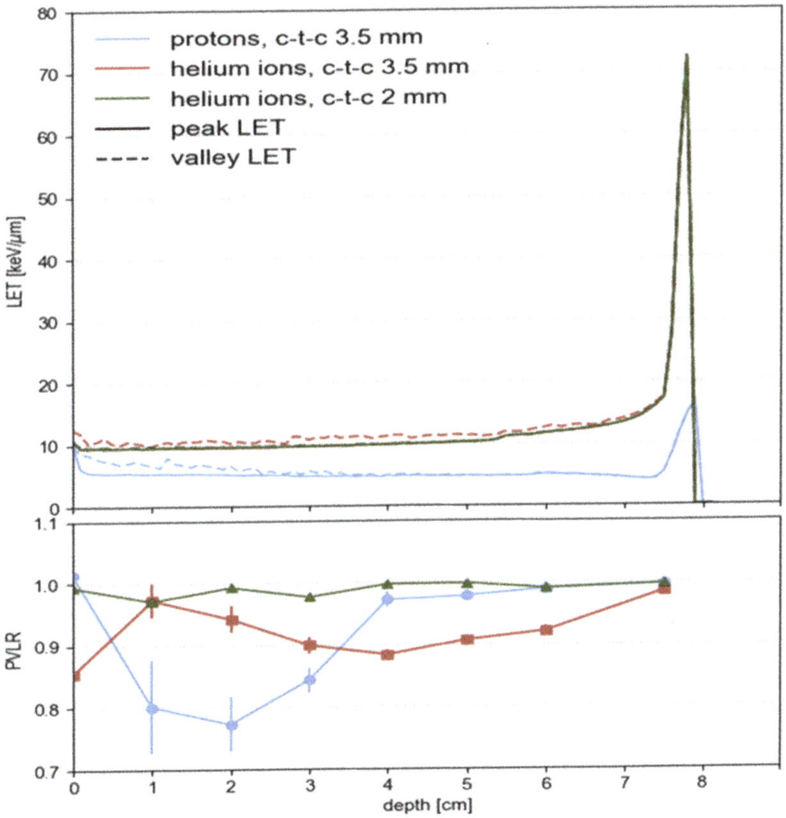


**Figure 21.4.** Depth–dose averaged LET profiles in the peak and valley regions and evolution of the peak-to-valley LET ratio as a function of depth [44] John Wiley & Sons, © 2019, American Association of Physicists in Medicine.

contribution of high-LET secondary particles to the valley doses, which are considered to be responsible for tissue sparing in SFRT. The participation of the different secondary species to the valley dose was assessed, including the function of the center-to-center distance, primary ion, and depth. Gonzalez *et al* showed that the dose in the valley regions is mainly composed of scattered primary ions (in which case, similar LET values can be expected in the peaks and valleys). The contribution of secondary species is lower than 20%, and δ-rays are the main participants at depths of up to 4 cm, which might benefit normal tissue sparing (figure 21.5).

A dosimetric experiment was carried out at the Heidelberg Ion Therapy Center [47], where two different detector systems (the PTW microDiamond detector and EBT3 Gafchromic films) were used to carry out dosimetric measurements of submillimetric field sizes in carbon and oxygen therapy. The general agreement between the two detectors confirms the reliability of those systems for small-field dosimetry in mixed LET irradiation when proper corrections are applied.

The confirmation of the potential of this innovative approach requires the realization of biological experiments. Thus far, only one experiment in carbon

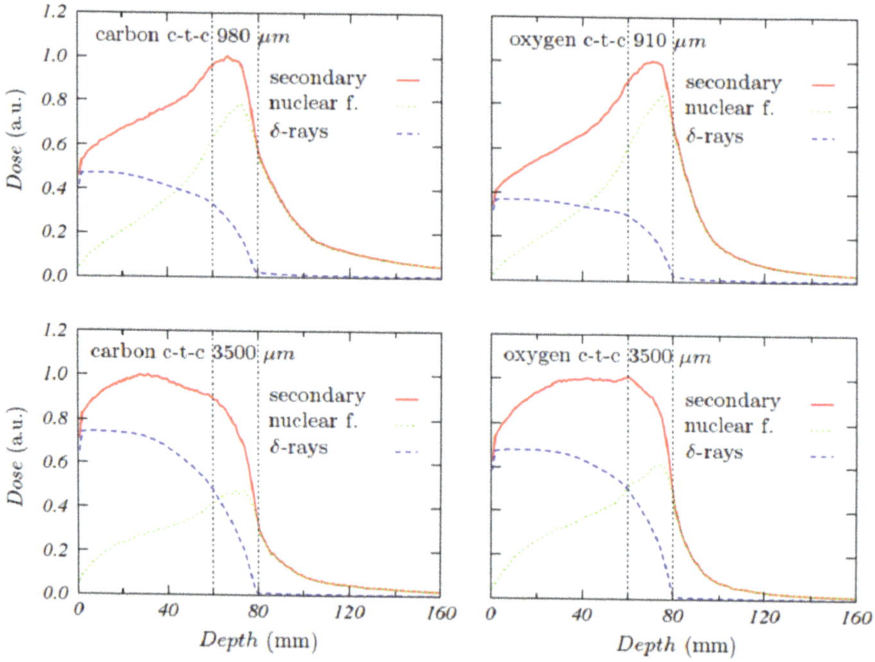


**Figure 21.5.** The contribution of the different species of secondary particle to the peak depth–dose curves for carbon (left column) and oxygen (right column) and the different center-to-center distances. The doses are normalized to the maximum of the total sum of secondary products [46] John Wiley & Sons, © 2019, American Association of Physicists in Medicine.

MBRT has been reported [49]. A single rabbit brain was irradiated with several arrays of 130 MeV/nucleon carbon 300 μm wide beams interlacing at the target, which showed a reduced impact on the non-targeted tissues. Further evaluations, including long-term follow-ups, statistically significant data, and dose escalation studies in clinical beams, are needed to confirm the clinical potentials of carbon MBRT and oxygen MBRT.

As in the case of protons, the combination of carbon ions and GRID therapy has also been explored. In a Monte Carlo simulation study, Tsubouchi *et al* [50] evaluated different crossfire geometries. The potential reduction of the impact on normal tissues needs to be balanced with the technical complexity of accurately irradiating tumors using these configurations. No conclusion was reached regarding the optimum beam width or center-to-center distance.

### 21.2.5 Very heavy ion SFRT

Due to their high LETs, heavier ions, such as neon or argon, produce a reduced oxygen enhancement effect. This could provide a benefit in the treatment of hypoxic tumors, which remains one of the major challenges in RT. Radiobiological findings in the laboratory have indicated that the resistant cells of hypoxic tumors could be effectively destroyed by beams of very heavy ions such as silicon and argon.

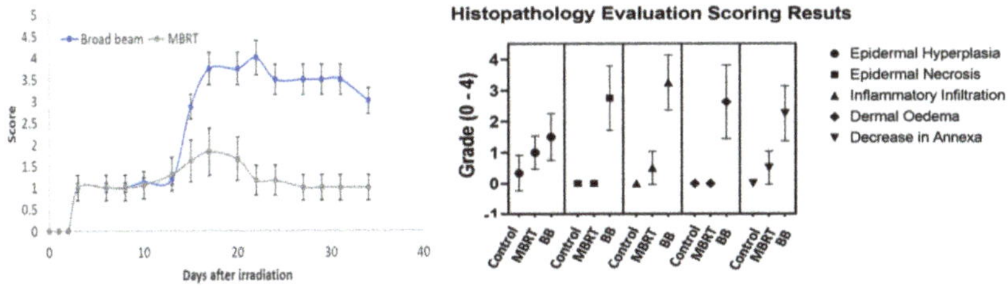


**Figure 21.6.** Left: evaluation of the average skin damage scores as a function of follow-up time and irradiation method. Mean and standard deviation values are represented in the plot. Right: histology evaluation scoring results showing mean values and standard deviations for the different irradiation modes. Reprinted from [53], with permission of MDPI.

However, clinical results with a few patients performed with argon in 1979 and with silicon in 1982 revealed late adverse effects, resulting in the discontinuation of these beams [51]. Nevertheless, the tissue sparing provided by the use of SFRT may further benefit from the remarkable effectiveness of these heavy ions, which could offer a new treatment method for aggressive radioresistant hypoxic tumors that are refractory. The high LET in the target would overcome hypoxia, while SFRT might limit the side effects that normally prevent the use of heavy ions in conventional irradiation settings.

The alliance of very heavy ions and MBRT was first proposed by Peucelle *et al* [52]. The advantageous dose distributions obtained in the first Monte Carlo studies [48, 52] encouraged the further exploration of extremely high PVDR values (>100), very narrow penumbras, and low valley doses, which were achieved in the first centimeters as well as in the fragmentation tail that spared the proximal normal tissues. Although the yield of secondary nuclear products increases with the atomic number, the actual dose deposited by the secondary nuclear fragments in the valleys becomes dominant only at the Bragg peak (tumor) position [52].

The first *in vivo* experiment was carried out at HIMAC-NIRS (Japan). Among the different ion species, neon ions were selected since, in addition to high LET values (close to 100 keV $\mu m^{-1}$), they were shown to offer the best balance between having a high PVDR and a high peak-to-valley LET ratio in normal tissues in the target region [48].

Three groups of mouse legs were irradiated with 230 MeV $A^{-1}$ of neon ions to compare the skin response: (i) one group received BB conventional irradiation (20 Gy, $N = 8$); (ii) a second group received neon MBRT at the same mean dose (20 Gy, $N = 8$); and (iii) a third group received neon MBRT with a peak dose equal to 20 Gy ($N = 8$). The animals were then followed up for four weeks. A significant difference was observed between the mice that received conventional and MBRT irradiations [53]; six out of eight mice in the BB group had to be sacrificed two weeks after irradiation, as they reached damage scores of four to five (ulceration, necrosis). In contrast, only dermatitis was observed in the MBRT groups (score, <2). This suggests a clear benefit of using neon MBRT in terms of normal tissue sparing. Figure 21.6 depicts the evolution of the skin damage scores as a function of time and irradiation method as well as the histological results.

## 21.3 Future perspectives

SFRT is rapidly moving toward the use of charged particles, due to their inherent advantages when combined with SFRT. Although some patients have been treated with proton GRID with a palliative intent [43], the final aim is to develop curative treatments for large and/or radioresistant tumors. This could be potentially achieved using techniques such as pMBRT [18]. The biological data collected thus far support the preparation of phase I clinical trials, which include the development of dosimetry protocols and treatment planning systems that provide sufficient accuracy (2%) for the dose determination of such narrow beams (0.5–1.0 mm).

In addition, the biological mechanisms involved in SFRT in general and in charged-particle SFRT are not completely understood. As previously indicated, the utilization of charged particles may also modify the underlying mechanisms or their relative weights with respect to photons. For example, there is increasing evidence that charged particles are more effective in activating the immune system and inhibiting angiogenesis [16]. In pMBRT, the immune system has been shown to play a central role in the antitumor response [37]. Some other potential effects include cell signaling effects, i.e. bystander-like effects [54], and the preferential effect on the tumoral versus normal vasculature [55]. These phenomena need to be further investigated using a comprehensive approach. Additionally, at present, it is unclear how these effects are translated when the type of particle or the spatial dose distribution is modified, as no systematic evaluation of the influence of the beam width and spacing on the tissue response to SFRT has ever been performed.

Future research should be focused on determining: (a) the underlying mechanisms, (b) how these effects are translated when the spatial distribution and/or type of particle is modified, and (c) the best way of prescribing the dose in charged-particle SFRT, i.e. in terms of peak, valley, average dose, or novel metrics.

## 21.4 Conclusions

Charged-particle SFRT is a novel cancer therapy approach that promises a high therapeutic index in difficult-to-treat cases. The results gathered thus far indicate that charged particles and SFRT are a promising combination. The normal tissue sparing that occurs in SFRT can be enhanced by the dosimetric and ballistic advantages of charged particles. Charged particles provide a more selective depth–dose deposition that that of photons along with a negligible dose deposition after the Bragg peak. Moreover, the reduced MSC of heavy ions results in high PVDR and low valley doses in normal tissues. All these factors spare normal tissues, which add to the already-known benefits of SFRT. However, the use of protons leads to a more homogenous dose distribution in the tumor than that of x-rays. The superior relative biological effectiveness of heavy ions can also effectively control tumors. In addition, the enhanced ability of heavy ions to activate the immune system, as compared to that of x-rays, can lead to a synergic effect with SFRT [16, 17].

The most evaluated technique thus far is pMBRT. It reduces neurotoxicity, which is of interest for brain tumor treatments, specifically in pediatric oncology. Several *in vivo* experiments have shown that pMBRT has equivalent or superior tumor control to that of standard proton therapy. pMBRT also offers the best balance between the thick beams employed in GRID and lattice therapy and the extreme conditions of x-ray MRT. Although it is a novel method, the biological data gathered from pMBRT thus far challenges the classical paradigm in RT and supports the preparation of phase I clinical trials, which is currently ongoing at Institut Curie. Finally, the normal tissue preservation provided by MBRT may allow an optimized and renewed interest in the use of very heavy ions for therapy, which are very effective for treatment of hypoxic tumors.

In conclusion, charged-particle SFRT may overcome some of the limitations of x-ray SFRT, which may allow this method to shift from mainly palliative to curative treatment as well as to offer an efficient treatment in difficult cases such as GBM.

## References


[1] Borras J M *et al* 2016 How many new cancer patients in Europe will require radiotherapy by 2025? An ESTRO-HERO analysis *Radiother. Oncol.* **119** 5–11

[2] Bernier J, Hall E J and Giaccia A 2004 Radiation oncology: a century of achievements *Nat. Rev. Cancer.* **4** 737–47

[3] Yan W *et al* 2020 Spatially fractionated radiation therapy: history, present and the future *Clin. Transl. Radiat. Oncol.* **20** 30–8

[4] Mohiuddin M *et al* 1999 High-dose spatially-fractionated radiation (GRID): a new paradigm in the management of advanced cancers *Int. J. Radiat. Oncol. Biol. Phys.* **45** 721–7

[5] Amendola B E *et al* 2019 Safety and efficacy of lattice radiotherapy in voluminous non-small cell lung cancer *Cureus* **11** e4263

[6] Slatkin D N *et al* 1992 Microbeam radiation therapy *Med. Phys.* **19** 1395–400

[7] Dilmanian F A *et al* 2006 Interlaced x-ray microplanar beams: a radiosurgery approach with clinical potential *Proc. Natl Acad. Sci. USA* **103** 9709–14

[8] Laissue J A, Blattmann H and Slatkin D N 2012 [Alban Kohler (1874–1947): inventor of grid therapy] *Z. Med. Phys.* **22** 90–9

[9] Zhang H *et al* 2020 Photon GRID radiation therapy: a physics and dosimetry white paper from the Radiosurgery Society (RSS) GRID/LATTICE, Microbeam and FLASH Radiotherapy Working Group *Radiat. Res.* **194** 665–77

[10] Zeman W *et al* 1959 Tolerance of mouse-brain tissue to high-energy deuterons *Science* **130** 1760–1

[11] Eling L *et al* 2019 Ultra high dose rate synchrotron microbeam radiation therapy. preclinical evidence in view of a clinical transfer *Radiother. Oncol.* **139** 56–61

[12] Fernandez-Palomo C *et al* 2020 Animal models in microbeam radiation therapy: a scoping review *Cancers (Basel)* **12** 527

[13] Sotiropoulos M *et al* 2021 X-rays minibeam radiation therapy at a conventional irradiator: pilot evaluation in F98-glioma bearing rats and dose calculations in a human phantom. *Clin. Transl. Radiat. Oncol.* **27** 44–9

[14] Prezado Y *et al* 2017 Transfer of minibeam radiation therapy into a cost-effective equipment for radiobiological studies: a proof of concept *Sci. Rep.* **7** 17295

[15] Bazyar S *et al* 2017 Minibeam radiotherapy with small animal irradiators; *in vitro* and *in vivo* feasibility studies *Phys. Med. Biol.* **62** 8924–42

[16] Tinganelli W and Durante M 2020 Carbon ion radiobiology *Cancers (Basel)* **12** 3022

[17] Potez M *et al* 2019 Synchrotron microbeam radiation therapy as a new approach for the treatment of radioresistant melanoma: potential underlying mechanisms *Int. J. Radiat. Oncol. Biol. Phys.* **105** 1126–36
[18] Prezado Y and Fois G R 2013 Proton-minibeam radiation therapy: a proof of concept *Med. Phys.* **40** 031712
[19] Zlobinskaya O *et al* 2013 Reduced side effects by proton microchannel radiotherapy: study in a human skin model *Radiat. Environ. Biophys.* **52** 123–33
[20] Schneider T 2020 *Advancing the Generation of Proton Minibeams for Radiation Therapy* Université Paris-Saclay https://theses.hal.science/tel-03105944
[21] Peucelle C *et al* 2015 Proton minibeam radiation therapy: experimental dosimetry evaluation *Med. Phys.* **42** 7108–13
[22] Dilmanian F A, Eley J G and Krishnan S 2015 Minibeam therapy with protons and light ions: physical feasibility and potential to reduce radiation side effects and to facilitate hypofractionation *Int. J. Radiat. Oncol. Biol. Phys.* **92** 469–74
[23] Guardiola C, Peucelle C and Prezado Y 2017 Optimization of the mechanical collimation for minibeam generation in proton minibeam radiation therapy *Med. Phys.* **44** 1470–8
[24] Lee E, Meyer J and Sandison G 2016 Collimator design for spatially-fractionated proton beams for radiobiology research *Phys. Med. Biol.* **61** 5378–89
[25] De Marzi L *et al* 2018 Implementation of planar proton minibeam radiation therapy using a pencil beam scanning system: a proof of concept study *Med. Phys.* **45** 5305–16
[26] Sotiropoulos M and Prezado Y 2021 A scanning dynamic collimator for spot-scanning proton minibeam production *Sci. Rep.* **11** 18321
[27] Schneider T *et al* 2020 Advancing proton minibeam radiation therapy: magnetically focussed proton minibeams at a clinical centre *Sci. Rep.* **10** 1384
[28] Schneider T *et al* 2021 Conceptual design of a novel nozzle combined with a clinical proton linac for magnetically focussed minibeams *Cancers (Basel)* **13** 4657
[29] Prezado Y *et al* 2011 Dosimetry protocol for the preclinical trials in white-beam minibeam radiation therapy *Med. Phys.* **38** 5012–20
[30] Guardiola C, De L, Marzi and Prezado Y 2020 Verification of a Monte Carlo dose calculation engine in proton minibeam radiotherapy in a passive scattering beamline for preclinical trials *Br. J. Radiol.* **93** 20190578
[31] Girst S *et al* 2016 Proton minibeam radiation therapy reduces side effects in an *in vivo* mouse ear model *Int. J. Radiat. Oncol. Biol. Phys.* **95** 234–41
[32] Lamirault C *et al* 2020 Short and long-term evaluation of the impact of proton minibeam radiation therapy on motor, emotional and cognitive functions *Sci. Rep.* **10** 13511
[33] Prezado Y *et al* 2017 Proton minibeam radiation therapy spares normal rat brain: long-term clinical, radiological and histopathological analysis *Sci. Rep.* **7** 14403
[34] Prezado Y *et al* 2019 Tumor control in RG2 glioma-bearing rats: a comparison between proton minibeam therapy and standard proton therapy *Int. J. Radiat. Oncol. Biol. Phys.* **104** 266–71
[35] Lamirault C *et al* 2020 Spatially modulated proton minibeams results in the same increase of lifespan as a uniform target dose coverage in F98-glioma-bearing rats *Radiat. Res.* **194** 715–23
[36] Prezado Y *et al* 2018 Proton minibeam radiation therapy widens the therapeutic index for high-grade gliomas *Sci. Rep.* **8** 16479

[37] Annaig Bertho E B, Juchaux M, Gilbert C, Lamirault C, Patriarca A, de Marzi L, Pouzoulet F and Prezado Y 2021 Role of the immune system in anti-tumoral resopnse to proton minibeam radiation therapy *Radiother. Oncol.* **161** 1
[38] Bertho A *et al* 2021 First evaluation of temporal and spatial fractionation in proton minibeam radiation therapy of glioma-bearing rats *Cancers (Basel)* **13** 4865
[39] Fernandez-Palomo C *et al* 2020 Complete remission of mouse melanoma after temporally fractionated microbeam radiotherapy *Cancers (Basel)* **12** 527
[40] Lansonneur P *et al* 2020 First proton minibeam radiation therapy treatment plan evaluation *Sci. Rep.* **10** 7025
[41] Henry T *et al* 2017 Proton grid therapy: a proof-of-concept study *Technol. Cancer Res. Treat.* **16** 749–57
[42] Gao M *et al* 2018 Spatially fractionated (GRID) radiation therapy using proton pencil beam scanning (PBS): Feasibility study and clinical implementation *Med. Phys.* **45** 1645–53
[43] Mohiuddin M *et al* 2020 Early clinical results of proton spatially fractionated GRID radiation therapy (SFGRT) *Br. J. Radiol.* **93** 20190572
[44] Schneider T, Patriarca A and Prezado Y 2019 Improving the dose distributions in minibeam radiation therapy: helium ions vs protons *Med. Phys.* **46** 3640–8
[45] Okada T *et al* 2010 Carbon ion radiotherapy: clinical experiences at National Institute of Radiological Science (NIRS) *J. Radiat. Res.* **51** 355–64
[46] Gonzalez W, Peucelle C and Prezado Y 2017 Theoretical dosimetric evaluation of carbon and oxygen minibeam radiation therapy *Med. Phys.* **44** 1921–9
[47] Martinez-Rovira I *et al* 2017 Carbon and oxygen minibeam radiation therapy: an experimental dosimetric evaluation *Med. Phys.* **44** 4223–9
[48] Gonzalez W and Prezado Y 2018 Spatial fractionation of the dose in heavy ions therapy: an optimization study *Med. Phys.* **45** 2620–7
[49] Dilmanian F A *et al* 2012 Interleaved carbon minibeams: an experimental radiosurgery method with clinical potential *Int. J. Radiat. Oncol. Biol. Phys.* **84** 514–9
[50] Tsubouchi T *et al* 2018 Quantitative evaluation of potential irradiation geometries for carbon-ion beam grid therapy *Med. Phys.* **45** 1210–21
[51] Castro J R *et al* 1994 Experience in charged particle irradiation of tumors of the skull base: 1977–92 *Int. J. Radiat. Oncol. Biol. Phys.* **29** 647–55
[52] Peucelle C, Martinez-Rovira I and Prezado Y 2015 Spatial fractionation of the dose using neon and heavier ions: a Monte Carlo study *Med. Phys.* **42** 5928–36
[53] Prezado Y *et al* 2021 A potential renewed use of very heavy ions for therapy: neon minibeam radiation therapy *Cancers (Basel)* **13** 1356
[54] Lobachevsky P *et al* 2021 Synchrotron X-ray radiation-induced bystander effect: an impact of the scattered radiation, distance from the irradiated site and p53 cell status *Front. Oncol.* **11** 685598
[55] Bouchet A *et al* 2015 Effects of microbeam radiation therapy on normal and tumoral blood vessels *Phys. Med.* **31** 634–41

**IOP** Publishing

Spatially Fractionated, Microbeam and FLASH Radiation Therapy
A physics and multi-disciplinary approach
**Hualin Zhang and Nina A Mayr**

# Chapter 22

# Ultra-high dose-rate electron FLASH therapy

**Peter G Maxim, Emil Schüler and Kristoffer Petersson**

FLASH promises to be the first fundamentally new radiobiological approach to improving the therapeutic index of cancer radiation therapy in decades. Preclinical studies of FLASH have demonstrated reduced normal tissue toxicity without compromising tumor control in several organ systems, tumor models, and species, using several radiation beam types (electrons, x-rays, and protons). Although the fundamental mechanisms underlying these biological effects remain to be determined, the repeated demonstration of this phenomenon has generated broad interest throughout the cancer radiobiology and radiation oncology communities due to its potential to substantially affect therapeutic outcomes. However, the routine clinical implementation of FLASH radiation therapy will require capabilities beyond current technologies, particularly in the case of FLASH dosimetry and the necessary beam control and monitoring systems.

In this chapter, we present the current technological state of FLASH, specifically, the electron radiation sources capable of delivering FLASH dose rates, along with some challenges for FLASH dosimetry. We also discuss recent developments related to the beam-monitoring and control systems that FLASH-capable systems will require and the challenges associated with the clinical translation of FLASH.

## 22.1 Introduction

Ultra-high dose-rate irradiation, dubbed 'FLASH' by Favaudon *et al* in 2014 [1], has recently gained attention because of the surprising observation in preclinical *in vivo* model systems of a markedly increased therapeutic index compared to that of conventional dose rate irradiation. FLASH radiation therapy (RT), which refers to radiation delivered in subsecond time scales, could represent a paradigm shift in curative RT, given preclinical evidence that FLASH can significantly spare normal tissues while remaining as effective as conventional irradiation in the treatment of tumor tissues [1–6].

doi:10.1088/978-0-7503-4046-5ch22

Although much remains to be learned about the mechanisms underlying the FLASH phenomenon, a rational approach to initial clinical testing, in parallel with preclinical investigations, is feasible and will contribute to mechanistic understanding. In addition, elucidation of the mechanisms responsible for the FLASH effect through preclinical and clinical translational research will inform more specific and innovative clinical trial designs in the future, such as optimal fractionation schemes, combinations with oxygen modulation, immunotherapy, or other potentially biologically synergistic approaches. However, the routine clinical implementation of FLASH RT will require capabilities beyond currently available technologies, particularly in the areas of dose monitoring and control.

In this chapter, we present the current technological state of FLASH, specifically the electron radiation sources capable of delivering FLASH dose rates, along with some challenges for FLASH dosimetry. We also discuss recent developments related to the beam-monitoring and control systems that FLASH-capable systems will require and the challenges associated with the clinical translation of FLASH.

## 22.2 FLASH dosimetry

One of the major challenges for FLASH RT is dosimetry at these extreme dose rates (a mean dose rate of >40 Gy $s^{-1}$). FLASH uses high doses per pulse, which results in short delivery times and makes accurate dosimetry particularly challenging. This is because current protocols and equipment are designed for conventional RT, in which the dose rates are much lower. Further, any calibration factors used in FLASH dosimetry must be traceable to primary standards to ensure accurate dosimetry. Unfortunately, no such primary standards for ultra-high dose rates are available at this time. Therefore, further research is needed to develop suitable dose-monitoring devices with clinically acceptable dose accuracy, reproducibility, and traceability.

### 22.2.1 Ionization chambers

Ionization chambers (ICs) are the standard dosimeters used for reference dosimetry in clinical RT due to their traceability to national and international standards which are implemented through recognized national and international protocols for the calibration of RT equipment [7, 8]. However, since FLASH utilizes ultrahigh dose rates, the direct application of these protocols introduces significant calibration errors; thus, the protocols cannot be used. The non-negligible effects of ion recombination need to be accounted for if ICs are to be used as reference dosimeters in ultra-high dose per pulse beams [9–13].

The efficiency with which ICs collect ions decreases in high dose rate beams; thus correction factors are needed, such as $k_s$ in the International Atomic Energy Agency (IAEA) 398 convention. In medical linear accelerators, these saturation effects result primarily from ion recombination, which depends on the dose per pulse, chamber design, and bias voltage; when the dose per pulse is <1 mGy, these corrections are minor (much less than 5%) [7, 9, 11, 12, 14]. However, they increase rapidly with the dose per pulse and become detrimentally large in ultra-high dose per pulse beams

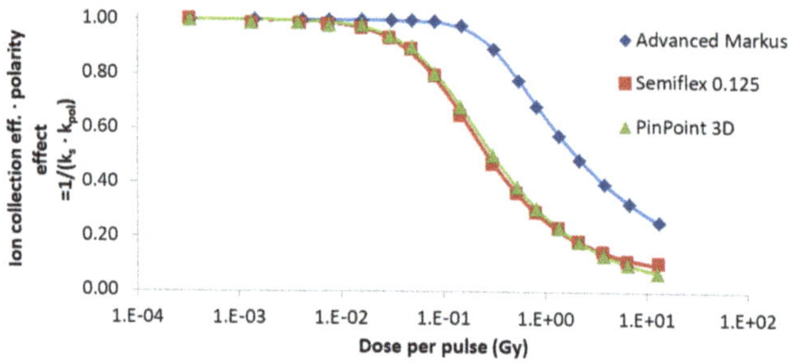


**Figure 22.1.** The effect of ion recombination in three types of ionization chamber (PTW-Freiburg GmbH, Freiburg, Germany) when the dose per pulse is varied in a 6 MeV electron beam.

(figure 22.1) [13, 15]. Thus, interest is growing in determining the requisite recombination corrections over a broader range of doses per pulse, i.e. from mGy to Gy, for various beam modalities [9, 16–19].

Ideal ICs for ultra-high dose rate dosimetry should suffer as little as possible from saturation effects in order to minimize the values of the associated correction factor and the uncertainty introduced by its calculation [13]. Recent studies show that the ion collection efficiency and the polarity effect can be reduced by increasing the electric field in the ionization chamber, either by applying a higher bias voltage or by decreasing the electrode distance [13, 20, 21]. Among systems that address this issue, the Advanced Markus IC (PTW-34045) has been well characterized by Petersson *et al* [13]. The authors determined appropriate correction factors for recombination ($k_s$) and polarity ($k_{pol}$), which resulted in a dose uncertainty of 2.8% for measurements in ultra-high dose rate beams. The authors further developed models specific to their irradiation setup that spanned a wide range of dose per pulse values (0.3 mGy–10 Gy) and demonstrated that the ion recombination effects were largely independent of the mean and intrapulse dose rates at up to $1.3 \times 10^3$ Gy s$^{-1}$ and $7 \times 10^6$ Gy s$^{-1}$, respectively, if the dose per pulse remained constant.

### 22.2.2 Radiochromic film

Gafchromic film (Ashland Inc., Covington, KY, USA) has been used extensively as a dosimetry system in FLASH-related studies. It is often considered the 'gold standard' against which to compare other detector systems. Gafchromic film is preferred for its flexibility, tissue equivalency, energy independence (>50–100 kV), and high spatial resolution. Gafchromic film has also been extensively characterized in high-dose-rate beams and is independent of dose rate for rates up to $9 \times 10^{12}$ Gy s$^{-1}$ [22–24]. However, Gafchromic film is limited by delays in the readout; ideally, the film should not be analyzed until 24 h after the irradiation to allow the polymerization rate to stabilize.

Another class of passive dosimeters used in FLASH dosimetry includes alanine and thermoluminescent dosimeters (TLDs) [15, 24–26]. While these detectors have similar characteristics to those of Gafchromic film, they only offer point dose

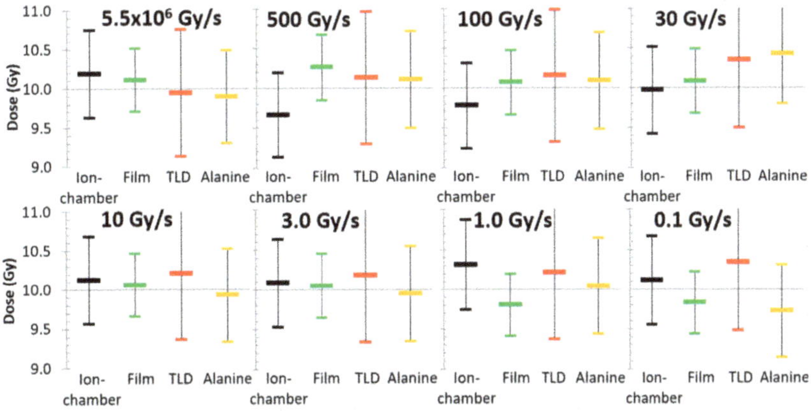


**Figure 22.2.** Absorbed dose measurements at the surface of a 30 × 30 $cm^2$ solid water phantom obtained using the Advanced Markus ionization chamber (Ion-chamber), Gafchromic EBT3 film (Film), a thermoluminescent dosimeter (TLD), and alanine pellets (Alanine) for a dose of 10 Gy delivered at various dose rates in a 1.7-cm-diameter circular field. Error bars represent the (expanded, $k$=2) uncertainties in the absorbed dose measurements. Reprinted from [25], Copyright (2017), with permission from Elsevier.

measurements. Nevertheless, their dose rate independence at up to $1.5 \times 10^9$ Gy $s^{-1}$ has rendered alanine and TLDs useful tools for use in FLASH beams [22, 25–27].

### 22.2.3 Alanine dosimeters

Alanine dosimeters are used in national laboratories and for industrial purposes [28]. Due to their low energy response and wide dose range, alanine dosimeters have also been used for dose verification in FLASH beams [29]. Doses ranging from 1 Gy to $1 \times 10^5$ Gy for 0.1–30 MeV electrons and photon beams can be measured with alanine dosimeters (International Standardization Organization). However, uncertainty increases at doses of <10 Gy due to a low signal-to-noise ratio [30]. While alanine dosimeters show a dose-rate dependence as a function of the delivered dose, the dependency is minimal for doses of up to $5 \times 10^3$ Gy [31]. For continuous and pulsed electron beams, alanine dosimeters are dose rate independent at mean dose rates of up to $10^2$ Gy $s^{-1}$ and instantaneous dose rates of up to $3 \times 10^{10}$ Gy $s^{-1}$, respectively [27], which makes them suitable for FLASH. A comparison by Jorge *et al* validated TLDs, alanine pellets, and films for absolute dosimetry against an Advanced Markus IC and found good agreement among these dosimeters for average dose rates of 0.078 Gy $s^{-1}$, 210 Gy $s^{-1}$, and 1050 Gy $s^{-1}$ [15]. Montay-Gruel *et al* had previously shown that an ion chamber, Gafchromic films, alanine pellets, and TLDs were able to provide reliable dosimetry (±5%) for 10 Gy delivered over a wide range of average dose rates (figure 22.2) [25].

### 22.2.4 Scintillation detectors

Scintillator- and Cherenkov-based dosimeters are also of particular interest for FLASH beams. Organic scintillation detectors are tissue equivalent and energy and dose rate independent, and allow the measurement of integrated doses to be performed in real time as well as the temporal resolution of individual linac pulses [32–34]. Inorganic scintillation detectors have similar characteristics, but their use of high-atomic-number materials precludes their tissue equivalence and energy independence. However, because these detectors are generally more radiation resistant and have higher light outputs and easier corrections for the stem effect than organic scintillators, they remain attractive for FLASH-beam dosimetry. For FLASH dosimetry, the signal generated is several orders of magnitude higher than that generated in conventional-dose-rate dosimetry. For this reason, the active volume could be made smaller to allow easier filtering of signals pertaining to stem-effect features, even with organic scintillators. Archer *et al* recently demonstrated the successful implementation of a 10 μm thick BC-400 film plastic scintillator coupled to a 1 mm diameter optical fiber in a synchrotron x-ray beam, which showed excellent performance at dose rates of up to $4.4 \times 10^3$ Gy $s^{-1}$ [35]. Two- and three-dimensional measurements with luminescent technology have also been successfully implemented [36–40].

To summarize, when this chapter was written, FLASH dosimetry still posed a challenge. However, active research by academic groups and industrial partners, coupled with the recognition of the American Association of Physicists in Medicine (AAPM) of the need to devise guidelines, are poised to make a positive impact in the near future.

## 22.3 Current eFLASH systems

The Kinetron (CGR-MeV, Paris, France) is a pulsed electron beam delivery system with a beam energy of 4–5 MeV; it can be operated in conventional RT modes (dose rate <0.03 Gy $s^{-1}$, dose per pulse ~$10^{-3}$ Gy) or in 'FLASH' irradiation modes with a pulse output reproducibility better than 5% [41, 42]. The accelerator, driven by an adjustable triode electron gun, can provide beam currents of 10–250 mA, pulse widths of 0.1–2.2 μs at full width at half maximum (FWHM), and macropulse pulse repetition frequencies (PRFs) of 10–250 Hz [41, 42]. Under typical treatment conditions, this flexibility enables the linac to achieve average dose rates between $10^{-1}$ Gy $s^{-1}$ and $10^3$ Gy $s^{-1}$.

The Oriatron eRT6 (PMB-Alcen, Peynier, France) is another experimental electron linac that allows output control based on fine control over several beam parameters of interest, including the number of electron pulses, PRF (5–200 Hz), and pulse width (0.05–2.2 μs) [43]. The eRT6 beam energy is nominally 6 MeV, and it can be adjusted to achieve a dose per pulse that is a factor of $10^4$ greater than those of conventional linacs while operating with similar PRFs and pulse widths [13, 43]. For example, Petersson *et al* achieved average dose rates on the order of $10^{-2}$–$10^3$ Gy $s^{-1}$, corresponding to a pulse (instantaneous) dose rate of $10^2$–$10^7$ Gy $s^{-1}$ and a dose per pulse of $10^{-4}$–$10^1$ Gy, assuming a pulse width of 1.8 μs and a PRF of 100 Hz [13]. In addition, the eRT6 delivers ultrahigh dose rates at standard 100 cm source-to-surface distances (SSDs) in a field size of 1.6–20 cm and has a therapeutic (R80) range of 1.8–2.3 cm [43]. Several studies with the eRT6 have demonstrated a reproducible FLASH effect using a pulsed beam comprising one to ten pulses (1.8–2 μs width) delivered in less than 200 ms together with pulse dose rates of more than $1.8 \times 10^5$ Gy $s^{-1}$ [2].

Other investigators have adapted existing clinical linacs for electron FLASH experiments [44–46]. Such modified linacs have been successfully used to deliver electron beams at dose rates exceeding 200 Gy $s^{-1}$, with the caveat that the small field size and short SSD are only suited to small animals. Lempart *et al* (2019) demonstrated a scheme that achieved an average dose rate of 30–300 Gy $s^{-1}$ (dose per pulse = 0.1–1.9 Gy; PRF = 200 Hz) using an Elekta Precise linac ($E \sim 8$ MeV), depending on the measurement point within the treatment head [45]. This system was subsequently improved to become suitable for the treatment of veterinary (canine and feline) patients; it now has a 10 MeV beam that achieves doses per pulse of 2.2 Gy and 1 Gy, corresponding to average dose rates of 440 Gy $s^{-1}$ and 200 Gy $s^{-1}$, at SSDs of 70 and 100 cm, respectively [20, 47]. Similarly, Schüler *et al* successfully delivered ultrahigh dose rates using a modified Varian Clinac 21EX [46]. After extensive tuning, they achieved 220 Gy $s^{-1}$ (a pulse dose rate of $1.7 \times 10^6$ Gy $s^{-1}$ at a depth of 1 cm) at the location of the mirror, which was chosen so that the depth–dose and field size characteristics remained suitable for small-animal experiments [46].

Compared to the commercial preclinical systems mentioned above, the modified linacs' higher beam energies (~8–20 MeV) lead to improved dose homogeneity, although they are limited to small field sizes and fewer beam parameter choices.

Simmons *et al* used the modified linac of Schüler *et al* [46] to demonstrate reduced intestinal toxicity with FLASH after total abdominal irradiation in mice [48]. In this study, the only parameter that varied between the FLASH beam and the conventional-dose-rate beam was the overall delivery time. Both beams used a pulse width of 2 μs with a dose per pulse of 1.75 Gy and a pulse dose rate of $8.75 \times 10^5$ Gy $s^{-1}$, delivering FLASH irradiations at average dose rates of either 200 Gy $s^{-1}$ or 300 Gy $s^{-1}$ for 20 MeV and 16 MeV beams, respectively, and 0.13 Gy $s^{-1}$ for conventional irradiation (for both 16 and 20 MeV beams). This was achieved by modulating the PRFs, which were set to 108 Hz for the 20 MeV FLASH beam and 180 Hz for the 16 MeV FLASH beam and by delivering five trains of two to three pulses (at a PRF of 18 Hz), each separated by 60 s, for a total delivery time of 240 s.

Several intraoperative electron radiation therapy (IOeRT) electron linacs have recently been developed to deliver FLASH in preclinical and subsequent clinical studies, e.g. the Mobetron (IntraOp Medical Inc., Sunnyvale, CA, USA) [49], the ElectronFlash, the LIAC FLASH produced by Sordina IORT Technologies (Vicenza, Italy), and the FLASHKNiFE produced by PMB-Alcen.

A limitation of clinical electron beams in the 4–20 MeV energy range is the shallow depth of their penetration in tissue. Therefore, other treatment devices/techniques are needed for FLASH to be clinically useful for more than superficial treatments with external beam RT or intraoperative RT (IORT). One solution would be to use very-high-energy electron (VHEE) beams with beam energies of

100–250 MeV. Such beams have good depth penetration and superior depth–dose profiles, sharp beam penumbras, and less sensitivity to tissue heterogeneity than conventional x-ray beams [23, 50, 51]. Furthermore, in addition to their dosimetric advantage, VHEE beams can be electromagnetically steered around the patient using a similar approach to that of volumetric modulated arc therapy, yet at FLASH dose rates that do not compromise conformity. However, these beams are currently limited to research accelerators that are either relatively large or otherwise impractical for clinical use.

## 22.4 Beam-monitoring systems

In clinical RT practice, delivery of the radiation is monitored and controlled by dual, redundant transmission chamber signals, which have been calibrated (using ionization chambers whose calibration is traceable to a standard laboratory, see the section above) to display monitor units (MUs) corresponding to a dose at a certain depth in water, e.g. 100 MU = 1 Gy at a depth of the dose maximum in water. However, these chambers have poor ion collection efficiency for the high-dose-per-pulse FLASH beams, making them unsuitable for monitoring FLASH deliveries. As previously mentioned, the drop in efficiency can be mitigated by increasing the bias voltage [20], and the signal can be further conditioned to enable control of the delivery [52]. However, a new transmission chamber design is likely needed (e.g. with a smaller electrode gap [21]) for transmission chambers in order to achieve similar precisions of beam monitoring and control to those used in clinical RT. Currently, in electron FLASH irradiation studies, beam control is managed through macropulse counting and stopping irradiation once the desired number of pulses has been delivered, either by built-in systems [43, 53] or by the use of an external pulse detector [44–46]. For pulse counting to be useful, the output from the linac must be reproducible over time, and the dose delivered must be proportional to the number of pulses. Further, the dose delivered by each pulse should ideally be the same, regardless of whether it comes first, last, or somewhere in the middle of a train of pulses, which is rarely the case [54].

For the clinical translation and implementation of FLASH, beam delivery should be controlled by the dose delivered, not the number of pulses delivered. An alternative to the use of transmission chambers is the use of charge induction toroids or charge collector plates [43, 53, 55]. When electrons pass through a toroid, a charge is induced. Similarly, if an electron beam interacts with an electrical conductor (e.g. a metal plate [53]), a charge is deposited. The induced/collected charge can measure the beam output on a pulse-by-pulse basis. Again, for this to be useful, the measured charge must be proportional to the delivered dose. These charge detectors are suitable for measuring pulsed ultrahigh-dose-rate electron beams, as they are independent of dose rate and have an improved signal-to-noise ratio with increases in beam current/output [43, 55]. Unfortunately, the precision and stability of the measured charge for a specific delivered dose are considerably worse than those we are accustomed to obtaining from transmission chambers in clinical practice [43, 55].

## 22.5 Clinical translation

The following is rather a philosophical question: can clinical testing of FLASH begin without a complete understanding of its biological mechanisms of action? A better understanding of these mechanisms based on preclinical studies would likely inform more optimal designs of clinical trials. Arguably, however, it is possible to design some rational clinical trials without an extensive understanding of the mechanisms involved, especially if one considers that our mechanistic understanding of even our current standard-of-care treatments is far from complete. With the thoughtful design of translational endpoints, clinical trials will facilitate our mechanistic understanding of new treatment modalities such as FLASH and may ultimately be essential for that understanding.

One potential strategy would be to start with phase 1 trials of FLASH electron beam therapy for superficial tumors such as skin cancers using existing electron-based FLASH technologies. Ideal tumors to evaluate would be those of small to moderate size and in locations amenable to surgical salvage (in case of incomplete tumor control) or reconstructive surgery or skin grafting (in cases of late skin injury or radionecrosis). For example, a dose of 20–25 Gy in a single fraction could produce a high enough tumor control probability and a low risk of skin injury. A phase 1 clinical trial is ongoing at Lausanne University Hospital (CHUV), and the results for their first patient have been published [29].

An implementation of FLASH-enabling technologies that would cover a wide range of target volumes without compromising conformity does not exist currently but would create opportunities for randomized clinical trials, such as matched FLASH vs. conventional-dose-rate treatments that are similar in every way except for the speed of the radiation delivery. However, without the knowledge require for the optimal use of FLASH, randomized trials conducted too early might mask its clinical benefits or prove a detrimental effect.

Nevertheless, such a capability would allow empirical testing of whether FLASH is advantageous in different clinical scenarios. One reasonable approach would be to conduct randomized phase 2 studies using standard-of-care regimens, including stereotactic ablative RT (SABR) or conventionally fractionated RT, for selected indications. Particularly attractive settings would be those in which: (1) there is currently a high incidence of measurable toxicity with the best standard of care, e.g. concurrent chemoradiotherapy for head and neck cancers or pediatric brain tumors in which whole-cranium irradiation is used; (2) there is a high incidence of otherwise readily measurable early or delayed tissue damage, e.g. lung fibrosis in computed tomography imaging after SABR; (3) anatomic sites are accessible (by endoscopy or direct visualization, e.g. bulky cervix cancer) and amenable to serial biopsies for mechanistic studies. The initial focus should be on scenarios for which the potential exists to observe a large effect size, especially on normal tissue sparing, should one exist. To date, preclinical or even historical clinical data have not suggested that higher dose rates cause adverse effects, and the technical objective of improved motion management through rapid treatment is valid regardless of the potential biological benefits.

As stated above, such technologies do not exist; thus, the major practical limitation to the clinical translation of FLASH is technological. To date, preclinical FLASH irradiation of small animals and small, superficial targets in larger animals has been possible using modified existing irradiation systems that can produce FLASH dose rates when limited to small volumes (of up to a few cubic centimeters), including electron linear accelerators [43, 45, 46], a synchrotron light source producing kilovoltage-energy x-rays [56], proton accelerators [6, 57–59], and certain ion accelerators [60]. However, recent advances in linear accelerator science and radiofrequency power generation and distribution technologies have led to prototypes of compact, high-efficiency linear accelerators suitable for producing high-energy x-rays (in the megavoltage energy range) or very-high-energy electrons (at energies exceeding 100 MeV) capable of treating large-volume and deep-seated targets at FLASH dose rates. In particular, Stanford University and the SLAC National Accelerator Laboratory (previously called the Stanford Linear Accelerator Center) are engaged in a program to develop a medical linear accelerator system based on these technologies, called pluridirectional high-energy agile scanning electronic radiotherapy (PHASER), which is designed to deliver highly conformal FLASH intensity-modulated RT to general radiation therapy targets at FLASH dose rates [61].

In conclusion, FLASH promises to be a paradigm shift in curative RT, given the preclinical evidence for a fundamentally improved therapeutic index. Although much remains to be learned about the mechanisms responsible for the FLASH phenomenon, a rational approach to initial clinical testing, in parallel with preclinical investigations, is feasible and will contribute to mechanistic understanding. New technologies for FLASH dosimetry and analogous FLASH-compatible beam control systems with sufficiently high accuracy and response times will be necessary to implement FLASH RT in the clinic safely.

## References


[1] Favaudon V, Caplier L, Monceau V, Pouzoulet F, Sayarath M and Fouillade C *et al* 2014 Ultrahigh dose-rate FLASH irradiation increases the differential response between normal and tumor tissue in mice *Sci. Transl. Med.* **6** 245ra93

[2] Bourhis J, Montay-Gruel P, Goncalves Jorge P, Bailat C, Petit B and Ollivier J *et al* 2019 Clinical translation of FLASH radiotherapy: why and how? *Radiother. Oncol.* **139** 11–7

[3] Montay-Gruel P, Acharya M M, Gonçalves Jorge P, Petit B, Petridis I G and Fuchs P *et al* 2021 Hypofractionated FLASH-RT as an effective treatment against glioblastoma that reduces neurocognitive side effects in mice *Clin. Cancer Res.* **27** 775–84

[4] Zlobinskaya O, Siebenwirth C, Greubel C, Hable V, Hertenberger R and Humble N *et al* 2014 The effects of ultra-high dose rate proton irradiation on growth delay in the treatment of human tumor xenografts in nude mice *Radiat. Res.* **181** 177–83

[5] Levy K, Natarajan S, Wang J, Chow S, Eggold J T and Loo P E *et al* 2020 Abdominal FLASH irradiation reduces radiation-induced gastrointestinal toxicity for the treatment of ovarian cancer in mice *Sci. Rep.* **10** 21600

[6] Diffenderfer E S, Verginadis I I, Kim M M, Shoniyozov K, Velalopoulou A and Goia D *et al* 2020 Design, implementation, and *in vivo* validation of a novel proton flash radiation therapy system *Int. J. Radiat. Oncol. Biol. Phys.* **106** 440–8

[7] Almond P R, Biggs P J, Coursey B M, Hanson W F, Huq M S and Nath R *et al* 1999 AAPM's TG-51 protocol for clinical reference dosimetry of high-energy photon and electron beams *Med. Phys.* **26** 1847–70

[8] McEwen M, DeWerd L, Ibbott G, Followill D, Rogers D W and Seltzer S *et al* 2014 Addendum to the AAPM's TG-51 protocol for clinical reference dosimetry of high-energy photon beams *Med. Phys.* **41** 041501

[9] Bruggmoser G, Saum R, Schmachtenberg A, Schmid F and Schule E 2007 Determination of the recombination correction factor kS for some specific plane-parallel and cylindrical ionization chambers in pulsed photon and electron beams *Phys. Med. Biol.* **52** N35–50

[10] Burns D T and McEwen M R 1998 Ion recombination corrections for the NACP parallel-plate chamber in a pulsed electron beam *Phys. Med. Biol.* **43** 2033–45

[11] Karsch L 2016 Derivation of a formula describing the saturation correction of plane-parallel ionization chambers in pulsed fields with arbitrary repetition rate *Phys. Med. Biol.* **61** 3222–36

[12] Kry S F, Popple R, Molineu A and Followill D S 2012 Ion recombination correction factors (P(ion)) for Varian TrueBeam high-dose-rate therapy beams *J. Appl. Clin. Med. Phys.* **13** 3803

[13] Petersson K, Jaccard M, Germond J F, Buchillier T, Bochud F and Bourhis J *et al* 2017 High dose-per-pulse electron beam dosimetry – a model to correct for the ion recombination in the advanced Markus ionization chamber *Med. Phys.* **44** 1157–67

[14] Boag J W and Currant J 1980 Current collection and ionic recombination in small cylindrical ionization chambers exposed to pulsed radiation *Br. J. Radiol.* **53** 471–8

[15] Jorge P G, Jaccard M, Petersson K, Gondré M, Durán M T and Desorgher L *et al* 2019 Dosimetric and preparation procedures for irradiating biological models with pulsed electron beam at ultra-high dose-rate *Radiother. Oncol.* **139** 34–9

[16] Di Martino F, Giannelli M, Traino A C and Lazzeri M 2005 Ion recombination correction for very high dose-per-pulse high-energy electron beams *Med. Phys.* **32** 2204–10

[17] Gotz M, Karsch L and Pawelke J 2017 A new model for volume recombination in plane-parallel chambers in pulsed fields of high dose-per-pulse *Phys. Med. Biol.* **62** 8634–54

[18] Laitano R F, Guerra A S, Pimpinella M, Caporali C and Petrucci A 2006 Charge collection efficiency in ionization chambers exposed to electron beams with high dose per pulse *Phys. Med. Biol.* **51** 6419–36

[19] Sutton J D and Littler J P 2017 Accounting for the ion recombination factor in relative dosimetry of flattening filter free photon radiation *Biomed. Phys. Eng. Expr.* **3** 017002

[20] Konradsson E, Ceberg C, Lempart M, Blad B, Bäck S and Knöös T *et al* 2020 Correction for ion recombination in a built-in monitor chamber of a clinical linear accelerator at ultra-high dose rates *Radiat. Res.* **194** 580–6

[21] Kranzer R, Poppinga D, Weidner J, Schuller A, Hackel T and Looe H K *et al* 2021 Ion collection efficiency of ionization chambers in ultra-high dose-per-pulse electron beams *Med. Phys.* **48** 819–30

[22] Karsch L, Beyreuther E, Burris-Mog T, Kraft S, Richter C and Zeil K *et al* 2012 Dose rate dependence for different dosimeters and detectors: TLD, OSL, EBT films, and diamond detectors *Med. Phys.* **39** 2447–55

[23] Bazalova-Carter M, Liu M, Palma B, Dunning M, McCormick D and Hemsing E *et al* 2015 Comparison of film measurements and Monte Carlo simulations of dose delivered with very high-energy electron beams in a polystyrene phantom *Med. Phys.* **42** 1606–13
[24] Jaccard M, Petersson K, Buchillier T, Germond J F, Duran M T and Vozenin M C *et al* 2017 High dose-per-pulse electron beam dosimetry: usability and dose-rate independence of EBT3 Gafchromic films *Med. Phys.* **44** 725–35
[25] Montay-Gruel P, Petersson K, Jaccard M, Boivin G, Germond J F and Petit B *et al* 2017 Irradiation in a flash: unique sparing of memory in mice after whole brain irradiation with dose rates above 100 Gy/s *Radiother. Oncol.* **124** 365–9
[26] Vozenin M C, De Fornel P, Petersson K, Favaudon V, Jaccard M and Germond J F *et al* 2019 The advantage of FLASH radiotherapy confirmed in mini-pig and cat-cancer patients *Clin. Cancer Res.* **25** 35–42
[27] Kudoh H, Celina M, Kaye R, Gillen K and Clough R 1997 Response of alanine dosimeters at very high dose rate *Appl. Radiat. Isot.* **48** 497–9
[28] Sharpe P H, Rajendran K and Sephton J P 1996 Progress towards an alanine/ESR therapy level reference dosimetry service at NPL *Appl. Radiat. Isot.* **47** 1171–5
[29] Bourhis J, Sozzi W J, Jorge P G, Gaide O, Bailat C and Duclos F *et al* 2019 Treatment of a first patient with FLASH-radiotherapy *Radiother. Oncol.* **139** 18–22
[30] Gondré M, Jorge P G, Vozenin M-C, Bourhis J, Bochud F and Bailat C *et al* 2020 Optimization of alanine measurements for fast and accurate dosimetry in FLASH radiation therapy *Radiat. Res.* **194** 573–9
[31] Desrosiers M F, Puhl J M and Cooper S L 2008 An absorbed-dose/dose-rate dependence for the alanine-EPR dosimetry system and its implications in high-dose ionizing radiation metrology *J. Res. Natl. Inst. Stand. Technol.* **113** 79–95
[32] Beaulieu L and Beddar S 2016 Review of plastic and liquid scintillation dosimetry for photon, electron, and proton therapy *Phys. Med. Biol.* **61** R305
[33] Beddar A, Mackie T and Attix F 1992 Water-equivalent plastic scintillation detectors for high-energy beam dosimetry: I. Physical characteristics and theoretical considerations *Phys. Med. Biol.* **37** 1883
[34] Beddar A S, Mackie T and Attix F 1992 Water-equivalent plastic scintillation detectors for high-energy beam dosimetry: II. Properties and measurements *Phys. Med. Biol.* **37** 1901
[35] Archer J, Li E, Davis J, Cameron M, Rosenfeld A and Lerch M 2019 High spatial resolution scintillator dosimetry of synchrotron microbeams *Sci. Rep.* **9** 1–7
[36] Ashraf M R, Bruza P, Pogue B W, Nelson N, Williams B B and Jarvis L A *et al* 2019 Optical imaging provides rapid verification of static small beams, radiosurgery, and VMAT plans with millimeter resolution *Med. Phys.* **46** 5227–37
[37] Vigdor S, Klyachko A, Solberg K and Pankuch M 2017 A gas scintillator detector for 2D dose profile monitoring in pencil beam scanning and pulsed beam proton radiotherapy treatments *Phys. Med. Biol.* **62** 4946
[38] Darne C, Alsanea F, Robertson D, Hojo Y, Sahoo N and Beddar S 2019 3D scintillator detector system for proton scanning beam therapy *Int. J. Radiat. Oncol. Biol. Phys.* **105** S89–90
[39] Darne C D, Alsanea F, Robertson D G, Sahoo N and Beddar S 2017 Performance characterization of a 3D liquid scintillation detector for discrete spot scanning proton beam systems *Phys. Med. Biol.* **62** 5652

[40] Goulet M, Rilling M, Gingras L, Beddar S, Beaulieu L and Archambault L 2014 Novel, full 3D scintillation dosimetry using a static plenoptic camera *Med. Phys.* **41** 082101

[41] Favaudon V, Lentz J M, Heinrich S, Patriarca A, de Marzi L and Fouillade C *et al* 2019 Time-resolved dosimetry of pulsed electron beams in very high dose-rate, FLASH irradiation for radiotherapy preclinical studies *Nucl. Instrum. Meth. A* **944** 162537

[42] Lansonneur P, Favaudon V, Heinrich S, Fouillade C, Verrelle P, De and Marzi L 2019 Simulation and experimental validation of a prototype electron beam linear accelerator for preclinical studies *Phys Med.* **60** 50–7

[43] Jaccard M, Duran M T, Petersson K, Germond J F, Liger P and Vozenin M C *et al* 2018 High dose-per-pulse electron beam dosimetry: commissioning of the Oriatron eRT6 prototype linear accelerator for preclinical use *Med. Phys.* **45** 863–74

[44] Rahman M, Ashraf M R, Zhang R, Bruza P, Dexter C A and Thompson L *et al* 2021 Electron FLASH delivery at treatment room isocenter for efficient reversible conversion of a clinical LINAC *Int. J. Radiat. Oncol. Biol. Phys.* **110** 872–82

[45] Lempart M, Blad B, Adrian G, Back S, Knoos T and Ceberg C *et al* 2019 Modifying a clinical linear accelerator for delivery of ultra-high dose rate irradiation *Radiother. Oncol.* **139** 40–5

[46] Schuler E, Trovati S, King G, Lartey F, Rafat M and Villegas M *et al* 2017 Experimental platform for ultra-high dose rate FLASH irradiation of small animals using a clinical linear accelerator *Int. J. Radiat. Oncol. Biol. Phys.* **97** 195–203

[47] Konradsson E, Arendt M L, Bastholm Jensen K, Børresen B, Hansen A E and Bäck S *et al* 2021 Establishment and initial experience of clinical FLASH radiotherapy in canine cancer patients *Front. Oncol.* **11** 658004

[48] Simmons D A, Lartey F M, Schüler E, Rafat M, King G and Kim A *et al* 2019 Reduced cognitive deficits after FLASH irradiation of whole mouse brain are associated with less hippocampal dendritic spine loss and neuroinflammation *Radiother. Oncol.* **139** 4–10

[49] Moeckli R, Gonçalves Jorge P, Grilj V, Oesterle R, Cherbuin N and Bourhis J *et al* 2021 Commissioning of an ultra-high dose rate pulsed electron beam medical LINAC for FLASH RT preclinical animal experiments and future clinical human protocols *Med. Phys.* **48** 3134–42

[50] Schuler E, Eriksson K, Hynning E, Hancock S L, Hiniker S M and Bazalova-Carter M *et al* 2017 Very high-energy electron (VHEE) beams in radiation therapy; treatment plan comparison between VHEE, VMAT, and PPBS *Med. Phys.* **44** 2544–55

[51] Svendsen K, Guenot D, Svensson J B, Petersson K, Persson A and Lundh O 2021 A focused very high energy electron beam for fractionated stereotactic radiotherapy *Sci. Rep.* **11** 5844

[52] Snyder M, Vadas J, Musselwhite J, Halford R, Wilson G and Stevens C *et al* 2021 FLASH radiotherapy monitor chamber signal conditioning *Med. Phys.* **48** 791–5

[53] Berne A, Petersson K, Tullis I D C, Newman R G and Vojnovic B 2021 Monitoring electron energies during FLASH irradiations *Phys. Med. Biol.* **66** 045015

[54] Ashraf M R, Rahman M, Zhang R, Cao X, Williams B B and Hoopes P J *et al* 2021 Technical note: single-pulse beam characterization for FLASH-RT using optical imaging in a water tank *Med. Phys.* **48** 2673–81

[55] Oesterle R, Gonçalves Jorge P, Grilj V, Bourhis J, Vozenin M C and Germond J F *et al* 2021 Implementation and validation of a beam-current transformer on a medical pulsed electron beam LINAC for FLASH-RT beam monitoring *J. Appl. Clin. Med. Phys.* **22** 165–71

[56] Montay-Gruel P, Bouchet A, Jaccard M, Patin D, Serduc R and Aim W *et al* 2018 X-rays can trigger the FLASH effect: ultra-high dose-rate synchrotron light source prevents normal brain injury after whole brain irradiation in mice *Radiother. Oncol.* **129** 582–8

[57] Patriarca A, Fouillade C, Auger M, Martin F, Pouzoulet F and Nauraye C *et al* 2018 Experimental set-up for FLASH proton irradiation of small animals using a clinical system *Int. J. Radiat. Oncol. Biol. Phys.* **102** 619–26

[58] Velalopoulou A, Karagounis I V, Cramer G M, Kim M M, Skoufos G and Goia D *et al* 2021 FLASH proton radiotherapy spares normal epithelial and mesenchymal tissues while preserving sarcoma response *Cancer Res.* **81** 4808–21

[59] Kim M M, Darafsheh A, Schuemann J, Dokic I, Lundh O and Zhao T *et al* 2021 Development of ultra-high dose rate (FLASH) particle therapy *IEEE Trans. Radiat. Plasma Med. Sci.* **6** 252–62

[60] Tessonnier T, Mein S, Walsh D W M, Schuhmacher N, Liew H and Cee R *et al* 2021 FLASH dose rate helium ion beams: first *in vitro* investigations *Int. J. Radiat. Oncol. Biol. Phys.* **111** 1011–22

[61] Maxim P G, Tantawi S G and Loo B W Jr 2019 PHASER: a platform for clinical translation of FLASH cancer radiotherapy *Radiother. Oncol.* **139** 28–33

**IOP** Publishing

Spatially Fractionated, Microbeam and FLASH Radiation Therapy
A physics and multi-disciplinary approach
**Hualin Zhang and Nina A Mayr**

# Chapter 23

# The use of synchrotrons in SFRT and FLASH therapy

**Audrey Bouchet and Marine Potez**

Since the beginnings of synchrotron spatially fractionated radiation therapy (SFRT) in 1995, many improvements have been made in order to optimize the irradiation parameters. As a result of testing the efficacy and safety of microbeams (<100 μm) and minibeams (>100 μm), multiple studies have agreed on the beneficial effects of synchrotron fractionated radiation for different tumor treatments and for the sparing of the surrounding tissues. The evaluation of the effects of synchrotron SFRT on the normal and tumoral tissues, mature and immature blood vessels, immune response, and molecular response has enabled this method to be considered for therapeutic application. This chapter aims to summarize the current knowledge about the mini- and microbeam radiotherapies delivered using synchrotron light. In addition to the spatial fractionation of the high dose, synchrotron SFRTs are also characterized by an ultrahigh dose rate, which can allow the sparing of normal tissues due to a biological FLASH effect. This latter property is currently pushing research toward the development of spatially homogeneous, ultrahigh-dose-rate radiotherapy in parallel with SFRTs.

## 23.1 Synchrotron radiotherapy: the dose–volume effect and the FLASH effect

As early as 1896, six months after the discovery of x-rays by Wilhelm Röntgen, the first attempts to use them to treat cancers were made by Victor Despeignes, a doctor from Lyon, France [1]. He was interested in using x-rays to try to cure a gastric lymphoma that he believed to be a stomach cancer. The tumor responded strongly to x-rays and showed a rapid decrease in volume. The response was perhaps too strong and probably led to the death of the patient due to tumor lysis syndrome. Discredited by a part of the scientific community, the results of Dr Despeigne were forgotten at first. Nevertheless, anticancer radiotherapy was born, an x-ray

doi:10.1088/978-0-7503-4046-5ch23

radiotherapy. More than a century later, failures in the modern radiotherapy of tumors are mainly due to the sensitivity of normal tissues surrounding the tumor, which does not allow the delivery of the dose required to control the tumor. Although radiotherapy is currently the most efficient treatment for several tumors, such as gliomas, it induces numerous adverse effects in normal tissues surrounding the lesion [2]. In the case of brain irradiation, radiation can lead to delayed but incapacitating or even lethal neurological complications.

To overcome this therapeutic dead end, alternative radiotherapy techniques were developed to take advantage of the physical characteristics of synchrotron sources [3] in the form of mini- and microbeam radiation therapies and most recently synchrotron FLASH. The former are based on the dose–volume effect, which postulates that the dose applied to healthy tissue can be increased by reducing the volume of irradiation. This concept has been pushed to the micrometer scale by the use of synchrotron sources and their exceptional properties: very low divergences and extremely high dose rates. This last characteristic, as we will see at the end of this chapter, is of primary interest in the context of the recently rediscovered biological FLASH effect.

## 23.2 Synchrotron radiation

The first particle accelerators were developed in the 1930s for particle physics applications. Their evolution in the 1940s improved the power of the first accelerators but limited their use, because the energy produced did not exceed 1 GeV. As early as 1943, Professor Marcus Oliphant proposed the concept of synchronizing a magnetic field (to move particles in a circular fashion) and an electric field (to accelerate them), which gave rise to the term 'synchrotron.'

These facilities, initially dedicated to the study of the collisions of charged particles and the resulting elementary particles, exhibit an enormous loss of energy in the form of radiation, which was first observed by Herb Pollock, Robert Langmuir, Franck Elder, and Anatole Gourevitch in 1947. This photon radiation, called synchrotron radiation (or synchrotron light), is curvature radiation because it is produced tangentially to the circular trajectories described by the charged particles. It was initially considered to be an unnecessary loss, even a nuisance [4, 5]. Since 1960, it has no longer been considered to be an artifact, and its exceptional characteristics have been exploited at facilities dedicated to the exploration of matter in general and the development of medical applications in particular [6, 7]. Now designed as facilities to host experiments by scientists from around the world, there are only a few synchrotrons in the world that can perform experiments dedicated to medical and biological applications. Among them, the European Synchrotron Radiation Facility (ESRF) at Grenoble in France has been the most powerful since its upgrade program—the Extremely Brilliant Source (EBS)—was finished in 2022.

The systems used to produce synchrotron light are not the subjects of this chapter, but for a better understanding of such systems, the reader is referred to the more

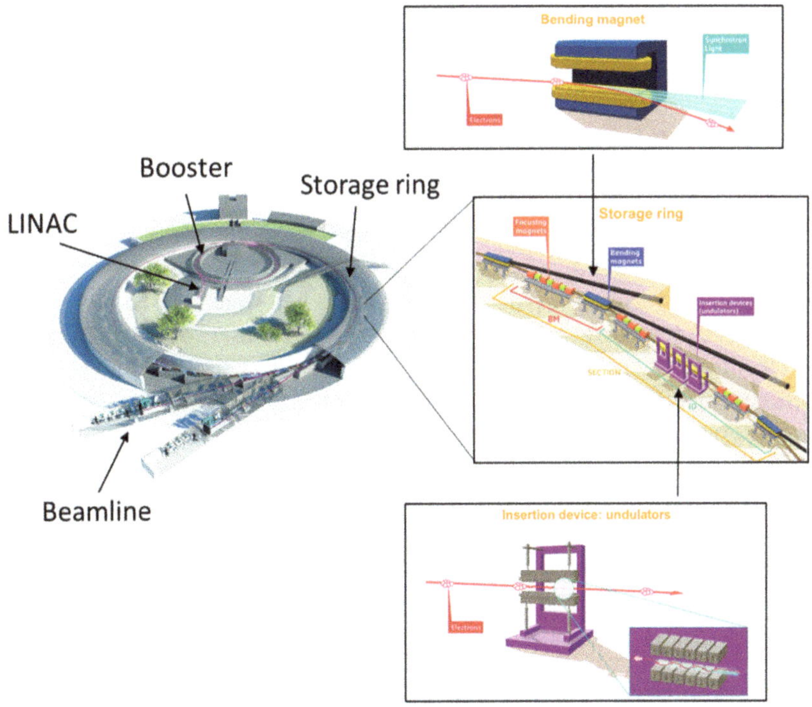


**Figure 23.1.** Diagram of a synchrotron in operation. The x-rays are produced by high-energy electrons as they circulate around the synchrotron. Synchrotron science depends on one physical phenomenon: when a moving electron changes direction, it emits energy. Electrons moving fast enough emit energy at x-ray wavelengths. Synchrotron machines accelerate electrons to extremely high energies and induce them change direction periodically. The resulting x-rays are emitted as thin beams, each directed toward a beamline next to the accelerator. Credit: ESRF.

detailed explanations available online on the website of the largest synchrotron, such as: https://www.esrf.fr/home/education/what-is-the-esrf/how-does-the-esrf-work.html.

In brief, these light sources produce brilliant x-rays (figure 23.1). To produce such intense radiation, electrons are emitted by an electron gun and accelerated linearly in the linac (LINear ACcelerator), bringing them to an energy of hundreds of MeV. They are then transferred to a circular accelerator hundreds of meters in circumference, the booster. This succession of accelerations brings the electrons up to the GeV energy range. When the electrons have reached this energy level, they are transported to a storage ring hundreds of meters in circumference. At this level, electrons travel at the quasi-speed of light inside a tube under ultrahigh vacuum conditions. The storage ring is composed of alternating curved and straight sections, each with a different type of magnet. In the curved sections, bending magnets allow the electrons to deviate by several degrees from their initial trajectory. This change of direction causes tangential emission energy, some of which, i.e. synchrotron radiation (x-rays), was initially considered to be an energy loss, but which is transmitted on beamlines for a plethora of applications (figure 23.1). This synchrotron light, which is extremely collimated, polarized, and brilliant, has constantly evolved so that the most performant synchrotron has a brilliance 14 times higher than that of a conventional x-ray tube in the 1950s [8].

## 23.3 Spatially fractionated radiation therapy with synchrotron radiation: minibeam and microbeam radiation therapy

The concept of the dose–volume effect has been used for x-ray therapy since the beginning of the last century with the clinical use of the first SFRT: the GRID therapy invented by Alban Köhler [9]. Delivering heterogeneous doses of radiation to voluminous tumors not amenable to surgery, GRID therapy only splits the beam at the subcentimeter scale. It was not until the late 20th century and the advent of third-generation synchrotrons that the concept of SRFT with x-rays was pushed to the microscopic scale by microbeam radiation therapy (MRT) [10] and then minibeam radiation therapy (MBRT) [11]. The highly brilliant synchrotron sources have the advantages of very small beam divergences and extremely high dose rates.

### 23.3.1 Microbeam radiation therapy (MRT)

Microbeams were proposed as a radiobiological tool by Curtis [12] in 1963, and their use was illustrated with deuteron irradiation few years later [13]. The absorbed dose of around 3000 Gy applied by a 25 μm beam caused only a loss of cell nuclei upon the passage of the microbeam, with no macroscopic damage to a mouse brain parenchyma. Maintenance of the cerebral vessels traversed by this microirradiation was also reported.

The use of MRT as a radiotherapy technique was initiated at the National Synchrotron Light Source (NSLS) of Brookhaven National Laboratory (BNL), Upton, New York, USA (patent no. 5339347 [14]) at the end of the 1980s; it was implemented at the ESRF in 1994 and later at several other centers worldwide. MRT uses the non-divergent, highly collimated, and very-high-dose-rate x-rays produced by a synchrotron.

The birth of this technique was reported in the reference review article written by Elke Bräuer-Krish, Jean Albert Laissue, and their collaborators: 'Per Spanne, a Swedish radiation physicist, Daniel N Slatkin and their colleagues attempted microtomography of the head of an anesthetized mouse using an around 30 μm-diameter pencil beam of synchrotron x-rays with absorbed doses under 10 Gy being delivered to the brain. As the contrast was poor, they remembered the high tolerance of normal tissues for microbeams reported by Curtis and thus increased the microbeam doses up to around 200 Gy. The mouse recovered normally. One month later, a careful search of the brain revealed no histopathological evidence of damage along the beam's path' [10]. MRT was born!

In recent decades, several 'multislit' collimators have been developed and perfected [15–17] (figure 23.2) to allow the incident beam (50–350 keV) to be spatially split into several quasi-parallel arrays of x-ray microbeams. These are a few tens of micrometers wide, delivering a peak radiation dose of several hundred Gy. They are separated by microplanar spaces a few hundred micrometers wider

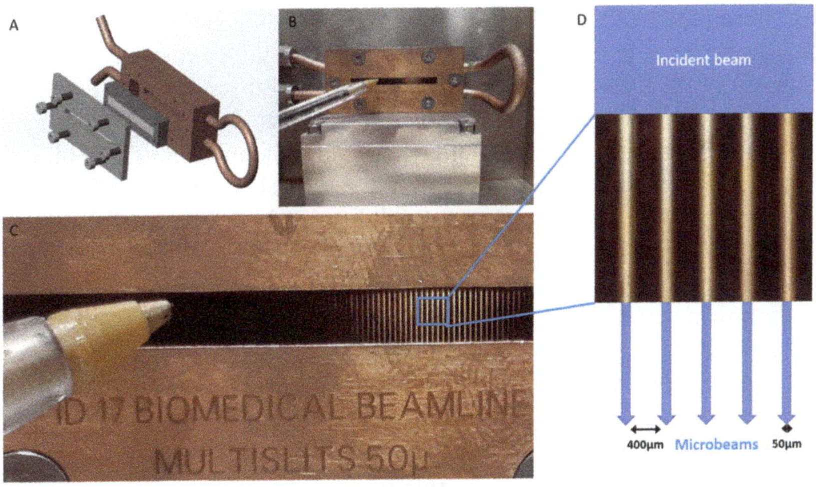


**Figure 23.2.** The single-stack multislit collimator (MSC) used at the ESRF—ID17 Biomedical Beamline, France, in 2022 to fractionate the homogeneous field into an array of 50 μm wide beams spaced at intervals of 400 μm center-to-center. (A) Technical drawing of the multislit collimator (reproduced with permission from [17] © International Union of Crystallography), (B) A picture of the current multislit collimator and (C and D) close-ups of the slits of this collimator, which allow the spatial fractionation of the incident synchrotron beam into a few tens of micron-scale quasi-parallel microbeams of 50 μm, spaced at 400 μm. Picture courtesy of Paolo Pellicioli, ESRF.

(100–400 μm center-to-center), from which tissues receive a valley dose of few Gy [3, 10, 14, 18–20].

The biological effects of synchrotron MRT on tissues have been widely described since its development. The normal tissue tolerance was the first parameter evaluated for synchrotron MRT, using doses of up to 10 000 Gy in rodent brains [19]. Shortly after, the efficacy of MRT on glioblastoma was tested with entrance doses of 625 Gy, and Laissue *et al* demonstrated the increased survival of animals following uni- or bidirectional irradiation with synchrotron microbeams [3]. Since these pioneer studies, the safety of MRT has been tested and demonstrated for multiple organs, such as immature and mature brains, the spinal cord, the skin, eyes, and optic nerves, bones and teeth, the testes, and the lungs [10]. The tumoricidal effect of synchrotron MRT has been widely evaluated and proven not only for different glioblastoma models (9L, F98, C6, and the human model U251) but also for mouse mammary carcinoma (EMT6.5, 67NR and 4T1), squamous cell carcinoma (SCCVII), melanoma (B16F10), and Lewis lung carcinoma (LLC1) (for review until 2020 [21], then [22–24]).

Due to the very small effect of synchrotron microbeams on normal tissues, the idea of using this type of beam on non-neoplastic diseases was illustrated in 2010 [25] with interlaced microbeams, which were later used on epileptic brains to suppress the neural synchronization caused by cortical transection [26, 27]. Synchrotron microbeams were also shown to be safe for microtransections of the corpus callosum [28], the sensorimotor cortex [29, 30], the hippocampus [31], and the visual brain cortex [30].

The preferential effect of MRT on tumor tissue while sparing normal irradiated areas has been attributed to the destruction of the immature vascular network found in tumors, while the mature vascularization of normal tissue is preserved [3, 19]. The maturation stage of the blood vessels is important, as shown by studies of a chick chorioallantoic membrane (CAM) model [32] and of hemi-amputation of the caudal zebrafish fin [33]. In tumors, immature blood vessels showed a modification in their number, composition, distribution, permeability, and perfusion following synchrotron MRT ([34–40], for review [41]).

Although the vascular response was the main parameter studied and understood in tissue following MRT (for review [41]), studies have also analyzed and showed implied cell death following DNA damage [42] and the bystander effect, a modification of gene expression [43, 44], and an implied radioinduced immune response (for review [21, 45]).

### 23.3.2 Minibeam radiation therapy (MBRT)

Minibeam radiation therapy (MBRT) was first proposed in 2006 by Dilmanian and colleagues [11]. Although MBRT was first developed using a synchrotron beam [11], it was established to address some technical and dosimetric challenges associated with MRT. Minibeams are defined as beams wider than 100 μm and up to 1000 μm. Their particularity is that they are produced by higher-energy photons, possibly from a special x-ray tube, without losing the specificity of the beams due to scattering, in contrast to microbeams. Moreover, wider beams are less sensitive to cardio-synchronous tissue pulsation, which induces beam smearing [46].

Dilmanian *et al* (2006) demonstrated that the rat spinal cord tolerated 680 μm thick synchrotron minibeams at 400 Gy for up to six months post irradiation [11]. Applied to healthy brains, parallel minibeams (as illustrated by figure 23.3) with a maximum dose of 170 Gy were well tolerated, while magnetic resonance imaging (MRI) revealed damage caused by crossed minibeams (figure 23.3) at doses of 120 and 150 Gy. Later studies showed limited damage to healthy brains, as evaluated by

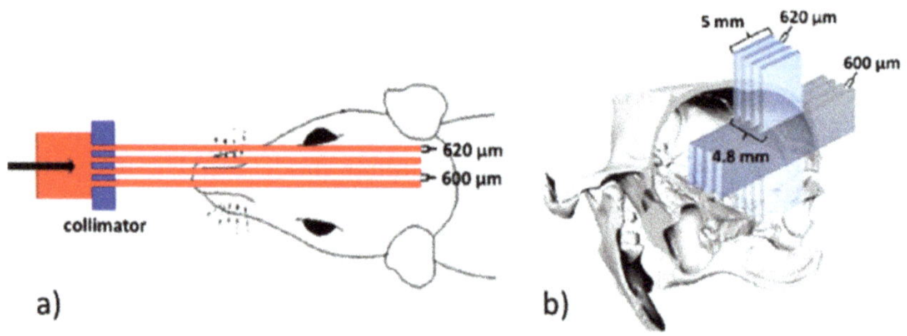


**Figure 23.3.** Minibeam radiation therapy irradiation geometries for rodent experimental tumor therapy studies: (a) single- incidence protocol: four beams 620 μm wide and 5 mm high, separated by 600 μm wide nonirradiated zones. (b) Dual interleaved incidence protocol: four beams in each incidence, 620 μm high and 5 mm wide, interleaved in the rat's right striatum. Reproduced [47], Copyright (2012), with permission from Elsevier.

MRI and behavior assessment [30, 47]. The beneficial effects of MBRT on tumors were also reported, showing increased survival in animals with glioblastomas and increased apoptosis and necrosis in the tumors [48–52].

Deeper studies are required to fully understand the effect of MBRT for clinical applications. But in contrast to MRT, MBRT has the advantage of not necessarily requiring a synchrotron beam to control tumors while inducing low damage in normal tissue. Multiple studies have reported the beneficial effects of MBRT using heavy ions [53] or protons [54], which are covered in other chapters of this book.

## 23.4 Synchrotron FLASH therapy: what do we know about this recent application?

More than ever, increasing the differential response between healthy and tumoral tissues is a major challenge in radiotherapy. Synchrotron SFRT is being developed with this aim. These unusual irradiation methods are generating growing interest in the scientific community. Several international sites have equipped their facilities with a medical line for preclinical tests.

Synchrotron SFRTs are well tolerated by healthy tissue, at least better than non-spatially fractionated conventional radiotherapies. In addition to its use of spatial fractionation, synchrotron SFRT can be distinguished from conventional irradiation by its extremely high dose rate (instantaneous dose rate: ~14 kGy $s^{-1}$ versus 30 mGy $s^{-1}$ in conventional radiotherapy). The biological effects of irradiation at such high dose rates and their differences from the effects induced by conventional dose rates are still unknown.

Since 2014 and the rebirth of radiotherapies based on the use of ultrahigh-dose-rate irradiation to obtain the FLASH effect [55], the dose rates produced by synchrotrons have been considered a crucial characteristic of the new radiobiological approach. Indeed, the FLASH effect has been defined as an *in vivo* phenomenon consisting in a relative absence of normal tissue toxicity with a similar antitumor effect at isodose to that of conventional-dose-rate irradiation. Considering this concept, the dose rate used to produce synchrotron mini- and microbeams may explain, at least in part, the sparing effect of normal tissue by SFRTs. The dose rates achieved by synchrotron radiation are of hitherto poorly exploited radiobiological interest. In addition, a potential FLASH effect obtained with synchrotron dose rates could justify the development of a spatially homogeneous (i.e. not spatially fractionated) radiotherapy mode, which would be easier to set up than synchrotron SFRT and which would benefit from the latter's technical, instrumental, and safety developments.

Very few studies have addressed the complicated challenge of understanding the involvement of the FLASH effect in synchrotron SFRTs or even the existence of a FLASH effect mediated by broad-beam synchrotron x-rays [56] (figure 23.4). Recent reviews by Eling *et al* (2019) [57] and Montay-Gruel *et al* (2021) [8] have reported on these topics.

Taken together, these recent studies suggest that the healthy tissue preservation and tumoricidal efficacy of synchrotron SFRTs should be considered as resulting

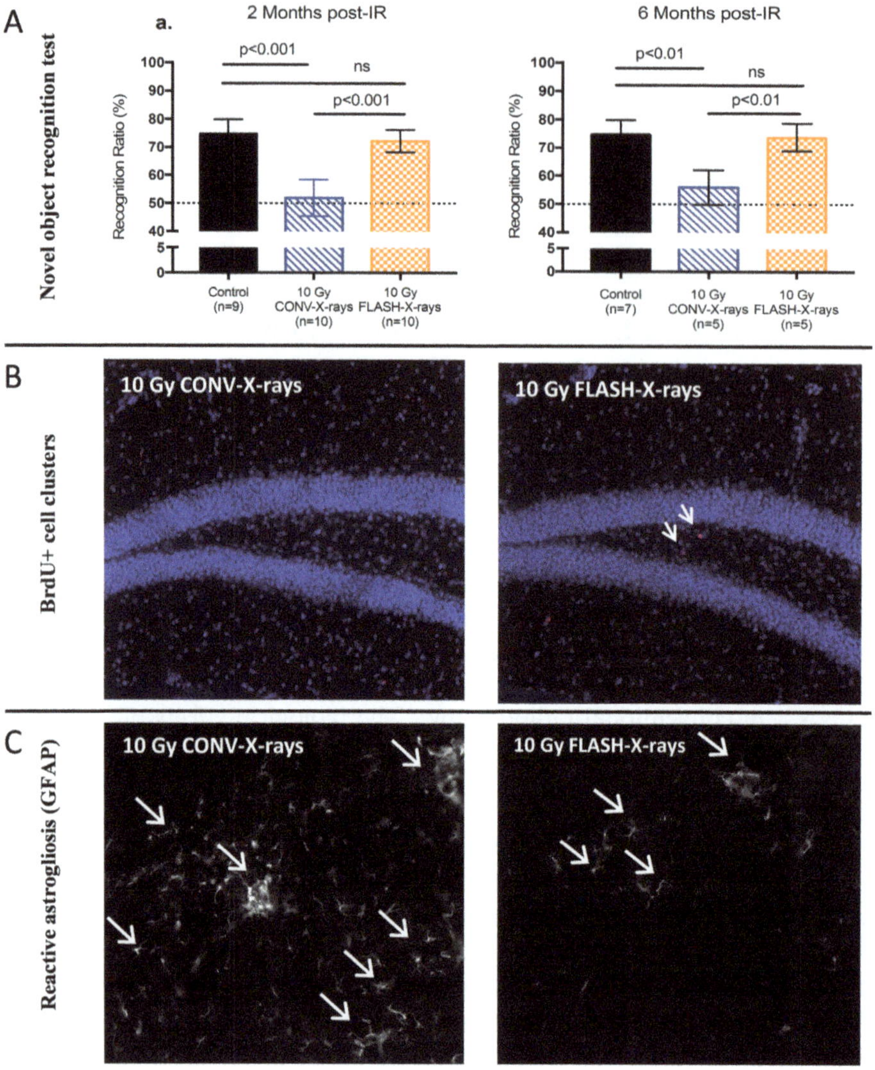


**Figure 23.4.** A comparison of the effects of an ultrahigh-dose-rate synchrotron broad beam and conventional-dose-rate irradiation on the mouse brain. (A) Evaluation of the recognition ratio (RR) at two (a) and six months (b) post irradiation for groups of mice that received sham irradiation (Control), 10 Gy whole brain irradiation with FLASH (FLASH-X-rays), and x-rays delivered at the conventional dose rate (CONV-X-rays). The bars represent mean values and whiskers the standard deviations. (B) Bromodeoxyuridine (BrdU) immunostaining of brain hippocampal sections performed two months post whole brain irradiation on mice irradiated with x-rays delivered at the conventional dose rate (CONV-X-rays) or with a single dose of 10 Gy with FLASH (FLASH-X-rays). The arrows point to BrdU positive clusters in the subgranular zone. Blue: 4',6-diamidino-2-phenylindole (DAPI); Red: BrdU. (C) Reactive astrogliosis assessment performed by glial fibrillary acidic protein (GFAP) immunostaining of brain striatum sections two months post whole brain irradiation on mice irradiated with 10 Gy with x-rays delivered at the conventional dose rate (CONV-X-rays) or with FLASH (FLASH-X-rays). The arrows point to GFAP-positive cells in the striatum. Reprinted from [56], Copyright (2018), with permission from Elsevier.

from both the benefits of spatial fractionation and the ultrahigh dose rates achieved by some synchrotrons. Both spatial and temporal parameters are difficult to dissociate for technical reasons, especially *in vivo*, and will require methodological ingenuity, as an example of which, the study by Steel *et al* is a first step for cell studies. Nevertheless, the FLASH effect, defined as a biological effect, is obtained using synchrotron beams that reach dose rates equivalent to those of the ESRF [56]. The development and study of the effects associated with homogeneous synchrotron radiotherapy (x-ray ultrahigh-dose-rate broad-beam irradiation) seem extremely promising and require a research field of their own. The description of beam parameters such as the mean dose rate, the instantaneous dose rate, the irradiated target volume and the total time of irradiation are more than ever essential for future studies, as recently emphasized [58].

## 23.5 Knowledge gaps and future perspectives

Although ultrahigh-dose-rate synchrotron SFRTs have been used for 25 years, the question of inducing a FLASH effect has only recently been raised. Many MRT studies have reported the maintenance of normal irradiated tissue, with good preservation of the normal brain features, such as myelin, neurons, oligodendrocytes, and vasculature. A recent study using a seamless ultrahigh-dose-rate synchrotron x-ray beam to induce a FLASH effect also confirmed the feasibility of using this type of irradiation to spare normal brain tissues [56]. However, proper studies of FLASH therapy and MRT using with comparable parameters and controls have to be established to validate the hypothesis that a FLASH effect is present in MRT or other synchrotron SFRTs.

Crucial differences in the setup and irradiation parameters (such as the field of irradiation and instantaneous dose rate, for example) exist between the high-dose-rate irradiations produced by electrons (in reference experiments) and those produced by synchrotrons. To avoid shortcuts or even interpretation errors, it is necessary to create an accurate description of the irradiation parameters such as the instantaneous dose rate, the size of the direct irradiation field, the total size of the target irradiation, the total time of irradiation, and thus the mean dose rate of the total irradiation field. It is important to further understand and evaluate the characteristic essentials required to induce a FLASH effect.

Although synchrotron MRT has been widely preclinically studied, a major gap remains concerning the application of this method to big animals for clinical trials. Only two studies in 25 years have shown the capacity of the ESRF to handle and irradiate big animals, such as pigs [59, 60]. To ensure the feasibility of using synchrotron MRT for human clinical trials, veterinary trials on cats and dogs are currently running. These trials will provide important technological and scientific information for the transition to preclinical trials on rodents and human trials. The accurate positioning of the patient, the specific treatment planning, the dosimetry, and guidance must be determined and tested to move toward clinical trials.

One of the main limitations of synchrotron SFRTs and now FLASH synchrotrons is the accessibility of such high-performance facilities. Although the ESRF has developed a beamline with important upgrades capable of accommodating clinical trials [10], the geographical limitation will remain. Thus, several international sites have equipped their facilities with a medical line for preclinical tests. Since 2005, the Japanese Spring 8 synchrotron has been able to perform SFRT experiments, and the Canadian (CLS) and Australian (Australian Synchrotron) facilities have been able to do so since 2008. In 2021, preclinical studies were conducted at the biomedical beamline SYRMEP of the Italian synchrotron facility ELETTRA [61]. Between 2013 and 2018, a group of laboratories from 16 countries was supported by the European Union under the framework of the COST Action (TD 1205, SYRA3), in which SFRT, and in particular, MRT, amply mobilized the scientific community [62]. Another option that could be used to counteract the low synchrotron accessibility would be to develop a compact source for the clinical application of SFRT and x-ray FLASH, such as the line-focus x-ray tube that has been demonstrated to be suitable for MRT [61, 63]. Multiple alternative sources of radiation that can be used to apply SFRTs to patients are currently being developed, which should help the expansion of these techniques for the treatment of patients with incurable tumors.

## 23.6 Conclusions

Since the development of SFRTs based on synchrotron beams, such as MRT or MBRT, great progress has been made in the optimization of the irradiation parameters, accurate dosimetry, and experimental setups. Our understanding of synchrotron MRT has also been widely developed using different tissues and for different purposes. It has recently been suggested that the FLASH effect obtained using ultrahigh dose rates is part of the explanation for the strong tolerance of healthy tissues to synchrotron MRT. Recent studies have shown the possible implications of FLASH in broad-beam synchrotron therapy, opening the way to synchrotron FLASH.

## References

[1] Foray N 2021 *Victor Despeignes ou le premier traitement du cancer par rayons X* (Paris: Les éditions Glyphe) https://www.editions-glyphe.com/livre/victor-despeignes-ou-le-premier-traitement-du-cancer-par-rayons-x/

[2] Schultheiss T E, Kun L E, Ang K K and Stephens L C 1995 Radiation response of the central nervous system *Int. J. Radiat. Oncol. Biol. Phys.* **31** 1093–112

[3] Laissue J A, Geiser G, Spanne P O, Dilmanian F A, Gebbers J O and Geiser M *et al* 1998 Neuropathology of ablation of rat gliosarcomas and contiguous brain tissues using a microplanar beam of synchrotron-wiggler-generated X rays *Int. J. Cancer* **78** 654–60

[4] Blewett J P 1946 Radiation losses in the induction electron accelerator *Phys. Rev.* **69** 87–95

[5] Elder F R, Gurewitsch A M, Langmuir R V and Pollock H C 1947 Radiation from electrons in a synchrotron [8]. *Phys. Rev.* **71** 829–30

[6] Gil S, Fernández M, Prezado Y, Biete A, Bravin A and Sabés M 2011 Synchrotron radiation in cancer treatments and diagnostics: an overview *Clin. Transl. Oncol.* **13** 715–20
[7] Suortti P and Thomlinson W 2003 Medical applications of synchrotron radiation *Phys. Med. Biol.* **48** R1
[8] Montay-Gruel P, Corde S, Laissue J A and Bazalova-Carter M 2021 FLASH radiotherapy with photon beams *Med Phys.* **49** 2055–67
[9] Laissue J A, Blattmann H and Slatkin D N 2012 Alban Köhler (1874–1947): inventor of grid therapy *Z. Med. Phys.* **22** 90–9
[10] Brauer-Krisch E, Serduc R, Siegbahn E A, Le Duc G, Prezado Y and Bravin A *et al* 2010 Effects of pulsed, spatially fractionated, microscopic synchrotron X-ray beams on normal and tumoral brain tissue *Mutat. Res.* **704** 160–6
[11] Dilmanian F A, Zhong Z, Bacarian T, Benveniste H, Romanelli P and Wang R *et al* 2006 Interlaced x-ray microplanar beams: a radiosurgery approach with clinical potential *Proc. Natl Acad. Sci. USA* **103** 9709–14
[12] Curtis H J 1963 The microbeam as a tool in radiobiology *Adv. Biol. Med. Phys.* **9** 207–24
[13] Curtis H J 1967 The use of deuteron microbeam for simulating the biological effects of heavy cosmic-ray particles *Radiat, Res, Suppl.* **7** 250–7
[14] Slatkin D N, Dilmanian F A and Spanne P O 1994 Method for microbeam radiation therapy *US Patent* US 5,339,347 https://image-ppubs.uspto.gov/dirsearch-public/print/downloadPdf/5339347
[15] Archer D W 1998 Collimator for producing an array of microbeams *US Patent* US 5771270 https://patentcenter.uspto.gov/applications/08813547
[16] Bräuer-Krisch E, Requardt H, Brochard T, Berruyer G, Renier M and Laissue J A *et al* 2009 New technology enables high precision multislit collimators for microbeam radiation therapy *Rev. Sci. Instrum.* **80** 074301
[17] Pellicioli P, Donzelli M, Davis J A, Esteve F, Hugtenburg R and Guatelli S *et al* 2021 Study of the X-ray radiation interaction with a multislit collimator for the creation of microbeams in radiation therapy *J. Synchrotron Radiat.* **28** 392–403
[18] Slatkin D N, Dilmanian F A, Nawrocky M M, Spanne P, Gebbers J O and Archer D W *et al* 1995 Design of a multislit, variable width collimator for microplanar beam radiotherapy *Rev. Sci. Instrum.* **66** 1459–60
[19] Slatkin D N, Spanne P, Dilmanian F A, Gebbers J O and Laissue J A 1995 Subacute neuropathological effects of microplanar beams of x-rays from a synchrotron wiggler *Proc. Natl Acad. Sci. USA* **92** 8783–7
[20] Slatkin D N, Spanne P, Dilmanian F A and Sandborg M 1992 Microbeam radiation therapy *Med. Phys.* **19** 1395–400
[21] Fernandez-Palomo C, Fazzari J, Trappetti V, Smyth L, Janka H and Laissue J *et al* 2020 Animal models in microbeam radiation therapy: a scoping review *Cancers.* **12** 527
[22] Laissue J A, Barré S, Bartzsch S, Blattmann H, Bouchet A M and Djonov V G *et al* 2021 Tolerance of normal rabbit facial bones and teeth to synchrotron X-ray microbeam irradiation *Radiat. Res.* **197** 233–41
[23] Schültke E, Bayat S, Bartzsch S, Bräuer-Krisch E, Djonov V and Fiedler S *et al* 2021 A mouse model for microbeam radiation therapy of the lung *Int. J. Radiat. Oncol. Biol. Phys.* **110** 521–5
[24] Trappetti V, Fernandez-Palomo C, Smyth L, Klein M, Haberthür D and Butler D *et al* 2021 Synchrotron microbeam radiation therapy for the treatment of lung carcinoma: a preclinical study *Int. J. Radiat. Oncol. Biol. Phys.* **111** 1276–88

[25] Serduc R, Brauer-Krisch E, Siegbahn E A, Bouchet A, Pouyatos B and Carron R *et al* 2010 High-precision radiosurgical dose delivery by interlaced microbeam arrays of high-flux low-energy synchrotron X-rays *PLoS One.* **5** e9028

[26] Pouyatos B, Serduc R, Chipaux M, Chabrol T, Bräuer-Krisch E and Nemoz C *et al* 2013 Synchrotron X-ray interlaced microbeams suppress paroxysmal oscillations in neuronal networks initiating generalized epilepsy *Neurobiol. Dis.* **51** 152–60

[27] Pouyatos B, Nemoz C, Chabrol T, Potez M, Bräuer E and Renaud L *et al* 2016 Synchrotron X-ray microtransections: a non-invasive approach for epileptic seizures arising from eloquent cortical areas *Sci Rep.* **6** 27250

[28] Serduc R, Bouchet A, Pouyatos B, Renaud L, Bräuer-Krisch E and Le Duc G *et al* 2014 Synchrotron x ray induced axonal transections in the brain of rats assessed by high-field diffusion tensor imaging tractography *PLoS One* **9** e88244

[29] Romanelli P, Fardone E, Battaglia G, Bräuer-Krisch E, Prezado Y and Requardt H *et al* 2013 Synchrotron-generated microbeam sensorimotor cortex transections induce seizure control without disruption of neurological functions *PLoS One* **8** e53549

[30] Fardone E, Bravin A, Conti A, Bräuer-Krisch E, Requardt H and Bucci D *et al* 2017 Rat sensorimotor cortex tolerance to parallel transections induced by synchrotron-generated X-ray microbeams *Sci. Rep.* **7** 14290

[31] Fardone E, Pouyatos B, Bräuer-Krisch E, Bartzsch S, Mathieu H and Requardt H *et al* 2018 Synchrotron-generated microbeams induce hippocampal transections in rats *Sci Rep.* **8** 184

[32] Sabatasso S, Laissue J A, Hlushchuk R, Graber W, Bravin A and Brauer-Krisch E *et al* 2011 Microbeam radiation-induced tissue damage depends on the stage of vascular maturation *Int. J. Radiat. Oncol. Biol. Phys.* **80** 1522–32

[33] Brönnimann D, Bouchet A, Schneider C, Potez M, Serduc R and Bräuer-Krisch E *et al* 2016 Synchrotron microbeam irradiation induces neutrophil infiltration, thrombocyte attachment and selective vascular damage *in vivo Sci. Rep.* **6** 33601

[34] Bouchet A, Potez M, Coquery N, Rome C, Lemasson B and Bräuer-Krisch E *et al* 2017 Permeability of brain tumor vessels induced by uniform or spatially microfractionated synchrotron radiation therapies *Int. J. Radiat. Oncol. Biol. Phys.* **98** 1174–82

[35] Bouchet A, Lemasson B, Leduc G, Maisin C, Bräuer-Krisch E and Siegbahn A E *et al* 2010 Preferential effect of synchrotron microbeam radiation therapy on intracerebral 9L gliosarcoma vascular networks *Int. J. Radiat. Oncol. Biol. Phys.* **78** 1503–12

[36] Bouchet A, Lemasson B, Christen T, Potez M, Rome C and Coquery N *et al* 2013 Synchrotron microbeam radiation therapy induces hypoxia in intracerebral gliosarcoma but not in the normal brain *Radiother. Oncol.* **108** 143–8

[37] Potez M, Bouchet A, Wagner J, Donzelli M, Bräuer-Krisch E and Hopewell J W *et al* 2018 Effects of synchrotron X-ray micro-beam irradiation on normal mouse ear pinnae *Int. J. Radiat. Oncol. Biol. Phys.* **101** 680–9

[38] Potez M, Fernandez-Palomo C, Bouchet A, Trappetti V, Donzelli M and Krisch M *et al* 2019 Synchrotron microbeam radiation therapy as a new approach for the treatment of radioresistant melanoma: potential underlying mechanisms *Int. J. Radiat. Oncol. Biol. Phys.* **105** 1126–36

[39] Eling L, Bouchet A, Ocadiz A, Adam J F, Kershmiri S and Elleaume H *et al* 2021 Unexpected benefits of multiport synchrotron microbeam radiation therapy for brain tumors *Cancers (Basel)* **13** 1–16

[40] Sabatasso S, Fernandez-Palomo C, Hlushchuk R, Fazzari J, Tschanz S and Pellicioli P *et al* 2021 Transient and efficient vascular permeability window for adjuvant drug delivery triggered by microbeam radiation *Cancers (Basel)* **13** 2103

[41] Bouchet A, Serduc R, Laissue J A and Djonov V 2015 Effects of microbeam radiation therapy on normal and tumoral blood vessels *Phys. Med.* **31** 634–41

[42] Bouchet A, Bräuer-Krisch E, Prezado Y, El Atifi M, Rogalev L and Le Clec'h C *et al* 2016 Better efficacy of synchrotron spatially micro-fractionated radiotherapy than uniform radiotherapy on glioma *Int. J. Radiat. Oncol.* **95** 1485–94

[43] Bouchet A, Sakakini N, El Atifi M, Le Clec'h C, Brauer E and Moisan A *et al* 2013 Early gene expression analysis in 9L orthotopic tumor-bearing rats identifies immune modulation in molecular response to synchrotron microbeam radiation therapy *PLoS One* **8** e81874

[44] Bouchet A, Sakakini N, Atifi M E, Le Clec'H C, Bräuer-Krisch E and Rogalev L *et al* 2015 Identification of AREG and PLK1 pathway modulation as a potential key of the response of intracranial 9L tumor to microbeam radiation therapy *Int. J. Cancer* **136** 2705–16

[45] Trappetti V, Fazzari J M, Fernandez-palomo C, Scheidegger M, Volarevic V and Martin O A *et al* 2021 Microbeam radiotherapy—a novel therapeutic approach to overcome radioresistance and enhance anti-tumour response in melanoma *Int. J. Mol. Sci.* **22** 7755

[46] Poncelet B P, Wedeen V J, Weisskoff R M and Cohen M S 1992 Brain parenchyma motion: Measurement with cine echo-planar MR imaging *Radiology* **185** 645–51

[47] Deman P, Vautrin M, Edouard M, Stupar V, Bobyk L and Farion R *et al* 2012 Monochromatic minibeams radiotherapy: from healthy tissue-sparing effect studies toward first experimental glioma bearing rats therapy *Int. J. Radiat. Oncol. Biol. Phys.* **82** E693–E700

[48] Deman P, Vautrin M, Stupar V, Barbier E L, Elleaume H and Esteve F *et al* 2011 Monochromatic minibeam radiotherapy: theoretical and experimental dosimetry for preclinical treatment plans *Phys. Med. Biol.* **56** 4465–80

[49] Prezado Y, Sarun S, Gil S, Deman P, Bouchet A and Le Duc G 2012 Increase of lifespan for glioma-bearing rats by using minibeam radiation therapy *J. Synchrotron Radiat.* **19** 60–5

[50] Livingstone J, Adam J F, Crosbie J C, Hall C J, Lye J E and McKinlay J *et al* 2017 Preclinical radiotherapy at the Australian Synchrotron's imaging and medical beamline: instrumentation, dosimetry and a small-animal feasibility study *J. Synchrotron Radiat.* **24** 854–65

[51] Gil S, Sarun S, Biete A, Prezado Y and Sabés M 2011 Survival analysis of F98 glioma rat cells following minibeam or broad-beam synchrotron radiation therapy *Radiat. Oncol.* **6** 37

[52] Gil S, Prezado Y and Sabés M 2013 Double-strand breaks on F98 glioma rat cells induced by minibeam and broad-beam synchrotron radiation therapy *Clin. Transl. Oncol.* **16** 696–701

[53] Prezado Y, Hirayama R, Matsufuji N, Inaniwa T, Martínez-Rovira I and Seksek O *et al* 2021 A potential renewed use of very heavy ions for therapy: neon minibeam radiation therapy *Cancers (Basel)* **13** 1–14

[54] Prezado Y, Jouvion G, Patriarca A, Nauraye C, Guardiola C and Juchaux M *et al* 2018 Proton minibeam radiation therapy widens the therapeutic index for high-grade gliomas *Sci. Rep.* **8** 16479

[55] Favaudon V, Caplier L, Monceau V, Pouzoulet F, Sayarath M and Fouillade C *et al* 2014 Ultrahigh dose-rate FLASH irradiation increases the differential response between normal and tumor tissue in mice *Sci. Transl. Med.* **6** 245ra93

[56] Montay-Gruel P, Bouchet A, Jaccard M, Patin D, Serduc R and Aim W *et al* 2018 X-rays can trigger the FLASH effect: ultra-high dose-rate synchrotron light source prevents normal brain injury after whole brain irradiation in mice *Radiother. Oncol.* **129** 582–8

[57] Eling L, Bouchet A, Nemoz C, Djonov V, Balosso J and Laissue J *et al* 2019 Ultra high dose rate synchrotron microbeam radiation therapy. Preclinical evidence in view of a clinical transfer *Radiother. Oncol.* **139** 56–61

[58] Vozenin M-C, Montay-Gruel P, Limoli C and Germond J-F 2020 All irradiations that are ultra-high dose rate may not be FLASH: The critical importance of beam parameter characterization and *in vivo* validation of the FLASH effect *Radiat. Res.* **194** 571–2

[59] Laissue J A, Blattmann H, Di Michiel M, Slatkin D N, Lyubimova N and Guzman R *et al* 2001 Weanling piglet cerebellum: a surrogate for tolerance to MRT (microbeam radiation therapy) in pediatric neuro-oncology *Proc. SPIE* **4508** 65–73

[60] Coquery N, Adam J-F F, Nemoz C, Janvier R, Livingstone J and Chauvin A *et al* 2019 Locomotion and eating behavior changes in Yucatan minipigs after unilateral radio-induced ablation of the caudate nucleus *Sci. Rep.* **9** 17082

[61] Schultke E, Fiedler S, Menk R H, Jaekel F, Dreossi D and Casarin K *et al* 2021 Perspectives for microbeam irradiation at the SYRMEP beamline *J. Synchrotron Radiat.* **28** 410–8

[62] Bravin A, Olko P, Schültke E and Wilkens J J 2015 SYRA3 COST action—microbeam radiation therapy: roots and prospects *Phys. Medica* **31** 561–3

[63] Bartzsch S and Oelfke U 2017 Line focus x-ray tubes-a new concept to produce high brilliance x-rays *Phys. Med. Biol.* **62** 8600–15

# Conclusions

**Charles L Limoli, Charles B Simone II, Nina A Mayr and Hualin Zhang**

The foregoing 23 chapters have provided an exciting and provocative backdrop for the evolving and emerging radiation modalities that offer the promise of improving patient outcomes, while cautioning about the need for robust technological development and rigorous research. The field of radiation oncology has advanced considerably over the years due to the development of imaging and beam delivery technologies that have improved the conformality of treatment plans, enabled high-precision treatment delivery, and ushered in the era of hypofractionation. Now, by taking advantage of the capability to further minimize the dose given to normal sensitive tissues collaterally interspersed with the tumor target, the tumoricidal dose can be escalated with an improved ability to maintain acceptable toxicities to dose-limiting normal tissues.

The GRID, Lattice and micro/minibeam SFRT modalities challenge the long-held belief that the radiation dose must be as uniform as possible within the target in order to optimize tumor control. Meanwhile, advances in biology and immunology have begun to offer hypotheses for the high response rates observed in SFRT and to provide a possible rationale for the application of heterogeneous dose distributions in a biologically heterogeneous tumor environment. Rigorous clinical trials are needed to substantiate or refute these hypotheses and evaluate them safely in clinical patients.

The preceding chapters also touch on several overlapping principles and technical challenges that must be resolved. The clinical implementation of GRID and Lattice SFRT with the original intent of minimizing normal tissue volume effects is now at the stage at which optimal spatially fractionated geometries must be defined and coordinated with dosimetric standards so that treatment outcomes can be critically evaluated and compared. The physics of SFRT plays a prime role in this complex endeavor. New tumor response modeling approaches that take into account the heterogenous intratumoral dose pattern will be needed. The next steps fall to clinicians testing and implementing specific variations of SFRT for definitive or

doi:10.1088/978-0-7503-4046-5ch24  

neoadjuvant treatment approaches through well-conducted prospective clinical trials in selected cancer types. Physical and dosimetric robustness and well-conceived translational science components, embedded in multi-institutional clinical trials, will be indispensable to broaden our comprehensive understanding of SFRT's mechanistic phenomena and underpinnings, its potential clinical benefits, and its limitations.

Mini/microbeam approaches, while more difficult to clinically translate at this time, provide unique higher-resolution insights into peak–valley dose–response relationships between tumors and normal tissues, and studies have largely pointed to the importance of vascular effects. At this time, it is uncertain whether or how higher linear energy transfer modalities may (or may not) improve SFRT, but as these technologies continue to develop, the generalized capability to partially and heterogeneously irradiate tumor volumes under the conditions of carefully controlled clinical trials has great potential to lead to improved patient outcomes and biological understanding, perhaps regardless of the beam types used.

FLASH radiotherapy, which involves ultrahigh-dose-rate beam delivery, holds much of the same promise as SFRT and faces similar—albeit distinctly different—technical challenges to overcome. As alluded to in the previous chapters, central to FLASH radiotherapy is the capability to achieve at least isoefficient tumor control while minimizing normal tissue toxicities. The key parameter here, different from SFRT, is the dose rate modulation for therapeutic gain. As the resultant 'FLASH effect' has and must be defined *in vivo*, the characterization of critical beam parameters is essential and will differ based on the beam modality involved. Similarly, the field is increasingly aware that the mean dose rate is an oversimplification of the necessary physical parameters, and that certain total dose, volume effects, and dose-rate thresholds required to mitigate normal tissue toxicities will depend on the beam properties and the irradiated tissue involved. The role of physics is crucial to the further exploration of these heterogenous dose concepts, and the value of preclinical research remains essential, as both the preclinical treatment outcomes and mechanism-based studies can guide clinical efforts to safely translate these novel treatments to patient care, with or even without a clearly defined mechanism of action. Salient to this point will be the rise and fall of multiple models proposed to explain the FLASH effect, largely focused on explanations that can account for normal tissue sparing or selective cancer cell killing. Currently, perhaps the more intriguing unanswered question is: why does FLASH radiotherapy kill tumors but spare normal cells?

As the fields of GRID, Lattice, Minibeam, Microbeam, and FLASH radiation continue to evolve at a rapid pace, many of these questions will be resolved and many more will undoubtedly surface. It has become ever more clear that the entire field of radiation oncology is at a juncture, with previously unforeseen opportunities to improve patient care developing rapidly before our eyes, and potential pitfalls that demand our vigilance. Careful and prudent implementation will require research at many levels across the disciplines of physics, engineering, biology, computer science, experimental and clinical radiation oncology, and others. Encouraging such conversations and collaborations has been an intent of this book. If different disciplines can work together effectively, the future of cancer therapy is poised to reap benefits.

# Glossary of spatially fractionated and FLASH radiation therapy

**Juergen Meyer, Yolanda Prezado, Hualin Zhang and Nina A Mayr**

Spatially fractionated and FLASH radiation therapy are emerging highly interdisciplinary modalities in various stages of development. The scientific investigation and clinical translation of these modalities span the disciplines of physics, biology, immunology, biophysics, engineering, and radiation oncology. In these fast evolving fields, terms to describe new methods, parameters, and specifications within and across these fields have also evolved at a fast pace. This evolution has often taken place in a decentralized way within a scientific discipline or subspecialty space and in various focus groups and institutions.

However, for any scientific field to advance, *a common language* is critical to communicate, exchange ideas, and effectively collaborate and contribute to the various fields within the scientific space and across disciplines. This is critically important to ultimately advance the understanding and the science of any new field. In a medical field, clarity and standardization of terms become even more acute because of the need for patient safety.

We have long noted that that the descriptive *terms and abbreviations* related to spatially fractionated and FLASH radiation therapy are sometimes not fully standardized and described, interpreted, and used in the same way.

This *glossary of terms* strives to provide a structured overview and definitions of the terms and pertinent abbreviations used in this textbook to help the reader navigate the book's content.

The terms and abbreviations presented in tables G.1 and G.2 have been derived from the respective literature and scholarly dialogue at scientific meetings and practice. The editors thank the book's contributors for their thoughtful input to this glossary. Collectively, we also worked to harmonize terms where applicable. Much of this harmonization and standardization effort has been underway across the field of heterogeneous dose irradiation through guideline efforts made by several scientific groups and organizations, although much work still needs to be done. The SFRT

doi:10.1088/978-0-7503-4046-5ch25

and FLASH terms are further supplemented by pertinent radiobiological concepts and models, experimental assays, and medical terms (tables G.3–G.5).

While we aimed to be as comprehensive as possible, this glossary is by no means complete and will undoubtedly be subject to further refinement as the community develops new insights and as the concepts, terminology, and technology used to deliver spatially fractionated and FLASH treatments continue to grow and evolve. It is the editors' hope that this glossary of terms and concepts will enhance the scientific interchange and help to improve patient care.

# Glossary

**Table G.1.** SFRT and FLASH terms.

| Abbreviation | Full Term, description |
|---|---|
| ctc | **Centre-to-centre distance**: sometimes also referred to as the peak-to-peak distance. The abbreviations 'CTC' and 'c-t-c' are also used. |
| cERT | **Conventional external-beam radiation therapy**: conventional 3D conformal or intensity-modulated radiation without intentional dose heterogeneity. |
| $D_{max}$ | **Maximum dose** of the plan |
| $d_{max}$ | **Depth of the maximum dose** |
| $D_{mean}$ | **Mean dose** |
| $D_p$ | **Prescription dose** *(units of Gy)* |
| $D_{peak}$ | **Peak dose** *(units of Gy)* |
| $D_{ref}$ | **Reference dose**: usually $D_{ref} = 2$ Gy. |
| $D_{valley}$ | **Valley dose** *(units of Gy)* |
| EOD | **Equivalent open-field dose** *(units of Gy)* |
| FLASH or FLASH-RT | **FLASH radiation therapy**: radiotherapy delivered at a dose rate several orders of magnitude higher than that of conventional radiotherapy, typically ⩾40 Gy $s^{-1}$. FLASH and FLASH-RT are used interchangeably. |
| FWHM | **Full width at half maximum:** the width between 50% of the peak values. This is also referred to as the peak width ($W_{peak}$). |
| GRID therapy | **GRID radiation therapy**: GRID-pattern dose-modulated nonuniform radiation therapy. Two-dimensional pattern, parallel beamlets, with a beamlet width from 1–2 cm and a ctc distance of 2–4 cm. |
| LRT | **Lattice radiation therapy**: three dimensionally dose-modulated, lattice-like nonuniform radiation therapy. 3D pattern, non-parallel beamlets, with a vertex diameter of approximately 1 cm and a ctc distance of 2–5 cm. |
| MBRT | **Minibeam radiation therapy**: for photon and proton beam small-field radiation therapy. Two-dimensional pattern, parallel beamlets, beamlet width 0.1–1.0 mm, ctc 1–4 mm. |
| MRT | **Microbeam radiation therapy**: synchrotron-beam based microbeam radiation therapy (typically). Field dimension is smaller than 0.1 mm. Two-dimensional pattern, parallel beamlets, beamlet width 20–100 μm, ctc 200–400 μm. |

| | |
|---|---|
| PHASER | **Pluridirectional high-energy agile scanning electron radiotherapy**: PHASER is a platform for the clinical translation of FLASH. |
| pMBRT | **Proton minibeam radiation therapy** |
| PVDR | **Peak-to-valley dose ratio**: alternatively, the valley-to-peak dose ratio (VPDR) is used. |
| SFRT | **Spatially fractionated radiation therapy**: general overarching term, which includes MBRT, MRT, GRID therapy and LRT. |
| UHDR | **Ultrahigh dose rate**: usually a dose rate of ⩾40 Gy $s^{-1}$. |
| VHEE; VHEE machine | **Very-high-energy electron** (>100 MeV); **very-high-energy electron machine**. |
| $V_L$ | **Lattice (or LRT) volume**: the $V_L$ contains the vertices and is created by connecting the outermost vertices, or by contracting the GTV with an inward margin. |
| VPDR | **Valley-to-peak dose ratio**: this term is an alternative for PVDR. |
| VTV | **Vertex tumour volume**: total volume of vertices within the gross tumour volume (GTV) |
| VTV/GTV ratio | **Volume of vertices /volume of gross target volume** |
| $W_{peak}$ | **Peak width**: the width between 50% of the peak values. This is also referred to as the full width at half maximum (FWHM). |

**Table G.2.** SFRT and FLASH physics and engineering terms.

| Abbreviation | Full Term, description |
|---|---|
| ACCT | AC current transformers |
| BB | Broad beam |
| BEDR | Bragg peak-to-entrance dose ratio |
| CNT | Carbon nanotube field emission technology |
| DCS | Atomic differential cross section |
| DMF | Dose modifying factor |
| $D_{pulse}$ | Dose per pulse |
| $DR_{av}$ | Average dose rate |
| ICS | Inverse Compton scattering |
| MC | Monte Carlo |
| MCS | Multiple Coulomb scattering |
| MSC | Multislit collimator |
| PRF | Pulse repetition frequency |

**Table G.3.** Biological metrics and modeling concepts.

| Abbreviation | Full Term, Description |
|---|---|
| EQD2 | **Equivalent dose delivered in 2 Gy fractions**: compares different fractionation schedules using a dose of 2 Gy per day as the reference (*units of Gy*). |
| EUD | **Equivalent uniform dose**: the dose distribution given to a region of tissue that has the same biological effects as a nonuniform dose distribution (*units of Gy*). |
| gEUD | **Generalized EUD**: an empirical, tissue-level concept for capturing the larger-scale functional aspects of heterogeneous dose distributions (*units of Gy*). |
| LET | **Linear energy transfer**: the amount of energy transferred to a tissue or material by an ionizing particle per unit distance (*units of* $keV\ \mu m^{-1}$). |
| LQ Model | **Linear–quadratic model** of radiation response: describes the relationship between cell survival and delivered dose. |
| MLQ Model | **Modified linear–quadratic model** of radiation response |
| NTCP | **Normal tissue complication probability:** a dose-dependent model that predicts the probability of complications in normal tissues. |
| RBE | **Relative biological effectiveness:** describes the biological effect of one type of radiation relative to another type of radiation, usually $^{60}Co$ γ-rays or MV x-rays. Varies with dose, particle type, and kinetic energy (and LET), the biological endpoint of interest and the cell-, tissue-, and tumour-specific response to radiation (*dimensionless*). |
| RWD | **RBE-weighted dose:** the product of absorbed dose and the RBE, which depends on multiple biological factors and the particle type and kinetic energy (i.e. LET) (*units of Gy*). |
| SF2 | **Surviving fraction at 2 Gy**: a measure of tumour radiosensitivity. |
| TCP | **Tumour control probability:** the probability that a given dose of radiation eradicates all tumour cells |
| USC Model | **Universal survival curve model**: a combination of the LQ model and the multitarget model, which provides an alternative description of clonogenic survival as a function of radiation dose. |

**Table G.4.** Biology terms.

| Abbreviation | Full Term, Description |
|---|---|
| APC | Antigen-presenting cell |
| ATP | Adenosine triphosphate |
| BATF3 | Basic leucine zipper transcriptional factor ATF-like 3 |
| CAR T cell therapy | Chimeric antigen receptor T cell therapy |
| cGAS/STING | Cyclic GMP-AMP synthase/stimulator of interferon genes |
| DAMP | Damage-associated molecular pattern |
| DNAase | Deoxyribonuclease |
| DSB | Double-strand break |
| dsDNA | Double-stranded DNA |
| GFAP | Glial fibrillary acidic protein |
| GJIC | Gap junction intercellular communication |

| | |
|---|---|
| HCT | Hematopoietic cell transplantation |
| HIF-1 | Hypoxia-inducible factor |
| HMGB1 | High-mobility group box 1 |
| ICD | Immunogenic cell death |
| IDO | Indoleamine 2,3-dioxygenase pathway |
| IFN | Interferon |
| IFNAR | IFN-α/β receptor |
| IFN-β | Interferon beta |
| IFNγ | Interferon gamma |
| IL-2 | Interleukin-2 |
| ISG | IFN-stimulated gene |
| miRNA | microRNA |
| NKG2D receptor | An activating receptor (transmembrane protein) belonging to the NKG2 family of C-type lectin-like receptors that is encoded by KLRK1 (killer cell lectin-like receptor K1) gene. |
| PIM | Peritumoral immune microenvironment |
| PRRs | Pattern recognition receptors |
| RAE-1 | Retinoic-acid early inducible-1 |
| RIBE | Radiation-induced bystander effect |
| SSB | Single-strand break |
| TRAIL | TNF-related apoptosis-inducing ligand |
| TREX1 | DNAase three prime repair exonuclease 1 |
| ZF | Zebrafish |

**Table G.5.** Medical terms.

| Abbreviation | Full Term, description |
|---|---|
| CR | Complete response |
| BOLD MRI | Blood-oxygen-level-dependent MRI |
| DSF | Disease-specific survival |
| HCT | Hematopoietic cell transplantation (only 1×) |
| NLR | Neutrophil-to-lymphocyte |
| OS | Overall survival |
| PBMCs | Peripheral blood mononuclear cells |
| pCR | Pathologic complete response |
| PR | Partial response |
| RIL | Radiation-induced lymphopenia |
| TdLNs | Tumour-associated draining lymph nodes |
| TOLD MRI | Tissue-oxygen-level-dependent MRI |

www.ingramcontent.com/pod-product-compliance
Ingram Content Group UK Ltd.
Pitfield, Milton Keynes, MK11 3LW, UK
UKHW051907100926
8556IPUK00005B/799

9 780750 340441